THE RED CELL

PRODUCTION, METABOLISM, DESTRUCTION:
NORMAL AND ABNORMAL

THE RED CELL

PRODUCTION, METABOLISM, DESTRUCTION:
NORMAL AND ABNORMAL

JOHN W. HARRIS, M. D.

Professor of Medicine, Western Reserve University
Department of Medicine at Cleveland Metropolitan General Hospital

PUBLISHED FOR THE COMMONWEALTH FUND

BY HARVARD UNIVERSITY PRESS

CAMBRIDGE, MASSACHUSETTS · 1963

TO MY MOTHER AND FATHER

FOREWORD

Two challenges to the student and teacher of medicine have been made sharply by Vannevar Bush,* physicist and statesman of science:

"(i) Medicine is largely empirical in spite of scientific progress in biochemistry and physiology: it has new and powerful tools but understands and controls them only vaguely: and its progress toward logical processes is slow because of the appalling complexity of its subject matter.

"(ii) The library, as we know it, can not cope with the task before it. Science has become bogged down in its own products, inhibited like a colony of bacteria by its own exudations. . . . The pile is mounting daily, science is becoming polyglot, duplication is rife: synthesis, crossing many fields, becomes increasingly difficult and more and more necessary. In such a morass, how are the great syntheses of the future to be brought to light?"

In preparing the following monograph, John W. Harris has had the courage to prepare a synthesis in a field of great complexity and bring it to the desk of the second-year student of medicine and to the teacher. Both find this monograph to be challenging in depth, filled with detail but rich in principles that are dynamic and applicable to the understanding of physiologic and pathologic processes. Observations of the clinical investigator have been coupled with those of biologic scientist, biophysicist, chemist, and physicist.

The advancement of knowledge in medicine is evident from inspection of this monograph with its 2,074 references. For example, the bursting new knowledge of abnormal hemoglobins had its origin only 13 years ago in the report by Linus Pauling and his colleagues on sickle cell anemia, a molecular disease. They gave the clues to both the biochemical and genetic differences in hemoglobin formation. The chapter on this field of globin synthesis is brief but has 225 references, 180 of which were pub-

* *For Man to Know*, Atlantic Monthly, pp. 37, 32, August 1955.

lished from 1955 to date. Probably no field of medicine offers more opportunity for student and teacher to synthesize principles of genetics, hemoglobin chemistry, biophysical behavior of hemoglobin molecules, and the consequences of such abnormalities as sickle cell hemoglobin in producing symptoms of pain and dangerous thromboses in the patient, anemia, and abnormalities in organs where thromboses occur.

The problems facing the student, teacher, and author have much in common. There is mutual desire to understand the scientific basis of medicine to help in the care of patients. The complex fields are greatly simplified when a principle is clearly defined, understood, and applied. The author who will study, correlate, and clarify principles makes a major contribution to us, especially when he presents the evidence to support his concepts. The hurried and harried reader may be required to omit the details, avoid the historic development of concepts, and go crashing toward the summary statements. This is the dilemma of enormous advances in knowledge.

John W. Harris has derived this monograph for students showing his faith in them and in their ability and desire to learn principles and the bases of the principles. In fact, this document has inspired the development of a program of cooperative research in teaching hematology in which several medical schools are participating. The question is raised, "Can the student take the responsibility to learn on his own initiative from the study of problems?" Obviously, any student and any faculty member is challenged to learn from the monograph by Harris.

From the practical point of view, the author has insisted that the dollar-cost of this volume be kept to a minimum to meet the needs of the student's pocketbook and the rapid obsolescence of any report in a rapidly advancing field.

Thomas Hale Ham, M.D.

PREFACE

The various sections of this work were developed for use in the second-year course of hematology at Western Reserve University School of Medicine and have been so used in approximately their present form for the past 3 years. They have been titrated for concepts and factual content so that under the conditions employed the ready grasp of the good student is somewhat exceeded while the outstanding student takes them in stride and supplements with source materials.

The attempt is made to report the current status of the body of knowledge relative to the various topics considered in such a way that the experimental approaches employed in reaching conclusions are illustrated and sufficient data are supplied to support the conclusions and indicate their limits of accuracy and dependability. It is entirely organized around and limited to the red cell—development, synthesis of component parts, function, metabolism, and destruction (normal and abnormal)—and is intended to extend into a specific model system (hematology) the student's knowledge of biochemistry, physiology, pathology, etc. Brief clinical descriptions are presented to provide frames of reference into which the illustrative pathophysiology and disease mechanisms can be placed and retained for subsequent clinical application. The bibliographies supplied are fairly extensive and selected to allow ready penetration beyond the outlines here reported; as such they have sometimes been cited with less regard for priority than for aptness of documentation, illustration, and usefulness in leading the inquirer further along a search.

To enable the student to take the responsibility for learning on his own initiative, so-called "Case Development Problems" have been employed as simple learning devices* in association with this text. A group of these

* Harris, J. W., Horrigan, D. L., Ginther, J. R., and Ham, T. H.: Pilot study in teaching hematology with emphasis on self-education by the student, J. Med. Educ. 37:719, 1962.

problems has been published by The Commonwealth Fund and is available as an inexpensive supplement.*

Credit for what is accurate must go largely to the following workers, who most helpfully reviewed various sections: Drs. Franklin G. Ebaugh, Jr., Clement A. Finch, Clifford W. Gurney, Ernst R. Jaffé, Wallace N. Jensen, Robert F. Schilling, Rudi Schmid, and Scott N. Swisher. Their corrections and suggestions are gratefully acknowledged. For any remaining inaccuracies, omissions, and misleading statements, the blame is wholly mine.

Special thanks are given to Mrs. Marie K. Gubics for her invaluable aid and unfailing patience in preparing the manuscript, not only in the several preliminary forms in which it has been used for teaching, but also for publication. David B. Harris was of material help in preparing the index. Mrs. Dorothy S. Obré and Roger A. Crane of The Commonwealth Fund have contributed greatly in the process of bringing the book to its final form.

John W. Harris, M.D.
Cleveland Metropolitan General Hospital

* Harris, J. W., and Horrigan, D. L.: Case Development Problems in Hematology: Series 1, The Red Cell, Problems 1–8, Harvard University Press, Cambridge, Mass., 1963.

CONTENTS

PART II.   GENERAL CONSIDERATIONS OF ANEMIA

PART III.   THE RED CELL: PRODUCTION

PART VII. THE RED CELL: UNDERPRODUCTION

REFERENCES

PART I] HEMOGLOBIN BIOSYNTHESIS

CHAPTER ONE

HEME BIOSYNTHESIS, THE PORPHYRIAS, AND PORPHYRINURIA

NORMAL HEME BIOSYNTHESIS[*]

Although the chemical structure of heme had been established by the work of H. Fischer in 1929 (44), prior to 1945 no certain information was available concerning the chemical precursors or the pathways of in vivo synthesis of the porphyrin ring of heme (ferroprotoporphyrin 9) (Figure 1.1). In that year Shemin and Rittenberg (169) made the chance observation that N^{15}-tagged glycine specifically labeled the heme of human hemoglobin by becoming a component of the porphyrin ring. At the present time the origin of each of the atoms in the heme moiety is accurately known.

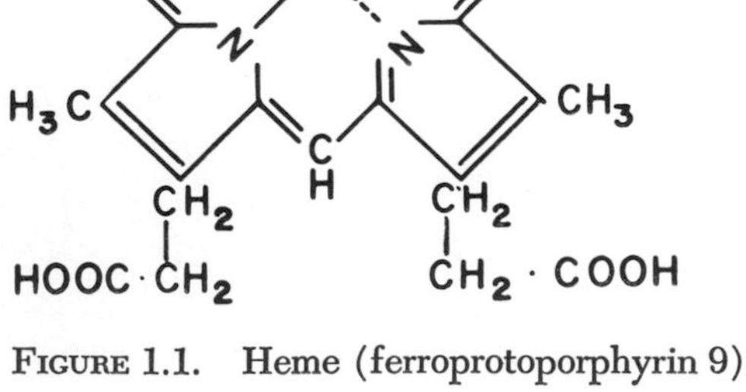

Most of the studies delineating the steps in porphyrin synthesis have for convenience employed systems leading to the production of hemoglobin. Available evidence warrants the conclusion that the steps of biosynthesis are the same whether the heme moiety is destined to become a component of hemoglobin, myoglobin, catalase, cytochrome, etc. in the appropriate body or tissue site (39, 55, 100, 115, 121, 131).

Although most mammalian cells (a notable exception being the normal mature erythrocyte) are capable of synthesizing heme, for technical reasons major portions of the work concerning the various steps of synthesis have employed nucleated duck or chicken erythrocytes. However, a number of the essential reactions have been shown to occur in human reticulocyte preparations, and enough information is now available concerning the abnormalities of heme synthesis in disease states to make certain that the sequence of events is comparable.

The established steps in the biosyn-

FIGURE 1.1.   Heme (ferroprotoporphyrin 9)

[*] General references and review articles: 39, 47, 58, 143, 145, 162, 183.

thesis of heme (Figure 1.2) will now be considered.

Condensation of Glycine and Succinate

By rigid chemical and physical analysis of heme, Shemin et al. (170–176) determined the precise location in the por-

phyrin ring of all the carbon atoms derived from α-C-labeled glycine when it was employed as a precursor; the origin of the remaining carbon atoms was established by similar analytic procedures employing labeled succinate or acetate.

Of the eight molecules of glycine re-

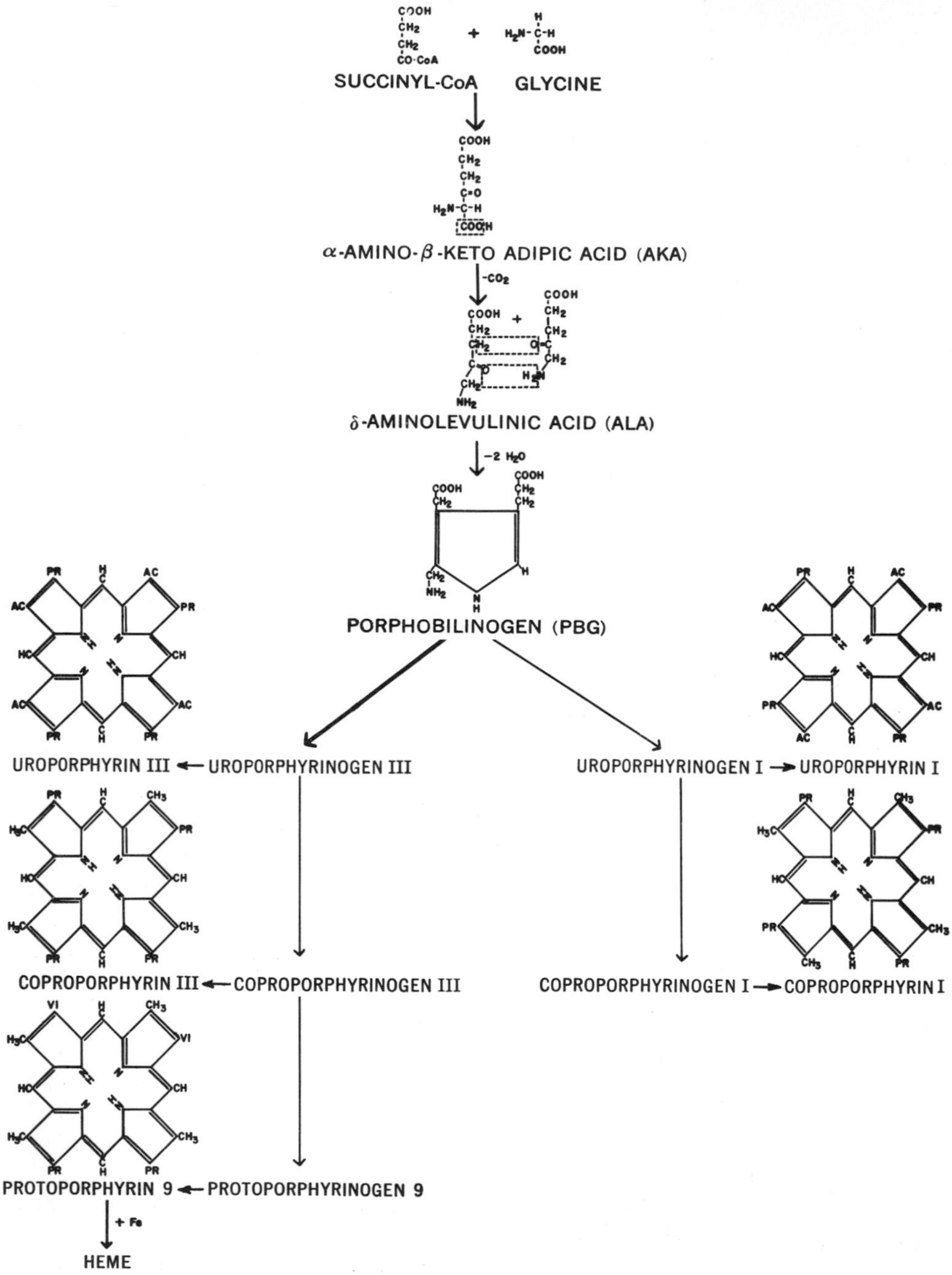

FIGURE 1.2.   Biosynthesis of heme

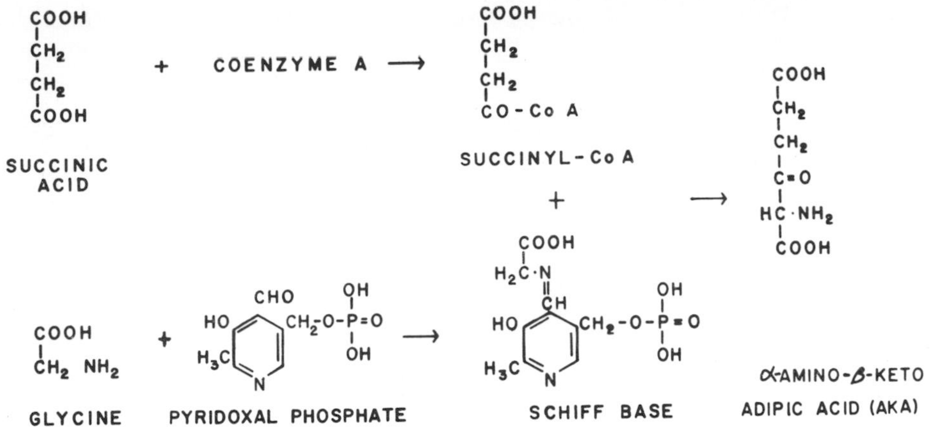

FIGURE 1.3.   Formation of α-amino-β-keto adipic acid

quired in the biosynthesis of heme, four of the eight nitrogen atoms (122, 170, 175) and eight of the sixteen carbon atoms (123, 170, 175) are utilized; none of the carboxyl carbons is utilized. Four of the eight utilized α-carbons of glycine are attached to the four nitrogen atoms; the other four constitute the methene bridges (=CH−) linking the pyrrole rings. The remaining twenty-six carbon atoms found in heme are derived from intermediates of the tricarboxylic acid cycle (acetate, α-ketoglutarate, citrate, succinate). Therefore, in the biosynthesis of heme 8 moles of glycine and 8 of a four-carbon intermediate of the tricarboxylic acid cycle are required. The four-carbon compounds have now been demonstrated to be succinate of succinyl–coenzyme A (98, 171, 175).

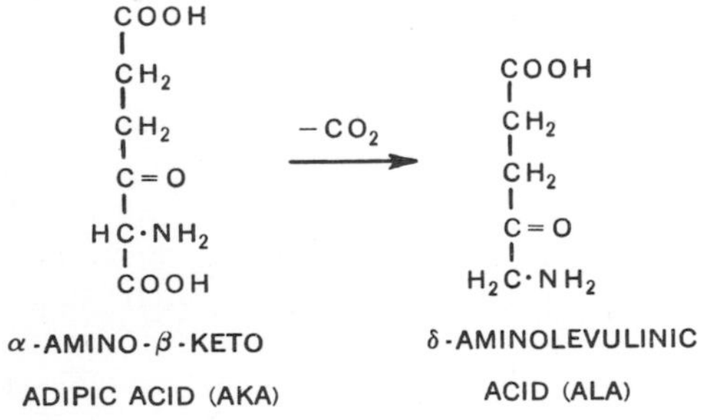

The initial step in the biosynthesis of heme involves the condensation of succinate and glycine. Both compounds require "activation" before they can participate in the specific reaction. "Activated succinate" consists of the thio-ester[*] of coenzyme A derived from the Krebs tricarboxylic acid cycle. Pyridoxal phosphate (vitamin B_6) is necessary for the condensation reaction and apparently participates by the activation of glycine. It has been proposed (69, 91, 176) that a reasonable mechanism is the formation of a Schiff base between glycine or a derivative and pyridoxal phosphate, thus activating the methylene group to condense with "active succinate." The two "activated" precursors condense under appropriate conditions to form α-amino-β-keto adipic acid (AKA) (Figure 1.3).

This latter compound (β-ketonic acid) is unstable and readily loses carbon dioxide to form δ-aminolevulinic acid (ALA) (Figure 1.4). This loss probably occurs spontaneously and is not enzymatically controlled. Although there is

FIGURE 1.4.   Formation of δ-aminolevulinic acid

[*] Rimington (145) has proposed a cycle involving lipothiamide and diphosphopyridine nucleotide (DPN) by which succinyl–coenzyme A is generated; consistent with this Brown (24) has shown that the addition of lipoic acid will stimulate the synthesis of ALA when δ–oxoglutarate is the substrate.

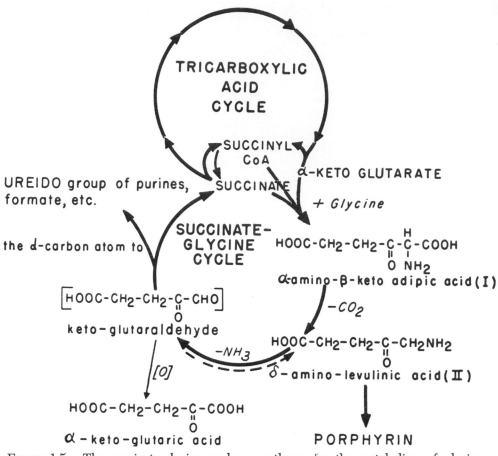

FIGURE 1.5.   The succinate-glycine cycle: a pathway for the metabolism of glycine. (From Shemin, D., et al., J. Biol. Chem. 215:613, 1955)

some evidence for its participation in heme biosynthesis (175), AKA has not been identified during the reaction. However, injected radioactive AKA results in formation of labeled heme.

The position of ALA as an obligatory intermediate in the synthetic chain has been firmly established by radioactive labeling experiments, trapping techniques (40, 153, 172), and, recently (98), by the demonstration of a net synthesis of ALA during the first stages of heme production.

It is interesting to note that Shemin (124, 175, 212) has found evidence that through the above "succinate" cycle glycine is utilized not only in the formation of porphyrins but also in the provision

of carbon fragments that enter into formate, serine, methionine, and the ureido groups of purines (Figure 1.5).

Concerning the production of ALA, Laver et al. (98) showed that particles* obtained from lysates of erythrocytes of anemic chickens could catalyze a net synthesis of ALA from glycine and succinate. This synthesis required the presence of oxygen and was enhanced by the addition of pyridoxal phosphate, coenzyme A, phosphate, and magnesium. When the particles were broken by freeze-drying or homogenization (56), succinyl–coen-

* The exact nature of the particles is not known: nuclei, cell membrane, mitochondria, etc.

zyme A (enzymatically generated or synthetically produced) had to be used.

Schulman and Richert (141, 163) showed that the red cells obtained from ducks deficient in vitamin B_6 had decreased ability to incorporate labeled glycine into heme, while heme synthesis from ALA proceeded satisfactorily. The addition of pyridoxal phosphate to the deficient system stimulated the synthesis of heme from glycine but not from ALA. As stated above, recent work indicates that vitamin B_6 is necessary for the activation of glycine required for its initial condensation with succinyl–coenzyme A. Numerous studies have shown that vitamin B_6 is necessary for normal hematopoiesis in several animals and man: an abnormality in the metabolism of this vitamin results in hypochromic anemia correctable only by vitamin B_6.

By in vitro experiments utilizing red cells from deficient ducks Schulman and Richert (163) also demonstrated that pantothenic acid is necessary for heme synthesis. As would be expected, since it is a component of coenzyme A, pantothenic acid is also required for the formation of ALA from glycine and succinate. Although it has not been demonstrated essential for human erythropoiesis, its deficiency is known to result in hypochromic anemia in various birds and animals.

By way of summarizing the complex reactions involved in the synthesis of ALA, it may be pointed out that a-ketoglutarate can serve as a precursor by entering a portion of the citric acid cycle. Here a-ketoglutarate is converted to succinate and "activated" through the formation of a thio-ester with coenzyme A. A cytochrome electron transfer system to oxygen and oxidative phosphorylation are also required. Since the citric acid cycle, the cytochrome electron transfer system, and the oxidative phosphorylation system are present in mitochondria, and since a particulate system is required for ALA

production, it is tempting to conclude that ALA is synthesized in relation to mitochondria. In a nonparticulate system in which the enzymes have been at least sterically disrupted, succinyl–coenzyme A must be added for ALA synthesis to occur.

Before it can react with succinyl–coenzyme A, glycine also must be activated. This apparently takes place by the formation of a pyridoxal phosphate derivative of glycine. The two activated compounds thus condense to form an intermediate (AKA) that by spontaneous loss of carbon dioxide yields ALA.

Under various experimental conditions it has been shown that the following factors are necessary for or augment the production of ALA: citric acid cycle, oxidative phosphorylation, cytochrome electron transfer system, pyridoxal phosphate, glycine, coenzyme A, DPN, ATP, magnesium ions, iron ions (23, 192), inosine, glutamine, and unidentified liver factors (56).

ALA is normally excreted in small quantities in human urine (111, 117). Its excretion is increased in certain acquired or inherited abnormalities of heme synthesis.

Condensation of Two Molecules of ALA to Form Porphobilinogen

Two molecules of ALA react under the influence of an enzyme, "ALA dehydrase" (56, 64, 158), present in normal human adult red cells as well as in many other tissues such as liver, kidney, and bone marrow, to form a substituted pyrrole, porphobilinogen (PBG) (Figure 1.6). The enzyme is soluble, has been purified, and is now known to be sulfhydryl-containing.* A particulate system is not required for its function, and the

* Originally it was described as copper-containing (85), but recent analyses of more purified preparations do not appear to support this finding.

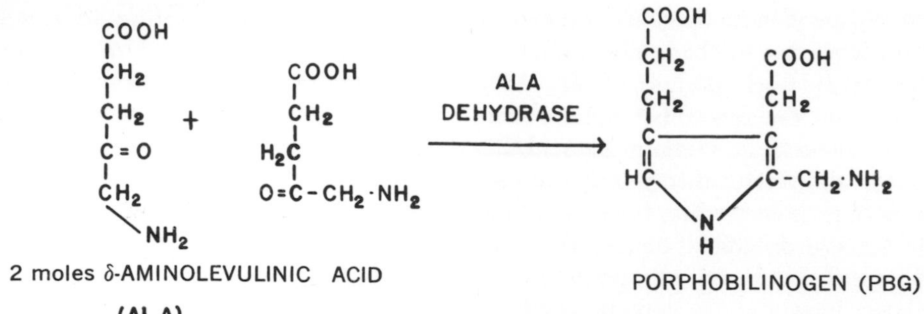

2 moles δ-AMINOLEVULINIC ACID

(ALA)   PORPHOBILINOGEN (PBG)

FIGURE 1.6.   Formation of porphobilinogen

enzyme has been shown to bind two molecules of ALA in the reaction.

PBG has been established as a specific precursor and obligatory intermediate of heme by labeling and trapping experiments (40). Chemically it is a substituted pyrrole. Described in 1934 by Waldenström (199), porphobilinogen has been demonstrated in large amounts in the urine of patients with certain diseases through its color reaction with Ehrlich's aldehyde reagent. However, its chemical composition was not established until 1953, when the studies of Cookson and Rimington were published (32). Contrary to predictions, it was conclusively

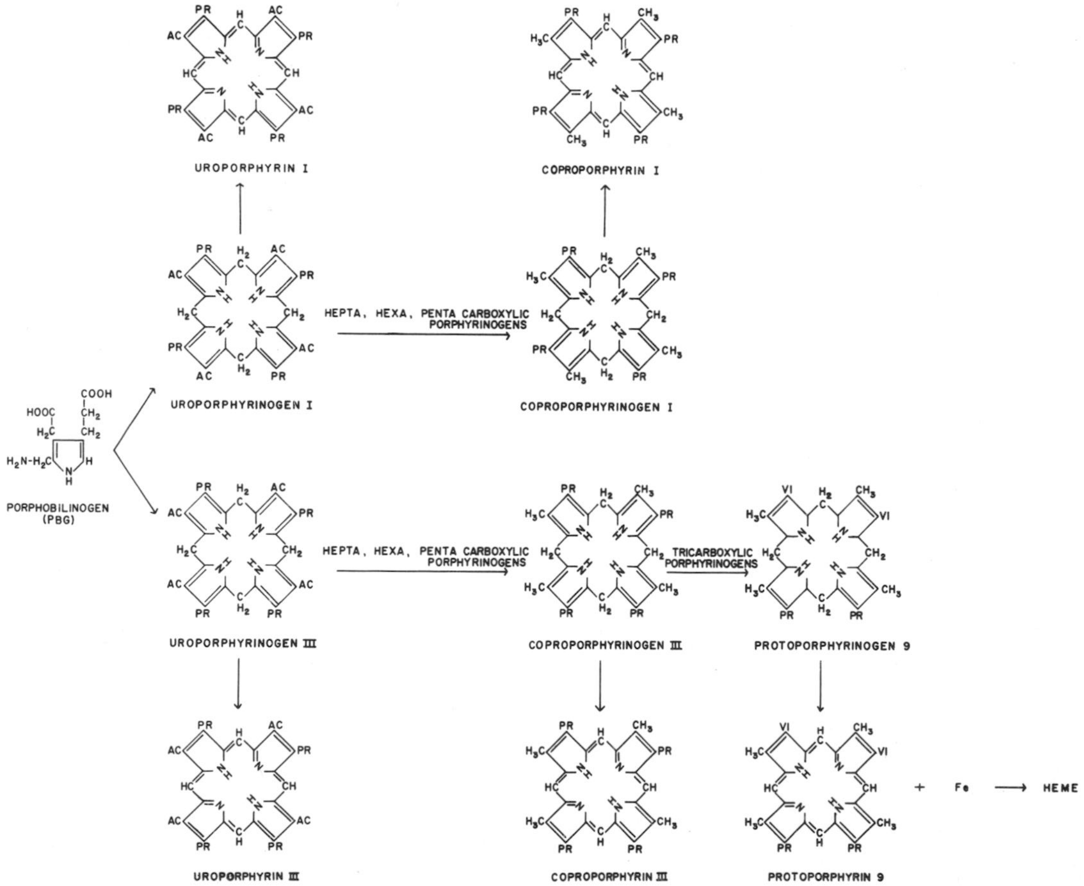

FIGURE 1.7.   Formation of tetrapyrroles from porphobilinogen

shown to be a monopyrrole. This monopyrrole furnishes all the atoms of the final heme product except, of course, iron. Normally a small amount of porphobilinogen is excreted in human urine (117). In some acquired defects of heme biosynthesis greater amounts are excreted, and in some inherited abnormalities of heme synthesis, very large amounts. In the latter instances the detection of PBG forms the basis of a (nearly) pathognomonic test.

Formation of Uroporphyrinogen from PBG

Under the influence of "porphobilinogenase," an enzyme purified and characterized by Lockwood and Rimington (101), four molecules of PBG react, ultimately forming the tetrapyrrolic ring compound, uroporphyrinogen (Figure 1.7).

At this point some information is supplied concerning the nomenclature of the various porphyrins and their isomeric configurations. The basic structure of the porphyrin skeleton consists of four pyrrole rings joined by four =CH—, or methene bridges. Substitutions may occur only at the eight carbons located at the β- positions, or outer corners, of the pyrrole rings: the substituents determine the nature of the particular compound. During the 15 years of Fischer's work upon pyrrole and porphyrin chemistry that culminated in the synthesis of heme, four artificial porphyrins (called the etioporphyrins) were synthesized. To these the isomeric configurations of all other porphyrins are conventionally referred. These etioporphyrins are tetrapyrrolic rings (porphyrins) with either methyl or ethyl substituents attached to the pyrroles, as indicated in Figure 1.8. The po-

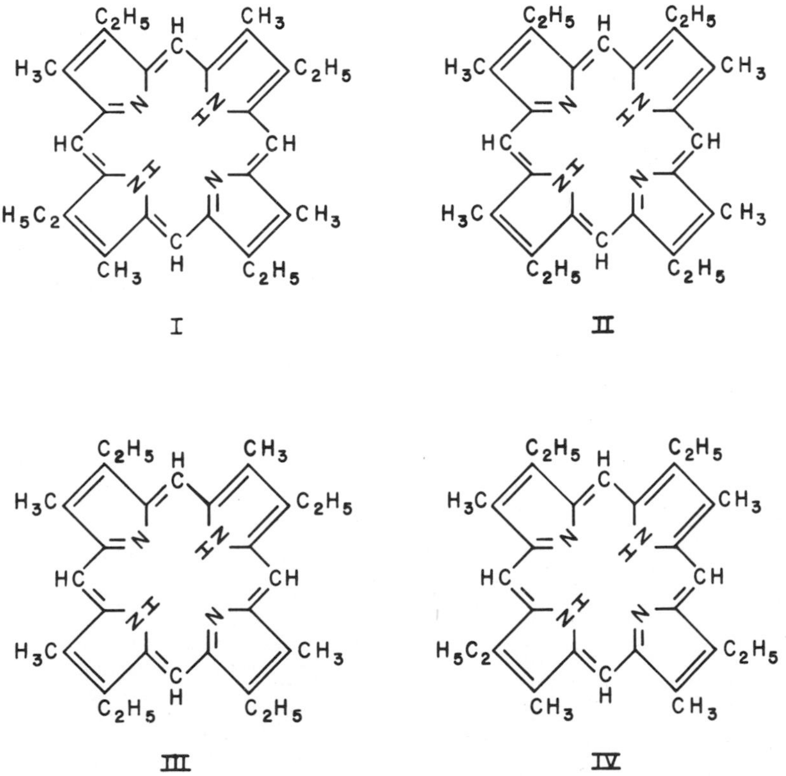

FIGURE 1.8. The four etioporphyrins (synthetic)

sitions of the substituents relative to each other give rise to the different isomeric configurations.

Only compounds of type I or III isomeric configuration have been identified in nature. Two types of substituents are found in uroporphyrinogen* (four acetic and four propionic acid residues) (Figure 1.7) so that four possible structural isomers exist. Protoporphyrinogen, however, has three types of substituents (two vinyl, four methyl, and two propionic acid residues) (Figure 1.7), and thus fifteen isomeric configurations are possible. The protoporphyrinogen that combines with iron to form heme is designated as the number nine (9) isomer and is derived from a type III porphyrin; it is usually referred to as protoporphyrinogen 9, type III isomer. Unlike uro- and coproporphyrinogens, the type I isomer of protoporphyrinogen has not been identified in nature (70), and heme compounds of the type I isomer have never been found.

Although several schemes have been proposed for the intermediate steps in the formation of the porphyrin ring from porphobilinogen, the exact mechanism is unknown and the possibilities will not be reviewed here (see Figures 3–5 in reference 145). On the basis of the isolation of an intensely radioactive polypyrrole during studies on heme-synthesizing duck cells, Wittenberg (210) has hypothesized that the enzyme porphobilinogen deaminase forms a linear tetrapyrrole. Two of these tetrapyrroles apparently condense and then split into two uroporphyrinogen III tetrapyrroles by exchanging single pyrrole rings. Thus, the type III porphyrin series is preferentially formed.

When PBG reacts under the influence of porphobilinogenase, the type III isomer series is formed. If the enzyme is heated, the type I isomer series results. This latter series is the one present in abnormal amounts in various diseases. This finding suggests that the enzyme porphobilinogenase is composed of more than one component. Two separate fractions have been prepared: a PBG deaminase and a uroporphyrinogen isomerase. One of the actions of PBG deaminase† is to remove the amino groups and combine the individual pyrroles into polypyrrolic methanes. The enzyme uroporphyrinogen isomerase does not react with PBG alone, but when it is added to a system containing PBG and PBG deaminase, uroporphyrinogen III is produced.

Numerous studies (20, 117) have established that the biosynthetic pathway from PBG to heme proceeds over a series of porphyrinogens (Figure 1.7). The "—ogen" compounds are colorless tetrapyrroles that contain six more hydrogen atoms than the corresponding porphyrins. In the presence of light and oxidizing agents the colorless "—ogen" compounds are readily converted to the colored porphyrins. In comparison with the total amount of heme synthesized, the fractions of the "—ogen" compounds that are oxidized to porphyrins and elude the biosynthetic pathway are small indeed (Table 1.2, normal values), attesting to the efficacy of light exclusion and intracellular reducing compounds.

Conversion of Uroporphyrinogen III to Coproporphyrinogen III

It is now well established by labeling, trapping, and net synthesis studies that in the synthetic series leading to heme, uroporphyrinogen precedes coproporphyrinogen (40, 125). The transformation of one to another takes place through successive removal of carboxyl groups from the side chains (Figures 1.2 and 1.7).

---

* Fischer's prefix designation used in naming the various porphyrins was based on their then-described major site of occurrence or source for isolation: "proto-" indicated widespread distribution; "copro-" fecal source; "uro-" urine source. With more sensitive methods for detection, the latter terms have become fairly unsatisfactory but by convention are still retained.

† The enzyme is heat-stable and acting alone converts PBG to uroporphyrinogen I.

Thus, uroporphyrinogen has as substituents four acetic acid and four propionic acid residues (eight COOH groups); coproporphyrinogen has four methyl and four propionic acid residues (four COOH groups), four carbons having been removed from the acetic acid side chains. Some of the intermediate compounds (hepta-, hexa-, and pentacarboxylic porphyrinogens) have been identified but not completely characterized; their place in human disease is not defined. Little is known about the enzyme(s) required to decarboxylate the porphyrins in the transformation of uro- to coproporphyrinogen (uroporphyrinogen decarboxylase(s)) except that it is unstable, requires a dialyzable and heat-stable factor, and is present in normal human red cells (20, 67).

Uroporphyrinogen and coproporphyrinogen are known to be in the direct synthetic chain. The uro- and coproporphyrinogen compounds which are direct precursors of heme are colorless, do not fluoresce, cannot bind metals, and are readily auto-oxidatively and photocatalytically dehydrogenated to form uroporphyrin and coproporphyrin. Mainly because of technologic limitations, the porphy*rin* compounds have until recently been the substances usually recovered, tested for, and characterized by those working with normal and pathologic urines. Because of the very nature of the methods employed, the precursors were changed in varying degrees to the various porphyrins. It is only recently that reliable data concerning the excretion of precursors have become, in part, available. Uroporphyrins I and III are not altered by the enzyme that converts uroporphyrinogen to coproporphyrinogen. Moreover, the enzyme is only about one-third as active in converting type I uroporphyrinogen as in converting type III uroporphyrinogen. Uroporphyrin and coproporphyrin are *not* in the direct line of heme synthesis but are, rather, terminal products of side reactions arising by auto-oxidation of the parent compounds. Uro- and coproporphyrins are not used by red cell hemolysates, but uro- and coproporphyrinogens (type III isomer only) are readily transformed into heme. Uro- and coproporphyrinogens I and III and uro- and coproporphyrins I and III are found in normal human urine in very small quantities but may be found in large amounts and in altered ratios in induced or inherited abnormalities of heme synthesis.

Conversion of Coproporphyrinogen III to Protoporphyrin(?ogen) 9

By successive decarboxylation, this time with added oxidation (dehydrogenation of two propionic acid side chains to form vinyl residues), the coproporphyrinogen compound is converted to protoporphyrin (?ogen) 9. This is apparently a specific reaction since, as mentioned above, only type III protoporphyrin 9 is found in nature. For the reaction, oxygen (or hydrogen acceptors) and intact or disrupted mitochondria are necessary. Hemolysates of human adult red cells, although unable to utilize glycine and acetate, readily transform ALA or PBG into uro- and coproporphyrinogens III. Addition of liver mitochondria results in the formation of protoporphyrin. Neither protoporphyrin or protoporphyrinogen has been demonstrated in human urine, but free protoporphyrin is regularly found in all human red cells (197, 211). Under conditions of abnormal heme synthesis the levels of free erythrocyte protoporphyrin may be markedly increased.

There is considerable debate at the present time whether iron is inserted into protoporphyrin or protoporphyrinogen. In experiments by Granick (68), Goldberg et al. (61), and Grinstein et al. (74) added protoporphyrin was well utilized for heme synthesis. However, there apparently is the possibility that the added protoporphyrin is' reduced to the "—ogen" compound before final utilization. On the basis of unpublished work from his laboratory, Rimington believes that "at the penultimate stage in the biosynthesis of heme, protoporphyrin appears from the reduced precursor either spontaneously or by a specific dehydrogenase" and that protoporphyrinogen is in the synthetic chain as a direct precursor of protoporphyrin. Other factors governing the insertion of iron into the protoporphyrin ring to form heme (ferroprotoporphyrin 9, type III porphyrin) will be discussed in Chapter 2, in the section on Iron Metabolism.

Approximately 300 mg of heme is produced daily by the bone marrow of an adult and utilized for hemoglobin formation. No satisfactory estimate of the total amount of heme produced by a normal individual is available because of the lack of precise information concerning turnover time of myoglobin,* the cytochromes, etc. The turnover time of liver catalase has been estimated as a few days (159) so that it is likely that second to bone marrow the liver is a major producer of heme and that the total-body biosynthesis of heme is considerably greater than 300 mg per day.

INHERITED ABNORMALITIES: THE PORPHYRIAS†

Utilizing as a background the established chain of events leading to the production of heme, it is of interest to consider some of the clinical disorders associated with or characterized by abnormalities in heme biosynthesis. As mentioned previously, there is evidence that the biosynthesis of heme is the same whether the pigment is ultimately to be hemoglobin, myoglobin, catalase, cytochrome, etc. There are thus several main body sites at which disordered heme biosynthesis can occur. Based on observations that in a certain disease most of the heme precursors are concentrated and undoubtedly produced in the developing red cells of the bone

marrow and that in other diseases the heme precursors are concentrated and probably produced in the liver (198), Watson has proposed the following abbreviated classification of the porphyrias (201).

A. Erythropoietic porphyria. A very rare disease in which there is excessive and abnormal formation of heme precursors in the developing red blood cells of the bone marrow. It is characterized by skin photosensitivity in the young; by excretion of abnormal amounts of various heme precursors; and usually by increased erythropoiesis, hemolytic anemia, and splenomegaly.

B. Hepatic porphyria. A disease in which there is excessive and abnormal formation of heme precursors in the liver. Inexplicably, this disorder can have several modes of clinical expression, all characterized by excretion of excessive amounts of various heme precursors. In one such expression, designated *intermittent acute hepatic porphyria,* the manifestations are predominantly abdominal pain and/or neurologic abnormalities. Another, designated *cutanea tarda hepatic porphyria* is characterized mainly by skin photosensitivity and frequently by hepatic dysfunction. Finally there is a *mixed* or *combined type of hepatic porphyria* characterized by photosensitivity *with* episodes of abdominal pain and/or neurologic abnormalities *and,* frequently, by evidence of liver dysfunction.

Not all authorities in the field are in agreement with this classification, some believing it to be based on evidence that is insufficient to support the main division. They maintain that some of the

* Akson et al. (2) have reported that studies employing labeled glycine to tag the heme and globin components of myoglobin indicate the existence of two populations of myoglobin, one with a half life of 20 days and the other with a half life of 80 to 90 days.

† General references and review articles: 4, 36, 41, 54, 62, 87, 116, 142, 162, 166, 180, 194, 195, 201, 204.

above-designated subtypes are indeed diseases of different etiology. However, the classification is useful for the cases seen and reported in this country (202). Watson's extended classification of porphyrias is given in Table 1.1.

Both types of porphyria (the erythropoietic and the hepatic) are believed to represent examples of those diseases resulting from constitutional faults, or inborn errors, of metabolism (194), in these instances abnormalities in heme biosynthesis and overproduction of various heme precursors. Family studies on human beings and animals warrant the conclusion that the errors of metabolism are often genetically governed. Indeed the newer, more sensitive analytic techniques have uncovered familial instances of *latent forms of porphyria.* As in an increasing number of other metabolic abnormalities of demonstrated or presumed enzyme insufficiency, a precipitating factor may or may not intervene to make the disease clinically overt.

Erythropoietic Porphyria

According to Watson, the basis for this disease is a constitutional fault in the biosynthesis of the heme of hemoglobin in the red cell precursors. It is associated with skin photosensitivity appearing at an early age; excessive excretion of various heme precursors; and frequently by increased hematopoiesis, hemolytic anemia, and splenomegaly (3). It is an excessively rare disease, a total of some forty-two clear-cut cases having been described. There is no significant sex preponderance (twenty-five females, seventeen males). Sixteen of these forty-two cases are familial, occurring in siblings of eight families but never in different generations of the same family. The disease has been seen in several different races. Although a governing autosomal recessive gene is the suspected genetic mechanism, there is no proof of this. Consanguinity has been found in three families, so affected patients are probably homozygous for the recessive gene. Rimington has demonstrated by father-daughter matings a recessive type of inheritance of a disease of cattle showing the "closest similarity" to human erythropoietic porphyria (142).

The clinical features of the disease are uniformly dominated by skin photosensi-

TABLE 1.1.   Extended classification of the porphyrias

I.   Erythropoietic porphyria and erythropoietic protoporphyria
II.   Hepatic porphyria
A.   Hereditary acute intermittent
1. Manifest
2. Latent
B.   Hereditary mixed or "variegate"
1. Cutaneous with little or no acute manifestations
2. Acute intermittent with cutaneous symptoms
3. Various combinations
4. Latent
C.   Hereditary cutaneous (?)
D.   Constitutional or idiosyncratic (cutanea tarda)
1. Resulting from chemicals, especially alcohol
2. Idiopathic
3. With systemic disease
E.   Acquired
1. Secondary to hepatoma
2. Secondary to hexachlorbenzene

Adapted from Watson, C. J., New England J. Med. 263:1205, 1960.

tivity that appears early: shortly after birth or within the first few years. This dermal sensitivity is manifested by the formation of vesicles or bullae in response to exposure to natural light. The lesions, therefore, occur most frequently on the head and extremities and may, because of repeated exposures and complications from secondary infections, result in scarring and mutilation of face (especially nose, eyelids, and ears) and hand (loss of fingers). Since the vesicles occur in response to natural light, they appear more frequently during the summer months, and have been named "hydroa aestivale." Increased pigmentation and hypertrichosis have frequently been described and are thought by some to be compensatory mechanisms. Red staining of the deciduous and permanent teeth (erythrodontia) is an inconstant finding, but red fluorescence of the teeth under ultraviolet light is always present. Pigmentation of the skeletal bones may be a most striking manifestation and is due to the adsorption or incorporation of porphyrins. At some time during the course of the disease the excretion of red-colored urine begins, usually to continue fairly constantly thereafter. Apart from the sensitivity to light, symptoms are usually not bothersome. Abdominal pains, hypertension, and neurologic symptoms characteristic of other forms of porphyria do not occur. Women with the disease have given birth to normal offspring (89). Typically, overt hemolytic anemia is present along with splenomegaly. This anemia is variable but usually mild. It is characteristically associated with reticulocytosis, hyperactive bone marrow, increased level of unconjugated bilirubin in the blood, and increased urobilinogen* excretion. Measurements of red cell survival time (the critical determination to establish the presence or absence of a hemolytic process) have yielded results consistent with normal (28), slightly increased, and markedly increased (73)

rates of erythrocyte destruction.

In this disorder the excretory abnormalities of heme biosynthesis are confined to the tetrapyrrolic, or porphyrin, compounds. The urinary excretion of ALA and PBG is not abnormal (179). As mentioned above, most of the methods employed in studying the porphyrins yield results in terms of the oxidized porphyrin compounds so that the amounts of true heme precursors are largely unknown. The urine contains a large amount of uroporphyrin I and a smaller amount of coproporphyrin I; the reverse ratio is found in the feces (3). Urinary protoporphyrin is not increased.

The most interesting observation concerning the pathophysiology of this disease has been the demonstration of large amounts of porphyrins in the developing red cells of the marrow (152, 160, 198). Fluorescence microscopy demonstrated excessive formation of porphyrins in the normoblast nuclei. Curiously enough, only a certain proportion of the normoblasts were demonstrably abnormal. Quantitative considerations indicated that large amounts of the excreted porphyrins had been released from intact, developing erythrocytes in the bone marrow. Moreover, the amounts present in the bone marrow greatly exceeded those in the liver. Since the porphyrins were believed to originate largely, if not entirely, in the developing nucleated erythrocyte, the disease was termed erythropoietic porphyria. The primary defect is associated with the overproduction of porphyrins of the type I isomer configuration, a defect which appears confined to the hematopoietic system. In a case recently described, needle-shaped, crys-

---

* Heme precursors are components of an *anabolic* process associated with hemoglobin *production;* bilirubin and urobilinogen result from *catabolic* processes *degrading* hemoglobin. There is no evidence at present that, once formed, hemoglobin can revert to any of its precursors or, conversely, that heme precursors can be metabolized through the bilirubin-urobilinogen cycle.

tal-like structures were formed in some of the abnormal normoblastic and non-nucleated red cells (187). Erythrocytes of patients with erythropoietic porphyria (143) can convert ALA and PBG to porphyrins of *both* type I and III isomers. The most likely site for the metabolic defect would appear to be in the enzyme that converts PBG to uroporphyrinogen. PBG deaminase converts PBG to uroporphyrinogen I only; uroporphyrinogen III requires the combined action of PBG deaminase and uroporphyrinogen isomerase. Overactivity of PBG deaminase or underactivity of the isomerase could account for the findings.

An additional abnormality noted by Schmid et al. (160) in the nuclei of some of the fluorescent normoblasts was the presence of benzidine-positive inclusions: hemoglobin or some closely related substance. Although the spleen was found to contain large amounts of porphyrins, these were believed present secondarily to splenic destruction of the circulating red cells. However, the rate of destruction of red cells was such that it did not seem reasonable that more than a small fraction of the excreted porphyrins came from destroyed circulating red cells. In the first case studied in this fashion significant splenic enlargement was present along with overt, severe hemolytic anemia. Splenectomy was done and resulted in dramatic improvement. The hemolytic anemia was cured, the porphyrin excretion declined markedly, and the photosensitivity disappeared (3). The child has developed normally and has had no recurrence of anemia or photosensitivity (201). These changes can probably best be interpreted as resulting from the abolition of a hemolytic process by splenectomy, which reduced the requirement for new red cells and consequently diminished bone marrow erythropoiesis and the biosynthesis of the heme of hemoglobin. Unfortunately, the responses of subsequent patients to splenectomy have

not been uniform (69, 187). Some apparently showed no significant change in any modality of the syndrome; others showed improvement in one or another modality without associative change elsewhere. In one case, despite reduction in porphyrin formation and excretion, photosensitivity and anemia persisted. Aside from the possibly beneficial effects of splenectomy, treatment is limited to general supportive measures and protection from sunlight by means of clothing, ointment, lotions, and avoidance of sunny climates.

Magnus et al. (110) have recently reported a patient with "erythropoietic protoporphyria—a new porphyria syndrome with solar urticaria due to protoporphyrinaemia." This patient did not excrete abnormal amounts of ALA, PBG, or porphyrins in the urine, but large amounts of coproporphyrins and protoporphyrins were found in the feces, and the erythrocyte concentration of coproporphyrin and protoporphyrin was markedly elevated. The erythrocytes had a slightly shortened survival time and fluoresced readily.

Intermittent Acute Hepatic Porphyria

In studies similar to those outlined above, Watson (198) demonstrated that in this disease the amounts of heme precursors in the liver were invariably increased while those in the bone marrow were consistently normal. This evidence was interpreted as indicating the liver to be responsible for the excessive formation and release of heme precursors. This fundamental fault occurs in a disease characterized by attacks of acute abdominal pain, neurologic disorders, and the excretion of a urine that darkens significantly on standing because of the conversion of abnormal amounts of porphyrinogens and other heme precursors into porphyrins, porphobilins, and other unidentified pigments. During the course of the disease the patient experiences remissions and exacerbations of varying degrees.

The disease is infrequent but not rare. A number of surveys have demonstrated its familial nature, many families having been described in which both parent and child had the disease in an active form (194, 195). Recent refinements in analytic techniques have allowed the detection of *latent forms* of the disease in relatives of afflicted patients by the demonstration of abnormal amounts of heme precursors in the urine (107). An unknown factor is how many of the presumably normal relatives might excrete abnormal amounts of precursors if suitably provoked.* It is generally considered that the condition is inherited as a Mendelian dominant character with varying degrees of clinical expression. All workers agree that the clinical disorder is more frequently seen in females than males (ratio approximately 60:40) for unknown reasons and is usually seen in the third or fourth decade of life.

The initial complaints are almost invariably abdominal pain and/or neurologic aberrations. The abdominal pain is usually colicky in nature, located mainly in the epigastrium and right lower quadrant, causing great distress and lasting seldom less than 48 hours, usually for several days, but rarely for months. The pain is most frequently accompanied by constipation and vomiting, but diarrhea may occur. The abdomen is usually soft; tenderness is not marked, and rebound tenderness is lacking. Intestinal spasms alternating with atonia and dilatation have been demonstrated by laparotomy, recording balloons, and radiography.

The neurologic manifestations are variable (38, 54, 62, 164). First, paralysis or paresis of limb musculature occurs secondary to lower motor neuron disease. The motor disturbance develops in a random fashion, and although usually bilateral, it may be asymmetric. In severe cases the trunk muscles and cranial nerves may also be affected. Bulbar signs may be associated with respiratory paralysis. Second, sensory disturbances frequently occur and consist of anything from analgesia to hyperesthesia and pain in almost any area but usually the lower limbs. Third, various cortical disturbances occur, such as epileptiform seizures and psychic aberrations. The latter may take the form of schizophrenia, manic or depressive states, or simply "peculiar behavior." A significant number of patients are diagnosed only after admission to and prolonged residence in a mental hospital.

Most patients have marked tachycardia during the acute phase of the disease, and indeed this is thought by some to represent a good index of the activity of the disease. Transient hypertension is frequent, sometimes with evident changes in the retinal arteries.

By and large the routine laboratory studies yield results well within normal limits unless the patient has suffered dehydration, fever, or convulsions. During acute attacks, marked hyponatremia may occur probably on the basis of inappropriate secretion of antidiuretic hormone (79a, 106). Along with the hyponatremia, serum hypo-osmolality, natruresis, and urine hypertonicity occur.

A significant finding is the presence in the urine of markedly increased amounts of ALA and PBG (77, 117); a hundred-fold increase of these heme precursors is not remarkable during an acute attack. The detection of an abnormal amount of ALA constitutes a very sensitive screening test since the level is fairly consistently elevated; the detection of an abnormal amount of PBG by a relatively simple, readily available method is nearly pathognomonic of intermittent acute hepatic porphyria (199, 204). The basis

* As will be pointed out, it is not feasible to employ barbiturates and other such agents in attempts to make manifest otherwise latent porphyrias, since severe and even fatal attacks may be produced. Interesting studies by Richards et al. (140) indicate that loading doses of glycine may provoke abnormal increases in ALA by individuals with latent porphyria without activating the disease process.

for the test is the easily demonstrable intense red color that develops from the interaction of PBG and Ehrlich's aldehyde reagent.* Analysis of the urine for content of various porphyrins has yielded seemingly controversial results. However, since it has been pointed out that most of the isolated porphyrins are actually formed from precursors *after* the urine is passed and are thus largely artifactual, depending on external factors such as pH, exposure to light and air, and presence of oxidizing substances, disparity of the analytic results is to be expected. Owing to this conversion of precursors to porphyrins and related compounds, freshly voided and normal-appearing urine darkens on standing in light and air. However, not all the color is due to porphyrin formation, since porphobilin, a brown amorphous oxidation product of PBG, also appears. The excretion of uroporphyrin(ogen) I is increased in the urine but coproporphyrin(ogen) I is present only in small amounts. Conversely uroporphyrinogen III is present in a small amount in the feces, but coproporphyrinogen III is increased. Most of the porphyrins are found as a metal complex, probably zinc. No good explanation has been offered for this finding or for the fact that in erythropoietic porphyria the free forms are found. Protoporphyrin(ogen) has not been demonstrated in the urine. Despite the fact that most of the tetrapyrrole heme precursors are excreted as the colorless, nonfluorescent precursors, the following attests to the fact that some porphyrin compounds may be present. The first-noticed symptom of a gasoline station night attendant subsequently shown to have intermittent acute hepatic porphyria was that his urine had a peculiar red glow when voided into one of the newly installed ultraviolet-light-sterilized toilets. It has been well documented that during remission there may be a marked reduction of the heme precursors in the urine, sometimes to the normal range.

As would be expected from the account of the initial symptoms, the course and prognosis of this disease are extremely varied. Its existence in latent form is now definitely established; a second type is characterized by occasional intermittent abdominal pain; a third by explosive attacks fatal in a matter of days, usually because of neurologic involvement. The disease pattern in some patients is nonprogressive and recurrent; in others the severity of attacks progresses steadily; some recover quickly and completely; some are left crippled or insane but over many years may completely regain physical and mental function. There is no doubt that certain chemicals may provoke a latent form into an overt one or precipitate an attack. Barbiturates are the worst offenders, but many other agents have been incriminated: Sulfonal, Trional, Phanodorn, Sedormid, ergot preparations, chloroquine, alcohol, etc. Emotional disturbance and pregancy apparently increase the susceptibility to attacks.

Concerning the pathogenesis of the signs and symptoms (59), it has been demonstrated that purified porphobilinogen is pharmacologically inactive except for the photosensitizing effect when it is converted in the body to porphyrins (54); however, the administration was

---

* The test for PBG consists in mixing 5 ml of urine (fresh) and 5 ml of Fischer's modification of Ehrlich's reagent (0.7 Gm of p-dimethylaminobenzaldehyde, 150 ml of concentrated hydrochloric acid, and 100 ml of distilled water). A large amount of PBG will usually form a red compound at this point in the test. Then 10 ml of saturated aqueous solution of sodium acetate is added, thoroughly mixed to develop the color fully, and tested with Congo red paper to a negative reaction (red). The red color due to any urobilinogen present forms maximally at this point. Then 5 ml of chloroform is shaken with the mixture and allowed to separate. PBG is not extracted by the chloroform; however, its red color remains in the *upper* aqueous layer; urobilinogen is extracted into the chloroform, and its red color therefore is *down* in the chloroform layer. For clarity in separation repeated extractions with chloroform may be made.

admittedly only for relatively short periods of time. ALA has marked but temporary photosensitizing action (167). Since there is no photosensitivity in this disease, the symptomatology obviously cannot be explained by these chemical alterations, especially in view of the growing number of patients reported to have typical and marked chemical abnormalities but no clinical activity. Even with patients known to have porphyria there is no good correlation between the amounts of ALA, PBG, and precursors excreted and the clinical signs and symptoms (1). There is increasing evidence that the liver is the site of the abnormal biosynthesis of heme; several studies have demonstrated increased concentrations of ALA, PBG, uro- and coproporphyrinogens I. When fresh tissue was analyzed employing precautions to prevent formation of porphyrins from precursors, the amounts of uro- and coproporphyrins were only insignificantly increased. Amino-aciduria has recently been described in this disease, but its role in pathogenesis is obscure (120).

In 1956 Gibson and Goldberg (54) demonstrated the extensive primary demyelinization that occurs throughout the nervous system, suggested that the clinical features may be explained entirely on a neurogenic basis, and hypothesized that the nerve damage is secondary to or associated with a disturbance of pyrrole-pigment metabolism in the nervous system related to that in the liver. Demyelinization can explain the paresis seen in peripheral nerve involvement, and foci of demyelinization in the cerebellar and cerebral white matter can explain the ataxia and mental changes. The few studies correlating pathologic findings with clinical manifestations have shown good agreement (183). It has been suggested that the gastrointestinal manifestations may be due to abnormalities in the preganglionic fibers that innervate the viscera. Retrograde changes have been de-

scribed in the nuclei of these fibers located in the cord and medulla. Watson has reported temporary relief from use of ganglionic blocking agents and prolonged relief from bilateral splanchnicetomy (201).

It is clear that major biochemical defects in this form of porphyria involve the apparent overproduction and increased accumulation of the heme precursors ALA, PBG, and porphyrinogens; evidence concerning the possible mechanisms of these abnormalities is presently lacking.

It has been proposed on the basis that glycine is used in the "succinate" cycle not only for this formation of porphyrins but also for the formation of purines (124, 175, 212; Figure 1.5) that the porphyrias might result from an imbalance in the production of heme precursors and purine compounds. There is some evidence that in experimental porphyria the synthesis of purines is decreased with consequent build-up of ALA and porphyrins (182). Since it has not been possible to attribute the symptomatology and pathologic findings to the accumulation of heme precursors, it has also been suggested that there may be a deficiency in the phosphorylated derivatives of adenosine. In experimental porphyria inosine has been shown to decrease liver porphyrins, increase hepatic heme, and stimulate the incorporation of radioiron into heme (103). Consequently it is of interest that therapeutic trials of adenosine monophosphate have been associated with reversal of clinical and biochemical abnormalities (9, 49) and that "very encouraging" results have been obtained by treating porphyria patients with inosine (151). The therapeutic trials of these compounds thought "to correct the basic metabolic defect" have been very limited, and further evaluation is obviously necessary.

Treatment is largely directed at relieving pain. Barbiturates must be avoided! Paraldehyde, chloral hydrate, and Demerol are reliable and of the most value. Chlorpromazine (119), ACTH, and cortisone have been reported to induce remission in some patients, but quite unpredictably. Many failures have occurred. Perhaps of more promise although certainly not adequately established as reliable therapeutic aids are chelating agents (132) such as BAL and EDTA (133). These have been reported to induce remissions, presumably by correcting an enzyme system block caused by zinc, copper, or other cations. This block is thought to result from depletion of chelation reserves related to the porphyrin pool. It is still safe to say there is no reliable, satisfactory, rational treatment for the porphyrias.

Cutanea Tarda Hepatic Porphyria

This disease is also associated with excessive formation of some heme precursors in the liver and is characterized mainly by skin photosensitivity and frequently by the development of hepatic dysfunction. Its hereditary transmission is thought governed by a dominant gene, but its expression appears to be more frequent in males than females. Although cases have been described that began in childhood, by and large the term "cutanea tarda" is an apt one, since the onset of manifestations ordinarily occurs in the fourth decade or later. The skin lesions are similar to, but not as severe as, those seen in erythropoietic porphyria; disfigurement seldom occurs. Bullous lesions are common and, although limited almost entirely to the areas exposed to light, frequently appear to be associated with trauma and heat. Considerable scarring and sometimes chronic ulceration result. The signs and symptoms may remain fairly stationary and follow a rather benign course. The skin lesions may also be eczematoid or urticarial. Some reports have noted that patients have an increased brownish pigmentation; others have commented on a peculiar violaceous hue of the face. Manifestations of hepatic disorder usually play an important role at some time during the course of the disease. Episodes of jaundice occur that early are not associated with other evidences of liver dysfunction detectable by laboratory tests. Later, results of tests for hepatic function are abnormal, and spider nevi and ascites may be present. Alcoholism has been noted perhaps significantly frequently in some series, and Watson has induced exacerbations of the excretory abnormalities by the administration of alcohol. An association with diabetes has been reported in some studies. Liver biopsy or autopsy examination may show varying degrees of fatty liver, parenchymal cell injury, and/or cirrhosis.

Fluoresence microscopy of liver preparations shows the abnormal light activity to be caused mainly by preformed uroporphyrin and secondarily by small amounts of coproporphyrin; the amount of PBG is small or negligible. This abnormal heme precursor pattern is also present in the urine. In contrast to intermittent acute hepatic porphyria, little or no increase in ALA and PBG excretion is found. The porphyrins are partly excreted as zinc complexes; a mixture of coproporphyrins is found with more type III than type I. The plasma porphyrin level is reported to be elevated (154). As usual, protoporphyrin excretion cannot be detected in the urine. The characteristic finding is the continuous excretion of high concentrations of coproporphyrin and protoporphyrin in the feces.

Except for the dermal photosensitivity there are no definite conclusions concerning the pathogenesis of the disease or the signs and symptoms. The skin lesions have been produced by exposure to artificial light of wave lengths corresponding to those absorbed maximally in the spectrum of the porphyrins (400 mμ) (109, 149a). Consequently the porphyrins have been implicated in the production of the skin lesions. Fluorescence of the lesions under ultraviolet light has been employed by some as a valuable diagnostic test.

Mixed Type of Hepatic Porphyria

In this type of porphyria, again thought governed by inheritance of a dominant gene, the manifestations are skin photosensitivity, episodes of abdominal pain, and neurologic aberrations which may or may not be concurrent with photosensitivity. These patients also frequently show evidence of liver disease. The onset of the clinical manifestations is usually in middle life, but a few childhood cases have been described. The signs and symptoms of this disease are the same as of the acute and cutanea tarda types. However, long and complete remissions have been observed, and the over-all prognosis is apparently somewhat better.

As might be predicted, the excretory pattern of the heme precursors varies according to the clinical manifestations. ALA and PBG are usually not found in the urine except when abdominal or nervous manifestations are present. When the photosensitivity is the dominant symptom, the excretory pattern is similar to that seen in cutanea tarda porphyria. In Table 1.2 an attempt is made to summarize the changes occurring in the amounts of the various heme precursors in the several types of porphyrias and lead poisoning.

The above oversimplification of the various porphyrias would be inadmissible without some stringently qualifying remarks and presentation of data. Although reports on several series of patients have come from different laboratories, some authorities do not believe the evidence concerning the site of origin of the heme precursors sufficient to support the pathophysiologic division proposed by Watson into the erythropoietic and hepatic types of porphyria. Moreover, opinions differ on the validity of the subdivisions of hepatic porphyria, a group based on Watson's hypothesis that the clinical findings are varied manifestations of a single underlying metabolic abnormality. Rimington believes that the disorders classified by Watson as subtypes of hepatic porphyria (intermittent acute and cutanea tarda hepatic porphyria) are in reality independent diseases of distinct etiology. Disorders classified by Watson as combined or mixed types, Rimington regards as representative of the cutanea tarda group with abdominal or nervous symptoms added to photosensitivity. This opinion is based on detailed studies of a number of patients (83) in whom he has demonstrated, in contradistinction to the findings in intermittent acute porphyria, high fecal output of porphyrins during the quiescent phase of the disease and "highly characteristic switch-over from a fecal to a urinary route of excretion of porphyrin with each attack" (108). In view of the hepatic dysfunction and jaundice that later develop, it is presumed that the switch-over results from temporary hepatic insufficiency of obscure etiology. Thus, Rimington believes that a disease distinct from the others exists, having high fecal porphyrin excretion in remission and characterized clinically by photosensitivity only. Severe attacks, however, may be accompanied by abdominal or nervous symptoms and high urinary excretion of porphyrin precursors.

Another recently restudied discrepancy between the findings of two workers is the following. Waldenström observed that in Sweden, where there is a high incidence of porphyria of the intermittent acute type with no admixture of the cutanea tarda type, patients characteristically excrete abnormal amounts of porphobilinogen during remission. In South Africa, where the disease has a high incidence among whites,*† within porphyric families the cutanea tarda type is more common in the male and the intermittent acute type in the female.†† In these groups PBG was excreted in excessive amounts only during attacks. Because of this discrepancy, a comparative study of Swedish and South African patients was done by Dean and published in 1959 (37). The results confirmed and extended the original observations from both countries demonstrating different patterns of heme precursor excretion. The Swedish group, with only acute episodes of abdominal and neurologic disorders, had high ALA and PBG excretion continuously, while the fecal excretion of porphyrins was normal or slightly raised during attacks. The South African group, with acute intermittent manifestations and/or skin sensitivity, had raised ALA and PBG excretion only during attacks, while increased fecal excretion of copro- and protoporphyrins persisted even during remission. The name variegate porphyria has been proposed for the disease of this group. It would seem, however, that the occurrence of two types of porphyria in one family supports Watson's proposed classification, and new terms only further confuse the issue. Obviously only precise knowledge of the biochemistry of the lesions will clarify the situation. It would be profitless to raise here the many points of difference and discrepancies encountered concerning methods of isolation, identification, and chemistry of various porphyrins, porphyrin complexes, and intermediates.

In all these inherited disorders of heme biosynthesis the number of different abnormal genes involved is unknown; the underlying mechanisms for the metabolic defects are obscure; and accurate evaluations have not been made concerning the modifying effects of environment, nutrition, drugs, etc. upon the clinical and chemical manifestations of the diseases.

Also, in view of the simplified presentation, it must be noted that excessive excretion of heme precursors may be encountered in a few other situations not necessarily known to be related to genetically determined inborn errors of metabolism. Considerable amounts of PBG or uroporphyrin or both together may occasionally be found in the urine of patients with carcinomatosis (201), primary hepatoma (184), Hodgkin's disease, systemic infections, nervous system disease, or advanced liver disease (201) in which the ordinary clinical manifestations of porphyria are lacking. Except for the possibility that a disease reveals an otherwise latent abnormality, the reason for these abnormalities is unknown. An "idiopathic coproporphyrinuria" has been described in which an otherwise normal individual excretes large amounts of coproporphyrin III but no PBG or uroporphyrins (14, 201). Instances of congenital transitory porphyria have been studied in newborns of porphyric mothers. The infants were asymptomatic and did well despite the various heme precursors in the blood and urine. These patients are particularly interesting in view of the lack of symptoms (4, 90).

An outbreak of a cutaneous type of porphyria has been reported recently in which blistering of exposed skin, pigmentation, scarring, hypertrichosis, hepatomegaly, but no abdominal pain or neurologic manifestations, occurred. The patients' urine was red colored and contained increased amounts of uro- and

---

* From metabolic and genetic studies on South African Bantu patients excreting heme precursors, it has been concluded that the disease is not a true porphyria but rather an acquired disease secondary to toxic factors (10, 37, 95).

† In 1688 two emigrants from Holland married and settled at the Cape of Good Hope; in the subsequent six generations 564 individuals of fifty-four family groups descending from this couple have been demonstrated to have this disease (34, 35, 51).

†† It should be noted that both types of inheritance have been described in this country (202).

TABLE 1.2. Summary of changes in amounts of various heme precursors occurring in patients with porphyria and with lead poisoning compared with normal persons

	ALA	PBG	Heme precursors Uro	Copro	Proto
			Porphyrin and/or porphyrinogen, isomeric configuration as specified		
Normal					
Bone marrow	—	—	N	N	N
Liver	—	N	N	N	N
Urine[a]	2 mg/24 hr	1–1.5 mg/24 hr	I>III; 20–60 μg/24 hr	I>III; 100–300 μg/24 hr	—
Feces	—	—	1–3 μg/24 hr	300–1000 μg/24 hr	30–45 μg/24 hr/Gm dry wgt (? exogenous source)
Red blood cells	—	—	—	1–2 μg/100 ml RBC	10–60 μg/100 ml RBC
Erythropoietic porphyria					
Bone marrow	—	—	↗↗↗ (I)	↗↗↗ (I)	↗↗ (III)
Liver	—	—	↗ (I)	↗ (I)	↗ (III)
Urine[a]	N	N	↗↗↗ (I)	↗ (I)	—
Feces	—	—	↗↗↗ (I>III)	↗↗↗ (I>III)	N
Red blood cells	—	—	↗↗↗ (I)	↗↗ (I)	↗ (III)
			{ Free form }		
Acute intermittent hepatic porphyria					
Bone marrow	—	N	N	N	—
Liver	↗↗	↗↗↗	↗↗↗	↗↗	—
Urine[a]	↗↗ 180 mg/24 hr	↗ 50–170 mg/24 hr	↗↗↗	↗↗	N↗
Feces	—	—	N↗	N↗	N↗
Red blood cells	—	—	N	N	↗
			{ Metal complex (Zn) }		

	Heme precursors		Porphyrin and/or porphyrinogen, isomeric configuration as specified		
	ALA	PBG	Uro	Copro	Proto
Cutanea tarda hepatic porphyria					
Bone marrow	—	N	N	N	N
Liver	—	↗	↗↗	↗	—
Urine[a]	N↗	N↗	N↗	N↗	—
Feces	—	—	↗↗↗	↗↗↗ (III)	↗↗↗ (III)
Red blood cells	—	—	N	N	N
Lead poisoning					
Bone marrow	—	—	↗↗ (I)	↗ (III)	↗↗
Liver	—	—	—	—	N
Urine[a]	↗↗↗	N↗	↗ (I)	↗↗↗ (III)	—
Feces	—	—	—	↗↗ (I>III)	—
Red blood cells	—	—	—	↗ (III)	↗↗

N normal amount; ↗ slightly increased amount; ↗↗↗ markedly increased amount; N↗ normal or slightly increased amount; — no data.
[a] A large fraction of the porphyrins present in the urine is excreted in the form of precursors ("-ogens"). ALA and PBG may also be converted nonenzymatically to porphyrins.

coproporphyrins, but no ALA or PBG. This disorder was fairly conclusively established as secondary to a chemical (hexachlorbenzene) used as a fungicide to treat wheat (161).

Experimentally it has been shown that the chronic administration of hexachlorbenzene to rats (48, 129) will produce weight loss, cutaneous and neurologic lesions, liver damage, and the increased excretion and tissue accumulation of porphyrins and porphyrin precursors. In view of the possible metabolic block hypothesized as basic to porphyria, it is of interest to note that treatment with adenosine monophosphate is reported (50) to effect a clinical improvement and decrease the excretion and tissue accumulation of ALA, PBG, and uroporphyrin.

Other methods are available whereby lesions akin to those of the erythropoietic and hepatic types of porphyria can be produced in experimental animals. A combination of lead (128, 165, and below, under Porphyrinuria) to block various steps in heme synthesis, phenylhydrazine to produce hemolytic anemia and consequent bone marrow normoblastic proliferation, and rose Bengal plus ultraviolet light for photodynamic insult produces intense fluorescence of normoblasts and urinary excretion of heme precursors. Feeding with Sedormid (157) produces increased porphyrin and PBG excretion in urine and increased concentrations in the liver. The animals usually die of gastric distention. In neither instance, however, is the urinary pattern of heme precursors analogous to that of the inherited disease.

ACQUIRED ABNORMALITY: PORPHYRINURIA*

Numerous studies have shown that the in vitro synthesis of heme can be markedly inhibited by lead at various stages of the synthetic chain. In patients with lead poisoning (plumbism, saturnism) there is evidence of profound alteration in

heme biosynthesis; abnormal quantities of heme precursors are excreted in the urine or are present in the circulating red cells.

Lead poisoning (7) occurs today in adults largely because of industrial exposure or accidents (6) and in children (27) because of pica and concomitant lead ingestion. Although it still occurs, lead poisoning due to improper storage or transport of water or other liquids (in lead containers and pipes) or the burning of battery cases as fuel for household heating (186) is infrequent.

Clinically, plumbism usually takes one of two forms: in the first the major manifestations resemble those of acute encephalopathy; in the other the predominating signs and symptoms are in the abdomen (lead colic) and/or extremities (lead palsy). Although there are exceptions, children almost invariably have signs of lead encephalopathy, while adults have colic and/or neuromuscular weakness (81). There seems little doubt that the nature of the lead compound and the speed of development of poisoning to some extent determine the symptoms. Tetraethyl lead has been proved to produce encephalopathy even in adults (21),† as does the inhalation of massive amounts of inorganic lead dust.

The average intake of lead per day from food, liquids, and air is approximately 0.4 mg. Of that presented to the gastrointestinal tract, approximately 8 per cent is absorbed. It is transported almost exclusively in association with the red cells (146), and 90 per cent is deposited in the bones. Although small

* General references and review articles: 5, 6, 7, 29, 84, 105, 200.

† Tetraethyl lead is associated with little change in blood lead concentration even when in the body in toxic amounts. Recent studies indicate that tetraethyl lead itself is inert. Because of lipid solubility it apparently goes preferentially to the liver, where one ethyl group is removed. The resulting triethyl lead is water-soluble and has a marked and preferential toxicity for brain and nervous tissue (33).

amounts are present in all viscera, the major part of that not deposited in bone is present in the liver and blood. Lead is apparently handled like calcium and is deposited in bone as insoluble phosphates. In growing bones especially the concentration is highest in the epiphyseal portions, where, in association with a dense deposition of calcium, x-ray examination may show transverse lines of increased opacity that are of diagnostic importance (193). Skeletal lead is biologically inert but not immobile. Under normal conditions it is slowly mobilized from the bone and excreted. With certain metabolic abnormalities (those usually associated with increased calcium turnover) and with chelation therapy, it may be more rapidly withdrawn from the bone. Lead is excreted by the kidney and bowel. The greater part of the fecal lead consists of ingested and unabsorbed lead. The renal excretion is determined by renal function and the concentration of lead in the blood. Probably because of its affinity for red cells very little lead is cleared from the blood, and without chelation therapy urinary excretion is small in amount. Because of this limited excretory capacity lead accumulates, and toxic effects result when the lead intake exceeds some 0.6 mg daily. An unusual mode of lead intake is the absorption through an otherwise impermeable skin of organic lead compounds. Very rapid and complete absorption may take place through the respiratory tract when volatile lead substances or insoluble lead dusts of suitable particle size are inhaled.

The encephalopathic signs and symptoms almost always predominate in lead poisoning in children (5). It occurs largely in children between the ages of 6 months and 4 years and has a definite seasonal incidence: the increase begins in the spring months, reaches a maximum in July and August, and tapers off in the fall months (Figure 1.9). The mortality rate may be as high as 40 per cent, and complete recovery (without mental retardation (53), behavior aberrations, and recurrent convulsive seizures) may be infrequent (26). The seasonal incidence is determined by several factors such as temperature, sunlight, and vitamin D, but mainly by the fact that during these months children of these ages are allowed out of doors, where they have access to paint chips, painted railings, etc. (8). This, coupled with pica, results in a tremendously increased lead intake. Frequently radiopaque material is demonstrable in the gastrointestinal tract, and paint chips may be recovered from the feces.

The clinical manifestations are usually irritability, anorexia, failure to gain weight, behavior disorders, hyperactivity progressing to mania, pallor, lassitude, headache, visual complaints, stupor, coma, and convulsions. Physical examination may be unrewarding but usually reveals a striking pallor,* oculomotor disturbance, reflex changes, signs of meningeal irritation and increased intracranial pressure, bradycardia, and lead line on the gums.

This picture may also be seen in adults with fast-developing lead poisoning, usually due to rapidly absorbed lead, e.g., tetraethyl lead or lead fumes and dusts. Most frequently, however, lead poisoning in adults is the result of a fairly prolonged, moderately increased intake and is manifested by weakness out of proportion to physique; anorexia; abdominal discomfort; colicky abdominal pain, sometimes of extreme intensity and, mistakenly, interpreted as necessitating surgical intervention (112); constipation; and obstipation. Neuromuscular abnormalities are sometimes present in the form of paresthesias, peripheral neuropathy, wrist drop, and foot drop. Physical

---

* Many children with lead poisoning also have iron deficiency, not infrequently associated with pica. Iron metabolism in lead poisoning will be commented on in Chapter 2.

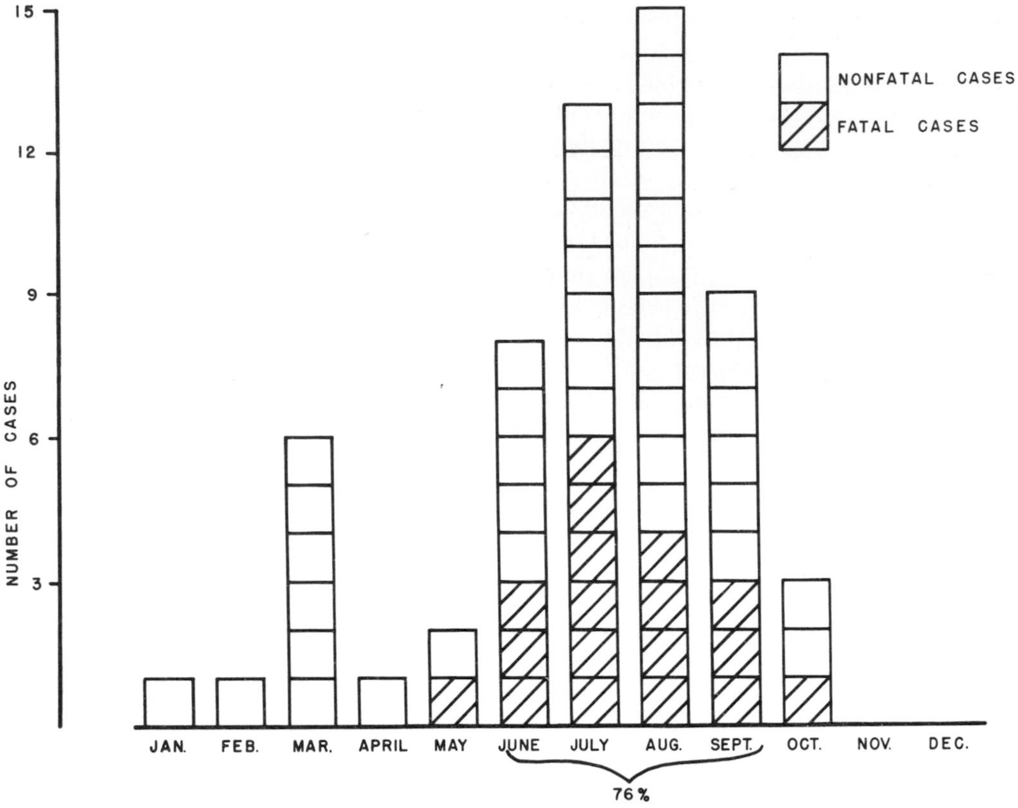

FIGURE 1.9.   Seasonal distribution of childhood lead poisoning in Cuyahoga County

examination is frequently unrevealing and usually at the most shows lead line;[*] neuromuscular weakness; and such nonspecific abdominal symptoms as a scaphoid contour, decreased peristalsis, guarding, or tenderness.

The mechanisms whereby the symptoms are produced are largely unknown, but the similarity to those seen in intermittent acute hepatic porphyria is intriguing, especially since both diseases are associated with abnormal heme biosynthesis and excretion of abnormal quantities of heme precursors. By fluoroscopy and direct observation during surgery, the bowel has been seen in intense contraction that cannot be attributed to a direct action of lead in the amounts known to circulate. However, as discussed under the porphyrias, none of the known heme precursors in the forms and amounts so far employed experimentally have reproduced the clinical findings. The lesions accounting for the brain damage (34, 137), the peripheral nerve changes, and the neuromuscular alterations have not been defined. Present opinion indicates that the muscular abnormality may be primary and the peripheral nerve changes secondary (84). Curiously, the morphologic finding of diagnostic importance (possibly pathognomonic) at autopsy (16, 96) is the presence of characteristic nuclear inclusion bodies in renal tubular cells and in hepatic cells, unassociated with any known functional abnormality. Amino-aciduria (63, 209) and glycosuria are frequently present

[*] This is most reliably demonstrated by inserting the corner of a white paper between the tooth and gum margin, thereby making it evident that the stippled dark line is on the gum margin.

(41, 46).* Myocardial changes have been detected (92).

The important hematologic findings are those of anemia—mild in the adult (149), very constant and frequently severe in the child (205)—characterized by normocytic, slightly hypochromic† red cells (46). The reticulocyte count is usually elevated to the 2 to 7 per cent range. Basophilic stippling (118), most evident and marked in the young, polychromatophilic cells, is frequently present to some degree; the stippling may be fine or heavy, few or many granules per cell. The stipples are thought to be composed of altered and precipitated ribonucleic acid or perhaps some abnormal globulin from the altered hemoglobin biosynthesis. The erythrocytes also have a normal or slightly *decreased* osmotic fragility. After 24 hours of sterile incubation they become abnormally *resistant* to osmotic stress even though the mechanical fragility becomes abnormally increased (79). Identical osmotic and mechanical fragility alterations can be induced by incubating normal cells with lead ($PbCl_3$). These changes can be inhibited or reversed by the addition of EDTA. It has been shown that treatment of cells with lead induces a largely irreversible leak of potassium cations by interfering with an energy-requiring "pump" (86, 130, 189, 200).

When red cells are removed from a patient with lead intoxication, labeled with Cr^{51}, and reinfused into the patient, their life span is significantly decreased (18 to 26 days of half life compared with a normal minimum of 30 days) (72). In the rare patient the erythrocyte half life may be markedly diminished (10 days), a finding that is consistent with some observations reporting overt hemolytic anemia, with hemoglobinemia and hemoglobinuria, in acute severe lead poisoning. If cells are obtained from a hematologically normal subject, treated with lead to produce the characteristic osmotic and mechanical fragility alterations, labeled with Cr^{51}, and reinfused into the donor, the erythrocyte life span is somewhat below normal (18 to 30 days of half life) (45). It would seem most reasonable to conclude that the hemolytic component in this disease is a direct consequence of the action of lead on the erythrocyte.

As indicated above, most patients with plumbism have mild anemia. With few exceptions, the shortening of the red cell life span is of such a degree that the bone marrow should be able to compensate for it, so that hemoglobin depression should not occur. This suggests that lead also inhibits the production of red cells by the marrow. Direct evidence for this has come from studies relative to heme and globin biosynthesis. The hematologic alterations of lead poisoning result from (a) direct effect of lead on the erythrocyte, a hemolytic component, and (b) inhibition of erythropoiesis.

The effects of lead on the various stages of the in vitro synthesis of heme (Figure 1.10) have been outlined in a previous section (52). Lead has been shown to inhibit the formation of ALA from glycine and succinate, the formation of PBG from ALA, and the incorporation of iron into protoporphyrin. Some of these blocks have been demonstrated in subcellular systems, some in cellular systems. Lead does not inhibit the uptake of iron by reticulocytes, but it does largely prevent the utilization of the iron for hemoglobin production. This is consistent with the electron microscopic demonstration of iron granules (ferritin, hemosiderin) in the marrow red cells of patients with plumbism (15). Figure 1.11 shows the abnormalities that have been

---

* Long-term follow-up studies made in Australia indicate that chronic renal damage may follow childhood poisoning (80).

† In children with superimposed iron-deficiency anemia the cells will, of course, be hypochromic and microcytic and show the usual morphologic variations from the normal.

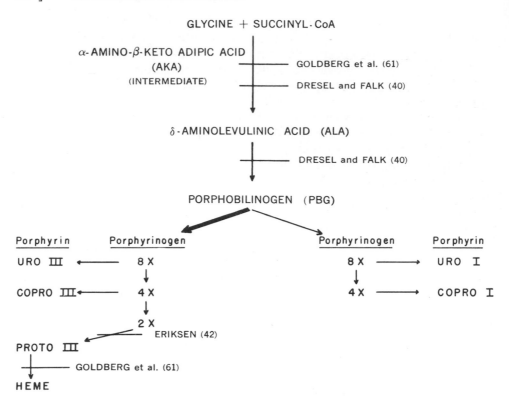

FIGURE 1.10.   Biosynthesis of heme. The horizontal lines followed by name and reference number indicate the site at which lead is thought to inhibit heme synthesis

	URINE	BONE MARROW	RBC
δ-AMINOLEVULINIC ACID	✓		
PORPHOBILINOGEN	✓		
UROPORPHYRIN I	✓	✓	
COPROPORPHYRIN III	✓		✓
PROTOPORPHYRIN III			✓

FIGURE 1.11.   Effect of lead poisoning on presence of heme precursors in urine, bone marrow, and red blood cells. Check indicates abnormally increased amount

demonstrated in the heme precursors of patients with lead poisoning: (a) ALA excretion in the urine is almost invariably markedly increased (78); this is an early, sensitive, and reliable indicator of lead poisoning, appearing early and persisting for a long time (75, 76, 185, 208); (b) porphobilinogen excretion is usually in the upper range of normal and in some instances has been moderately elevated; (c) type III coproporphyrin is usually increased in the urine (82, 134, 213); this has been a fairly consistent finding in patients with lead poisoning, and is now widely used as a screening test;* (d) uroporphyrin I is increased in the marrow; (e) the protoporphyrin is markedly increased in the circulating red cells (148, 197, 211), so much so that they can be detected as fluorocytes when the blood is examined under the fluorescence microscope (207). Thus it seems likely that lead blocks the in vivo synthesis of heme at several points in the sequence.†

By means of studies (88) of the rate at which labeled glycine is incorporated into heme and globin, it has recently been shown that the biosynthesis of globin is retarded in lead poisoning and that the inhibiting effect of lead on globin biosynthesis may be greater than the effect on heme production. Varying degrees of amino-aciduria have been demonstrated in plumbism, so permeability and transport alterations as yet not elucidated may also play significant roles in these findings.

Iron metabolism (13, 22, 22a) is unaffected down to the subcellular level. The iron is cleared from the plasma at a rapid or normal rate and transported to the bone marrow. There it is taken up by and incorporated into the developing red cell, but from then on its utilization is abnormal. It therefore appears only slowly in the hemoglobin of the peripheral blood; this constitutes more evidence for impaired erythropoiesis.

The diagnosis of lead intoxication is suggested by a history of exposure to lead. However, not all exposures to lead are hazardous. Clinical signs and symptoms must be evaluated. The presence of stippled erythrocytes indicates an abnormal intake of lead but does not necessarily indicate a significant degree of poisoning from lead. Moreover, erythrocyte stippling is sometimes minimal or lacking in evident lead poisoning and appears in other hematologic abnormalities such as Cooley's anemia, pernicious anemia, iron deficiency, etc. Excessive excretion of lead in the urine coupled with abnormal concentration of lead in the blood are necessary for a definitive (one might even say legal) diagnosis of lead poisoning. (The demonstration of increased amounts of the heme precursors in the urine, bone marrow, and red blood cells is strong supporting evidence and certainly is indicative of biochemical abnormality.)

The treatment of lead poisoning consists first of all in cessation of exposure. Since the other forms of therapy entail a certain risk, e.g., renal damage from EDTA (25), removal from exposure may be the only treatment required in instances of mild intoxication. The lead will slowly leave the bone and be excreted. However, it takes years for the lead con-

---

* The test is accomplished as follows: 5 ml of *freshly* voided urine is acidified with 5 drops of glacial acetic acid; 5 ml of ether is added and the mixture shaken vigorously. The tube is allowed to stand for a few minutes to allow separation of the layers and then viewed in front of the Woods (ultraviolet) light. A coruscating *red* fluorescence in the ether layer indicates the presence of coproporphyrin III and is strong presumptive evidence of lead poisoning. The red color of the positive test is in marked contrast with, and need not be confused with, the lambent green fluorescence of the normal. It should be remarked that occasionally the tube must be held in front of the light for a few minutes until fluorescence develops. This may be due to transformation of the precursors to the porphyrin compound (206).

† The evidence points to the bone marrow as the source of heme precursors. Schmid has shown that no alteration in liver catalase occurs in lead poisoning.

tent of the body to return to normal. For immediate control of the colicky cramps, intravenous calcium gluconate is rapidly and fairly reliably effective. It may be given in repeated doses or as a continuous drip. For the alleviation of signs and symptoms of increased intracranial pressure, intravenous administration of hypertonic urea may be effective (71). In some instances surgical decompression is necessary (30, 71a). BAL, EDTA, and penicillamine have been employed as deleading agents (99, 168). Although urinary excretion is augmented by all, BAL may combine with lead to form a toxic compound, resulting in acute exacerbation of symptoms. Penicillamine is effective only in a minor way. EDTA forms a nontoxic complex with lead and enhances its excretion manyfold. This rapid deleading is presently the treatment of choice, but the possible nephrotoxic effects of the drug must be borne in mind. Neither BAL nor EDTA reacts with tetraethyl or triethyl lead (33). Recent balance studies have demonstrated that solutions of ammonium chloride and sodium citrate, previously thought to be deleading agents, are no more effective than comparable amounts of fluids which increase urine flow (84); specific metabolic mobilization does not occur.

Bibliographic references for Chapter 1 begin on page 363.

CHAPTER TWO

IRON METABOLISM AND IRON-LACK ANEMIA

A firm grasp of the general principles of iron metabolism and a working knowledge of the details of iron metabolism are essential for insight into the pathophysiology of practically all the major hematologic diseases. Moreover, a significant distortion of some phase of iron metabolism occurs in many situations in which the abnormality is not primarily or predominantly hematologic, e.g., infection and inflammation (60), and in many situations in which erythropoiesis is deranged as a secondary effect of the basic disorder, e.g., renal diseases (62).

In this country iron-lack anemia is the most common of the treatable anemias; on a world-wide basis it is very probably the most prevalent type (181). Occurring in every age group—infancy, adolescence, the childbearing age, middle age, and old age—it accounts for few deaths but plays an important role in contributing to the valetudinarian condition and substandard work performance of millions.

IRON METABOLISM*

Early studies concerning iron metabolism were made using inorganic compounds that were usually administered in unphysiologic amounts. In attempted balance studies quantitation was done by methods not capable of yielding the accuracy required. While much more valuable information was obtained than might be expected, especially with respect to medicinal preparations, it is really only with present-day methods and tracer techniques that physiologically relevant observations and measurements have been possible.† In the following discussion, therefore, major emphasis will be upon the conclusions and results of those studies that have employed physiologic amounts of iron in naturally occurring forms, so that a first approximation may be made concerning nutrition and iron metabolism.

Body Content of Iron

The total-body iron content of the normal adult is somewhere between 2 and 6 Gm, depending chiefly on body size and hemoglobin level (130). Vanishingly small amounts, if any, are present as inorganic iron compounds or in ionized forms. At a

---

* General references and review articles: 18, 26, 34, 45, 47, 58, 67, 68, 79, 87, 95, 128–130, 144, 148, 163, 170, 173, 181.

† Josephs (95) has pointed out that unlike the technique employing radioactive labels, balance studies had the advantage of extending over prolonged periods of time so that variations due to such physiologic changes as intestinal mobility were smoothed out. Moreover, uptake from the whole diet was assayed, not from just one food. These points should be taken only as criticisms of the radioactive techniques, for they do not allow the balance studies to surmount the insensitivity inherent in the method.

TABLE 2.1.   Allocation of iron in body of 70–Kg man

Compound	Total in body (Gm)	Iron factor (Gm/Gm)	Total iron in compound (Gm)	Per cent of total body iron	Function
Hemoglobin					
Peripheral blood	650.0	0.0034	2.21	64.0	O_2 transport
Bone marrow	25.0	0.0034	0.09	2.5	O_2 transport
Myoglobin	40.0	0.0034	0.14	4.0	O_2 transport and "storage"
Parenchymal or cellular					
Cytochrome	0.8	0.0043	0.0034	0.097	O_2 utilization
Catalase	5.0	0.009	0.0045	0.13	H_2O_2 destruction
Peroxidases	—	—	—	—	H_2O_2 destruction
Storage iron					
Ferritin	2.0	0.23	0.46	13.0	Fe storage
Hemosiderin	1.5	0.37	0.56	16.0	Fe storage
Transport iron	6.5	0.0004 to 0.0012	0.004	0.12	Fe transport
Total iron			3.47		

Adapted from Drabkin, D. L., Physiol. Rev. 31:362, 1951.

physiologic pH the solubility product of ferric iron is 10^{-36}; to overcome the problems inherent in the metabolism of this element, special complexing agents have been evolved. Moreover, the toxic effects of free iron are many and violent as judged by enzymatic, cellular, or total-body reactions (173). Consequently iron is precisely handled and firmly bound to a protein while in transport and tightly chelated to a protein while in storage.

As indicated in Table 2.1, there are two general types of iron compounds found in the body. In the first type, iron is present in a porphyrin ring; the resulting heme complex is, in turn, attached to a protein that gives to the total molecule its specific function. In the second type, the iron is directly chelated to the protein; no heme is present. The former compounds are concerned with the transport, storage, and activation of oxygen (hemoglobin, myoglobin, cytochrome); the latter are concerned with the transport and storage of iron (iron-binding protein, ferritin,* hemosiderin). It has

been pointed out that iron is quantitatively the single most important biocatalytic element in the entire realm of animal enzymology.

The major proportion (approximately two-thirds) of body iron is found in the circulating hemoglobin and the myoglobin. Very small amounts are present in the respiratory enzymes and transporting iron-binding protein. The remaining body iron is stored in the liver, spleen, bone marrow, and muscle as ferritin and hemosiderin. In terms of absolute amounts of iron, hemoglobin occupies a most important position. Moreover, because of the rapid turnover of hemoglobin (3 million red cells produced and broken down per second; 6.3 Gm of hemoglobin containing 21 mg of iron synthesized and degraded each 24 hours), the amount of iron handled by the body for hemoglobin metabolism puts the latter in a dominant role in the total-body iron economy. To

* There is evidence that ferritin also has some vasomotor regulatory function: "VDM," or vasodepressor material (67).

develop and maintain the various iron fractions listed above, precise mechanisms are present, some of which can be described on the basis of substantial evidence.

Nutritional Iron Balance

One of the most important considerations to evaluate is iron balance: amount taken into the body versus amount excreted. It is only recently that acceptable approximations of this balance could be arrived at in terms of nutrition: how much *food iron* is ingested per day and how much of the ingested iron is absorbed? Because iron is a ubiquitous element and therefore a ubiquitous contaminant, the difficulties of long-term balance studies done by quantitative analysis were practically insurmountable and required confirmation by other approaches. It is necessary to be able to label the naturally occurring food iron so that it can be identified, traced, and quantitated. This was first achieved by Moore (124–127), and his findings have now been confirmed by several different workers (37, 61, 140, 146, 158, 165, 175). Chickens were injected with radioactive iron so that their eggs subsequently contained a traceable label built into a naturally occurring source of food iron. By means of the label, iron could be followed through absorption, utilization (for hemoglobin synthesis), storage, and, ultimately, excretion. The unabsorbed radioactive iron could also be measured. Similar studies have been made by labeling the naturally occurring iron of liver, meat, milk, eggs, and various vegetables. These foods can then be prepared as in the average American diet, for example, to obtain a true evaluation of iron nutrition.

The over-all conclusion of these studies is that a normal individual absorbs 5 to 10 per cent (usually considerably under 10 per cent,* very seldom over) of ingested iron. Since the average diet contains some 10 to 15 mg of elemental iron

per day, somewhat less than 1 to 1.5 mg of iron is absorbed into the body per day. This then is the figure for the positive side of the balance and has been repeatedly confirmed both by determining the amount of iron built into the circulating hemoglobin and by obtaining the difference between the amounts ingested and excreted.

Contrary to previous teachings, a small amount of iron is excreted per day exclusive of shed blood (50, 89). All cells are known to contain iron enzymes. Therefore, when leukocytes and epithelial cells are discharged in body secretions, when cells are desquamated from the skin or intestinal mucosa (50 to 80 Gm per day), or even when hair and nails grow, some iron is lost to the body. A small quantity of iron is excreted in the bile and not reabsorbed. Labeled iron is also regularly found in sweat,† but whether it is truly excreted from sweat glands or derived from desquamated epithelial cells has not been established. The

---

* The average figure for 133 experiments on normal subjects was 6.5 per cent. Strictly speaking, one should not speak of a percentage absorption of iron without including the amount of ingested iron, since the percentage absorbed depends upon the absolute amount ingested. At high levels of iron ingestion the absorption is low and at low levels it is very high. When some 50 μg of iron was fed to normal individuals, the absorption ranged from 40 to 60 per cent (20). The amounts employed by Moore give the figures most physiologically and nutritionally relevant but admittedly become susceptible to inaccuracies because of the technical errors incurred by dealing with low values of absorption.

Probably the most accurate results are obtained from whole-body counting. This technique measures the amount retained in the body and obviates the need for feces collection and calculations based on excretion (84, 154).

† A discordant note stands out here in contrast to the otherwise remarkably harmonious results obtained in different laboratories by different methods of investigating the nutritional balance of iron. Dermal iron loss is estimated as considerable (6.5 mg per day) by some workers employing chemical analysis (90) and radioiron turnover (21). It is presently impossible to reconcile this figure with the studies of Moore (130) and Finch (57).

total loss by all routes as measured by radioactive tracer techniques* has been calculated to be 0.5 to 1.5 mg per day. For the adult male, the intake of about 1 to 1.5 mg of iron per day adequately balances the loss of 0.5 to 1.5 mg per day. However, in the case of a growing individual with expanding iron compartments or a female of childbearing age, further considerations must enter. The menstrual blood flow of 35 to 70 ml every 27 days in a normal woman with a hemoglobin level of 14 Gm per 100 ml contains 16 to 32 mg of iron. The average daily *additional* loss (over and above the daily base line of 0.5 to 1.5 mg) amounts to 0.5 to 1 mg. Here the iron balance is precarious indeed unless augmented absorption compensates for the increased losses (see below).

Iron Absorption

Iron exists in foods mainly as ferric hydroxide complexes, trivalent iron directly chelated to proteins, amino acids and organic acids, or heme iron complexed to protein.† Many studies with iron salts have shown that the human being absorbs iron chiefly or entirely in the divalent state (123). Therefore, for absorption from most compounds to occur, iron must be split from its complex and chemically reduced. This begins in the stomach and continues in the intestines. The amount absorbed by the stomach is unknown but is probably very small. Absorption is greatest in the upper part of the small intestine and decreases progressively in the more distal segments of the ileum (30, 51), a gradient that has never been adequately defined or explained: it may be due in part to the increasing amounts of insoluble iron salts (phosphates, carbonates, phytates) that are formed in addition to an intrinsic change in the mucosa.

Although for years it has been thought that the presence of free hydrochloric acid in the gastric juice reduces the iron to the divalent state and thereby aids absorption (68, 79), the studies made on food iron indicate no demonstrable role for hydrochloric acid and/or pH in augmenting the absorption of iron from such organic compounds (128).

Most of the iron enters the blood stream directly and not by way of lymphatics (51, 127). The mechanisms of absorption into, and transportation across, mucosal cells are almost completely unknown.

Granick (69) has proposed the following hypothesis concerning the mechanism and regulation of iron absorption by the mucosal cell. An iron-protein complex, ferritin, can be recovered from the intestinal mucosa following the oral administration of iron. With continual iron administration, the intestinal ferritin steadily increases in amount to "saturation levels." Ferritin is formed by a combination of a protein called apoferritin with iron. According to this theory apoferritin is the acceptor substance necessary for iron absorption and is constantly being made and broken down within the cells. However, when apoferritin is combined with iron, degradation stops; the complex becomes stable and is the normal form in which iron is stored. Ferritin has a molecular weight of 465,-

* An accurate value can be obtained only when a steady state exists and total mixing of the labeled iron with all iron compartments has occurred. This probably takes well over a year. Moore's observations were made up to 150 days after feeding, a few up to 320 days. Finch derived the value of 0.6 mg of iron excreted per day in studies done 3 to 5 years after administration of labeled iron. These are probably the most accurate figures available. The turnover rate was calculated on the daily absorption or excretion of iron. The actual figures presented were: males 0.61 ± 0.08; nonmenstruating females 0.64 ± 0.05; and menstruating females 1.2 ± 0.11 mg per day.

† Under the food-fortification program in the United States practically all grain and cereal products have iron added in various inorganic forms. Tests conducted on bread indicate that during the baking process the various compounds are reduced to a single type, of which some 10 per cent is absorbed (165).

000 and contains some 17 to 23 per cent iron by weight as ferric hydroxide–phosphate compounds in clusters of micelles. The molecule of ferritin is made up of a protein shell approximately 54 Å in diameter which is shown by electron microscopy to contain electron-dense areas 24 Å in diameter representing the iron clusters. Electron microscopy also reveals that the intestinal mucosal cells possess a brush border, the fingers of which measure 5,000 by 500 Å and are distributed some 300 per cell surface. These are probably the sites of iron absorption. Granick visualizes (Figure 2.1) that the apoferritin molecules form a portion of the membrane of the brush border. Each molecule has entry pores, which become filled with iron when apoferritin is changed to ferritin. When a small number of iron molecules are present in the gut, ferrous iron enters the mucosal cell through the entry pore of an apoferritin molecule, is oxidized to the ferric state, and then diffuses to the capillary side of the cell where it is reduced to the ferrous form. In the plasma it is oxidized to the trivalent form and chelated to the iron-binding protein. When larger numbers of iron molecules enter the cell, some become bound to apoferritin, resulting in

the formation of ferritin. Still larger numbers result in maximal, or saturation, levels of ferritin and the accumulation of ferric iron in the luminal portion of the cell so that the molecular entry pores of apoferritin become plugged and remain so, preventing further iron absorption until the iron is cleared at the capillary end of the cell. The entire transport system operates by concentration gradients made possible by the ease with which iron can be converted from the ferrous to the ferric state. Granick has stated that the assumption of an oxidation-reduction potential that is greater in the front, or luminal, portion of the cell, and a reducing mechanism that is more active in the rear, or capillary, area of the cell might account for the concentration gradient across the cell.

The theory was originally proposed to account for the following group of experimental observations. There is a one-way transfer of iron across the gut wall; the only demonstrated gastrointestinal losses occur by sloughing off of mucosal cells, by loss of leukocytes, or by excretion in the bile without reabsorption. Iron is absorbed more readily in the ferrous than the ferric form in human beings. When *large* amounts are fed, ab-

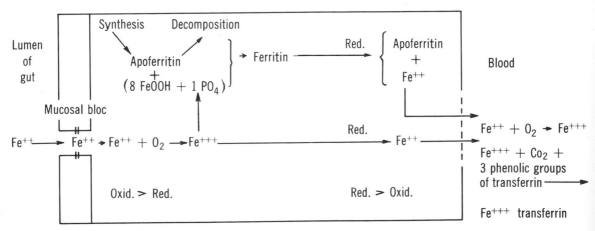

FIGURE 2.1.   Diagram to illustrate mechanisms proposed by Granick to account for absorption or rejection of iron by mucosal cells of the gastrointestinal tract. (From Granick, S., *in* Metabolism and Function of Iron (report of Nineteenth Ross Pediatric Research Conference), p. 17, Ross Laboratories, Columbus, Ohio, 1956)

sorption takes place while the ferritin complex is building up in the cell. Absorption then decreases despite the high concentration of iron in the mucosa, and if labeled iron is now administered, little or no absorption is demonstrable. A so-called "mucosal block" has occurred. This block persists until the ferritin has been cleared from the cells. Finally, since there is no established mechanism controlling the rate of iron absorption, the mucosal cell presumably regulates the absorption or rejection of iron from the gastrointestinal tract by the mechanism outlined.

It is evident that the existence of a mucosal block becomes critical to the entire theory. Considerable doubt concerning this was generated by Wöhler and Heilmeyer's (179) observations that fed radioactive iron continued to accumulate in newly formed ferritin of liver cells during the period of time when the mucosal block should be strongest because of maximal content of ferritin in the gastrointestinal mucosa. A careful analysis of the problem by Brown et al. (29) employing two different radioisotopes of iron makes it extremely doubtful that at *reasonably physiologic levels of iron administration* any such block of iron absorption actually occurs. These considerations (combined with those developed below)* make it appear more likely that in the mucosal cell as elsewhere in the body ferritin is a convenient, nontoxic form of iron storage rather than a regulator of iron absorption. Actually it is somewhat of a relief to realize that one does not have to believe in the existence of a sort of super-Intelligence or Maxwell's demon residing in the mucosal cell and determining on the basis of total-body requirement how much iron is to be absorbed or rejected.

Evidence for an active transport system that carries iron across the mucosal cells has been presented by Dowdle (46). In experiments with rats it was demon-strated, using everted sacs prepared from the small intestine, that radioactive iron could be be transported from the mucosal to the serosal surface against a concentration gradient. This active transport was dependent upon oxidative metabolism and the generation of phosphate bond energy, and was limited in capacity. Although the relation of the active transport process to in vivo iron absorption cannot be defined at this time, it is of interest to note that the active transport process was found to be maximal in the proximal duodenum and to be diminished in the more distal segments. This distribution of energy-dependent transport activity corresponds with the previously demonstrated absorption gradient for iron mentioned above: little absorption from the stomach, maximal absorption in the proximal duodenum diminishing to low levels in the distal ileum. Moreover, the addition of ascorbic acid enhanced markedly the active transport of radioactive iron in vitro as it is known to do in vivo.

Ferritin may be a mediator in iron transport across the mucosal cell, but it would now appear established that ferritin neither blocks nor controls iron absorption.

As mentioned above, the exact mechanism by which iron passes through the mucosal cell and into the blood stream is unknown. Nevertheless, there are a number of factors and conditions known to influence iron absorption (25–28, 107). The factors that have been regarded as most important in regulating

---

* Moore (130) lists six points of evidence against the existence of a physiologically significant mucosal block: (a) block obtained with large doses of iron is partial and transient, (b) absorption increases with dose over range from 0.001 to 300 mg, (c) absorption is high in many situations when tissue iron is high and erythropoiesis is increased, (d) absorption is high in iron overload and hemochromatosis, (e) absorption is high in vitamin B_6 deficiency, and (f) presence of recently induced mucosal ferritin does not stop increase of liver ferritin.

iron absorption are: (a) iron stores and iron enzymes, (b) erythropoietic activity, (c) hypoxia, and (d) level of unsaturated iron-binding protein.

Numerous studies have established that the absorption of iron is increased above normal when a deficiency of iron is present. Moreover, the increase in absorption may occur when the iron stores are decreased but before the appearance of anemia. The constituents of the diet are of importance. Reducing substances favor the absorption of iron. Ascorbic acid when fed (but not when given parenterally) in large amounts enhances the absorption of labeled food iron two- (140) to threefold (124, 128). It is not clear whether this is done by keeping the iron reduced to the ferrous state or by forming chelates of low molecular weight that are readily absorbed. Substances such as phosphates, carbonates, and phytates, that favor the production of insoluble compounds and precipitates, may reduce iron absorption. Diets low in phosphates enhance absorption. Pancreatic secretion is influential, since in long-term observations duct ligation results in iron overload. Moreover, patients with long-standing pancreatic insufficiency have excess iron stores (44). Patients with total or partial gastrectomy absorb food iron poorly (33, 83). This may result from lack of local secretory factors or disturbed intestinal motility. Studies on dogs have demonstrated no effect of bile on the absorption of iron (178). Defective iron absorption occurs, presumably because of altered mucosal factors, as a part of the general picture of the malabsorption syndromes such as sprue, celiac disease, idiopathic steatorrhea, myxedema, infection, etc. (33, 49). The opposite situation, increased iron absorption, occurs in pyridoxine deficiency and idiopathic familial hemochromatosis, wherein continued increased absorption takes place despite excessive iron stores. In untreated pernicious anemia and various hemolytic anemias increased absorption also takes place despite overladen iron depots. The consistent association of increased erythropoiesis and increased iron absorption has been repeatedly demonstrated. However, recent studies on rats (118) have shown increased absorption independent of erythropoiesis. It has been suggested that anemia (68), with its concomitant low oxygen-carrying power, might affect the redox level in the mucosal cell and favor transfer of iron to the plasma and thereby enhance absorptive capacity. However, patients with iron-deficiency anemia absorb similar amounts of iron before and after transfusions to normal hemoglobin levels, and iron-depleted dogs absorb iron equally well under high oxygen tension as under atmospheric oxygen tension (128). Anemia and oxygen tension per se cannot be in *direct* control of absorption.

All this may seem very involved and negative, but it is important to point out how little is known about the positive aspects and controls of the actual mechanisms of iron absorption, although recent evidence indicates the existence of an active transfer system for transporting iron across the mucosal cells.

From the above considerations two generalizations arise that have clinical and some experimental backing: iron-deficient subjects absorb more iron than normal subjects; and when red cell formation is stimulated, the absorption of iron is usually greater than normal. How this is brought about is unknown.

Iron Transport

Once across the mucosal cell, the iron is picked up by a specific transport protein (70, 103, 145, 148, 149, 168, 176). This is a β_1-globulin with a molecular weight of 90,000, variously termed transferrin, β_1-metal-combining globulin, siderophilin, iron-binding protein, or iron-binding globulin. It is known that each molecule of the protein will bind two atoms of iron and thereby assume a salmon-pink color. The iron is in the trivalent form, tightly chelated in complexes with three phenolic groups and one bicarbonate ion. The complex is very stable at a physiologic pH and in vitro may be dissociated only at very low pH values (100, 148). Normally iron-binding protein is present in quantity sufficient to bind about 300 μg of iron per 100 ml of plasma.* Normally it is only one-third saturated with iron.

The half life of the iron-binding protein has been estimated as approximately 12 days by Gitlin et al. (65). Employing crystalline material labeled with radioiodine, Katz (97) described a slow diffusion from the intravascular space (comparable to that of albumin) so that equilibrium was reached in 4 to 5 days, when some 55 to 62 per cent of the material was extravascular. From this point on the iron-binding protein disappeared at a single exponential rate, with a half life of 6.7 to 8.4 days. By a similar technique Jarnum and Lassen (93) calculated the half life of transferrin to be 8.7 days, and Awai and Brown (4), 8 to 10.4 days. These values make it most unlikely that the protein enters cellular compartments with its iron at storage or utilization loci; rather, it probably gives up its iron at strategically placed acceptor sites and promptly returns to the circulating plasma (103–105). If the protein is bound at the site of delivery, it must have a very brief stay before being released back to the vascular space. Again the mechanism whereby the protein gives up its iron is unknown. As will be pointed out below, the dissociation constant of iron and iron-binding protein is such that at physiologic pH values little or no iron is released.

Although not firmly established, it seems most likely that iron-binding protein is a true carrier of iron in the way that hemoglobin is the carrier of oxygen,

and that the complex by itself has no enzymatic or metabolic function.†

The mechanism controlling the amount of iron-binding protein present in the plasma is unknown. It has been postulated that the level is regulated by (a) erythropoiesis, (b) erythropoietic factor, or (c) tissue oxygen supply. By varying these factors independently in animals, Morgan (132) concluded that iron-binding protein is under the influence of tissue oxygenation, hypoxia resulting in significant increases in circulating levels.

An abnormally high iron-binding capacity (greater than 450 μg per 100 ml) is regularly observed in iron deficiency independent of the cause. The highest values observed have been in the last trimester of pregnancy not necessarily complicated by overt iron deficiency. Low values invariably occur in acute and chronic infection. It is curious to note that for unknown reasons it is the only globulin fraction that is decreased; all other components are usually increased in infectious diseases. The evidence obtained by Jarnum and Lassen (93) indicates that in acute infection the lowered level is due to hypercatabolism, while in chronic infection it is due to hypoanabolism.

Recent electrophoretic studies of the β-globulins binding iron reveal that there are at least nine genetically controlled variants of human transferrins, or iron-

* This is obviously a simplified, approximate value easily remembered. Actually the range of normal (usually 200 to 450 μg per 100 ml) must be determined in each laboratory for the particular method employed, of which there are many (148). Iron-binding protein is routinely quantitated not in terms of the absolute weight of protein but in terms of the *amount of iron* it is capable of binding and is conventionally referred to as the iron-binding capacity of the serum. An iron-binding capacity of 300 μg per 100 ml equals 0.24 mg of iron-binding protein per 100 ml of plasma.

† Another function of this compound has been examined by Martin and Jandl (112), who demonstrated inhibition of virus multiplication probably by decreased synthesis, not by binding to the virus or virucidal action.

binding proteins, differing in electrophoretic mobility (168). They all are antigenically related and bind and deliver iron in equivalent fashion for utilization and storage. Although the report leaves much to be desired in the way of definitive data, one patient was described in 1956 who possibly was deficient in iron-binding protein (152). In the past year two additional, well-documented instances (designated congenital atransferrinemia)* have been reported (80–82).

The normal concentration of iron in the plasma (100 μg per 100 ml, or about 4 mg in the total plasma volume) is the result of many effects and represents the balance between the iron delivered to the circulating blood from the gastrointestinal tract, hemoglobin breakdown, and iron stores, and that removed by heme biosynthesis, cell metabolism, excretion, and deposition into stores. The plasma iron is thus in a dynamic state, and its concentration is subject to significant variations. In the normal person there is a distinct diurnal variation (75, 106, 137), the highest values being present in the morning and the lowest in the late evening. Variations from 140 μg per 100 ml at 8 A.M. to 40 μg per 100 ml at 10 P.M may occur. It is evident that for meaningful, reproducible results blood for iron determinations must be obtained at standard times. Plasma iron values are, however, known to have a minimal diurnal variation in diseases such as iron lack or overload, hemolysis, infection, vitamin B_{12} lack, etc. (137). Recent adequately controlled studies have not confirmed prior observations that the iron level varied with ACTH and cortisone administration.

Many observations have established the patterns of the concentrations of iron-binding protein and plasma iron in various diseases (54, 110, 131, 148). The patterns are usually as represented in Figure 2.2, and the v⸱ ⸱s are conventionally reported in a series of four figures: plasma iron concentration; total iron-binding capacity; unsaturated iron-binding capacity (amount of iron-binding protein not carrying iron—it must be remembered that the amount is expressed in terms of the micrograms of iron it is capable of binding when saturated); and per cent saturation (proportion of iron-binding protein that is saturated with iron). In iron-lack anemia the plasma iron concentration is low, the total iron-binding capacity high, the unsaturated iron-binding capacity high, and the per cent saturation very low. In infection the plasma iron content is low, the total iron-binding capacity somewhat depressed, and the per cent saturation moderately decreased. In iron overload the plasma iron content is high (unless infection or neoplasia is present), the iron-binding capacity is slightly depressed, and the per cent saturation nearly complete. These patterns are frequently of help in differential diagnosis or as confirmatory points but, since they are susceptible to change by many modifying circumstances, are not as valuable as might be desired.

It was formerly proposed that the degree of unsaturation of the iron-binding capacity governed the rate of iron absorption from the gut. In favor of this were the experimentally determined affinity constant of 10^{27} (at pH 7) for the equation $Fe^{+++} + Transferrin \rightleftarrows Fe^{+++} - Transferrin$ (68) and the enhanced absorption known to occur in iron-deficiency anemia and pregnancy. However, it has been shown that increasing the iron-binding capacity by infusion of purified material does not increase iron

* Characterized by decreased level of iron-binding protein in the parents and absence in the child; hypochromic anemia; tissue iron overload; half life of injected transferrin between 3 and 5 days; rapid clearance (T/2=5 minutes) of injected radioiron from the plasma with distribution to *all* storage sites; delayed reappearance in peripheral red cells (12 per cent at 8 days); greater-than-normal gastrointestinal iron absorption (81).

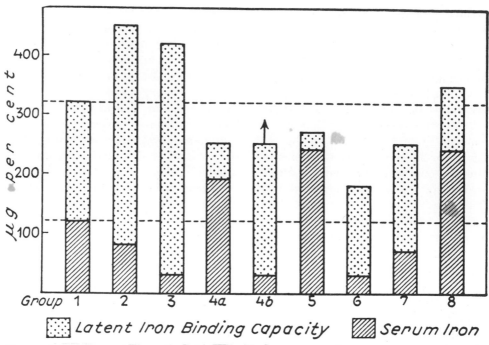

Figure 2.2. Serum iron and total iron-binding capacity of serum in various disturbances of iron metabolism. (1) Healthy adults. (2) Late pregnancy. (3) Chronic iron deficiency. (4a) Hemolytic, pernicious, aplastic, and myelophthisic anemias; fetus at parturition. (4b) Hemolytic and pernicious anemias during remission. (5) Hemochromatosis and transfusion hemosiderosis. (6) Acute infections. (7) Chronic infections, malignant tumors, myelomatosis, uremia, leukemia, hepatic cirrhosis, acute or subacute liver atrophy. (8) Acute hepatitis (second to fifth week). Lower horizontal dashed line represents normal level of globulin-bound iron in human serum; upper dashed line represents normal level of iron-binding capacity of human serum. (From Laurell, C. B., Pharmacol. Rev. 4:371, 1952)

absorption. Moreover, several conditions exist during which iron absorption is normal or increased in spite of very low unsaturated iron-binding capacity and elevated plasma iron concentration (untreated pernicious anemia, hemolytic anemias in general, hemochromatosis, etc.). Therefore, it is unlikely that either the plasma iron concentration or the iron-binding capacity plays a major or determinant role in governing iron absorption.*

Mitchell et al. (101) have proposed that the iron-binding protein exists in two phases: one circulating in the plasma for transport purposes, the other sequestered owing to orientation of the iron-laden protein to receptors at cell sites where iron is being absorbed, utilized, and stored. This concept is based largely upon the reported finding of a lowering of the level of circulating iron-binding protein in iron-depleted subjects immediately following a substantial dose of orally administered ferrous sulfate. According to this proposal, iron-binding protein is specifically concerned with the transport of iron across cell membranes, not by crossing the membrane itself but

* Recent work by Hallberg (73) employing constant perfusion of iron into the gastrointestinal tract to maintain a gradient has provided an interesting approach to evaluating factors that influence the *rate* of iron absorption and has again raised the possibility that absorption is influenced by the iron-binding capacity of the circulating blood.

by spending some time at the cell surface during passage of the iron.

Ferrokinetics

The measured patterns of iron and iron-binding capacity mentioned above give a fairly static picture of what obviously is an extremely active transport mechanism. A more dynamic picture may be obtained by the use of tracer amounts of radio-active isotopes of iron (5, 19, 24, 48, 85, 86, 142, 143). When the proper amount of radioactive iron is added to plasma in vitro, the element is firmly chelated to the unsaturated iron-binding protein. This complex can then be administered intravenously, and the travels and destinations of the iron can be followed by appropriate sampling or by detection of radioactivity employing externally applied directional scintillation counters.

For the normal it may be simply stated that initially all the administered iron is in the plasma; 7 to 10 days later, almost all (90 per cent plus) is to be found in the circulating red cells. The intermediate stages of this over-all reaction have been explored in detail, and the studies have yielded much information of physiologic, pathologic, and clinical interest.

Following injection into a normal person, the rate of disappearance of the labeled iron-protein complex from the plasma can be determined by serial sampling of the peripheral blood. During a 5- to 8-hour period there is a rapid exponential decrease in the radioactive iron, indicating the clearance of 50 per cent of the iron from the circulating plasma in approximately 90 minutes.* This 50 per cent clearance, or turnover, value varies considerably in different diseases (Figure 2.3). However, after the 5- to 8-hour period the rate of clearance diminishes, and after approximately 2 days a slower exponential rate is established (Figure 2.4). These changes have been taken as evidence for a feedback of labeled iron into the plasma. It should be pointed out that this feedback makes itself seen in the clearance curve only at a time when the great majority (90 per cent plus) of the iron has been cleared from the plasma, since the values are plotted on a logarithmic ordinate. Except for precise investigational purposes these latter changes are usually not detected or employed (the previously mentioned 50 per cent clearance time is accurate enough for the usual clinical purposes), but in terms of mechanisms and pathophysiology they are very significant, as will be explained.

When the plasma iron content and the plasma volume are known, the clearance rate obtained by radioactive techniques can be employed to calculate the absolute amount of iron passing through the plasma per unit of time. Studies on normal individuals indicate that 32 mg of iron leaves the plasma daily; this is referred to as the plasma iron turnover (PIT) and is variously expressed as "mg per 24 hours" or "mg per Kg per hour." It must be remembered, however, that a significant diurnal variation in the plasma iron level has been demonstrated and that diurnal variations in the time required to clear iron from the plasma have also been shown to exist (26). Despite the fact that the changes are somewhat complementary, so that the plasma iron turnover in absolute amounts per 24 hours tends to remain constant, a certain precision is lacking from the figures that is not usually calculable.

External tracking of the radioactive iron by collimated scintillation detectors

---

* It has been satisfactorily demonstrated that there is no exchange of iron with peripheral mature red cells or hemoglobin (71). The bonds linking protoporphyrin, iron, and protein together are irreversible as long as the molecule remains intact, so that iron, incorporated into hemoglobin at the site of biosynthesis, remains an integral part of the molecule until the erythrocytes are destroyed and hemoglobin catabolism takes place. The amount of nonhemoglobin iron in the normal adult red cell is negligibly small.

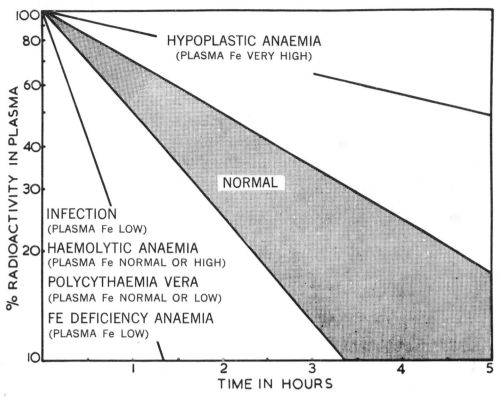

FIGURE 2.3. Patterns indicating rates of clearance from plasma of radioiron bound to transferrin in various situations. (From Bothwell, T. H., et al., Brit. J. Haemat. 2:1, 1956)

has demonstrated that virtually all the injected iron moves rapidly from the plasma to the bone marrow (Figure 2.5). Initial counting, immediately following injection, detects the radioactive iron contained in the circulating plasma. As the iron leaves the plasma and accumulates in the marrow, the counting rates monitored over the splenic and hepatic areas decrease as the counting rate over the sacrum (representing an active marrow area) increases. The counting rates then indicate that the iron, which has almost all been transferred to marrow, remains there for approximately 24 hours. During the next 4 to 6 days the radioactive iron leaves the marrow and simultaneously appears in the hemoglobin of the circulating red cells. In the normal person 90 per cent plus of the injected amount of labeled iron has appeared in the circulat-

ing red cells by 8 to 10 days. From serial samplings of the peripheral blood the rate at which the iron appears in the circulating erythrocytes can be determined and the percentage of the administered iron utilized for hemoglobin production calculated (per cent iron utilization). This information is of considerable value in various clinical situations (Figure 2.6) and also in terms of pathophysiologic mechanisms. If during the time of appearance of the iron in the peripheral red cells the external monitoring is continued, the counting rates over the organs will be found, in the normal person, to return to the initial postinjection values.

It was originally proposed (85, 86) that a quantitative determination of hemoglobin synthesis could be made employing the plasma iron turnover values, the per cent iron utilization, and the known

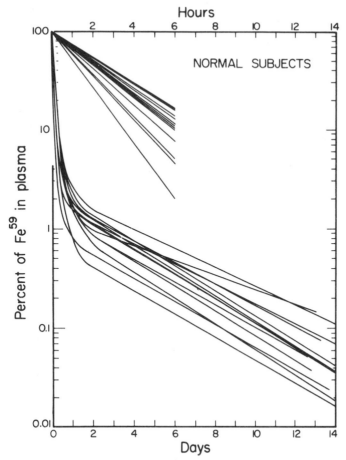

FIGURE 2.4.   Percentage of radioiron remaining in plasma of normal subjects at various times after intravenous injection, showing rapid and slow exponential components. (From Pollycove, M., and Mortimer, R., J. Clin. Invest. 40:753, 1961)

content of iron in hemoglobin (3.4 mg of iron in 1 Gm of hemoglobin). However, the values thereby derived were considerably greater than those obtained by other calculations or those predicted from the known life span of the red cell. Consequently it became important to determine the nature and extent of the feedback mentioned above in connection with the description of plasma iron clearance. Had the proposed quantitation of hemoglobin synthesis worked out in agreement with other calculations, it would have implied a linear progression of the iron from plasma to marrow to erythrocytes without significant devia-

tion. However, considerable error was evident in such calculations, and a feedback, or deviation, of the iron was indicated by the clearance studies. Since virtually all the plasma iron was considered to go to the bone marrow, it was evident that the source of the feedback would be in the marrow. On the basis of collateral evidence, conclusions have been drawn concerning the source of the feedback.

Iron is known to be present in the bone marrow as hemosiderin and ferritin complexes; they normally exist in approximately equal proportions (63, 74, 96, 159). Of the normal total-body iron stores, the liver contains about one-third;

EXTERNAL COUNTING OF LIVER AND SPLEEN

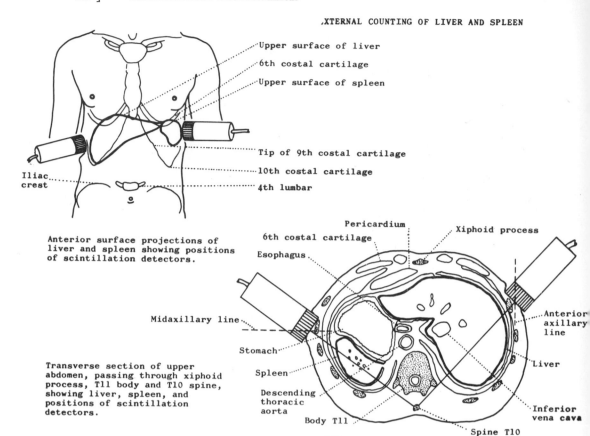

Upper surface of liver

6th costal cartilage

Upper surface of spleen

Tip of 9th costal cartilage

10th costal cartilage

4th lumbar

Iliac crest

Anterior surface projections of liver and spleen showing positions of scintillation detectors.

Pericardium

6th costal cartilage

Xiphoid process

Esophagus

Midaxillary line

Anterior axillary line

Stomach

Liver

Spleen

Transverse section of upper abdomen, passing through xiphoid process, T11 body and T10 spine, showing liver, spleen, and positions of scintillation detectors.

Descending thoracic aorta

Body T11

Inferior vena cava

Spine T10

EXTERNAL COUNTING OF SACRUM

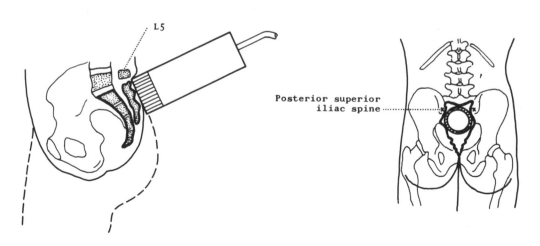

L5

Posterior superior iliac spine

Sagittal section through pelvis showing sacrum and position of scintillation detector.

Posterior surface projection of sacrum showing position of scintillation detector.

FIGURE 2.5.   Tracing of radioactive iron by means of externally applied directional scintillation counters. (From Pollycove, M., and Mortimer, R., J. Clin. Invest. 40:753, 1961)

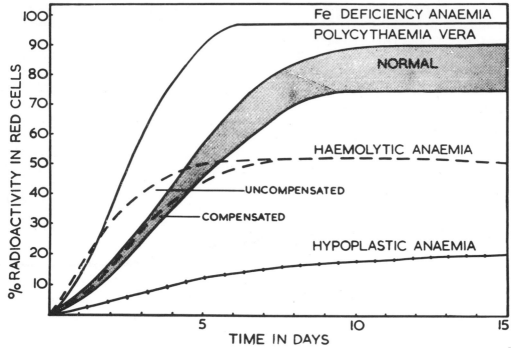

FIGURE 2.6. Patterns of radioiron reappearance in peripheral red cells. (From Bothwell, T. H., et al., Brit. J. Haemat. 2:1, 1956)

considerably less is present in the bone marrow; both have about a fifty-fifty distribution between hemosiderin and ferritin. If the plasma iron were transferring to the stores, which would then serve as the feedback source, a significant build-up of radioactivity in the liver would be expected as well as in the marrow. But this was not detected in man. Moreover, other observations indicate that release of iron from storage sites is normally delayed beyond the critical period of observation.* Finally, if the marrow's uptake of iron from the plasma, which is almost complete in 8 hours, were occasioned by irreversible fixation of radioactive iron in the developing erythrocytes, then the release of iron from the marrow and its appearance in the circulating red cells should correspond to the division and maturation time of the erythrocytes into which the iron was fixed. Since the total time required for division and maturation is estimated at from 2.5

to 3 days, the reappearance of the iron in the circulating red cells should be complete in approximately 3 days. And since observation has shown that 7 to 10 days is required for maximal iron incorporation, the assumption of irreversible fixation in developing erythrocytes cannot be accurate. Accordingly Pollycove (143) has proposed the existence of a *labile erythropoietic iron pool* which is intermediate between the plasma iron and the iron that is irreversibly fixed and destined for incorporation into red cell hemoglobin. He has also proposed that the labile erythropoietic iron pool is located at or in the membrane of the developing erythrocytes.

Iron may be transferred directly from transferrin to young, developing red cells by a specific mechanism. Most of the iron

* In patients with iron excess (hemochromatosis) such depositions of iron from the plasma into hepatic and marrow stores, with subsequent feedback from both sources, have been detected.

so attached to the membrane is destined in the normal individual for incorporation into the red cell and utilization for hemoglobin biosynthesis. However, some of the iron has been shown to be reversibly fixed and can return from the membrane to unsaturated iron-binding protein. Studies made in dogs 8 hours after most of a tracer amount of labeled iron had accumulated in the marrow showed that about one-half the marrow iron was nonhemoglobin iron associated chiefly with the erythrocyte membrane; the remainder was hemoglobin iron and located inside the red cell. Sondhaus and Thorell (164) have shown that (in salamander cells) the ratio of nonhemoglobin iron to hemoglobin iron is greater than 20 in the youngest cells of the erythrocyte series and reduced to 2 in the later stages. In normal adult human erythrocytes the iron is almost entirely in the hemoglobin, with only extremely small amounts detected as nonhemoglobin iron. Accordingly Pollycove has suggested that the labile erythropoietic iron pool is bound to the membrane of the maturing erythrocyte, and that from that site the iron may be fed back into the plasma or moved onward for incorporation into the red cell and hemoglobin biosynthesis.

Although neither the anatomic location nor the chemical state of the labile erythropoietic iron pool has been established with certainty, by analysis of the kinetic curves of iron turnover Pollycove has estimated that in the normal person the feedback amounts to 11 mg per day and that the labile erythropoietic pool is 85 mg in size. Since the total amount of iron leaving the plasma per day was computed at 32 mg, allowing for the 11 mg per day feedback, 21 mg per day was calculated as the amount of iron fixed irreversibly in the maturing erythrocytes. Calculations from this (1 Gm of hemoglobin equals 3.4 mg of iron) should yield the amount of hemoglobin synthesized per day: 6.3 Gm. This value is in line with

other types of observations and is consistent with a red cell life span of 117 days. However, these conclusions based on "ferrokinetic"* studies overlap the general problem of erythropoiesis. "Erythrokinetics" must be approached from other aspects besides ferrokinetics and will accordingly be considered more appropriately in a later chapter.

In iron lack, the body is apparently functioning to utilize most effectively every bit of available iron; consequently iron is removed from the plasma more rapidly than normal, rapidly processed through the marrow, and practically all of it is incorporated into the hemoglobin of the newly formed red cells. In hemolytic states the labeled iron is very rapidly cleared from the plasma and soon appears in the newly formed erythrocytes, but because of premature removal of the cells from the peripheral blood by the hemolytic mechanism, the apparent maximal value reached is usually less than

* Ferrokinetic studies demonstrating the rates of turnover and exchange, the manner of ebb and flow, and the existence of labile and relatively fixed pools of iron within the body represent considerable advances in the understanding of the physiology and pathology of iron metabolism. In the extensive mathematical analysis of the kinetics models constructed, it is most encouraging to note how well biologic data of this sort can survive when tested on the rack of mathematics. But certain factors difficult at present to evaluate militate against too final an acceptance of the derived figures: the plasma iron disappearance curves after a few hours become complicated by additional variables and are subject to interpretation in extrapolation; there are sizable errors and variables inherent in the present methods for determining plasma iron content and the plasma volume; the diurnal variations in plasma iron content and plasma iron turnover are difficult to iron out in calculations; the amount of nonhemoglobin iron in the red cell at the moment it is delivered to the peripheral blood is unknown, and although it is presumed negligible, it is demonstrably not so in certain diseases; the turnover and demand for iron of other heme-containing pigments or iron-requiring enzyme are largely unknown; and the precise quantitation of intramarrow red cell destruction (ineffective erythropoiesis) is unknown, although again it is demonstrably considerable in certain diseases (42) and there is evidence for its existence in the normal individual.

normal. If the hemolytic mechanism involves splenic sequestration and destruction of the red cells, there is an associated excessive build-up of radioactivity over that organ. In conditions of bone marrow failure (aplastic or aregenerative anemias), the clearance of iron from the plasma may be slow, with very little incorporated into hemoglobin (10 to 15 per cent in 9 to 12 days). Here the tagged iron can usually be traced from the bone marrow to the iron stores of the liver.

A most important point in iron metabolism in terms of body economy will bear repeating here. When the red cell containing labeled hemoglobin comes to the end of its life span, the hemoglobin is liberated from the cell, the heme moiety is degraded through the urobilinogen cycle, and excreted. Contrariwise, the iron is tenaciously retained, transported through the plasma by the iron-binding protein, and very nearly all of it is preferentially reutilized for new hemoglobin formation. The iron is thereby put through its erythropoietic cycle again and again, illustrating most efficient conservation.

The mechanism is unknown whereby physiologic amounts of iron (whether ingested, administered parenterally, or derived from the in vivo destruction of erythrocytes) are allowed to bypass storage depots and yet be guided to the marrow for preferential utilization in erythropoiesis. Nevertheless, it is very clear (a) that such is the situation; (b) that the mechanism is most effective and efficient since practically 100 per cent utilization of iron for hemoglobin formation is demonstrable; and (c) that this is a critical point in body conservation of iron, ferrokinetics, and erythrokinetics. The available information strongly suggests that the phenomenon is occasioned by unique properties of the iron-binding protein at normal saturation levels, the developing red cells, and interactions between the

two. In myeloid metaplasia, a condition in which active erythropoiesis may occur mainly in extramedullary areas such as the spleen and liver, tracer studies indicate that labeled iron bound to transferrin is delivered to the liver and spleen for incorporation into hemoglobin (167). Iron-binding protein complexed with iron attaches to developing erythrocytes with considerably greater avidity than does the protein devoid of iron. How the normally saturated transferrin that is carrying iron avoids giving up its metal to sites other than the bone marrow is unknown. But there is evidence to show that iron not bound to its specific transport protein leaves the circulation with extreme rapidity and is deposited in practically all body areas but especially those with concentrations of reticuloendothelium such as spleen and liver. The same is true for transferrin-bound iron when the per cent saturation of the iron-binding protein is abnormally high. It is also of considerable interest to note that the patients with atransferrinemia have iron-refractory hypochromic, microcytic anemia with tissue iron overload and that administered radioiron clears rapidly from the plasma, is distributed to all storage areas, and is poorly utilized for red cell production. With this in mind, it is difficult to avoid the conclusion that the remarkably specific and efficient unloading of iron from normally saturated transferrin at sites of active erythropoiesis while shunning other sites is due to a peculiar interaction between the metal-containing transport protein and an intramarrow reactant associated with the developing red cell.

To summarize the radioactive tracer techniques: (a) the rates at which iron is cleared from plasma and incorporated into newly formed red cells can be determined; (b) the amounts of iron cleared from the plasma and incorporated into newly formed red cells can be measured; and (c) the anatomic sites to which iron is delivered, the sites where it builds up, and the sites from which it is utilized can be mapped out, and the pathways of iron transport and metabolism thereby determined.

Ferrokinetic measurements (plasma iron clearance rates, red cell iron utilization rates and percentages, external scintillation counting, etc.) have yielded much valuable information concerning the pathophysiology of bone marrow function and iron transport in many different hematologic and nonhematologic disorders.

Iron Storage

The facts that in the normal person injected iron is rapidly cleared from the plasma and from 90 to 100 per cent of the administered iron is delivered to the bone marrow and incorporated into the hemoglobin of new red cells give valuable information concerning the state of iron stores. Iron does not have to go first to the stores in the liver and spleen. Indeed, the circulating iron does not mix uniformly with the iron stores but rather forms part of a "labile pool" preferentially used for hemoglobin production. This in turn means that labeled iron cannot be used as a means of measuring the size of iron stores; since uniform mixing does not occur, estimate of pool size by this means is impossible. Recent studies by Finch (57) indicate that dispersion of isotopic iron within the total miscible iron pool* does not occur until at least 1 year has elapsed. Moreover, this miscible pool is appreciably smaller than the estimates of total nonhemoglobin iron derived by other methods (see below). It seems probable that a portion of the storage iron is not miscible in normal individuals even over prolonged periods.

When present in normal total amounts (600 to 1,500 mg), iron is stored intracellularly as ferritin and hemosiderin in the liver, spleen, bone marrow, muscle, and other tissues. It is distributed approximately equally between the ferritin and hemosiderin compounds (159), and about one-third of the total stored iron is in the liver. Ferritin is the compound formed by combination of iron and apoferritin and found in mucosal cells of the gastrointestinal tract; it is discussed above in the section on Iron Absorption. Ferritin molecules are submicroscopic in size and are not stained by Prussian blue.† Ferritin is water-soluble and contains a variable amount of iron: 17 to 23 per cent by dry-weight measurement. All the iron can be removed without demonstrably damaging the protein capsule (apoferritin). Electron microscopic studies (Figure 2.7) originally were interpreted as indicating a core of four closely adjoining electron-dense particles and a peripheral shell (53). A more recent analysis indicates the presence of six clusters of electron-dense particles positioned at the apices of a hexad (Figure 2.8; 99). The electron-dense particles, 24 Å in diameter, represent the ferric hydroxide–phosphate aggregates, or micelles, and the peripheral shell, 54 Å in diameter, the protein portion. The iron aggregates have the approximate composition $[(FeOOH)8 (FeOPO_3H_2)]$ and are situated in the body of the protein molecule rather than on the surface. Mazur et al. (113) have demonstrated that a small number of ferrous ions are present on the surface of ferritin, stabilized by the surface sulfhydryl groups. When the sulfhydryl groups are oxidized to disulfide linkages, the ferrous ions are also oxidized and become attached to the

* This was estimated from the exaggerated drop of the concentration of radioactive iron in the peripheral red cells occuring during the first year of observation as the iron was diluted into the miscible tissue pool during the process of recycling and conserving iron.

† Recent observations by Shoden and Sturgeon (161) indicate that with more precise observational techniques ferritin does take the Prussian blue iron stain, as would be predicted from its known components and relation to hemosiderin (see below).

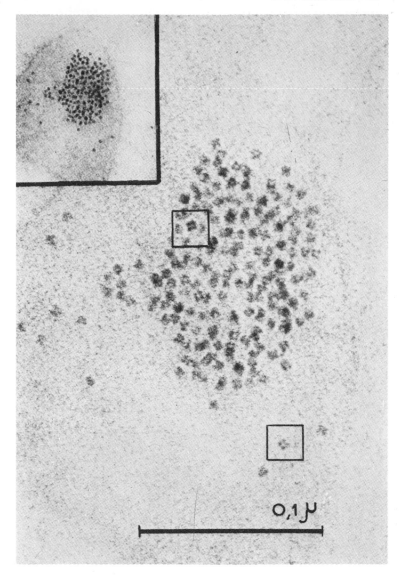

FIGURE 2.7.   Ferritin molecules as revealed by the electron microscope. (From Bessis, M. C., and Breton-Gorius, J., Blood 14:423, 1959)

internally situated iron micelles. Surface ferrous ions will dissociate from the ferritin molecule in the presence of a suitable iron-binding agent. Reducing substances and relative hypoxia facilitate the removal of iron from ferritin; oxidizing agents and aerobic conditions enhance the binding of iron.

By means of the injection of labeled amino acids, precise studies by Loftfrield and Eigner (109) show that the over-all

biosynthesis of a ferritin molecule by the rat liver takes 4 to 5 minutes. This time includes peptic bonding, steric arrangement, cross linking, folding, and complexing with iron (the latter not necessarily to full saturation) (Figure 2.8). Evidence indicates that apoferritin is the precursor of ferritin and that the presence of iron stimulates the rapid biosynthesis of apoferritin. Amino acid analysis of purified apoferritin and ferritin shows the protein

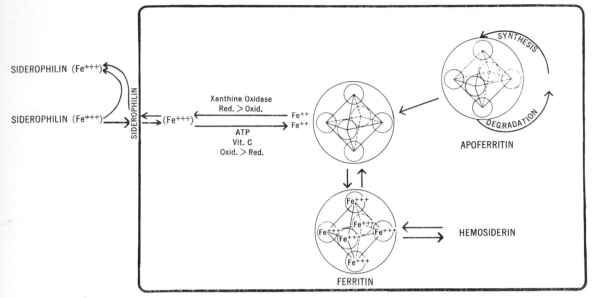

FIGURE 2.8.   Outline of proposed mechanisms for incorporation of iron into and mobilization from storage compounds

matrix to be the same in both compounds, and electron microscopic analysis indicates a structural identity between apoferritin and ferritin from which the iron has been removed. Some tissue sections show numerous organic shells with varying degrees of iron content (9).

The mechanism whereby iron is incorporated into the tissue for storage has been investigated by Mazur et al. (115). When labeled iron bound to iron-binding protein is followed in vivo in rats, about 20 per cent goes to the liver; one-half of this is found in the ferritin, and its distribution among the ferritin molecules of varying iron content indicates that it is first incorporated into iron-poor molecules that with time are converted to molecules with high iron content. The incorporation of labeled iron bound to iron-binding protein* into ferritin of liver (Figure 2.6) is dependent upon energy-producing oxidative metabolic reactions, specifically the biosynthesis of adenosine triphosphate. In addition to ATP, ascorbic acid is required; neither alone will effect the transfer reaction. The suggested mechanism is the formation of a complex

including two molecules of ATP, one molecule of ascorbic acid, and the protein-bound iron. ATP is thought to stimulate the oxidation of ascorbic acid in the presence of iron, thereby reducing the iron to the ferrous state. This liberates it from the protein bond and allows its transfer to acceptor sulfhydryl groups on the ferritin surface. Evidence that the mechanism is operational in vivo is provided by studies on intact rats showing the the rate of incorporation of iron into liver and spleen ferritin varies with oxidative metabolism and is decreased in scorbutic animals (116).

On the basis of animal and tissue studies Mazur et al. (114) have proposed that the adaptive enzyme xanthine oxidase is required for mobilization of iron from the ferritin stores (Figure 2.6). In vitro, ferritin is reduced by xanthine oxidase and small amounts of iron are liberated. It has been demonstrated that anoxia results in an increase in the substrates of the enzyme and that the administration of hy-

* Markedly different results have been obtained employing ferric citrate.

poxanthine, xanthine, and purines, nucleotides, or nucleosides increases the
plasma iron of animals. It has therefore
been hypothesized that ferritin iron is
released from the liver to the plasma after
reduction by xanthine oxidase, but there
is no critical evidence to show this to be
the actual in vivo mechanism.

Mazur has pointed out that there is an
interesting inverse relation between the
biochemical mechanism of iron release
from, and iron incorporation into, ferritin.
The release of iron is favored by decreased oxygen supply to the cell: this
results in an accelerated breakdown of
molecules including ATP, yielding elevated cell levels of hypoxanthine and xanthine, and a consequent increase in oxidation of the substrates by xanthine oxidase,
a process demonstrated to induce the reduction and release of ferritin iron. The reverse reaction of incorporation of iron
into ferritin is dependent upon energy-
yielding reactions for the continued biosynthesis of ATP, which, together with
ascorbic acid, releases iron from its iron-
binding protein for addition into ferritin.

The iron in ferritin is in a unique magnetic state. It is the only normally occurring biologic iron compound possessing a
magnetic susceptibility equivalent to
three unpaired electrons per iron atom
(67). Ferritin is reported to have potent
vasodepressor and antidiuretic activity in
some circumstances and has been implicated in some instances of irreversible
shock. Heilmeyer and others, for example,
have demonstrated the presence of ferritin
and hemosiderin in the peripheral blood of
patients with iron overload in irreversible
shock (173). Nevertheless, it should be
pointed out that the intravenous injection
of ferritin is without effect on the blood
pressure of normal individuals, and it has
been proposed that the irreversible shock
in hemochromatosis may be due to an
endotoxin sensitivity associated with deranged iron metabolism (94).

The term hemosiderin is a misnomer
that originated when the compound was
thought to be a degradation product of
hemoglobin. Hemosiderin is a normal
constituent of most tissues. Hemosiderin
granules are much larger than ferritin
molecules. They are microscopically visible, contain up to 37 per cent iron by dry-
weight measurements, take the Prussian
blue stain, have a different rate of electrophoretic migration, and are insoluble
in water. Because of these differences,
hemosiderin was originally thought to be
a different compound from ferritin. However, the recent studies by Richter (150,
151) and others on the basis of electron
microscopy, x-ray diffraction, paramag-
netic susceptibility, and antigenicity have
clarified their relation. Hemosiderin granules are now believed to be large aggregates of ferritin molecules with a higher
content of iron. They consist of innumerable closely packed, electron-dense
particles embedded in orderly fashion in
less electron-dense matter. Bordering the
dense aggregates typical individual or
small groups of ferritin molecules are
seen (Figure 2.7). Intracellularly the
dense aggregates are often found in the
form of discrete organelles bordered by
membranes and are called by Richter
"siderosomes." He postulated that ferritin and hemosiderin are synthesized in
the organelles that may be derivatives of
mitochondria (see below). Despite the
similarities between ferritin and hemosiderin demonstrated by the above techniques, chemical and spectrophotometric
analyses show porphyrin and other pigments to be present in very small amounts
in hemosiderin but not in ferritin (161,
162, 177, 180). Moreover, hemosiderin induced under different conditions varied
appreciably in porphyrin and pigment
content, and it is therefore evident that
physicochemically hemosiderin is not a
homogenous compound.

Functionally there are some significant
differences between the two compounds.
Normally the liver and bone marrow

storage iron is composed of approximately equal amounts of ferritin and hemosiderin. However, with iron overload, an increased proportion is hemosiderin. If iron is administered to rabbits, the ferritin iron reaches a peak concentration after which any further increase in tissue iron is quantitatively reflected by an increase in hemosiderin iron. This is of considerable clinical importance since it supports the interpretation that the presence and degree of iron overload can be estimated by the number of hemosiderin granules found in preparations from liver biopsy or bone marrow aspiration. It has been demonstrated that administered radioactive iron is first incorporated into the ferritin and only later appears in the hemosiderin granules. Conversely, following repeated venesection to remove hemoglobin iron and cause mobilization of iron stores for new hemoglobin formation, ferritin iron is more rapidly utilized than is the iron of the hemosiderin granules.

It would be of considerable clinical and physiologic value to have available an easily and widely applicable method of estimating the size of the iron stores. These are generally agreed to consist of approximately 1 Gm of iron distributed in compartments with different metabolic activities. Estimates in terms of absolute weight have been made on the basis of chemical analysis of tissue. Most of these determinations have been made in animals and the values translated to the human being. Nevertheless, the values obtained by this method are in fair agreement with those estimated by Finch, Haskins, and others (56, 57, 78, 88) employing a method which assayed the iron in terms of how much was available for erythropoiesis.

Normal subjects were repeatedly bled, and the amount of iron removed in the blood (500 ml of blood contains approximately 250 mg of elemental iron) was determined. Initially the subjects re-established their prebleeding hemoglobin levels by the rapid formation of new hemoglobin. The hemoglobin production was at such a rapid rate that the vast majority of the iron so utilized must have been obtained from the stores and not from newly absorbed iron. However, after repeated venesections, the subjects were unable to re-establish their hemoglobin levels as rapidly as before and finally could not regenerate hemoglobin more rapidly than predicted on the basis of dietary iron intake and absorption. At this point it was assumed that the iron stores ordinarily available for erythropoiesis had been depleted. By this method the stores of normal males were calculated to consist of 1,000 to 1,500 mg of iron available for erythropoiesis over a 3- to 4-month span.

It was also found that patients expected to have deficient iron stores tolerated phlebotomy poorly, while those with increased iron stores could tolerate weekly bloodletting for very prolonged periods. As mentioned above, the size of iron stores estimated by this method is significantly larger than the size of the miscible iron pool as determined by radioactive iron dilution techniques (57). There is a difference of approximately 600 mg, indicating that some of the storage iron is in a metabolically relatively inert form but can, nevertheless, be mobilized for hemoglobin production if necessary. There is some reason to think that the metabolically inert, difficultly mobilizable iron is contained in the grosser hemosiderin granules. If a patient with iron overload (hemochromatosis) is repeatedly bled to the point where his hemoglobin no longer is regenerated, liver biopsy or bone marrow aspiration may demonstrate an occasional large hemosiderin aggregate. With time, this iron is made available and the hemoglobin regenerated. With continued venesections, the point is ultimately reached at which there is no stainable iron in the tissue,

Iron-lack Anemia   [53

and the hemoglobin is formed from ingested iron.

A semiquantitative estimate of iron stores can be made from the number of stainable iron granules present in a smeared-out fragment of bone marrow. No appreciable amount of stainable iron is found in specimens obtained from iron-deficient subjects. At present this is undoubtedly the most readily available method for estimating the state of the iron stores as absent, normal, or increased. The other, more indirect, methods that have been evaluated (plasma iron content, iron tolerance curve, radioactive iron studies, bone marrow iron content, presence of sideroblasts, etc.) are subject to so many varying influences that it is difficult to be certain of a reliable interpretation.

A depleted iron store is the *sine qua non* of iron deficiency, and only this. All anemias, other than those associated with iron lack, have *increased* iron stores. Consequently increased iron stores may result from many causes: idiopathic familial hemochromatosis due to abnormal absorption; transfusion hemosiderosis resulting partly from the iron derived from repeated transfusion; tissue hemosiderosis resulting from the transfer of iron from its former location in the hemoglobin of the peripheral blood to the tissues, as in untreated pernicious anemia, chronic or acute hemolytic anemia, chronic infection and inflammation, etc. But depleted iron stores are indicative of iron deficiency regardless of the causes or complications.

It has been stated repeatedly that red cell production and hemoglobin biosynthesis play a dominant role in iron metabolism. This is especially true when the conservation and reutilization of iron in metabolism are added into the assessment. Elsewhere the problems of heme biosynthesis, globin biosynthesis, and the requirements for cell maintenance while these processes are taking place have been considered. The mechanisms whereby iron is taken into the developing red cell and incorporated into heme during the biosynthesis of hemoglobin and the completion of a functioning red cell unit will now be discussed.

Iron Transfer

Two mechanisms have been described by which iron enters into the developing red cell and is made available for the formation of hemoglobin. Ironically enough, the one that appears best documented in terms of in vivo processes seems less likely to play a major role in iron uptake than the one based almost purely on in vitro analyses. The former method was elucidated by Bessis et al. (8, 10–12a), who studied by means of the electron microscope human bone marrow preparations that reasonably could be expected to indicate processes as they function in vivo. The electron microscope employed had a resolving power of about 10 Å. As detailed above, the structure of ferritin molecules and hemosiderin granules can be identified and analyzed with this technique. The reticulum cells of bone marrow are found to contain numerous ferritin molecules scattered through their cytoplasm and clustered together as hemosiderin crystals or granules. In the marrow these iron-laden reticulum cells were surrounded by immature developing red cells: erythroblasts (Figure 2.9). By a process called "ropheocytosis" the ferritin and hemosiderin granules are transferred to the red cell. Ropheocytosis is somewhat akin to pinocytosis, the mechanism whereby a liquid droplet is incorporated into a cell by depressing the cytoplasmic membrane, thus forming a vacuole. In the iron transfer, the iron granules adhere to the membrane of the developing red cell, but always in an area of submicroscopic size. This area is then seemingly drawn in by the cytoplasm and an invagination, 500 Å in size, is

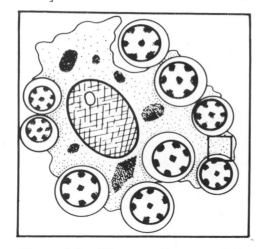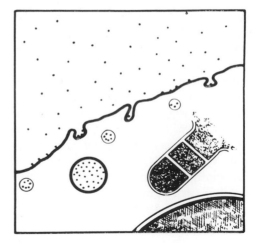

FIGURE 2.9.   Diagrammatic representation (based on electron microscopic view) of one mechanism whereby developing erythrocytes may obtain iron. Developing red cells clustered about an iron-laden reticulum cell are shown on left; ropheocytosis and mitochondrial rupture are shown on right. Single round dots represent ferritin molecules; clustered dots in reticulum cell represent hemosiderin granules. (From Bessis, M. C., and Breton-Gorius, J., Blood 14:423, 1959)

formed. By bringing together the two edges of the depression, a vacuole results, with the particles of iron adhering to the inner membrane. The membrane and liquid contents of the vacuole are reabsorbed, and the ferritin molecules are left in the cytoplasm. Here they concentrate into clusters of varying sizes. Large clusters may be visible under the light microscope, and the presence of iron may be demonstrated by specific staining reactions. These cells are termed "sideroblasts." In the more mature cells there is gradual disappearance of the iron clusters and ferritin molecules as hemoglobin appears. In certain hematologic abnormalities associated with defective heme biosynthesis (thalassemia, B_6 abnormalities, certain refractory anemias also called sideroblastic anemias, etc.) mitochondria are seen that are engorged with ferritin. Here the iron-laden molecules lose their characteristic structure, the mitochondrial membrane is burst apart, and the iron is liberated into the cytoplasm. A similar handling of ferritin by mitochondria has been demonstrated to occur in the normal subject before iron is incorporated into hemoglobin. On the basis of the evidence presented by Bessis et al. (8, 10–12) there is no doubt that such a process exists. However, the question has been raised that the operational sequence may actually be the reverse of that described and that this is rather a method for ridding erythrocytes of excess iron. There seem to be no critical data available to settle this objection even though pinocytosis in other situations appears always to indicate intake and not expulsion of particles. It is difficult to balance the quantitative advantages against the physical disadvantages of the system as an in vivo mechanism for iron transfer.

As described in the chapters on heme and globin biosynthesis, numerous observations have documented the fact that when reticulocytes are incubated in vitro with labeled iron, iron is taken into the cell and incorporated into newly formed hemoglobin (55). It is evident therefore that red cells can obtain iron existing in forms other than ferritin as described above. Iron is preferentially transferred from the iron-binding protein to immature heme-synthesizing cells (135). When studied by radioautography, the time course of iron uptake (166) is found to be continuous throughout differentiation; the proerythroblasts, however, show a markedly higher uptake than later stages. It seems clear that the major part of the iron complement of the red cell is acquired during its most primitive stages (3).

From the in vitro studies published by Jandl et al. (91), Jandl and Katz (92), Allen and Jandl (2), and Clark and Walsh (38), the following mechanism may be described. Iron-saturated transferrin is preferentially bound to young red cells with an affinity four to five times that of transferrin lacking iron. The cell-bound transferrin is in equilibrium with unbound transferrin while the iron remains attached to the cell. Iron is transferred from iron-binding protein by competitive binding to specific receptors on the cell surface. That is, the transfer of iron is not maximum until 25 per cent of the iron-binding protein is saturated; nonspecific unloading occurs at saturations greater than 60 per cent. The receptors for both transferrin and iron on the cell surface may be destroyed by proteolytic enzymes (trypsin and chymotrypsin) or partially blocked by antibody coating of the cell. Once bound to the specific receptor the iron is not elutable by washing or by chemical chelating agents (EDTA). The function of the receptors is dependent upon metabolic energy either for synthesizing the sites or for facilitating the release of iron from the sites to the cell interior. Their function may be blocked by various poisons (cyanide, azide) and supported or increased by glucose and oxygen. The uptake of iron by the receptors is not blocked by the action of lead. This would indicate that the uptake of iron by the receptors is not dependent upon heme biosynthesis (which is blocked by lead) and is consistent with the previously mentioned

electron microscopic findings of abnormal iron accumulations inside immature cells in lead poisoning. Thus a very specific mechanism exists for the transport of circulating iron to, onto, and into the developing red cell.

Sequential studies have shown that the specific activity (with reference to radioactive iron) of the stroma increases and then declines before the specific activity of the hemoglobin reaches its peak in the normal person (52). In some disorders associated with defective heme biosynthesis, the specific activity of the stroma remains above that of the hemoglobin peak. Also pertinent here are the recent observations of Lochhead and Goldberg (108) that heme can be formed in cell-free systems from labeled iron derived either from plasma iron-binding protein or liver proteins (presumably ferritin).

Iron accepted by the reticulocyte membrane from the plasma is first associated with the particulate fractions of the cell stroma, mitochondria and microsomes (2, 55, 147). From here it is gradually released to a transient nonhemoglobin protein phase before it is incorporated into hemoglobin. Mazur et al. (117) have recently reported that within the developing erythrocyte labeled iron is first incorporated into ferritin, which acts as a carrier or precursor, before it is incorporated into heme. The mechanism for incorporation of the iron into red cell ferritin is the same as into liver cell ferritin, and any procedure inhibiting its incorporation into ferritin decreases its incorporation into heme. By kinetic studies it has been concluded (2) that the entire process from the initial binding of iron by surface receptors to incorporation into hemoglobin takes only 6 to 8 minutes. In suitable concentrations lead blocks the transfer of iron from the particulate fractions to the nonhemoglobin protein.

It is difficult at present to assess which route of iron transport into the maturing red cell plays the major role. The fact that labeled iron attached to iron-binding protein is rapidly cleared from the circulating plasma and can be detected in circulating red cells in approximately 2 hours does not necessarily rule against the formation of a ferritin intermediate, since the formation of the compound in a matter of minutes has been demonstrated by labeled amino acids (109). The incorporation of granules of ferritin into cells tightly packed in solid masses in erythropoietic foci has much to recommend it. However, as mentioned previously, were ferritin to form a source of iron intermediate between plasma and red cells, delivery of iron from plasma to hepatic ferritin as well as to bone marrow ferritin would be expected. This is reported not to occur normally in man. On the other hand uptake of iron from circulating plasma obviates the mechanical difficulties that might well be encountered because of the demands of proximity.

This brings us to the last step in the transport of iron, namely the mechanism by which iron is inserted into the porphyrin ring. This phase of heme biosynthesis is of considerable interest to clinicians since there are several types of anemia in which iron incorporation appears to be deranged.

The most obvious example is iron-lack anemia, where the essential component is just not available. The evidence for impaired incorporation of iron into protoporphyrin in lead poisoning has been cited, and in the section dealing with thalassemia, work will be described indicating a partial block in the combination of iron and protoporphyrin. In these conditions there is a significant increase in the free erythrocyte protoporphyrin. On the basis of morphologic studies the probability seems good that in the miscellaneous group of so-called sideroachrestic anemias and in the anemias associated with pyridoxine abnormalities there is a similar impairment in the utili-

zation of iron that is present in the cell in such overabundance. In most of these situations there is also evidence for defects in the synthesis of globin and/or the heme precursors. It is impossible presently to estimate how much iron accumulates because of a primary defect or block of iron incorporation into the protoporphyrin of hemoglobin.

The enzymatic insertion of iron into protoporphyrin to form heme has been studied by Schwartz et al. (156, 157) in cell-free systems by determining the requirements for the production of heme from protoporphyrin and iron. One or more enzymes are required that can be partly inactivated by heating and inhibited by sulfhydryl blockers or EDTA (133). This "heme synthetase system" has a pH requirement for optimal activity (pH 7.4) and requires reduced glutathione, cysteine, and globin for optimal activity. When the most suitable concentrations of protoporphyrin and iron are present, the amount of heme synthesized depends upon enzyme concentration. The enzyme system has a very high specificity since iron is not enzymatically inserted into the porphyrin ring until the vinyl side chains are formed on the porphyrin ring, resulting in protoporphyrin.* The enzyme system is found in the particulate cell fraction; the work by Nishide and Labbe (134) and Labbe and Hubbard (102) indicates that most of it is in the mitochondria. Kinetic studies suggest that preincubation of the enzymes with protoporphyrin and DPN results in the formation of an intermediate which then chelates the iron. The few assays for enzymatic activity on human red cells indicate the enzyme is present only in reticulocytes (66).

At present the order in which the three components bind together has not been

---

* In aqueous solutions, at physiologic pH and temperature, iron can be *nonenzymatically* complexed into coproporphyrinogen and protoporphyrinogen.

definitely established. The iron may be inserted into the protoporphyrin, and the resulting heme may then complex with globin. Recent work indicates that heme may dissociate from globin at neutral pH, and both may thereby exist in equilibrium so that they can exchange with other apoproteins (153). Conversely, globin may complex with protoporphyrin to form a complex then receptive to the insertion of iron. It has also been proposed (69a) that iron combines with a protein (not ferritin but possibly a part of the globin) which unites with protoporphyrin to form heme and the complete hemoglobin molecule.

It should be pointed out that iron functions not only as a building block in the biosynthesis of heme but also as a cofactor in the biosynthesis of δ-aminolevulinic acid. In terms of the effect of iron depletion upon the biosynthesis of heme Vogel et al. (172) have demonstrated a lower rate of production from labeled glycine when erythrocytes from iron-deficient ducklings were employed than when normal cells were used. The addition of iron in vitro augmented the heme production from glycine only in the deficient cells. Starting from δ-aminolevulinic acid, both deficient and control cells were able to produce more protoporphyrin but only small amounts of heme unless iron was added. Following this iron repletion the amount of heme increased and the protoporphyrin decreased. Iron deficiency therefore has two effects upon heme biosynthesis: a decreased production of δ-aminolevulinic acid and a decreased formation of heme from protoporphyrin.

Iron-lack Anemia

In dealing with any anemia one must constantly be aware that it is not sufficient to establish the presence of a low level of circulating hemoglobin and the classification into which the anemia falls. One must recognize that anemia is a manifestation of an underlying disease. Anemia is not a disease or diagnosis; anemia is a readily and accurately determined manifestation of a disease. This is most evident in the anemia due to iron lack in adults. In this situation the presence of iron-lack anemia is usually quite readily established and accurately classified. The proximate cause of the anemia (namely, the iron lack) can be easily corrected by appropriate therapy, thereby allowing the hemoglobin to regenerate to normal levels. The anemia is classified, treated, and abolished. But the disease process responsible for the iron lack, and thus for the anemia, has not been affected by the treatment. The basic disease process must be sought out and dealt with. In the adult this is all too frequently a malignant tumor of the gastrointestinal tract. It is evident that correction of the hemoglobin deficit will be of little long-term benefit to the patient. In all instances, the ultimate as well as the proximate cause of the anemia must be determined and appropriately treated.

Iron lack or iron deficiency* results from a depletion of iron normally available to meet metabolic requirements. If the deficit is severe enough, anemia occurs. This anemia responds specifically to the administration of iron, and *only* iron, in an orderly, predictable sequence of events. It is the *only* type of anemia in which such treatment is effective. On the basis of the general principles of iron metabolism outlined above, the situations in which iron-lack anemia are seen may be accurately delineated.

A. Since intake and absorption of iron are limited, the anemia would be expected to occur during periods of increased iron demand such as exist in in-

---

* The nonspecific term "iron lack" is preferred to the more usually employed "iron deficiency" since by common usage deficiency connotes an insufficiency resulting from a nutritional, or intake, inadequacy. This immediately tends to put one on potentially dangerous ground in dealing with iron-lack anemia.

fants at about one to two years of age. Body growth is so rapid that the iron stores and supplies are outstripped; the expansion of the vascular tree is so rapid that the infant in effect "bleeds into his own expanding blood volume." Iron lack might well be expected during the growth spurt that takes place during adolescence and, of course, during pregnancy (especially with twinning or closely spaced pregnancies) when fetal iron demands are preferentially met.

B. Iron-lack anemia would also be expected to occur when iron loss exceeds absorption long enough to deplete the iron stores and impair hemoglobin production. This situation is apt to occur with chronic blood loss (usually from the gastrointestinal or genitourinary tract and caused by hemorrhoids, peptic ulcer, tumor, uterine fibroids, etc.). The loss may be continuous or intermittent, like the menstrual blood loss in females of child-bearing age. Malabsorption over prolonged periods of time may sufficiently upset the balance, but since the excretion of iron per day is in the range of 1 mg, true deficiency secondary to poor intake would require an inordinate length of time and in this country is, for practical purposes, never seen in adults.

The signs and symptoms of iron-lack anemia are those common to all anemias: pallor, easy fatigability, anorexia, weakness, lassitude, palpitations, dyspnea on exertion, angina on effort, ankle edema, etc. The onset is insidious and the progression very slow, usually measured in many months to years. Probably because of this, physiologic adjustments are made in many organs so that a severe hemoglobin deficit may be accompanied by a remarkable paucity of symptoms. Gastrointestinal disturbances may play a significant role. In children, pica (craving for unnatural articles of food, dirt, paint, etc.) is not infrequent and is said to be abolished by adequate iron administration. Constipation is a fairly common complaint, but mild diarrhea also occurs. A frequent complaint is that the fingernails break and crack easily and are paper-thin. The nails may assume peculiar shapes, with a central depression and raised borders, called spoon nail, or koilonychia. A smooth tongue with papillary atrophy may or may not be associated with discomfort or pain (glossitis). In exceptional cases almost all the mucous membranes may be involved, with resultant stomatitis, vaginitis, proctitis, etc. Cheilosis is not unusual. When the glossitis is accompanied by a sore mouth and dysphagia, the Plummer-Vinson (or Patterson-Kelly) (182) syndrome is said to be present. Disturbances of menses are frequent; either cessation of flow (not unusual in any type of anemia) or profuse flow may occur. Retinal hemorrhages are unusual and papilledema is very rare (155). With the exception of instances of remarkably prolonged anemia in children, who may have the "hair-on-end" skull lesion classically described in the hereditary hemolytic anemias, skeletal changes are not seen (32). Signs of peripheral neuropathy, usually minor, may occur in the form of numbness and tingling of extremities (often referred to as pins-and-needles sensation). Although all the above symptoms and manifestations are seen, the majority of patients have only nonspecific complaints of a tired, run-down feeling.

The physical findings are usually limited to those associated with the hemoglobin depression (pallor, tachycardia, cardiomegaly) and are commensurate with the depression. The lingual atrophy, or glossitis, and spoon nail mentioned above are usually late developments. Minimal or moderate splenomegaly occurs in less than 10 per cent of adults but is seen more often in children, in whom the more marked enlargement may be due to the frequent concomitant infections.

Hematologically, well-developed iron-lack anemia is characterized by erythrocytes poorly filled with hemoglobin (low mean corpuscular hemoglobin concentration, or hypochromasia); small in size (low mean corpuscular volume, or microcythemia); and showing considerable variation in size and shape. It is a hypochromic (MCHC 25 to 30 per cent), microcytic (MCV 55 to 74 cu μ) type of anemia. The central pallor usually seen in the erythrocyte because of the discoid form is exaggerated. This exaggeration can vary from a barely discernible change to one so marked that the cell has only a thin rim of hemoglobin at the periphery. Tiny microcytes and elongated or elliptical cells are seen. There is very little sign of new cell formation; the reticulocyte count is usually low. The level of circulating hemoglobin is depressed disproportionately more than the red cell count and the hematocrit. In a significant anemia, the red cell count may be within normal limits and the hematocrit only moderately lowered because many small, poorly filled cells are present. The leukocyte and platelet counts are usually within normal limits, although with prolonged iron lack (and perhaps associated with splenomegaly) both may be depressed. The differential count is unremarkable. The icterus index and bilirubin level are low, indicating catabolism of only a small amount of hemoglobin.

The routine chemical tests and organ function tests are ordinarily within normal limits except for changes consistent with chronic blood loss, e.g., guaiac-positive feces. Gastric atrophy and achlorhydria* (6, 43) are late developments, as are fibrous adhesions in the upper esophagus (webs of the Plummer-Vincent syndrome). The reversibility of these abnormalities depends to some extent upon the duration of the iron lack (1). Bone marrow examination shows normoblastic hyperplasia with decreased cellular hemoglobin in the majority of the normoblasts. Otherwise no significant alterations are seen on routine preparation and staining. The plasma iron content is low, usually less than 35 μg per 100 ml, and values near zero are not unusual. The total plasma iron-binding capacity is elevated (350 to 500 μg per 100 ml) and the proportion of iron-binding protein that is saturated with iron, the per cent saturation, is thereby markedly depressed (2 to 10 per cent). The erythrocyte protoporphyrin is elevated (35).

The above is, of course, the picture of well-developed iron-lack anemia. Any gradation between this and the normal may be seen. This is best illustrated by tracing the sequence of events in the development of iron-lack anemia (40, 41, 59, 76, 141, 183). First of all by one or more of several mechanisms the individual's iron balance becomes negative (Figure 2.10). To counteract the negative balance, iron is mobilized from body stores to meet metabolic requirements, chiefly for the maintenance of hemoglobin production. This process continues until the stores have been depleted (liver, spleen, marrow, etc.). During the depletion of the iron stores and before detectable changes occur in the following aspects of iron metabolism, the absorption of iron is increased (146). The iron-binding capacity of the plasma increases above the normal range, and the plasma iron concentration then falls below the normal range. Sideroblasts (normoblasts with aggregation of iron in the cytoplasm) are no longer seen in the marrow. It is most important to realize that up to this point there has been no impairment of heme biosynthesis, that there is *no anemia*, and that the red cells are *normal in*

* There have been a number of studies reporting achlorhydria and gastric atrophy in iron-lack anemia and suggesting a causative relation, i.e., decreased iron absorption because of achlorhydria. However, Moore's studies, mentioned above, show no effect of pH and hydrochloric acid upon the absorption of *food* iron, and recent surveys show no increased achlorhydria in iron-lack anemia as opposed to other anemias in comparable age groups (31).

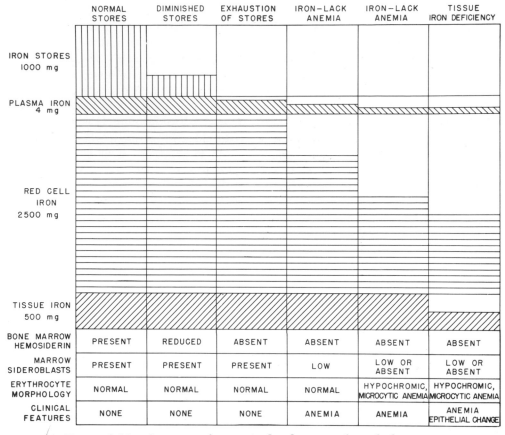

	NORMAL STORES	DIMINISHED STORES	EXHAUSTION OF STORES	IRON–LACK ANEMIA	IRON–LACK ANEMIA	TISSUE IRON DEFICIENCY
IRON STORES 1000 mg						
PLASMA IRON 4 mg						
RED CELL IRON 2500 mg						
TISSUE IRON 500 mg						
BONE MARROW HEMOSIDERIN	PRESENT	REDUCED	ABSENT	ABSENT	ABSENT	ABSENT
MARROW SIDEROBLASTS	PRESENT	PRESENT	PRESENT	LOW	LOW OR ABSENT	LOW OR ABSENT
ERYTHROCYTE MORPHOLOGY	NORMAL	NORMAL	NORMAL	NORMAL	HYPOCHROMIC, MICROCYTIC ANEMIA	HYPOCHROMIC, MICROCYTIC ANEMIA
CLINICAL FEATURES	NONE	NONE	NONE	ANEMIA	ANEMIA	ANEMIA EPITHELIAL CHANGE

FIGURE 2.10.   Sequence of events in development of iron-lack anemia

size, shape, and hemoglobin content. Nevertheless, it is evident that at this point a serious *iron lack* exists and that the negative balance, caused by increased loss of iron or decreased intake of iron, must have been going on for a considerable period of time. Undoubtedly then there are more patients with iron lack than with *iron-lack anemia.* When heme biosynthesis is retarded because of lack of iron as an essential building block,* the amount of erythrocyte protoporphyrin increases, the amount of circulating hemoglobin falls below normal, and anemia is present. However, the available evidence indicates that for at least several months this is a normochromic, normocytic type of anemia. Finally, the marrow, perhaps attempting to compensate for defective hemoglobin pro-

duction, puts out many small, poorly filled cells, and the anemia acquires the hypochromic, microcytic characteristics previously described (36).

What, then, are the best criteria upon which to establish the presence of iron lack? Obviously the earliest and best way would be to demonstrate that the iron stores had been decreased below normal or depleted. Unfortunately there is at present no easy and reliable method for doing this. Satisfactory estimates of iron stores can be made from liver biopsy and bone marrow aspiration. These are presently the most reliable tests for obtaining information about the state of the iron stores (13, 14, 18). Several extensive

* It has been demonstrated that the iron content of the hemoglobin in iron-lack anemia is normal (15).

comparative studies on the reliability of the various tests that have been at one time or another *proposed* as indicators of the status of iron stores (determination of plasma iron concentration, iron-binding capacity, iron turnover, iron absorption, and demonstration of hypochromic, microcytic erythrocytes) consistently show this to be so (13, 14, 23, 76, 171). But liver biopsy and bone marrow aspiration are not widely applicable, and, except for special investigative purposes, are not used unless other circumstances suggest the possibility of altered iron stores. By their nature they cannot be used routinely as screening tests to indicate the status of the iron stores and thereby attain the earliest possible indication of a negative iron balance. If the plasma iron concentration is low and the iron-binding capacity increased, one can safely assume that iron stores have been depleted. But both these values are so readily altered by other influences (infection, inflammation, protein depletion, recent ingestion of iron, diurnal variations, lack of steady state in erythropoiesis, etc.) that they are not reliable enough to be uniformly satisfactory. The presence of hypochromic erythrocytes is readily determined by the calculation of red cell indices and examination of a stained film of the peripheral blood. But as already indicated, hypochromasia is a late change, and by the time this is present whatever pathologic process is responsible for the negative iron balance has been in existence for a considerable period of time. Irreversible damage may have been done or the lesion may be inoperable.

How reliable is the finding of hypochromic, microcytic erythrocytes as an indication of iron lack? Or stated in another way: What conditions other than iron lack are associated with hypochromic, microcytic peripheral blood? Thalassemia* (Cooley's anemia and trait, Mediterranean anemia and trait) is a condition that by red cell indices and morphologic criteria may be indistinguishable from iron lack. Except for certain population groups this a relatively unusual disorder and is usually fairly readily detected because it is a hemolytic disorder with (a) persistently elevated levels of reticulocytes and bilirubin, (b) a familial tendency, (c) a normal or, more usually, elevated plasma iron content, and (d) a lack of response to iron therapy. Chronic infection, inflammation, lead poisoning, and rheumatoid arthritis occasionally give rise to hypochromic, microcytic anemia, but in these situations the primary causes are usually clinically obvious. This type of anemia has been described in infants secondary to copper deficiency and/or protein abnormality, but again this is rare and may well be suspected because of the additional finding of edema. A hypochromic, microcytic anemia responsive to vitamin B_6 (pyridoxine) has been described in a small number of individuals. Here the plasma iron concentration is elevated, and a number of patients have shown other signs of abnormal iron metabolism (hemochromatosis, pigmentation). A few patients have been described with an anemia responding to a factor in crude liver extract as well as to vitamin B_6. A few instances of a familial hypochromic, microcytic anemia have been described in this country; this is a very rare sex-linked disorder that may or may not be responsive to pyridoxine. Increasing numbers of patients, but still comparatively few, with hypochromasia, microcytosis, hyperferremia, and tissue iron overload not responsive to any known agent have been designated as having sideroachrestic anemia.

Listing the various hematologic disorders associated with hypochromic, microcytic anemia (the differential diagnoses) makes it at once evident that aside

* Alone or in combination with an abnormal hemoglobin, most frequently E or S.

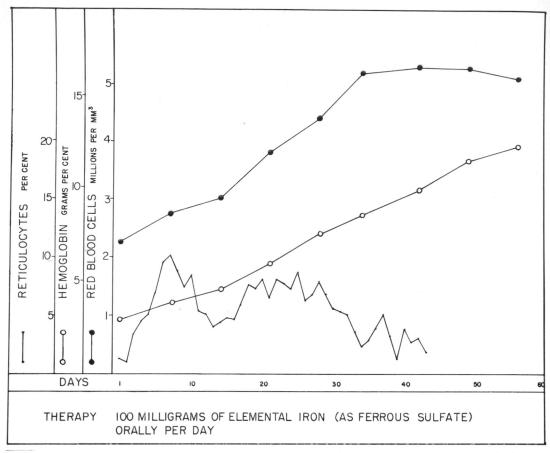

FIGURE 2.11.   Characteristic hematologic response of patient with severe iron-lack anemia to administration of iron

from iron lack the basic cause will be either obvious or readily detected, or else the condition is so rare as to be almost negligible. It therefore can be stated with assurance that if hypochromic, microcytic anemia is shown to be present, it should be considered due to iron lack. The final proof will come from a *specific orderly response* to iron therapy and only to iron therapy (40, 119, 120, 139). The specific orderly response (Figure 2.11) consists of an elevation above base line of the percentage of reticulocytes in the blood beginning on or about the third day after the start of adequate therapy, reaching a peak about the eighth to tenth day, and declining thereafter. A significant elevation in the hemoglobin level usually begins shortly after the reticulocyte peak,

is invariably present (more than 2 Gm per 100 ml) by 3 weeks after the start of therapy, and continues until normal values are reached: a satisfactory rate of increase is 0.2 Gm of hemoglobin per 100 ml of blood per day.* Frequently, in infants and adults a response that is readily discernible both clinically and subjectively occurs somewhere near the third or fifth day of therapy (increase in appetite and general well-being, increase in activity, feeling of returning strength, etc.). Since this change occurs before the hemoglobin rise, it has long been suspected that other iron-requiring enzymes

* The traditional intolerance of iron preparation due to gastrointestinal upsets has been studied by Kerr and Davidson (98), who concluded it to be iatrogenic.

depleted because of iron lack are promptly replenished or activated. Some experimental evidence has been provided to substantiate this.

For many years it was postulated that the tissue iron enzymes were inviolate even with severe iron depletion. However, the observations of Cohen and Elvehjem (39) suggested a decrease in the cytochrome-c content of tissues of iron-depleted rats. The observations were confirmed and extended by Gubler, who demonstrated low levels of cytochrome-c and myoglobin in deficient animals. Morphologic abnormalities have been demonstrated not only in the erythrocytes of iron-depleted human beings but also in the epithelial and mucosal cells, so that it is most reasonable that body-wide distribution of iron is affected (64). This concept finds confirmation in the recent demonstration of a marked decrease in the iron content of both cell-rich and cell-free thermally induced sweat.

Recently Beutler (18) has undertaken a systematic evaluation of iron enzymes in animals and man. The amount of cytochrome-c in liver and kidney was readily reduced, but the catalase content of liver and erythrocytes was unaffected. Intermediate degrees of reduction were found in cytochrome oxidase and succinic dehydrogenase. Whether or not the enzymes are depressed below critical functional levels that might limit steps in the involved metabolic pathway is not known. The oxygen consumption of tissue slices with markedly reduced cytochrome-c remains within normal limits, and the oxygen consumption of iron-deficient humans is not appreciably influenced by iron repletion (18).

In summary, a hypochromic, microcytic type of anemia is strong evidence of iron lack. A specific response to iron therapy will establish the fact. However, iron lack may exist (with or without anemia) without hypochromic and microcytic changes in the erythrocytes. Pres-

ently this is best documented by changes in storage iron and, less reliably, by changes in the plasma iron and iron-binding protein. The most important point to resolve is: What is the etiology of the disorder resulting in iron lack? In considering the basic factors concerned in iron balance, the special situations relative to increased iron demands in infancy, adolescence, and pregnancy (especially repeated pregnancies) have been mentioned. Because of precarious iron balance, it would be expected that menstruating females would be especially vulnerable to the development of iron lack. This is particularly true since it has been shown that most women cannot estimate menstrual blood loss within 50 per cent or more of the accurately determined amount (127). Menstrual flow may double without awareness of a change by the individual. Based on the considerations mentioned here and previously, iron lack is not an unexpected occurrence in infants, adolescents, and women of childbearing age. What then of its etiology in the adult male and the postmenopausal female whose iron intake normally exceeds or equals the loss, i.e., where a satisfactory iron balance would be expected? There is no question but that a long-standing malabsorption syndrome may result in iron lack with all its various manifestations. Usually, however, the malabsorption is obvious because of a variety of clinical and laboratory manifestations. May iron-lack anemia develop in an adult male or postmenopausal female on a nutritional basis, because of dietary lack? In the first place a diet significantly lacking in iron is difficult to obtain in the United States partly because of the food-fortification program. The diet would be so limited that it would be next to impossible to subsist on it for any considerable period of time. In Table 2.2., adapted from Moore and Dubach (127), are supplied the figures and calculations from which have been de-

TABLE 2.2. Calculation of time required for development of iron deficiency on nutritional grounds alone, in two hypothetical patients

	Adult male Hgb 15 Gm/100 ml Blood volume 5,000 ml		Postmenopausal female Hgb 14 Gm/100 ml Blood volume 4,000 ml	
When normal				
Total Hgb iron	2,500 mg		1,900 mg	
Storage iron	1,000 mg		500 mg	
Total		3,500 mg		2,400 mg
After development of iron deficiency (Hgb 7.5 Gm/100 ml)				
Total Hgb iron	1,250 mg		950 mg	
Storage iron	0		0	
Total		1,250 mg		950 mg
Deficit in Hgb and storage iron (with this degree of hypochromic anemia)		2,250 mg		1,450 mg
Time required to produce deficiency if no iron is absorbed and 1 mg is excreted per day		2,250 days (6.3 years)		1,450 days (4 years)

Adapted from Moore, C. V., and Dubach, R., J.A.M.A. 162:197, 1956.

rived the length of time required to produce iron-lack anemia if dietary intake stopped completely but excretion continued at the determined rate. For the adult male (losing 1 mg of iron per day) 6 years or more would be required, and for the postmenopausal female, 4 or more years. Actually, it is known that with the depletion of iron stores, excretion is appreciably reduced and absorption increased by compensating mechanisms (141). Taking these factors into account, the figures should probably be extended to 8 and 6 years, respectively. The development of iron-lack anemia in the adult male and postmenopausal female because of lack of ingestion of iron is therefore for practical purposes just about impossible. For a negative iron balance to occur, *iron loss must be increased*. This is possible only by blood loss. It cannot be too strongly emphasized that the presence of iron lack and iron-lack anemia commits the physician to a diligent search, repeated and prolonged if necessary, for the source and cause of the blood loss. Usually this is located in the gastrointestinal or genitourinary tract as a chronic occult process. All too often the basic cause is a malignant growth. For this reason it is unfortunate that a readily applicable test to determine the state of iron stores is not available so that a decrease could be detected early and the lesion responsible for the negative iron balance sought out and dealt with. Despite the fact that hypochromic, microcytic iron-lack anemia is a late development, it is a very reliable indicator of a specific derangement of iron metabolism.

Bibliographic references for Chapter 2 begin on page 373.

CHAPTER THREE

GLOBIN BIOSYNTHESIS
AND SICKLE CELL DISEASE

GLOBIN BIOSYNTHESIS*

The importance of globin in the body economy is made strikingly obvious from the facts that under normal conditions about 8 Gm is made per day (representing some 14 per cent of dietary protein intake), that globin production takes such precedence that it can be manufactured at the expense of other body proteins, and that slight abnormalities in its structure may give rise to fatal diseases.

By various relatively mild chemical procedures hemoglobin may be readily split into its component parts, heme and globin. Several types of analysis have established that globin is made up of 574 amino acid residues drawn from 19 different amino acids. In precisely ordered sequences these amino acids are built into the polypeptide chains that make up globin. Hemoglobin molecules possess a dyad of symmetry and are composed of identical halves. Every half-molecule is in turn composed of two different peptide chains (alpha, 141 amino acids, and beta, 146 amino acids; 81a), each of which has a heme radicle attached. The four peptide chains (two alpha and two beta) are tightly coiled in a highly specific helical fashion and arranged in definite configurations within the intact molecule.

Nutritional Requirements

By means of the following carefully controlled experimental conditions, Whipple and associates (209, 210) established the basic nutritional requirements for in vivo globin production. While dogs were maintained on a constant diet, blood was daily removed from them in amounts necessary to keep the circulating hemoglobin at a desired low level. In this artificially produced steady state the amount of hemoglobin formed per day by the marrow equaled the amount removed by daily bloodletting plus the endogenous blood destruction. The relation of any change of diet to hemoglobin production could then be quantitatively evaluated in terms of the altered amounts of blood that had to be withdrawn to re-establish the original steady state. It was demonstrated, for example, that various proteins differ in their biologic efficiency with respect to hemoglobin production (i.e., grams of hemoglobin produced per gram of protein fed). Hemoglobin itself was most effective, followed by plasma pro-

* General references and review articles: 6, 24, 27, 60, 73, 79, 83, 86, 91, 93, 100, 102, 103, 126, 127, 141, 144, 154, 168, 175, 188, 190, 192, 193, 198, 220.

teins, liver protein,* and casein. Vegetable proteins, frequently deficient in essential amino acids, were relatively inefficient. By this means it was also shown that amino acids can be utilized for hemoglobin production in place of preformed proteins. Consequently it was possible to conclude that globin is continuously formed anew from labile proteins or amino acid pools.†

Except under the most unusual circumstances, in man (8, 176) pure protein deficiencies or specific amino acid deficiencies do not result in anemia. This is presumably because other nutritional factors (vitamin B_{12}, folic acid, iron, etc.) or infections become limiting before the dietary defect and protein depletion of the body produce their full effects.

The later studies by Whipple and associates (43, 76, 209) on dogs with renal-bilary fistulae demonstrated that during the metabolism of intravenously administered hemoglobin the heme moiety is almost completely catabolized and excreted, whereas almost all the iron and the globin portions are reutilized in the synthesis of new hemoglobin. However, radioactive labeling (12) indicated that the globin is not preferentially reutilized for the formation of new erythrocytes, as is iron, but rather enters into the general dynamic exchange of body proteins, thereby in turn making available for hemoglobin production equivalent amounts of amino acids. Moreover, experiments labeling globin specifically indicated that while in the intact erythrocyte the protein (a histone) is outside general metabolic processes and exists for an average life of 100 to 120 days, the life span of heme and the red blood cell.

Both heme and globin must therefore be synthesized *de novo* in the developing red cell.

Globin Biosynthesis

Investigations on organs by Casperson, on tissues by Brachet (27), and on cells and cell-free systems by Zamecnik (220) have revealed that ribonucleic acid (RNA) is intimately concerned with the production of protein: specifically, that microsomal particles†† are the sites of protein production.

By means of microspectrophotometric techniques and interference microscopy of single erythrocyte precursors at different stages of maturation in the bone marrow, Thorell (197) has shown that hemoglobin is produced at a time when the cell is rich in cytoplasmic RNA and that hemoglobin accumulates as the RNA concentration is falling (Figure 3.1). When RNA is depleted, no further hemoglobin biosynthesis occurs. Maximal hemoglobin production occurs at the normoblastic stage of development while the cytoplasm is changing from a basophilic to an orthochromatic color. A small amount of biosynthesis takes place at the reticulocyte stage; none occurs in the adult cell. *Adult* red cells are unique in that they have no endoplasmic reticulum or microsomal particles (152, 217). Although electron microscopy does not reveal an endoplasmic reticulum in the *immature* red cell (31, 33, 36, 123), RNA granules are plentiful and mitochondria are present. Holloway et al. (84) have shown that the amount of RNA in erythrocytes varies with the number of reticulocytes present. Concentrating reticulocytes fiftyfold increases RNA thirtyfold; desoxy-

---

* This is the finding that led ultimately to Minot's demonstration of the efficacy of feeding liver in the treatment of pernicious anemia and the subsequent identification of folic acid and vitamin B_{12}.

† Recent evidence (32) obtained by parenterally administered labeled polypeptides suggests the utilization of short peptide chains.

†† "Microsomal particles" will be used to indicate the ribonucleoprotein particles (ribosomes, RNA granules) plus (when present) the supporting structures that make up the endoplasmic reticulum, disrupted by preparative processes but brought down by ultracentrifugation. Additional physicochemical characteristics are given in the footnote to p. 68.

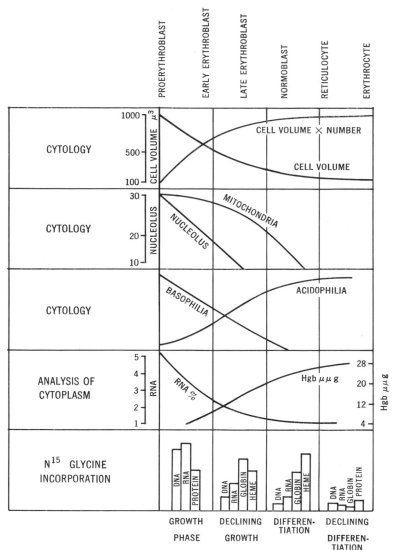

FIGURE 3.1.   Composite representation of red cell maturation with respect to terminology, biochemistry, and physiology

ribonucleic acid (DNA) concentration increases only fourfold.

While the *nucleated* forms of erythrocytes synthesize many different proteins and enzymes, of the soluble proteins produced by *reticulocytes* 98 per cent or more is hemoglobin. This makes the reticulocyte a cell admirably suited for the study of the production of a single protein, hemoglobin, in terms of the cell's component parts.

In 1948 London et al. (121) observed that red cells from a patient with sickle cell anemia take up labeled glycine in vitro and incorporate it into the *porphyrin ring*. Subsequent studies showed this a property of the immature, non-nucleated, but not necessarily reticulated, cells obtained from human beings (normal and abnormal) or animals (122). Studies of histidine uptake and incorporation demonstrated that *globin* formation also occurs in immature erythrocytes (180).

In 1949 Walsh et al. (203) demonstrated that under certain in vitro conditions reticulocytes obtained from normal individuals and from patients with sickle cell anemia or pernicious anemia take up radioactive iron from the incubation media and that the iron is incorporated into both stroma and hemoglobin of the cells. Since it had previously been shown that external iron does not exchange with either hemoglobin or cell iron, these observations indicate the production of new hemoglobin by immature erythrocytes. The observations have now been extended to many situations (see Chapter 1 and section on Iron Metabolism in Chapter 2) and are well confirmed and established. The original observations of iron uptake were not at that time extended to determine which part of the cell (structural protein, RNA granules, mitochondria, etc.) first became labeled. However, in 1958, employing rabbit reticulocytes, Rabinovitz and Olson (156) showed that some iron does go to the microsomal particles before being incorporated into hemoglobin.

In 1956 Rabinovitz and Olson (155), and in 1958 Dintzis et al. (48), incubated reticulocytes with various labeled amino acids and demonstrated that the amino acids became associated with the microsomal (RNA) granules, where they were bound but only for a short period of time. The label subsequently disappeared from the microsomal particles and appeared in the soluble protein of the cell cytoplasm. This protein was identified as hemoglobin, and by removal of the heme moiety, the labeled amino acids were shown to have been incorporated into the globin.* When several amino acids were incubated with reticulocytes, they entered the cell and became bound to the RNA granules, not in the ratios added to the incubation mixture, but rather in the same ratios that are known to exist in hemoglobin. The strong presumption then is that in association with the RNA

granule the amino acids are built into a prehemoglobin that is peptide in nature. By calculations involving uptake and release time, molecular weight of the particles, and the amount of non-RNA protein in the particle, it has been concluded that one RNA particle is capable of producing one polypeptide chain or one-fourth of a hemoglobin molecule per 1.5 minutes (48).

By means of a *cell-free system* composed of microsomes from rabbit reticulocytes, plus an energy-dependent enzyme system derived from *either* reticulocytes *or* rat liver cell,† Dintzis et al. (48) for the first time achieved an actual net production of hemoglobin. A properly balanced amino acid mixture increased the uptake of labeled leucine and valine by the RNA granules, and after 60 minutes, 50 to 60 per cent of the radioactivity had moved from the RNA granules to the soluble protein, of which 82 per cent contained heme and behaved electrophoretically like hemoglobin. Again the ratios of C^{14}-tagged leucine, isoleucine, and valine taken up by the RNA granules were the same as in hemoglobin (171). Rabinovitz and McGrath (158) demonstrated that the incubation of a valine analogue with reticulocytes completely inhibited the incorporation of other amino acids into hemoglobin. This

---

* Dintzis defined the properties of the microsomal particles and found three components: 82 per cent with sedimentation constant of 78 S; 9 per cent, 120 S; and 9 per cent, 50 to 60 S. The molecular weight was 4.1×10^6, and the protein/RNA ratio of the granules was approximately unity. Very little label was incorporated into or made a component part of the structure of the RNA granule itself. By electron microscopy the granules were found to be spheres 340 Å in diameter and by molecular weight calculations consisted of four RNA chains per granule.

† It is important to point out that the specificity of the protein synthesized is dependent not upon the amino acid–activating systems or energy-donating systems but upon the messenger RNA, which carries the information from the genetic DNA.

indicates that amino acid incorporation requires the participation of component amino acids and is therefore consistent with the true synthesis of a protein.

Recently it was shown that C^{14}-labeled RNA granules obtained from reticulocytes transferred their radioactivity to hemoglobin when they were incubated in the presence of unlabeled amino acids and soluble enzymes (4). By alternating periods of incubation with labeled valine and periods employing nonlabeled valine, Bishop et al. (22) obtained evidence that the polypeptide chains of hemoglobin are synthesized by starting at the N-terminal amino acid (N-terminal valine for a- and β-chains) and sequentially adding amino acids in precise order as determined by the template on the RNA granule until the chain is complete and release from the RNA granule takes place.

Concerning the time relations of heme and globin biosynthesis, i.e., whether or not they are produced simultaneously, present data are conflicting. Evidence obtained by Thorell (197) indicates that globin biosynthesis precedes heme and is nearly complete by the time heme formation begins. Additional evidence (49, 70, 111, 140, 145) employing microspectrophotometric and other techniques has been obtained by following the rates of incorporation of labeled glycine into both heme and globin. All the workers agree that with the presently available estimates of amino acid pool size, cell kinetics, etc., a strict interpretation of data is not possible, but most advance the tentative view that heme and globin biosynthesis occur independently, with a slightly prior production of globin. Granick (63) has proposed that heme synthesis may well be tied to, or coordinated with, globin synthesis by the simple process of amino acid utilization. For example, cysteine (and other amino acids) is known to inhibit heme biosynthesis. If the amino acid concentration were high in the developing cells, heme biosynthesis would not proceed until the level was reduced below a critical value through utilization of the amino acids as building blocks for globin biosynthesis. It is now known that the rates of biosynthesis of heme and globin can be altered by various factors such as starvation, ionizing radiation, lead poisoning, etc. (106, 160). In the latter instance, although heme biosynthesis is inhibited, globin biosynthesis is retarded to a greater degree.

The various enzymatic steps involved in the biosynthesis of heme and the intracellular location of the steps have been discussed in Chapter 1. Likewise, the specific mechanisms by which iron is taken up by the developing cell and enzymatically inserted into the porphyrin ring to complete the heme complex have been discussed in Chapter 2. We come now to the point of convergence of these three components of hemoglobin: iron, porphyrin, and globin. Evidence indicates that the RNA granule is the focal point at which the final product is assembled and from which the finished product is released.

The production of globin is one of the most clearly delineated of all protein syntheses, and the mechanisms involved are therefore of great interest and importance. Moreover, since it has now been firmly established that several genetically determined diseases (the molecular diseases) are characterized by abnormal globins, there is an unusually fine opportunity to examine the various known steps in the production of globin keeping in mind the now generally accepted hypotheses concerning heritable disorders. Desoxyribonucleic acid (DNA) is believed to make up the genetic material of cell nuclei by means of which characteristics are passed on to and through subsequent generations.

The double-stranded DNA macromolecule resembles a ladder twisted into a helix in which the sides consist of alternating units of a sugar (desoxyribose) and a simple phosphate compound, and the rungs—each attached to the sugar units—consist of a pair of complex organic bases, either adenine linked to thymine or guanine linked to cytosine. The sequence of the organic bases in DNA encodes the information according to which proteins and enzymes are made in such a way that their characteristics may be phenotypically expressed. The genetic information contained in the base sequence of DNA is carried from the nucleus by messenger RNA that is formed there (89). According to recent evidence that apparently breaks the code of the base sequence of the messenger RNA (39), a group of three bases (or a multiple of a group of three) determines the site at which a given amino acid is to be located in the final polypeptide chain or protein. Through this "template action" determined by the code of its base sequence, DNA's messenger imparts the genetic information to the proteins and enzymes that are assembled in association with it. But as detailed above, proteins are formed in association with the RNA granule or ribosome, a single-stranded macromolecule containing a sugar (ribose), phosphate, and any of four complex organic bases—guanine, cytosine, adenine, and uracil. It now seems clear that the ribosome is the machine responsible for synthesizing protein but cannot so function until the necessary information or template is supplied to it by messenger RNA, which apparently coats the ribosome.

Amino acids are transported into the maturing erythrocyte (3). They are there "activated" by a specific enzyme coupling them with adenosine triphosphate and then joined to another special form of RNA (soluble or transfer RNA). Each amino acid is "recognized" by a different transfer RNA, which carries it to the ribosome now coated with the RNA messenger template. The transfer RNA molecule is then released. From various data[*] it is clear that the specificity of the resultant hemoglobin is determined by the RNA messenger and not the amino acid–activating enzymes or the soluble RNA. Because of the code contained on the RNA granule through its covering of messenger RNA, the various amino acids are precisely oriented in sequence, perhaps also in steric arrangement, and linked into peptide chains. The amino acid sequence and steric arrangement determine the specific characteristics of the resulting polypeptide chain. At a proper time in globin production, protoporphyrin is conjugated with the peptide chain, and iron is inserted to form heme. The completed product emerges in the soluble protein fraction of the cell as the intact hemoglobin molecule.[†]

SICKLE CELL DISEASE

Sickle cell anemia is a heritable disease characterized by a hemoglobin that belongs to an *abnormal* molecular species. With the above account of protein biosynthesis as background, a consideration will be made of sickle cell disease with respect to (a) the genetic mechanisms involved, (b) the hitherto arcane nature of the hemoglobin abnormality, and (c) the pathophysiologic and clinical consequences of the abnormality.

---

[*] In cell-free systems producing hemoglobin by means of reticulocytes, activating enzymes may be supplied from liver cells and soluble (transport) RNA from *Escherichia coli* (23, 202).

[†] It is, of course, possible that each RNA granule is responsible for assembling one (or two) polypeptide chain along with its complement of porphyrin and iron. Such a situation would account for the labeling results outlined above. The completed hemoglobin would then result from association of its component portions after release from the RNA granule. For evidence that this type of association is possible, see the section on recombination of abnormal hemoglobins, below.

Genetic Mechanisms, Clinical Manifestations, and Laboratory Findings

Sickle cell disease* is the generic term applied to all disorders characterized by red cells containing an abnormal hemoglobin designated hemoglobin S. The clinical manifestations of the various subgroups of this main heading are determined largely by (a) the amount of hemoglobin S present in the red cells; (b) the type and amount of any other hemoglobin coexisting in the same cell (normal hemoglobin, another abnormal hemoglobin); (c) the presence of any additional red cell abnormality (hereditary spherocytosis, thalassemia, etc.); and (d) unknown modifying factors.

In this country the hemoglobin S variant is essentially peculiar to Negroes, in whom it is found in an incidence of about 8 per cent (142). The incidence of the sickle abnormality in Africa varies from tribe to tribe and in some reaches 45 per cent (143). It has also been found in communities in India, Greece, Italy, Turkey, Arabia, and Persia (Figure 9.11; 143).

The disorder was first described by Herrick in an East Indian medical student studying in Chicago in 1910 (80). It was singled out and named because the bizarre crescent shape of some of the erythrocytes was thought to resemble a sickle blade (Figure 3.2). Later it was shown that all the red cells from similar patients would, upon deoxygenation, assume the sickled form because of an abnormality residing in the erythrocyte, not in the plasma (73). It was later noted that some subjects whose cells could be made to sickle were essentially asymptomatic, while in others the disease was severe and usually fatal before the third decade (13). Sickle cell disease was therefore divisible by clinical criteria into a benign form, the sickle cell trait, and an aggressive, debilitating form, sickle cell

anemia. Owing to extensive surveys, it is now recognized that the abnormality is familial and hereditary and that while 8 to 11 per cent of Negroes (in this country, 1,887,000 persons) carry the abnormality, only 1 in 40 of these (0.2 per cent, or 47,100) have the anemic form of the disease (143).

The hereditary features of the disease are well explained by the assumption that the genetic determinant for the production of hemoglobins (a) is an allele for that determining the production of hemoglobin A; (b) is an incomplete dominant, and (c) is not sex-linked (Figure 3.3). In the heterozygous state (one normal and one abnormal gene) a certain proportion of hemoglobin S is present, and sickle cell trait results. If both abnormal genes are present, no normal hemoglobin is formed, only hemoglobin S and a variable though usually small proportion of fetal hemoglobin, and sickle cell anemia results (142). This genetic mechanism has been well substantiated by extensive

* A disorder in which production of normal adult hemoglobin is partly or completely suppressed and partly or completely replaced by production of one or more of the many hemoglobin variants (including fetal hemoglobin) is called a "hemoglobinopathy." There is no disputing the fact that such a situation is abnormal, but it is not clear that it is permissible to apply the terms "disease" or "hemoglobinopathy" to all the conditions meeting the above definition. Basic to any disease process is an existing or potential physiologic (or intellectual) disadvantage not found in the normal. As far as is presently demonstrated some individuals with hemoglobin types or proportions differing from the normal are symptom-free and at no disadvantage. Indeed, in some situations they appear to enjoy a distinct advantage. It has been concluded (8) that in the presence of hemoglobin S the morbidity and mortality from malaria is significantly decreased, especially in young children. The abnormal hemoglobin in the heterozygous sickle cell trait may confer enough protection against malaria to account for the persistence in some areas of Africa of the high incidence of homozygous sickle cell anemia, a condition that would otherwise be expected to be disappearing because of its high mortality and morbidity rates and because it decreases fertility.

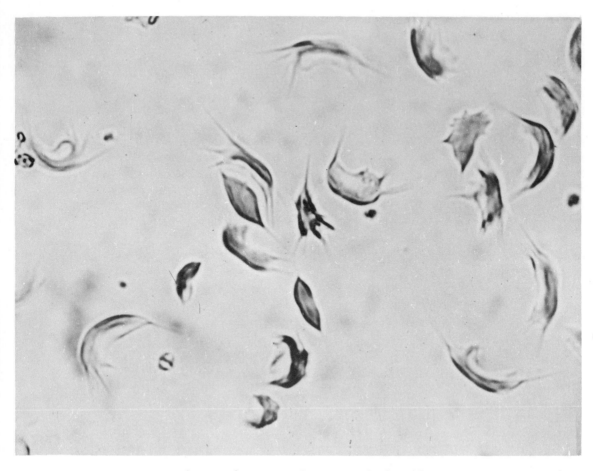

FIGURE 3.2.   Sickled erythrocytes in deoxygenated whole blood from patient with sickle cell anemia. Phase microscopy × 750. (From Harris, J. W., Proc. Soc. Exper. Biol. & Med. 75:197, 1950)

studies of the offspring of mothers with sickle cell anemia (all children must have at least sickle cell trait), the parents of children with sickle cell anemia (both parents must have at least sickle cell trait), and the expected number of offspring with the various possible hemoglobin types resulting from matings of one or both parents with sickle cell anemia and/or trait (142). It is also supported by the determined biochemical abnormalities and the modes of inheritance of other abnormal hemoglobins.

The difference in clinical manifestations has now been found due largely to the amount of hemoglobin S present in the cells. Erythrocytes from a patient with sickle cell trait usually contain from 20 to 40 per cent hemoglobin S, the remainder being normal adult hemoglobin. Erythrocytes from patients with sickle cell anemia contain approximately 80 to 100 per cent hemoglobin S (94). For practical purposes, in the laboratory the types and amounts of pigments present are usually determined by hemoglobin electrophoresis. But the amounts and types of hemoglobins determined by biochemical means do not *necessarily* reflect the complete genetic picture. The *genotype* cannot always be inferred from the *phenotype*. Although sickle cell anemia

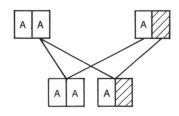

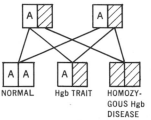

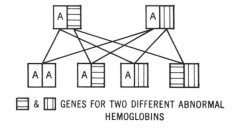

FIGURE 3.3.   Schematic representations of hereditary aspects of hemoglobin diseases on basis of population genetics. Only the detection of the gene is denoted in the diagrams, which are not intended to indicate hemoglobins in quantitative or qualitative fashion: genotype, not phenotype, is represented

and trait have of necessity been diagnosed clinically and biochemically, it is now well recognized that an accurate, "certified" diagnosis can be made only on clinical and biochemical grounds *supplemented* by genetic observations. An electrophoretic pattern showing a great predominance of hemoglobin S with a small admixture of hemoglobin F does not necessarily indicate homozygosity for the abnormal "S gene." It may sometimes indicate the presence of heterozygosity for the S abnormality plus a modifying factor, usually thalassemia, suppressing the production of hemoglobin A.

Sickle Cell Trait

Except under unusual circumstances sickle cell trait is a benign, asymptomatic condition, compatible with a normal life span, and discovered only through tests by means of which erythrocytes contain-

ing hemoglobin S are made to assume the sickled form, through hemoglobin electrophoresis, or through family study. Several studies have been made to determine the incidence of sickling in different age groups, since a decreased incidence in the older age groups would indicate a higher-than-normal death rate for those carrying the trait. The studies have so far been contradictory or inconclusive (168). No other hematologic abnormalities are detected by routine examination; the circulating hemoglobin levels are normal as are the size and shape of the red cells. No abnormal reticulocytosis is present, and red cell survival time, determined by various methods, is normal. Heme pigment anabolic and catabolic processes are qualitatively and quantitatively normal. The leukocytes, platelets, and bone marrow cells are normal in number and proportion. There are no deviations from the normal with respect to physical examination. Except for the fact that in an occasional patient specific gravity of the urine does not much exceed 1.010 (127, 169), the usual laboratory determinations are normal. Rarely, a patient has vascular occlusive phenomena or a hemolytic process when unique anatomic or functional conditions exist (117, 117a, 130).

Recent observations in the clinic and at the postmortem table indicate that extensive in vivo sickling can be fatal in individuals with sickle cell trait (130, 147) if extreme hypoxia or intravascular pooling with stasis of blood occurs. Such conditions have been observed in marked respiratory depression (acute alcoholism, deep anesthesia) or spinal anesthesia with dilatation of the splanchnic vasculature. Spontaneous hematuria, sometimes prolonged, may be seen, usually from the left kidney; cerebrovascular manifestations, thromboses, and subarachnoid hemorrhages have been described with no other explanation (40, 178). Splenic infarction (191) and splenic hypersequestration of radioactively labeled erythrocytes (116) have been demonstrated in volunteers in whom hypoxemia similar to that experienced at altitudes of about 7,000 ft was induced in an attempt to reproduce the clinical signs and symptoms that have been seen (rarely) in patients flying at high altitudes in nonpressurized cabins. However, it must be emphasized that these manifestations are rare and that for practical purposes sickle cell trait is an incidental finding of importance because of its genetic implications.

Sickle Cell Anemia

In contradistinction to the above, the history of patients with true sickle cell anemia almost invariably reveals a continuously aggressive illness, punctuated by repeated episodes, usually of a vascular occlusive type (204) with or without myelosuppressive effects (temporary failure of the marrow to produce erythrocytes). Signs and symptoms are usually due to chronic anemia; rapid, episodic aggravation of the anemia; pain in the joints, extremities, or abdomen; aseptic necrosis of bone; cerebrovascular accidents; pulmonary infarctions; etc. The complete clinical picture cannot be discussed in detail here; only a few of the most significant and more frequently encountered manifestations will be considered.

Although exceptions have been seen and documented, it is most unusual for the newborn to have trouble from sickle cell anemia. This is due to the high complement of fetal hemoglobin present in the erythrocytes at birth and the consequent low percentage of hemoglobin S (205) that to a large degree prevent the occurrence of the sickling phenomenon. The disease is usually detected during the first few years of life because of severe anemia or a painful crisis manifesting itself as a swollen, hot, tender hand or foot (67, 98, 173–175), recently designated the hand-foot syndrome (206). Growth and development are only slightly retarded in the studies made up to the age of adolescence (212). Once the disease becomes established, it pursues a relatively constant course, combining the signs, symptoms, and limitations of persistent anemia with the episodic and unpredictable intercurrence of various types of crises.* Patients adjust remarkably well to their low hemoglobin levels, but the usual history describes a child not being able to keep up with companions or an adult unable to do a full day's work or short periods of strenuous work without immediate undue or

---

* The term crisis is used to cover such widely divergent situations that it is very difficult to define. Hemolytic crisis, hyperhemolytic crisis, aplastic crisis, splenic crisis, abdominal crisis, painful crisis, etc. are all in the literature. By and large the term refers to any fairly rapidly developing manifestation or complication of sickle cell disease: a "sickle cell crisis."

adverse effect or prolonged fatigue. Patients almost invariably have moderately icteric sclerae; frequently have scars on the lower extremities from indolent ulcers usually located about the malleoli; and are often underdeveloped, with disproportionately long extremities and "spidery" fingers (190).

A typical "painful crisis" may have an apparently spontaneous onset, may accompany a viral or bacterial infection or follow exposure to cold (218). However, not every episode of infection or exposure to cold is necessarily associated with a crisis. Pain of mild (requiring no medication or an occasional aspirin at home or at work) to extreme (hospitalization and repeated massive doses of narcotics) severity may be present in an extremity, back, chest, or abdomen. In the adult it may be accompanied by no overt manifestations; in the child, especially if an extremity or joint is involved, it is frequently accompanied by increased local heat, swelling, and tenderness. With abdominal pain, the complaints and physical findings may mimic almost any surgical complication, from diffuse peritonitis to local inflammation. Since painful episodes involving the abdomen are frequently accompanied by fever, leukocytosis, nausea, and vomiting, the diagnostic possibilities are many and always serious (127, 177). A helpful and reliable finding that may be used to stay the hand of the surgeon is the persistence of normal bowel sounds and regular bowel movements despite other symptoms. The signs and symptoms may abate and disappear in a few hours, may reappear after an interval, or may persist for a few days or even weeks. Abdominal crises usually disappear leaving no residual clinical indications of damage. If a hip joint, an extremity, or the thorax has been involved, bony changes will frequently been seen if persistently searched for by x-ray in the ensuing weeks (167). These usually take the form of aseptic

necrosis. A carpal or tarsal bone, for example, will all but disappear, later to regenerate. Apparently if a critical area is involved, such as the head of the femur or radius, or the tibial tubercle, regeneration is hampered by weight bearing and use, and significant deformity may result (183, 196). Neurologic manifestations are fortunately infrequent, but are usually severe with resulting paresis, hemiplegia, signs of generalized encephalopathy (65, 127), and many types of retinal alterations (58, 59, 62, 109, 149). Vascular changes in the conjunctival vessels (55) consist mainly of venous sacculations and microaneurysms. Pain in the chest may be associated with transient friction rubs and x-ray findings consistent with infiltration or infarction. Cor pulmonale may occur if vascular occlusions in the pulmonary circulation are extensive (110). Pulmonary embolus due to bone marrow infarction may be seen, usually as a terminal event, and documented at autopsy by the finding of altered bone marrow in the pulmonary vessels (146, 179).

The cardiac changes have been characterized as those of severe chronic anemia carried to the extreme (137, 184, 216). Practically all patients have significant cardiomegaly, with loud pulmonary and mitral systolic murmurs; some have almost any type of diastolic murmur but no proved valvular deformity. The sounds are usually of good quality, and the pulmonary second sound is usually accentuated, even in patients with no demonstrable pulmonary hypertension (115, 194).

Most adults have some hepatomegaly and evidence of abnormal liver function (24, 53). The progressive liver damage seen during life probably results from actual infarcts and vascular occlusions, so that with increasing age liver impairment becomes more and more evident. Renal damage, also progressive with age, results from glomerular congestion and enlargement, then ischemia and fibrosis progressing to glomerular obliteration (19). The spleen is usually palpable in infants and children, but seldom is palpable by the time of adolescence or later. Owing to repeated episodes of infarction and scarring, only a small nubbin of fibrous tissue may remain. A palpable spleen in a postadolescent patient is to be taken as strong evidence against true sickle cell anemia and for practical purposes excludes the diagnosis. Presumably the repeated insults to the liver and spleen account for many but by no means all the episodes of abdominal pain. Pigment cholelithiasis is found in increased incidence and may become symptomatic (104). The serious nature of the complications that may arise during pregnancy demands that the patients be watched very closely during all trimesters and delivery. The incidence of pre-eclampsia and stillbirth is increased, and although no adequate statistics are available, fetal loss and maternal mortality are probably increased (7, 44, 78) to the range of 44 and 22 per cent respectively (163).

Chronic leg ulcers and scarring, usually over the lateral malleoli, occur in somewhere near 10 per cent of patients (127). The ulcers may be present steadily or intermittently for years or heal spontaneously at any time. Although many types of treatment have been tried, they respond reliably only to transfusions, when nearly normal hemoglobin levels are achieved.

One of the most serious complications is the so-called aplastic or aregenerative crisis (Figure 3.4). Usually in association with a viral or bacterial infection, the bone marrow becomes physiologically hypoplastic and, essentially, ceases to function as an effective erythropoietic organ while the infection persists (81, 101, 148, 187). A rapid decrease in hemoglobin ensues that may reach fatal levels in a few days, as illustrated by a recorded hemoglobin value of 0.5 Gm per

100 ml for a pregnant woman just before death (the hemoglobin content of the fetal blood was 19 Gm per 100 ml). It should be emphasized that painful crises, unless accompanied by a prolonged febrile course, are not associated with increased severity of the anemia or consistent changes in the plasma bilirubin content (47) and conversely that aplastic or aregenerative crises need not be accompanied by painful episodes.

There is some evidence that patients with sickle cell anemia are especially susceptible to infections. Certainly they react poorly, and the incidence of salmonella osteomyelitis is significantly increased (46, 85, 185, 214). Whether this increased incidence is due to pathophysiologic or socioeconomic factors is presently impossible to tell.

It can be readily appreciated that an individual subject to chronic symptomatic anemia and intercurrent crises has a most difficult time becoming a productive citizen. Most patients with true sickle cell anemia do not live beyond the third decade; a large proportion die during early childhood. Few are able to maintain gainful employment for considerable periods of time. It must, however, be remembered that many grades of severity are seen and that the course is unpredictable. Someone with twenty to thirty hospitalizations in 5 to 10 years may subsequently have many years without complications and, of course, vice versa.

The laboratory findings are those of severe anemia: the hemoglobin content of the blood is usually 5 to 9 Gm per 100 ml with a proportional drop in hematocrit and red cell count so that normocytic and normochromic red cell indices result. Examination of a stained film of the peripheral blood shows considerable variation in size and shape of the red cells; from 0.5 to more than 20 per cent of the red cells are sickled; target forms, microcytes, macrocytes, and a few spherocytes also are seen. The proportion of

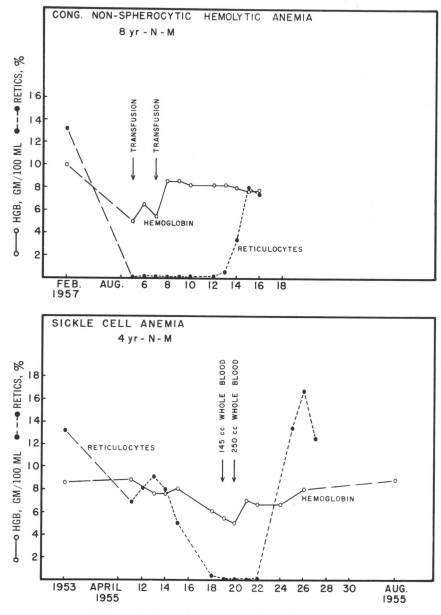

FIGURE 3.4. Aplastic crisis in hemolytic anemia

reticulocytes is elevated, usually to from 10 to 15 per cent, corresponding roughly with the polychromatophilia seen in preparations stained by Wright's method. Normoblasts are frequently present as are cells with basophilic stippling or Howell-Jolly bodies. The most convenient and accurate test to confirm a suspicion of sickled cells in the peripheral blood smear involves the exposure of fresh cells to a potent reducing agent, usually isotonic sodium metabisulfite, to deoxygenate the hemoglobin and produce the characteristic sickling changes (45). A more exact biochemical diagnosis can be made by the *additional* use of hemoglobin electrophoresis, a relatively simple technique now almost universally available in clinical laboratories.

Moderate leukocytosis is usually present (12,000 to 17,000 cells per cubic millimeter) with a mild shift toward immaturity of the granulocytes. The platelet count may be moderately elevated. Examination of the bone marrow shows a marked normoblastic hyperplasia, and active red marrow can be found in areas of the skeleton usually occupied by yellow fatty marrow. Staining for iron consistently reveals considerable overload in older children and adults, even those who have not required transfusions.

The total heme pigments (benzidine-reacting) circulating extracellularly in the plasma have been found elevated in several reported series (42, 107, 213). Although it was originally presumed that this elevation was mainly due to extracellular hemoglobin, recent studies by Lathem and Jensen (114) demonstrate that the amount of hemoglobin is low (average, 3 mg per 100 ml) but that the amount of methemalbumin* (a compound *usually* indicating intravascular destruction of erythrocytes) is elevated (average, 17 mg per 100 ml). (The normal level is too low to quantitate by method employed.) The free haptoglobins* (proteins found in normal plasma that specifically bind and transport extracellular hemoglobin) are usually absent (68, 113). Most patients are ahaptoglobinemic except with a superimposed infection, inflammation, or crisis. The small amount of hemoglobin that is present in the plasma is not bound to protein. The icterus index is elevated owing to an increased level of nonconjugated bilirubin;* an acholuric jaundice results. Because the amount of free hemoglobin in the plasma does not exceed the renal threshhold, hemoglobinuria is not present. The fecal urobilinogen content is elevated. Aside from the bony changes,† cardiomegaly, evidence of liver dysfunc-

tion, and lack of renal concentrating ability, mentioned above (108, 169, 211), other laboratory findings usually contribute little useful information.

Treatment of the disease is largely palliative. Except in the unusual circumstances of a coexisting deficiency (iron lack in children) or metabolic abnormality (relative depletion of folic acid, erythrocyte maturation abnormality, or aplastic crisis; 101, 148, 153a), the usual hematopoietic agents are of no value. Splenectomy is of moderate benefit in some children in whom it can be shown that the spleen is destroying the patient's or transfused cells at a significantly elevated rate (118). The many proposed therapeutic regimens involving administration of cobalt, Diamox, oxygen, ACTH, and corticosteroids, and those involving alkalinization, are almost unquestionably of no value, and some are even contraindicated. Sedatives, analgesics, narcotics, parenterally administered fluids, physiotherapy, and occupational rehabilitation are to be used generously but carefully. Transfusions are to be avoided if possible because of the danger of ultimately producing or aggravating iron overload, hepatic damage through transfusion hepatitis, and subgroup incompatibilities. They are, of course, mandatory during an aplastic crisis.

Pathogenesis

The pathogenesis of the disease is most interesting because almost certainly the main features can be explained on the basis of the available evidence. It has been pointed out that this is an inherited disease, one of the inborn errors, and

---

* Further discussion of the nature, significance, and occurrence of these compounds will be found in Chapter 9.

† In addition to deformation resulting from prior aseptic necrosis, there may be irregularities of the bony trabeculae, widening of the medullary cavities, areas of sclerosis, and thickening of the diploë of the skull (61, 134, 136).

must then have arisen as a mutation or alteration in the DNA genetic material. Consequently, the RNA messenger is abnormal and by template action produces an abnormal protein, hemoglobin S.* The abnormality has been shown to consist of one amino acid out of place, a substitution of valine for the normal glutamic acid. This least possible change in protein structure (unless abnormal folding also occurs) probably is a consequence of a point mutation within the DNA gene (or cistron). The protein abnormality results in sickling on deoxygenation. The sickle change results in fragile cells that are easily destroyed. Blood viscosity changes of sufficient magnitude to produce vascular occlusive phenomena follow sickling. Thus occur the chronic anemia of increased destruction and the signs, symptoms, and pathologic changes of the disease process.

ANATOMY AND PATHOLOGY OF THE HEMOGLOBIN S MOLECULE. The genetic mechanisms of sickle cell disease have been briefly considered above. The next step is to examine the abnormal hemoglobin molecule and its behavioral peculiarities. In 1949 Pauling (150) showed by free-boundary electrophoresis that hemoglobin S belonged to an abnormal molecular species possessing a mobility, isoelectric point, and surface charge different from normal adult hemoglobin. This demonstration of a molecular basis for a disease had great intrinsic as well as heuristic import. Indeed, at present it is difficult to say which aspect of the work is the more important. For although preceded by Hörlein and Weber's demonstration in 1948 of an abnormal globin in a type of familial methemoglobinemia, Pauling's demonstration undoubtedly was the starting point of much recent investigative work of major importance. At the present time more than thirty different hemoglobins have been satisfactorily described (Table 3.2), "new" clinical syndromes have been recognized, and "old"

clinical syndromes clarified by more accurate diagnostic criteria.

The erythrocytes from patients with classic sickle cell anemia were demonstrated to contain 90 to 100 per cent hemoglobin S, while those from patients with the trait contain approximately equal proportions of normal and sickle hemoglobin. This was consistent with, and at the time even anticipated, the homozygous and heterozygous types of inheritance proposed on classic genetic grounds.

Extensive chemical analyses have failed to reveal any abnormality of the heme moiety (151). Electrophoresis of the renatured globin derived from hemoglobin S demonstrated the abnormality to reside in the protein moiety. Repeated attempts at chemical analyses by various methods in several different laboratories failed to show significant abnormalities in the amounts of the various amino acids composing the approximately 600 units present in globin. It was not until Ingram in 1958 employed the known action of trypsin (91) in attacking arginine and lysine carboxyl bonding in peptide chains that positive results were obtained. Ingram denatured hemoglobin by heat and digested the coagulum with trypsin. The polypeptide digest was subjected to electrophoresis and subsequently chromatographed in the cross dimension. On the basis of calculations made from the numbers of arginine (fourteen) and lysine (forty-six) residues known present in hemoglobin, it was predicted that some fifty to sixty polypeptide chains would result from the digestive treatment. But since, as has been pointed out, the hemoglobin molecule is composed of two equal portions, only twenty-five to thirty different polypeptides should appear on the "fin-

---

* Other proteins may also be abnormal in this disease. Myoglobin has been tested by several criteria and no abnormality demonstrated (188). Amino acid sequence and steric arrangement would, of course, be the most conclusive criteria, but have not yet been examined.

gerprint" pattern.* This proved to be the case. When the fingerprints from hemoglobins S and A made under rigidly comparable conditions were analyzed, one peptide chain was found to be different— the "sickle peptide" (Figure 3.5B)—now also designated β^{TpI} (the number one, I, peptide derived from the β-polypeptide chain by tryptic, Tp, digestion). Its migration was such that one excess positive charge was indicated on the sickle peptide in contrast with its corresponding peptide derived from normal hemoglobin. These peptides were eluted from the paper, concentrated, and analyzed for their amino acid sequences. In the normal (Figure 3.6), the sequence is valyl-histidyl-leucyl-threonyl-prolyl-*glutamyl*-glutamyl-lysine; in the sickle peptide it is valyl-histidyl-leucyl-threonyl-prolyl-*valyl*-glutamyl-lysine. These sequences have now been confirmed by other workers (82, 91). Thus, in the sickle peptide glutamic acid has been replaced by valine. This change explains the difference in charge and electrophoretic migration of the sickle peptide. And since the hemoglobin molecule is composed of two equal parts, the substitution also explains the higher net positive charge of the parent protein (hemoglobin S) than of hemoglobin A and the observed differences in electrophoretic migrations previously noted.

Analytic studies of the number of peptide chains present in hemoglobin show that there are four N-terminal residues in the molecule. Each N-terminal residue is composed of a valine group (162, 190). Although the number of C-terminal residues has not been satisfactorily established for hemoglobin, available evidence indicates that branching of the peptide chains probably does not occur (170). Consequently hemoglobin must be composed of four polypeptide chains, each with an N-terminal valine. By various procedures it has been possible to separate two different peptide chains and to

determine the terminal amino acid sequence of each. One, arbitrarily designated the α-chain, has the sequence valyl-leucyl-; the other, designated the β-chain, has the sequence valyl-histidyl-leucyl-.

Since hemoglobin is composed of two equal portions,† it has been concluded that only *two different* peptides are present: two α-chains and two β-chains. The hemoglobin molecule is therefore known to be composed of four peptide chains (two α- and two β-chains) arranged in two equal parts. By a series of dissociation experiments, to be detailed later, it has been demonstrated that the amino acid abnormality of hemoglobin S is located on the β-chain. Shelton (170) has recently found that the terminal amino acid sequence of the β-chain is valyl-histidyl-leucyl-threonyl-prolyl-. This is precisely the same sequence found by Ingram and others for the sickle peptide now designated ^{TpI}. It is therefore most probable that the abnormally situated amino acid in hemoglobin S can be pinpointed at the sixth position from the end of the β-chain. There is no evidence of abnormality in the remainder of the molecule.

MECHANISM OF THE SICKLING PHENOMENON. Since the charge difference between the two hemoglobin types can be explained by the amino acid substitution, it is also likely that the abnormality is located at the surface of the molecule and can account in some degree for the behavioral abnormalities of hemoglobin S that underlie the sickling phenomenon. These behavioral abnormalities of hemoglobin S have been studied in stroma-free solu-

---

* A portion of the hemoglobin ("resistant core") was not susceptible to trypsin digestion. This did yield to chymotrypsin digestion. No abnormalities have been found in these polypeptide chains (91).

† Evidence for this comes from x-ray crystallographic analysis whereby the peptide chains are pictured (Figure 8.2), digestion experiments and N-terminal residue determinations mentioned above, and "dissociation" experiments (see p. 100).

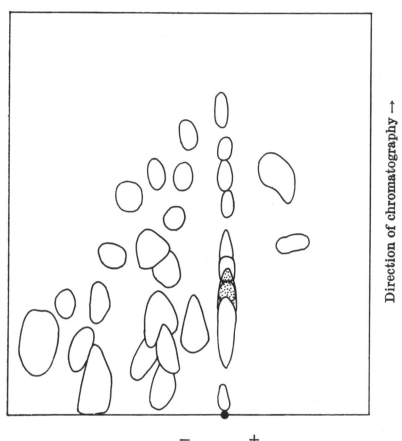

Direction of chromatography →

−   +

Normal hæmoglobin

FIGURE 3.5A.   "Fingerprint pattern" of normal hemoglobin. Outline tracings of polypeptide fragments derived from hemoglobin by tryptic digestion. Spatial dispersion of
the polypeptide fragments is result of subjecting the digest to electrophoresis followed by
cross-dimension chromatography. (From Ingram, V. M., Nature 178:792, 1956)

tions of varying concentrations of purified hemoglobin (71). When a solution
containing hemoglobin S in a concentration of approximately 20 Gm per 100 ml is
progressively deoxygenated, an increase
in viscosity occurs evidencing molecular
aggregation, long-chain polymer formation, and a resulting increased internal
friction which impedes flow. When a
solution containing hemoglobin S in a
concentration of 30 Gm per 100 ml is
employed (a concentration comparable
to that found in the intact erythrocyte),
the solution forms a semisolid gel upon
deoxygenation. Examination of the gel

under the phase and polarizing microscope reveals it to contain small, rigid,
boat-shaped objects that polarize light.
These are known as tactoids (nematic
fluid crystals) (Figure 3.7). Their presence indicates that the long chains of
hemoglobin polymers have attracted one
another into an orderly parallel orientation. All these deoxygenation-induced
changes can be reversed by reoxygenation and do not occur in comparable solutions of normal (or other abnormal) hemoglobins. The conditions under which
the hemoglobin polymers form and are
dispersed suggest a specific intermolecu-

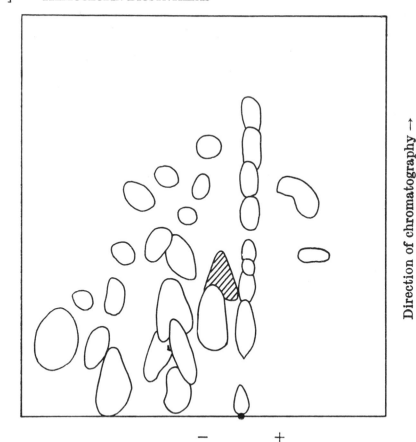

Sickle cell hæmoglobin

FIGURE 3.5B.   "Fingerprint pattern" of sickle hemoglobin. Position of abnormal poly-peptide fragment (the sickle peptide, now designated β^{STpI}, see Table 3.3) is indicated by cross-hatched area. Its displacement relative to position of comparable peptide of the normal indicates dissimilarity in charge and composition. (From Ingram, V. M., Nature 178:792, 1956)

lar linkage of the hydrogen-bond type reinforced by other low-energy bonds such as exist between antigens and anti-bodies (73).

It is probable that specific complemen-tary surfaces exist on the globin. To ac-tivate or uncover them so that mutual attraction between molecules may take place, oxygen must be removed from the iron. Again owing to the anatomy of the hemoglobin molecule, there must be two such sites per molecule so that chains of hemoglobin molecules are formed. Since the individual molecules are known by x-ray diffraction studies and direct

micrography by the electron microscope (37) to be slightly asymmetric (64 by 55 by 50 Å), it is to be predicted from the known behavior of other globular pro-teins that the long chains will be spiral and not strictly linear. This spiral, or heli-cal, polymer is the type known to form tactoids.

Since the *intact* sickled cell is known to be rigid and to polarize light, it seems reasonable to conclude that hemoglobin polymerization, orientation, and tactoid formation is the architectural basis of the sickling phenomenon (Figure 3.8). Find-ings entirely consistent with this process

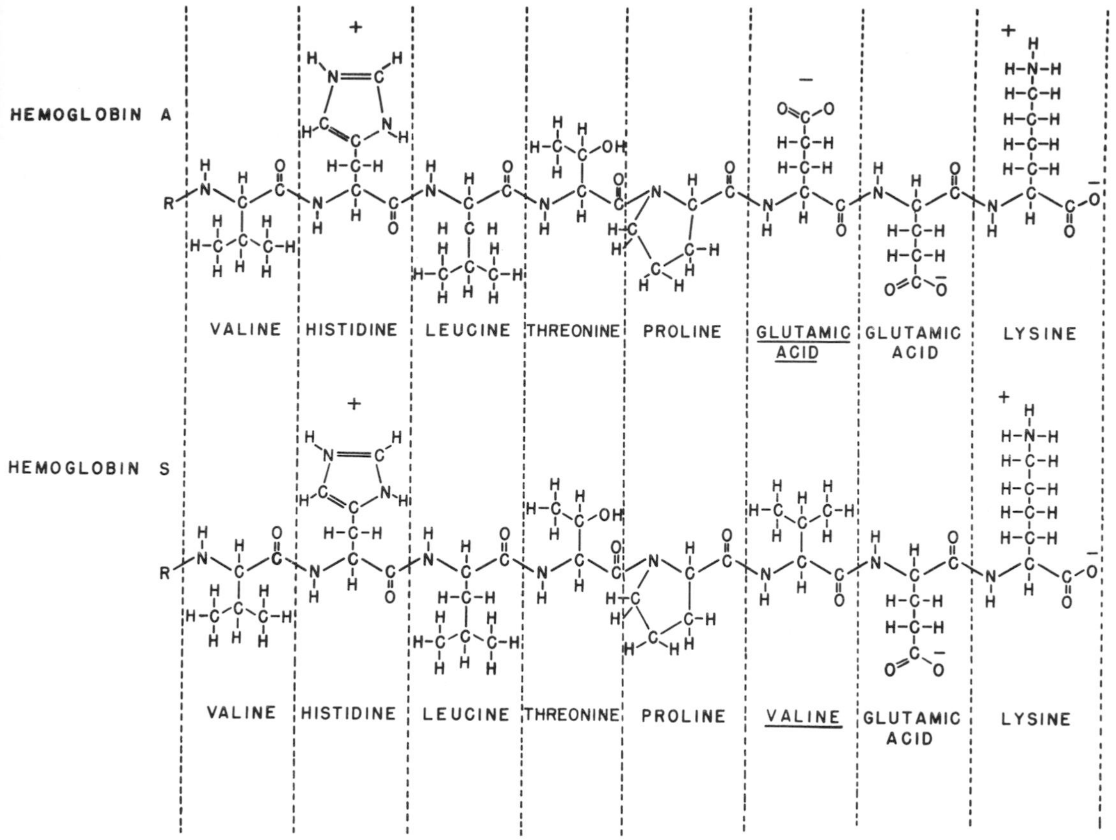

FIGURE 3.6.   Amino acid sequence of the sickle peptide, β^{STpI}, and its corresponding normal peptide, β^{ATpI}

have been described by electron microscopy. Repeated examinations at timed intervals during the sickling process have demonstrated the formation and orientation of rods of hemoglobin in a three-dimensional framework (161).

It has also been observed that deoxygenation of hemoglobin S induces a marked change in its solubility: it becomes many times less soluble than deoxygenated normal hemoglobin (73). However, crystallization of hemoglobin owing to its insolubility when deoxygenated is not the basis of the sickling phenomenon, since x-ray diffraction studies, electron microscopy of thin sections of sickled cells (20), and other physical measurements provide no evidence for actual three-dimensional crystals in the intact sickled cell.*

Physicochemical measurements indicate that upon oxygenation and deoxygenation significant alterations in the general configuration of the hemoglobin

* It has been reported that sickling occurs in hemoglobin I disease (9). It should be noted that the tests which resulted in the sickling of cells containing hemoglobin I used double-strength metabisulfite for prolonged periods of time and that the shape distortions were atypical and not reversible. However, there are also reports of an abnormal fetal hemoglobin that can produce the sickle distortion of the erythrocyte and of an abnormal nonhemoglobin S that is capable of producing sickling (153). All these are extremely rare exceptions to the rule that a positive sickle test indicates the presence of hemoglobin S. Most curious is the fact that nearly all species of deer have "sickle cell disease" on the basis of a hemoglobin that will form tactoids in solution (135) and the sickle shape distortion in the intact cell (199) but apparently at *high* oxygen tensions and at an alkaline pH.

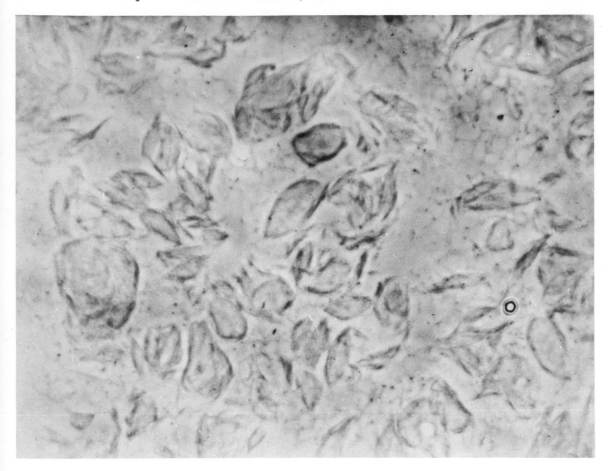

Figure 3.7. Hemoglobin tactoids formed in stroma-free solutions of deoxygenated sickle hemoglobin. Phase microscopy × 775. (From Harris, J. W., Proc. Soc. Exper. Biol. & Med. 75:197, 1950)

molecule take place: a gross change in size and shape probably based on spreading or recoiling of the peptide chains (219). This configurational change forms a ready basis for some of the unique behavioral characteristics of hemoglobin S but is especially applicable to the oxygen reversibility of the hemoglobin S polymer and tactoid formation through abolition of the complementary nature of the critical surface areas by the mechanism of steric hindrance.

Physiologic consequences of the sickling phenomenon. The basic mechanism of the sickling phenomenon has been outlined above; the effects of sick-ling upon the intact cell and the consequences of sickling on the whole blood will now be discussed. Figure 3.9 shows that as oxygen is removed from blood samples obtained from patients with *sickle cell anemia* more and more cells assume the sickled form until the vast majority are distorted. Most of the cells sickle in ranges of oxygen tension or hemoglobin saturation that are physiologic. If the cells from patients with *sickle cell trait* are similarly studied, very few, if any, sickled forms are seen in the physiologic ranges of oxygen tension. It is not until the extremely low ranges are reached that the shape change is induced.

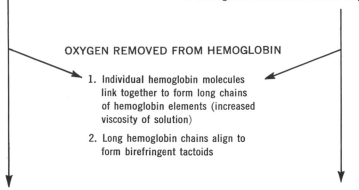

INTACT ERYTHROCYTE

1. Hemoglobin in the oxygen saturated state
2. M.C.H.C. = 30 Gm / 100 ml
3. Biconcave discs
4. Not birefringent (polarizing microscope)
5. Hemoglobin molecules at random dispersion

HEMOGLOBIN SOLUTION

1. Hemoglobin in the oxygen saturated state
2. Hemoglobin = 30 Gm / 100 ml
3. Low viscosity liquid
4. Homogeneous solution
5. Not birefringent (polarizing microscope)
6. Hemoglobin molecules at random dispersion

OXYGEN REMOVED FROM HEMOGLOBIN

1. Individual hemoglobin molecules link together to form long chains of hemoglobin elements (increased viscosity of solution)

2. Long hemoglobin chains align to form birefringent tactoids

1. Hemoglobin in the oxygen unsaturated state
2. Sickled forms
3. Birefringent (polarizing microscope)
4. Hemoglobin molecules in orderly arrangement

1. Hemoglobin in the oxygen unsaturated state
2. Hemoglobin tactoids present
3. Viscous semisolid gel
4. Tactoids are birefringent (polarizing microscope)
5. Hemoglobin molecules in orderly arrangement

THE SICKLED ERYTHROCYTE IS ESSENTIALLY
A HEMOGLOBIN TACTOID COVERED BY THE DISTORTED CELL MEMBRANE

FIGURE 3.8.   Mechanism of the sickling process

At complete deoxygenation very nearly all the cells assume the sickled form.* This difference in the behavior of erythrocytes from patients with sickle cell trait as opposed to those from patients with sickle cell anemia was first described by Sherman in 1940 (182). The observations have been frequently confirmed since then with added controls. For example, sickling is facilitated by lowering the pH of the suspending medium (mainly because of the effect upon the oxygen dissociation curve). Moreover, cells from a patient with sickle cell anemia are more susceptible to pH changes than those from a person with sickle cell trait (112).

In 1940 (69) it was noted that when *oxygenated* blood from a patient with sickle cell disease was centrifuged in the Wintrobe hematocrit tube the discoidal erythrocytes packed normally in the usual period of time. However, when the blood was *deoxygenated* and the cells thereby changed from the discoidal to the sickled form, the erythrocytes did not pack normally even after prolonged centrifugation. The hematocrit reading of the deoxygenated blood was greater than that of the oxygenated sample. From these observations Castle hypothesized that it was not possible to pack the sickled forms properly on centrifugation because they

* The fact that very nearly all (98 per cent or more) the erythrocytes from patients with sickle cell trait become distorted indicates that the 30 to 40 per cent of hemoglobin S present in the blood is distributed among all cells *in company with* the 70 to 60 per cent of normal hemoglobin and not confined to 30 to 40 per cent of the cells as their only intracellular pigment.

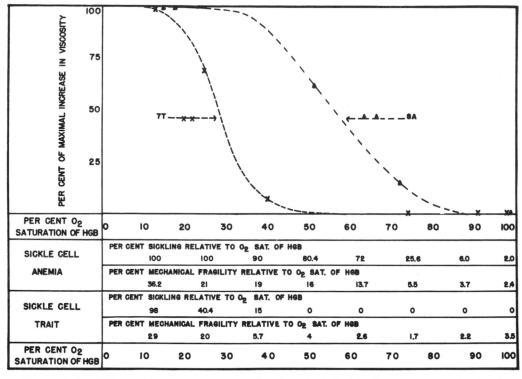

PER CENT O₂ SATURATION OF HGB	0	10	20	30	40	50	60	70	80	90	100
SICKLE CELL	PER CENT SICKLING RELATIVE TO O₂ SAT. OF HGB										
	100	100	90	80.4	72	25.6	6.0	2.0			
ANEMIA	PER CENT MECHANICAL FRAGILITY RELATIVE TO O₂ SAT. OF HGB										
	36.2	21	19	16	13.7	5.5	3.7	2.4			
SICKLE CELL	PER CENT SICKLING RELATIVE TO O₂ SAT. OF HGB										
	98	40.4	15	0	0	0	0	0			
TRAIT	PER CENT MECHANICAL FRAGILITY RELATIVE TO O₂ SAT. OF HGB										
	29	20	5.7	4	2.6	1.7	2.2	3.5			
PER CENT O₂ SATURATION OF HGB	0	10	20	30	40	50	60	70	80	90	100

FIGURE 3.9.   Effect of deoxygenation on viscosity of whole blood, percentage of sickled cells, and erythrocyte mechanical fragility in sickle cell anemia and sickle cell trait. (From Harris, J. W., et al., A.M.A. Arch. Int. Med. 97:145, 1956)

were "like haywire." He predicted that deoxygenated sickle cell anemia and sickle cell trait blood would show increased viscosity of flow in a capillary tube. Since then it has been demonstrated by different observers that the time required for a blood sample to pass through an Ostwald viscometer tube is indeed significantly increased when the cells are in the sickled form (72). With complete reduction of the blood to induce maximum sickling and shape distortion, increases in viscosity of from 43 to 115 per cent over values for the oxygenated blood samples are observed. When the cells assume the rigid, bizarre sickled forms with consequent enmeshing and entangling of the distorted erythrocytes, the internal friction of the suspension is increased and flow is impeded. Artificial mixtures of sickled and normal cells demonstrate a straight-line relation

between the viscosity increase and the number of cells in the sickled form. No detectable viscosity change occurs in samples of normal blood subjected to the same variations in oxygen saturation. The change in viscosity is therefore directly related to the increase in the number of sickled forms and very probably to the degree of sickling. All these changes noted in the blood from patients with sickle cell anemia, trait, and variants, are completely reversible by reoxygenation.

It is important to note that the increase in viscosity demonstrated in blood from patients with sickle cell anemia begins *in the physiologic ranges of oxygen saturation;* blood from persons with sickle cell trait starts to become more viscous only in the lower ranges of *artificial* oxygen tensions. The possible hematologic and clinical consequences of these differences are several. Most evident is the production of a vicious cycle in which, within the physiologic range of oxygen tensions, the following events may be assumed to take place. In the capillaries of various organs, particularly those with slow blood flow, oxygen is given up by the blood. Concomitant with the ensuing increase in the number of sickled forms, the viscosity of the blood increases so that circulation is impeded first at the distal ends of the capillaries, with the result that more and more oxygen is removed from the red cells in the capillaries by continuing tissue requirements. As stasis is prolonged, the *hydrogen-ion concentration* of the tissue and blood increases, causing further removal of oxygen from the hemoglobin and additional facilitation of the sickling process. This may eventually result in the formation of a static mass of sickled cells in the capillaries and venules.

It should, however, be noted (Figure 6.2) that there is little difference between the viscosity of completely *deoxygenated* blood from a patient with sickle cell anemia at a hematocrit of 25 per cent and that of fully *oxygenated* normal blood at a hematocrit of 50 per cent. Moreover, at hematocrit values of less than 25 per cent there is a very minor, perhaps physiologically insignificant, increase in viscosity upon deoxygenation. The physiologic consequences of sickling in vivo may, therefore, be small except at sites of erythrocyte concentration. This concept of the disturbance in the circulatory physiology implies that the two most important factors serving to trigger the vicious cycle are hemoconcentration and the oxygen tension or hemoglobin saturation at which the *first change* in whole-blood viscosity occurs. It has, therefore, been proposed that the physiologic consequences of the vicious cycle so defined explain in large part the striking vascular occlusive manifestations of sickle cell anemia. All these considerations have been made on the basis of "bulk viscosity" of whole blood. Jandl et al. (97) have recently pointed out that pathologic processes may evolve from the viscosity changes of individual cells. Milipore filters with capillary diameters of 5 μ, which permit the passage of normal discoidal cells, obstruct the passage of isolated sickled cells and then in turn the passage of discoidal cells. Moreover, deoxygenated sickled red cells cannot be forced through the filter even at perfusion pressures of over 120 mm Hg. It is possible that single sickled cells may occlude vessels and be sequestered even in blood vessels of high-pressure systems and so take a part in the pathophysiology of the hemolysis and vascular occlusions in sickle cell disease.

Extreme susceptibility to mechanical trauma of cells while in the sickled form has been reported by several observers (73, 112). The increased mechanical fragility is almost directly related to the number of cells in the sickled form. Employing erythrocytes from patients with sickle cell anemia, it has been demonstrated that the marked increase in mechanical fragility takes place in the physiologic range of oxygen tension or hemoglobin unsaturation of venous blood. In cells from patients with sickle cell trait the change can be induced only at the oxygen tensions or saturations produced under artificial laboratory conditions (73; Figure 3.9).

In all instances it has been shown that the mechanical fragility of erythrocytes is significantly increased at oxygen tensions somewhat higher than those required to produce the initial increase in the number of sickled cells (Figures 3.10 and 3.12). This suggests that deoxygenation initiates in the red cells some alteration which is not immediately reflected in any gross, detectable shape change but which does result in increased mechanical fragility. Conceivably this change could be caused by the intracellular formation of limited numbers of hemoglobin polymers or small tactoids of hemoglobin not large enough to distort the external appearance of the cell but capable of increasing the susceptibility of the cell stroma to disruption by mechanical trauma. Perhaps polymers are formed by combination of hemoglobin with the lipoproteins of the cell membrane, thereby increasing its susceptibility to rupture. The possibility also exists that with steric distortion the membrane is no longer able to derive from the internal enzyme system the support needed to maintain its integrity.

While the *oxygenated red cells* of patients with sickle cell trait are not abnormally susceptible to mechanical trauma, those of patients with sickle cell anemia are slightly but significantly more susceptible. This finding suggests (as will be developed below) that these latter cells have been deleteriously affected during their life spans. Sterile incubation for 24 hours increases the mechanical fragility of the erythrocytes of patients with sickle cell anemia. These findings concerning susceptibility to mechanical injury are subject to much the same interpretation as are the data presented below on the alterations in erythrocytes subjected to osmotic fragility tests.

The conventional osmotic fragility test can be used to demonstrate certain morphologic abnormalities of red cells. In addition, the incubation technique (performing the same osmotic fragility test after the cells have been sterilely incubated for 24 hours) can reveal cellular defects that may not be disclosed by the ordinary test. A major portion of the erythrocytes of patients with sickle cell anemia demonstrate *increased resistance* to osmotic stress, while a small proportion show *increased fragility* (Figure 3.10). Both abnormalities are enhanced by incubation: the resistant cells become even *more resistant* after incubation and the fragile cells become even *more fragile*. Those cells showing increased osmotic fragility in both the conventional test and

after incubation are the more spherical. Increase in spheroidicity of normal erythrocytes is produced in vitro by incubation. It has been hypothesized that the unincubated erythrocytes showing increased osmotic fragility have in the patient been selectively sequestered and, in effect, incubated in vivo. Further laboratory incubation accentuates the changes. Erythrocytes from patients with sickle cell trait react to osmotic pressure in a manner intermediate between the reactions of normal subjects and of patients with sickle cell anemia.

The erythrocytes' abnormal osmotic and mechanical fragility, immediately present in the blood of patients with sickle cell anemia, are believed to be the effect of in vivo sequestration, incubation, and conditioning.

When these in vitro observations are applied to the pathophysiology of sickle cell disease, it is at once apparent that sickling, increased mechanical fragility, and changes in whole-blood viscosity can be produced in sickle cell trait, but *only* when the usual limits of physiologic oxygen tension are exceeded. The changes, therefore, would be expected to have no in vivo counterpart or relevance. By and large, sickle cell trait is a benign, asymptomatic condition that results in significant disease only under exceptional circumstances. Such exceptional circumstances, which may result in decreased oxygen tension, are readily found during airplane flight. There are now numerous reports (191) showing that splenic infarction has occurred under these conditions in persons with sickle cell anemia, those with sickle cell–hemoglobin C disease, and those proved to have sickle cell trait. Hematologically, patients with uncomplicated sickle cell trait have no anemia, no significantly increased erythrocyte osmotic or mechanical fragility, no irreversibly sickled cells, and no shortened red cell life span. In marked contrast, patients with sickle cell anemia exhibit a

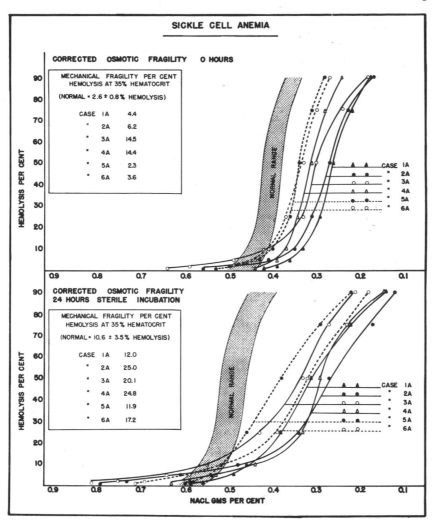

FIGURE 3.10. Erythrocyte osmotic and mechanical fragility in patients with sickle cell anemia. Top portion of chart shows results before incubation; lower portion shows results after 24 hours' sterile incubation of the blood sample. (From Harris, J. W., et al., A.M.A. Arch. Int. Med. 97:145, 1956)

variety of clinical manifestations and continually show the red cell abnormalities described above: increased osmotic and mechanical fragility, irreversibly sickled cells, and shortened erythrocyte life span. Even within the physiologic range of oxygen tension the deoxygenation of the hemoglobin is sufficient to result in molecular orientation, shape distortion, and sickling. In organs where the blood flow is slow, and particularly in sites of erythrocyte concentration such as the spleen,

sufficient numbers of erythrocytes sickle to produce an increased blood viscosity. This increase in viscosity impedes blood flow further, thereby triggering the vicious cycle outlined earlier. Physiologic consequences of this vicious cycle are multiple but the most important are: (a) a mechanism whereby plugs or masses of sickled erythrocytes become solid enough to occlude vessels and cause the vascular occlusive episodes characteristic of the disease; (b) a mechanism whereby the red cells become susceptible to mechanical trauma and consequently disrupted by the motion of the circulation; (c) a mechanism whereby erythrostasis can be effected; and (d) a mechanism whereby the cells deplete their reserves or sources of cell-maintaining energy and so become prone to destruction.

The evidence for the third point is indirect and is based on the observation that some of the circulating erythrocytes of sickle cell anemia are characterized by abnormal osmotic and mechanical fragility and because some are in the irreversibly, or permanently, sickled form. It has been shown that after sterile incubation there is a significant increase in erythrocytes' osmotic and mechanical fragility, and, as has been shown by Shen (181), sterile incubation of cells in the sickled form for varying periods of time results in the production of a number of cells that are irreversibly sickled despite reoxygenation. These changes constitute evidence that the processes of sequestration and conditioning are in operation in the patient with anemia.

Considerable direct evidence to support this hypothesis has been reported by Weisman et al. (208), who employed radioactive labeling techniques and differential agglutination methods. It was shown by studies done at the time of splenectomy that selective sequestration of the abnormal erythrocytes does in fact take place. Accordingly, if in a period immediately before splenectomy erythrocytes from a patient with sickle cell anemia were transfused to a hematologically normal patient or, conversely, normal cells were transfused into a child with sickle cell anemia, in both instances the spleen at the time of operation contained a greater proportion of sickle cell anemia erythrocytes than was found in the peripheral blood. Moreover, the cells that had been thus selectively concentrated in the spleen were markedly more susceptible to osmotic stress and mechanical

injury, and were more spheroidal, presumably because of "conditioning" that resulted from stasis. In sharp contrast to this, it was demonstrated that the erythrocytes from patients with sickle cell trait did not undergo selective sequestration in the spleen or increased osmotic fragility.

Lichtman et al. (118) have shown by needle puncture that in sickle cell anemia the spleen pulp contains a large percentage of sickled forms and that a large proportion of these are in the irreversibly sickled state.

There is a notable lack of evidence indicating that sickle cell anemia is accompanied by a marked increase in intravascular red cell destruction. Nevertheless, Crosby's finding (41, 42) of a significantly increased level of extracellular heme pigment in the plasma and the finding of a depleted haptoglobin level (79) make it probable that some intravascular destruction, presumably secondary to the erythrocytes' increased mechanical fragility, takes place. Fragmentation of the brittle sickled cells has been observed both in vitro and in vivo in the spleen. Moreover, the increased osmotic fragility observed by Weisman following erythrostasis in the spleen was of such magnitude that hemolysis by osmotic forces may account for the destruction of some of the red cells. Finally, the concept of erythrolytic factors in tissues, proposed by many workers, or the induced deficiency of cell-maintaining energy sources appears applicable to sickle cell anemia particularly because of the evidence for capillary blockage with prolonged erythrostasis.

Since autosplenectomy usually has taken place through repeated infarction in adults with sickle cell anemia, studies were made to determine whether or not selective sequestration occurs in other areas of the body (Figure 3.11). It is of interest to note (96) that the red cells of one patient had a half life of 11 days in the patient herself, by the Cr^{51} method,

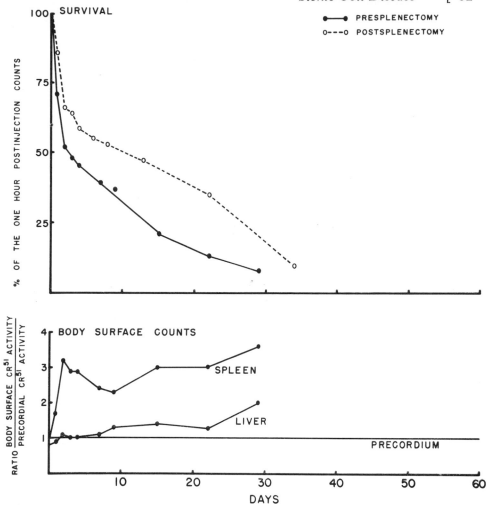

FIGURE 3.11.   Autosurvival of Cr51-labeled erythrocytes in child with sickle cell anemia and splenomegaly, before and after splenectomy

and that the patient's red cells tended to be sequestered in the liver, a site of low-pressure blood flow, with no apparent concentration in the area of the spleen. However, when the patient's red cells were transfused into a normal recipient with intact spleen, the half life of the cells was only 6 days. Moreover, in this recipient radioactivity appeared predominantly over the area of the spleen as well as of the liver. Several groups have now shown that when patients with sickle cell disease are subjected to lowered oxygen tensions, the number of sickled cells found in the peripheral blood increases

(116). When the cells of the subjects had previously been labeled with radioactive chromium, a significant build-up of the radioactivity occurred in the area of the spleen and/or liver, indicating selective sequestration (116).

Further evidence that the cellular and whole-blood changes described above have physiologic relevance is provided by the studies of Kass (105), who showed that partial remission, with achievement of near normal hemoglobin values, could be induced in sickle cell anemia by prolonged corticotropin (ACTH) therapy. This study demonstrated that a decrease in the sickling of the red cells at physiologic oxygen tensions of gas mixtures occurred coincident with the following changes: a decrease in the whole-blood viscosity corresponding to the decreased sickling, a decrease in the number of irreversibly sickled cells in the peripheral blood, a return to normal of the erythrocyte osmotic and mechanical fragility, a fourfold decrease in the per cent of reticulocytes, and fivefold decrease in the fecal urobilinogen.

These conclusions are also supported by the observations of Beutler and Mikus (21), who inhibited the sickling phenomenon by the in vivo induction of methemoglobin and demonstrated a lengthening of the erythrocyte survival time and an increase in the level of circulating hemoglobin.*

The severity of the anemia associated with sickle cell disease is, of course, dependent upon the balance established between erythrocyte destruction and production. Because of this balance, only incompletely evaluated at present, it is evident that measurements concerning factors contributing to the rate of erythrocyte destruction can have only a general correlation with the degree of anemia and that many exceptions are to be expected because of variations in the rate of production. In addition, factors other than the concentration of hemoglobin S have been shown to affect the sickling process. One of these, the pH variation, has been studied by Greenberg and Kass (64), who have demonstrated in some instances the induction of painful crises in a patient with sickle cell anemia by the administration of an acidifying agent and the termination of the crisis so produced (as well as spontaneous crises) by the administration of alkali.

Because of variations in the interactions of hemoglobin S with its companion intracellular pigment and because of the influence of other factors which determine the extent of interactions among the hemoglobin molecules, it is unlikely that the ease with which sickling can be induced is determined *solely* by the concentration of the intracellular reduced hemoglobin S. Indeed, the evidence indicates that the auxiliary factors mentioned and others as yet undefined play a significant role in the sickling process. Nevertheless, it has been demonstrated and confirmed by different workers that relative to oxygen tensions the erythrocytes of sickle cell anemia sickle much more readily than do the trait erythrocytes. Similarly, the oxygen tensions at which tactoid formation can be induced in solutions of various combinations of hemoglobins correlate fairly closely with the tensions of oxygen at which sickling can be induced in the intact cells. There is, therefore, a rough correlation between the amount of hemoglobin S present in a cell and the oxygen tension at which tactoid formation and sickling can be induced. The physiologic, clinical, and hematologic consequences of these observations in terms of sickle cell disease are that the sickling changes in erythrocytes of patients with sickle cell anemia take place in the physiologic range of oxygen tension; not so in erythrocytes of patients with sickle cell trait, for these can be made to change shape only at oxygen tensions well below the physiologic range (Figures 3.12 and 3.13).

The above account of the pathophysiology of sickle cell disease is evidently more than a little tendentious. From the above in vitro studies and their projected in vivo interpretations patients obviously could not survive, largely because of static masses of sickled erythrocytes in the many body areas of very low oxygen content. Consequently studies were made

---

* It should be pointed out that this is of investigative interest and *not* of therapeutic value. If the administration of the methemoglobin-inducing agent (para-amino propriophenone) is prolonged, increased red cell destruction occurs because of an additional effect of the agent itself.

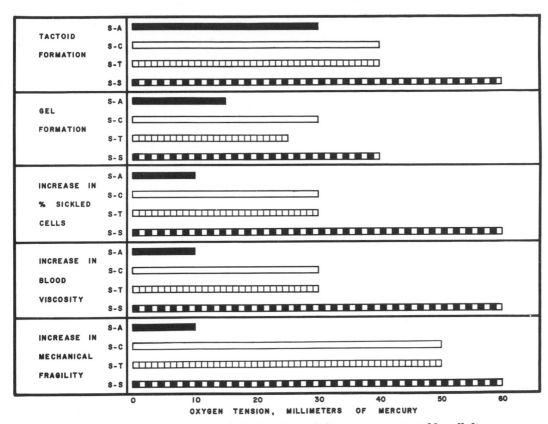

FIGURE 3.12.   Oxygen tensions at which biophysical changes occur in sickle sell disease. (From Griggs, R. C., and Harris, J. W., A.M.A. Arch. Int. Med. 97:315, 1956)

1. As oxygen is abstracted from blood
2. Cells go into the sickled form.
3. With increase in number of sickled forms
4. The viscosity of the whole blood increases
5. And the mechanical fragility of sickled cells is markedly increased.
6. With increased viscosity the flow of blood slows, and
7. More oxygen is taken from the cells by the metabolic demands of the tissues.

THUS STARTING

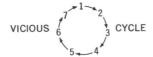

VICIOUS   CYCLE

8. Sickled cell thrombi formed because of marked increase in viscosity account in large part for clinical manifestations, and
9. The marked increase in sickled cell mechanical fragility for hemolytic manifestations.

SICKLE CELL TRAIT

These changes can be made to take place only below the physiologic levels of venous oxygen saturations. Therefore: No hemolysis and normal life span of trait erythrocytes.

SICKLE CELL ANEMIA

These changes take place at physiologic levels of venous oxygen saturations. Therefore: Continuing hemolysis and short life span of erythrocytes.

FIGURE 3.13.   Mechanism of erythrocyte destruction in sickle cell disease

by Jensen et al. (99) attempting to determine by means of venous catheterization the actual in vivo condition of the erythrocytes in the critically hypoxic areas of patients with sickle cell anemia.

During the course of circulation in an individual with sickle cell anemia, the red cells are exposed to widely varying and rapidly changing oxygen tensions. Any shape change that the cell may undergo (as a result of deoxygenation) is dependent upon (a) the degree of oxygen unsaturation to which it is exposed, (b) the length of time the oxygen tension is reduced, and (c) the rate at which the sickling change occurs. It was found that in venous blood samples with midrange oxygen saturations, the proportions of sickled cells varied from 10 to 32 per cent and correlated fairly well with those predicted by the in vitro experiments. However, major deviations from the predicted proportions occurred at the lower ranges of oxygen saturation, suggesting the existence of important modifying factors in the in vivo sickling process. For example, in the coronary sinus (where the oxygen tension is very markedly reduced) the percentage of sickled cells was approximately 20. This is in marked contrast to the in vitro studies described above, where at oxygen tensions comparable to that of coronary sinus blood, the majority of the cells would be in the sickled form. In the in vitro studies the cells were exposed to low oxygen tensions for relatively long periods of time (30 minutes to 4 hours); in the circulating blood the red cells are exposed to oxygen unsaturation for approximately 15 seconds. Moreover, in anemia there is a significantly accelerated rate of blood flow and a shift of the oxygen dissociation curve to the right (17). Studies by Ponder (quoted in 73) and Allison (5) both in vitro and in vivo, indicate that 2 to 3 minutes is required for the sickling change to develop and an equal length of time to reverse the process. These con-siderations probably provide the explanation whereby sickle cell anemia is compatible with life. Although the red cells frequently encounter oxygen tensions in the body which are capable of producing sickling, the majority of the cells become reoxygenated before mechanical distortion can occur. However, if a cell becomes trapped in some area of venous stasis and is deoxygenated for a sufficiently long time, sickling takes place. If it is again returned to the general circulation, minutes would be required for it to reassume the discoid form. Prolonged stay in the sickled form may result in irreversible sickling, and in the sickled form the cell is more fragile and subject to sequestration in other organs.

Summary

It is possible by assembling a remarkable array of genetic, chemical, physical, physiologic, and biologic information to outline what certainly must be the major factors responsible for the occurrence of the clinical entities grouped under the heading sickle cell disease. In doing this one can go almost step by step from the mutation to the production of a chemically abnormal hemoglobin which, because of behavioral abnormalities induced by deoxygenation, results in the sickled distortion of the erythrocyte. As a consequence of this deformity, changes take place in the cell and in the whole blood that can account for the existence of a chronic hemolytic anemia and the vascular occlusive phenomenon that characterize the clinical course of the disease: an abnormal DNA, a crucial amino acid out of place, a diseased individual.

Variants of Sickle Cell Disease

In collecting evidence to substantiate the homozygous-heterozygous genetic mechanism proposed to account for the inheritance of sickle cell disease, good agreement was obtained among several extensive surveys. However, a few exceptions were encountered even after the exclusion of impaternity. By and large these were patients whose clinical picture was similar to that of true homozygous sickle cell anemia but who had one parent not showing the sickling phenomenon. Further studies on these patients and their families demonstrated that instead of nullifying the above hypothesis, supporting evidence was actually provided, since these patients indeed possessed the sickling anomaly *plus* another hematologic defect. In the original patients described either a third type of adult hemoglobin, designated hemoglobin C, or the hematologic abnormality thalassemia was found. Since then, extension of genetic, hematologic, and biochemical investigations has determined the existence of more than thirty types of hemoglobins. Because many can occur in various combinations with each other or in conjunction with various other hematologic abnormalities, the disease spectrum possible is truly staggering.

A number of patients have been identified in whom hemoglobin S occurs in combination with another abnormal hemoglobin. Studies have been made (66) on the red cells and hemoglobin solutions from the patients most commonly encountered in this country, namely those with sickle cell–hemoglobin C disease, sickle cell–thalassemia disease, and the sickle cell–fetal hemoglobin combination that occurs in the infant with sickle cell anemia. In the sickling process hemoglobin S can complex to form polymers with hemoglobins A and C but not with hemoglobin F. In vitro studies have shown that the degree of sickling and viscosity changes in whole-blood samples and the tactoid formation, gel formation, and viscosity changes in hemoglobin solutions are roughly proportional to the concentration of hemoglobin S (Figure 3.12). Consequently, to produce physical alterations in the red cells or hemoglobin solutions obtained from patients with

sickle cell–thalassemia disease (67 to 82 per cent hemoglobin S), oxygen tensions are necessary that are lower than those needed to produce similar alterations in sickle cell anemia (75 to 100 per cent hemoglobin S). Still lower oxygen tensions are required to produce the same changes in blood from patients with sickle cell–hemoglobin C disease (50 per cent hemoglobin S). In sickle cell trait blood (25 to 45 per cent hemoglobin S) even lower oxygen tensions are needed.

These in vitro studies can be *roughly* correlated with clinical manifestations (86, 164, 188, 190, 192, 193). Those individuals most likely to have symptomatic disease have red cells containing a concentration of hemoglobin S sufficient to develop physical alterations at physiologic oxygen tensions. Clinically there is a gradation of decreasing severity of manifestations from sickle cell–thalassemia disease to sickle cell–hemoglobin C disease to sickle cell trait, but many areas of overlap are present.

Although significant differences have been described among the various disorders associated with hemoglobin S, no attempt will be made here to give details. Table 3.1, concerning *some* of the hemoglobinopathies, will give an idea of the complexity of the situation at present. Indeed at the rate new hemoglobins and new combinations are being described, it bids fair rapidly to get beyond the mind of man to retain all the types, subtypes, combinations, and manifestations. Because of this a few more pertinent and significant facts must be brought up relative to hemoglobin structure and genetics that are now serving to bring order to a complex area.

Several lines of biochemical and biophysical evidence concur in establishing that the protein of normal adult hemoglobin is made up of two different peptide chains, each occurring in pairs, and specifically arranged so that when combined with the four heme moieties the

Table 3.1. Summary of clinical and laboratory features of the major hemoglobinopathies

Major Hgb types	Per cent Hgb F[a]	Clinical severity	"Crises"	Spleno-megaly	Hemolytic anemia	Sickling	Micro-cytosis	Hypo-chromasia	Per cent target cells	Aniso-cytosis	Poikilo-cytosis	Reticulo-cytosis	Incidence, occurrence, and major biophysical abnormality of the abnormal hemoglobin
Adult normal AA	<2	0	0	0	0	0	0	0	0–2	0	0	N	
Newborn (1866) AF	50–85	0	0	0	+	0	0	0	0	+	+	N or ↗	Hgb P: first 2–3 months intra-uterine, life (?) Hgb F: alkali-resistant, solubility > A
Hgb S trait (1949) AS	<2	0	±0	0	0	+	0	0		0	0	N	Hgb S: electrophoretically abnormal, slower than A, tactoid formation→sickling, 8–11% American Negroes
Hgb C trait (1950) AC	<2	0	0	±	0	0	0	0	0–40	0	0	N	Hgb C: electrophoretically abnormal, slower than S, associated with target forms, 2–3% American Negroes, 6–21% of Gold Coast population
Hgb D trait (1951) AD	<2	0	0	0	0	0	0	0	0–10	0	0	N	Hgb D: electrophoretically like S,[b] no sickling, 0.5% American Negroes, major foci in Punjab (2%) and Algeria (2%)
Hgb E trait (1954) AE	<2	0	0	0	0	0	+	0	0–4	0	0	N	Hgb E: electrophoretically abnormal, between S and C, southeast Asia, peak in Thais (14%), Indonesia (4–6%), Ceylon, India, Burma, Indo-China
Hgb G trait (1954) AG	<2	0	0	0	0	0	0	0	0	0	0	N	Hgb G: electrophoretically like F,[b] not alkali-resistant, sporadic reports
Hgb I trait (1955) AI		0	0	0	0	0	0	0	0	0	0	N	Hgb I: "fast hemoglobin," faster than A, several U.S. families, Algeria
Hgb J trait (1955) AJ	<2	0	0	0	0	0	0	0	0	0	0	N	Hgb J: "fast hemoglobin," between A and I, sporadically in U.S., Liberia, Algeria, India

Major Hgb types — trait	Major Hgb types	Per cent Hgb F[a]	Clinical severity	"Crises"	Splenomegaly	Hemolytic anemia	Sickling	Microcytosis	Hypochromasia	Per cent target cells	Anisocytosis	Poikilocytosis	Reticulocytosis	Incidence, occurrence, and major biophysical abnormality of the abnormal hemoglobin
Hgb K trait (1955)	AK	<2	0	0	0	0	0	0	0	0	0	0	N	Hgb K: "fast hemoglobin," between A and J, Algeria, India
Hgb L trait (1957)	AL	<2	0	0	0	0	0	0	0	0	0	0	N	Hgb L: electrophoretically between S and G, Pakistan
Lepore trait (1958)		<2	0	0	?	?	0	0	0	+	+	+	↑	"Lepore Hgb" 12%
Sickle cell–Hgb C	SC	0–8	–to 3+	–to 2+	+to 3+	+to 3+	+	±	0	20–85	2+	2+	↑	See text
Sickle cell–Hgb D	SD	<2	2+	+	2+	2+	+	±	0	±	2+	2+	↑	Very rare
Sickle cell–Hgb G	SG	<2	?	±	±	0	?	?	0	? +	0	0	?	Very rare
Sickle cell–Hgb E	SE	2+	–	±	+	+	+	+	0	0–9	+	+	N or ↑	Very rare
Hgb C–Hgb D	CD						0			–				Very rare
Hgb Q–Hgb H[c]	QH	<2	2+	?	±	+	–	2+	2+	+	2+	2+	N	? Thalassemia also
√ Sickle cell anemia	SS	2–24	4+	4+	±	4+	+	0	0	5–30	3+	3+	↑	0.2% American Negroes
Homozygous C	CC	0–7	1+	0	+	+	0	0	0	40–100	+	+	↑	1 in 6,000 American Negroes
Homozygous D	DD	<2	0	0	±	±	0	+	0	60–80	+	+	N	Very rare
Homozygous E	EE	2–6	+	0	±	+	0	2+	0	25–60	2+	+	↑	Rare
Homozygous G	GG	<2	0	0	0	0	0	0	0	0	0	0	N	Rare

[a] Three different fetal hemoglobins have been described all with similar electrophoretic behaviors, one of which is composed of four γ-chains.

[b] Although the same electrophoretic behavior is seen in each, three different hemoglobins D have been described according to location of the abnormality and amino acid sequence: Dα, Dβ, Dγ. Similarly three hemoglobins G have been recognized: G Philadelphia and Honolulu (both α-chain abnormalities), and G San José (β-chain abnormality).

[c] Hemoglobin H is now known to be composed of four β-chains; no α-chains are found. It is found mainly in the Far East and may only occur in association with thalassemia. The hemoglobin is unstable and spontaneously denatures. Many of the abnormal hemoglobins have been observed to occur in combination with thalassemia. For a discussion of the genetics, biochemistry, and clinical manifestations, see section on Thalassemia, Chapter 9.

complete molecule is composed of two equal halves. By various chemical and physical manipulations, it has been possible to separate the two different polypeptide chains and demonstrate different amino acid sequences in each. In addition to the heme groups, normal adult hemoglobin is composed of two α-polypeptide chains and two β-polypeptide chains. With reasonable certainty the sequence for the 141 amino acids in the α-chain is known as is the sequence for the 146 amino acids in the β-chain. As recently announced they are illustrated in Table 3.2. It has been proposed that in designating hemoglobins the following nomenclature be adopted (60). A Greek letter with no subscript or superscript is employed in speaking of a polypeptide chain in general; when the α-polypeptide chain derived for normal adult hemoglobin is to be designated, α^A is employed. Similarly for the β-polypeptide chain, β^A is employed. Since the polypeptide chains occur in pairs in the intact molecule, normal adult hemoglobin, Hgb A, is written $\alpha_2{}^A\beta_2{}^A$.

In addition to this major component of the hemoglobin found in normal blood, minor components are also present in the forms of fetal hemoglobin and the so-called A_2 component. Studies have now indicated that fetal hemoglobin, following the general rule, is made up of two different polypeptide chains arranged in pairs. One of the chains is the same as that found in hemoglobin A, the α^A chain. The companion chain is, however, quite different in amino acid composition and sequence and has been called the γ^F (gamma) chain. Fetal hemoglobin (Hgb F) is accordingly written $\alpha_2{}^A\gamma_2{}^F$. The presence of the two γ^F chains confers the unique properties upon the intact molecule.

Similarly the other minor component of normal blood, hemoglobin A_2 has been shown to consist of two α^A-chains, the same as those occurring in hemoglobin A,

but again the companion chains are different from either the β- or the γ-chains and are designated as δ (delta). Hemoglobin A_2 (Hgb A_2) is accordingly written $\alpha_2{}^A\delta_2{}^{A_2}$.

The blood of a normal individual, therefore, contains a main hemoglobin component, Hgb A, $\alpha_2{}^A\beta_2{}^A$; and two minor components, Hgb F, $\alpha_2{}^A\gamma_2{}^F$, and Hgb A_2, $\alpha_2{}^A\delta_2{}^{A_2}$.

In considering an abnormal hemoglobin, it is evident that an abnormality can reside in either polypeptide chain or in both together. That this does in fact occur is evidenced by the digestion studies of Ingram revealing in hemoglobin S only one amino acid out of place and that in the sickle peptide which occurs in the β-chain.

In keeping with the nomenclature employed up to this point, the β-chain in hemoglobin S is designated as β^S and Hgb S is written $\alpha_2{}^A\beta_2{}^S$. This indicates that the abnormality is found in the β-chain. But in this instance much more is known about the location and nature of the abnormality. The location of an abnormality in a given polypeptide chain can be indicated by giving the number of the abnormal peptide fragment as determined by trypsin digestion and fingerprint pattern. The polypeptide fragments are indicated as TpI-XIV for the α-chain and TpI-XV for the β-chain; Tp indicates the method of trypsin digestion, and the Roman numeral indicates the position of the fragment on the intact α- or β-polypeptide chain, as indicated in Table 3.2. Hemoglobin S may then be designated $\alpha_2{}^A\beta_2{}^{STpI}$. When the precise location of the abnormality and substituted amino acid is known this may be indicated in the superscript, Hgb S: $\alpha_2{}^A\beta_2{}^{6\ val}$. In order of increasing specificity relative to the amino acid abnormality, sickle hemoglobin may be designated: hemoglobin S; $\alpha_2{}^A\beta_2{}^S$, $\alpha_2{}^A\beta_2{}^{STpI}$, and $\alpha_2{}^A\beta_2{}^{6\ val}$. Following this system of nomenclature the various normal and abnormal hemoglobins are listed in Table

TABLE 3.2. Amino acid sequence of α– and β–polypeptide chains of hemoglobin A

AMINO ACID SEQUENCE OF α–POLYPEPTIDE CHAIN OF HEMOGLOBIN A

TpI   TpII   TpIII
       10   20

Val-Leu-Ser-Pro-Ala-Asp-*Lys*-Thr-Asg-Val-*Lys*-Ala-Ala-Try-Gly-*Lys*-Val-Gly-Ala-His-

TpIV   TpV
       30   40

Ala-Gly-Glu-Tyr-Gly-Ala-Glu-Ala-Leu-Glu-*Arg*-Met-Phe-Leu-Ser-Phe-Pro-Thr-Thr-*Lys*-

         TpVI   TpVII TpVIII
       50   60

Thr-Tyr-Phe-Pro-His-Phe-Asp-Leu-Ser-His-Gly-Ser-Ala-Glu-Val-*Lys*-Gly-His-Gly-*Lys*-

                        TpIX
       70   80

Lys-Val-Ala-Asp-Ala-Leu-Thr-Asp-Ala-Val-Ala-His-Val-Asp-Asp-Met-Pro-Asp-Ala-Leu-

           TpX   TpXI
       90   100

Ser-Ala-Leu-Ser-Asp-Leu-His-Ala-His-*Lys*-Leu-*Arg*-Val-Asp-Pro-Val-Asp-Phe-*Lys*-Leu-

                  TpXII
       110   120

Leu-Ser-His-Cys-Leu-Leu-Val-Thr-Leu-Ala-Ala-His-Leu-Pro-Ala-Glu-Phe-Thr-Pro-Ala-

              TpXIII   TpXIV
      130   140

Val-His-Ala-Ser-Leu-Asp-*Lys*-Phe-Leu-Ala-Ser-Val-Ser-Thr-Val-Leu-Thr-Ser-*Lys*-Tyr-*Arg*

AMINO ACID SEQUENCE OF β–POLYPEPTIDE CHAIN OF HEMOGLOBIN A

TpI   TpII
       10   20

Val-His-Leu-Thr-Pro-Glu-Glu-*Lys*-Ser-Ala-Val-Thr-Ala-Leu-Try-Gly-*Lys*-Val-Asg-Val-

TpIII   TpIV
       30   40

Asp-Glu-Val-Gly-Gly-Glu-Ala-Leu-Gly-*Arg*-Leu-Leu-Val-Val-Tyr-Pro-Try-Thr-Glu-*Arg*-

          TpV   TpVI
          50   60

Phe-Phe-Glu-Ser-Phe-Gly-Asp-Leu-Ser-Thr-Pro-Asp-Ala-Val-Met-Gly-Asg-Pro-*Lys*-Val-

TpVII   TpVIII   TpIX
               70   80

Lys-Ala-His-Gly-*Lys*-*Lys*-Val-Leu-Gly-Ala-Phe-Ser-Asp-Gly-Leu-Ala-His-Leu-Asp-Asg-

            TpX   TpXI
         90   100

Leu-*Lys*-Gly-Thr-Phe-Ala-Thr-Leu-Ser-Glu-Leu-His-Cys-Asp-*Lys*-Leu-His-Val-Asp-Pro-

                 TpXII
       110   120

Glu-Asg-Phe-*Arg*-Leu-Leu-Gly-Asp-Val-Leu-Val-Cys-Val-Leu-Ala-His-His-Phe-Gly-*Lys*-

TpXIII   TpXIV
       130   140

Glu-Phe-Thr-Pro-Pro-Val-Glu-Ala-Ala-Tyr-Glu-*Lys*-Val-Val-Ala-Gly-Val-Ala-Asg-Ala-

         TpXV
Leu-Ala-His-*Lys*-Tyr-His

Complete amino acid sequence of the α– and β–polypeptide chains of hemoglobin A ($\alpha_2^A \beta_2^A$). During trypsin digestion of the heat-denatured hemoglobin, the polypeptide chains are broken at the sites of arginine and lysine carboxyl bonding; these sites are indicated by the italic type. The polypeptide fragments resulting are labeled TpI through XV to indicate trypsin digestion procedure (Tp) and position in the intact chain.

3.3 according to their known polypeptide chain structure and location of abnormality.

Most of the abnormal hemoglobins have been discovered by employing electrophoretic techniques. By and large, filter-paper electrophoresis at a pH of 8.6 has been used in routine studies and population surveys. It must be remembered that electrophoresis depends mainly on the charge carried by the protein molecule at the pH of the buffer and to a much lesser extent on the supporting and suspending media. Alterations in amino acid sequences will be revealed by electrophoresis only if the substituted amino acid confers a charge difference on the polypeptide. The prediction that such "hidden" abnormalities existed was fulfilled by studies on hemoglobin D, which, by fingerprint and amino acid sequence techniques, has been demonstrated to have three variant forms, D_a, D_β, and D_γ, even though all had identical migration patterns on electrophoresis.

The list of criteria by which hemoglobins are now identified has been summarized by Jonxis and Huisman (102) in a laboratory manual: alkali denaturation; electrophoresis (free-boundary, filter paper/glass plate, inverted-V, starch block, starch gel, agar gel, acrylamide gel); solubility; column chromatography (carboxymethyl cellulose, Amberlite); fingerprinting; association-dissociation. Spectral absorption curves of oxygenated hemoglobin and acid and alkaline methemoglobin, and oxygen dissociation curves have also indicated abnormalities. For many years it has been known that with the exception of the fetal type, hemoglobin is very poorly antigenic; consequently identification of the various hemoglobins by immunologic techniques has not been possible. Recent studies indicate that hemoglobins A, C, and S do not appear antigenic and the little antigenicity previously ascribed was due to the presence of minor components such as F and A_2 (77).

Because of the difficult nature of the techniques employed, it has not been possible to locate by polypeptide chain and amino acid sequence analysis the location of all hemoglobin abnormalities. Fortunately another technique, based on an observation made by Field and O'Brien (54) is available that has been employed to indicate which polypeptide chain carries the abnormality.

When hemoglobin is exposed to a media of low pH, it is dissociated into two fragments the molecular weights of which, as determined by the ultracentrifuge, are approximately one-half that of the intact molécule. If the pH of the media is returned to neutrality, reassociation of the fragments occurs and the original compound is re-established (38, 79, 94, 170, 189, 200, 201). If hemoglobins derived from man and dog, for example, are put together in solution and exposed to a low pH, dissociation of the molecules takes place followed by randomization of the half-molecules. When the pH of the solution is restored to neutrality, recombination of fragments takes place, but now in addition to repristination of the two original hemoglobins, two new hybrid molecules emerge from the moil (165). Before pH manipulation, electrophoresis demonstrated two hemoglobin peaks; after pH manipulation, four peaks were evident, the two original and two* new ones consisting of chimeric molecules half canine, half human.

Evidence now indicates that the half units produced by exposure of hemoglobin to low pH are dissimilar—one unit composed of two a-chains and the other

---

* One of the two peaks is formed by the hemoglobin resulting from the combination of the a-chains of the human hemoglobin and the companion canine chains; the other peak is formed by the hemoglobin resulting from the human β-chains and the companion canine chains.

of two β-chains. By employing a human hemoglobin whose defect is known to exist in the β-chain (hemoglobin S, for example) and the unknown abnormal human hemoglobin, the dissociation-reassociation procedure can indicate through the types of recombinants formed which chain carries the abnormality in the test hemoglobin. In this manner it has been possible, for example, to demonstrate or confirm that the abnormalities of hemoglobins S, C, and G are on the β-chain and the abnormalities of hemoglobins I and Ho2 are on the α-chain. In addition it has been shown that in fetal hemoglobin the α-chains are the same as in adult hemoglobin and that the companion chains account for the differences found between them.

These chemical findings relative to the normal and abnormal hemoglobins have forced a re-evaluation of the previously proposed mechanisms governing the inheritance of the various hemoglobins. Since the α-chains are the same in hemoglobins A, A_2, F, and S, and the hemoglobins differ one from another because of the companion chains β-, γ-, δ-, β^S (or $\beta^{6\ val}$), it is evident that the proposal that one gene governs the production of one complete hemoglobin molecule is no longer tenable. It is more in line with current genetic information that one gene locus (or cistron in more modern terms) is responsible for the production of one polypeptide chain. Evidence is available to indicate the genetic identity of the α-chain determinants in hemoglobins A, A_2, and F (11, 207). Since the pattern of inheritance of hemoglobins is not sex-linked, there will be one gene locus on each of two autosomal chromosomes (allelomorphs). Accordingly each normal individual will have two sets of factors governing the production of hemoglobin A, and his genotype is designated as Hgba^A/Hgba^A:Hgbβ^A/Hgbβ^A.

It must be remembered that each normal individual is making not only hemoglobin A but also fetal hemoglobin and several minor hemoglobin components (A_2, A_3, etc.). Although it is probable that at least one of the minor components (A_3) is a degradation product of hemoglobin A, some of the others cannot be either precursors or degradation products of the main component. This is evident since they contain isoleucine, an amino acid not present in hemoglobin A. All the hemoglobins must accordingly be under genetic control, and a more proper designation for the genotype of a normal individual than the one given above is Hgba^A/Hgba^A; Hgbβ^A/Hgbβ^A; Hgbγ^F/Hgbγ^F; Hgb$\delta^{A}2$/Hgb$\delta^{A}2$, etc. The production of hemoglobins in a normal individual might then be conceived as shown in Figure 3.14 A.

The genotype for a person with an abnormal hemoglobin can be changed from the normal in either α- or β-polypeptide chain in terms of the major hemoglobin component. Moreover, the individual can be either heterozygous or homozygous for the abnormality (Figure 3.14 B and C).

It should be pointed out again here that the polypeptide chains, whether normal or abnormal, appear always to exist in *pairs* of *like* chains. Thus, the main hemoglobin components formed in sickle cell trait are either $\alpha_2^A\beta_2^A$ or $\alpha_2^A\beta_2^S$ and *not* $\alpha_2^A\beta^A\beta^S$.

This system is certainly cumbersome and complex but it is unquestionably more accurate and brings order to an area that had become unwieldy. From the data provided in Table 3.2 indicating the polypeptide locus of the amino acid abnormality, the prediction can be made concerning the genetic patterns seen— allelic or nonallelic with respect to companion hemoglobins. On the one gene— one hemoglobin basis it was difficult or impossible to explain the occurrence of patients with four different hemoglobins (10, 131). On the above schema they are

TABLE 3.3.   Human hemoglobins: Normal and abnormal

Normal hemoglobins	**ADULT** Hgb A: $\alpha_2^A \beta_2^A$
	FETAL Hgb F: $\alpha_2^A \gamma_2^F$
	MINOR FRACTION OF ADULT Hgb A$_2$: $\alpha_2^A \delta_2^{A_2}$
Abnormal hemoglobins Abnormal hemoglobins in which the polypeptide chain is normal but the hemoglobin is composed of four identical polypeptide chains	Hgb Barts: γ_4^F Hgb H: β_4^A
Abnormal hemoglobins Abnormal hemoglobins in which an amino acid defect has been localized to a single polypeptide chain	Hgb A$_2^1$: $\alpha_2^A \delta_2^{A_2^1}$
	Hgb C: $\alpha_2^A \beta_2^C (\alpha_2^A \beta_2^{A \; 6 \, lys})$
	Hgb Dα: $\alpha_2^D \beta_2^A$
	Hgb D$_{\alpha \text{ St. Louis}}$: $\alpha_2^{D \text{ St. Louis}} \beta_2^A$
	* Hgb Dβ: $\alpha_2^A \beta_2^D$
	Hgb Dγ: Hgb D$_{Punjab}$: $\alpha_2^A \beta_2^D (\gamma_2^A \beta_2^{D \; T-13\,(glu \to leu)})$
	Hgb E: $\alpha_2^A \beta_2^E (\alpha_2^A \beta_2^{A \; 26 \, lys})$
	Hgb F$_{St. Louis}$: $\alpha_2^D \gamma_2^F$
*Each member of these pairs has an amino acid abnormality in the same chain, but at a different location in that chain	* Hgb G$_{Philadelphia}$: $\alpha_2^G \beta_2^A (\alpha_2^{G \; 68 \, lys} \beta_2^A)$
	Hgb G$_{Honolulu}$: $\alpha_2^G \beta_2^A (\alpha_2^{G \; 27 \, glu \, NH_2} \beta_2^A)$

<table>
<tr><td rowspan="5">Abnormal hemoglobins</td></tr>
</table>

Abnormal hemoglobins	* Hgb G Galveston: $\alpha_2^{A}\ \beta_2^{G\ Galveston}$
	Hgb G San José: $\alpha_2^{A}\ \beta_2^{G(\ A\ \ 7\ gly)}\ (\alpha_2^{A}\ \beta_2^{\ \ })$
	Hgb I: $\alpha_2^{I}\ \beta_2^{A}\ (\alpha_2^{16\ asp}\ \beta_2^{A})$
	Hgb I$_2$: $\alpha_2^{I_2}\ \delta_2^{A}$

Abnormal hemoglobins in which an amino acid defect has been localized to a single polypeptide chain

Hgb J: $\alpha_2^{A}\ \beta_2^{J}$

Hgb K: $\alpha_2^{K}\ \beta_2^{A}$

Hgb M Boston: $\alpha_2^{M}\ \beta_2^{A}\ (\alpha_2^{T\text{–}7\ (his\rightarrow tyr)}\ \beta_2^{A})$

---

* Hgb M Saskatoon: $\alpha_2^{A}\ \beta_2^{M}\ (\alpha_2^{A}\ \beta_2^{T\text{–}7\ (his\rightarrow tyr)})$

* Hgb M Milwaukee: $\alpha_2^{A}\ \beta_2^{M}\ (\alpha_2^{A}\ \beta_2^{T\text{–}9\ (val\rightarrow glu)})$

Hgb N: $\alpha_2^{A}\ \beta_2^{N}$

Hgb O: $\alpha_2^{A}\ \beta_2^{O}$

Hgb P: $\alpha_2^{A}\ \beta_2^{P}$

Hbg Q: $\alpha_2^{Q}\ \beta_2^{A}$

Hgb S: $\alpha_2^{A}\ \beta_2^{S}\ (\alpha_2^{A}\ \beta_2^{6\ val})$

Hgb Hopkins No. 2: $\alpha_2^{Ho2}\ \beta_2^{A}$

Hgb Lepore (? "Pylos"): $\alpha_2^{H}\ \delta_2^{L}$

*Each member of these pairs has an amino acid abnormality in the same chain, but at a different location in that chain

Abnormal hemoglobins

$$\text{Hgb Norfolk: } \alpha_2^{N} \beta_2^{A} (\alpha_2^{57\ asp} \beta_2^{A})$$

$$\text{Hgb Zürich: } \alpha_2^{A} \beta_2^{Z} (\alpha_2^{A} \beta_2^{63\ arg})$$

Adapted from Chernoff, A. I., Mod. Med. 29:63, 1961.

designated as doubly heterozygous: $Hgb\alpha^{A}/Hgb\alpha^{G}$; $Hgb\beta^{A}/Hgb\beta^{S}$ yielding polypeptide chains α^{A}, α^{G}, β^{A}, β^{S} and the experimentally demonstrated hemoglobins $\alpha_2^{A}\beta_2^{A}$ (hemoglobin A), $\alpha_2^{A}\beta_2^{S}$ (hemoglobin S), $\alpha_2^{G}\beta_2^{A}$ (hemoglobin G), and $\alpha_2^{G}\beta_2^{S}$ (new component).

A final implication inherent in the above account concerning the biosynthesis of hemoglobin is that the hemoglobin molecule need not be produced as a completed product from the RNA granule but that polypeptide chains may be separately released from RNA templates and after release combine with companion chains to form the completed hemoglobin molecule more under biochemical than genetic control.

Bibliographic references for Chapter 3 begin on page 382.

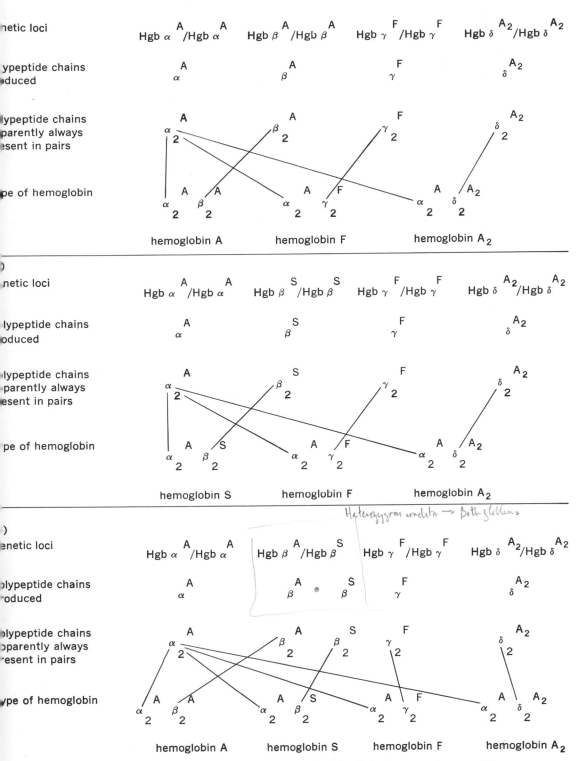

FIGURE 3.14.   Schematic representation of genotypes for (A) person with normal hemo-globin, (B) person with homozygous sickle cell anemia, and (C) person with heterozy-gous sickle cell trait. Note that in homozygous sickle cell anemia *no* hemoglobin A can be formed

PART II] GENERAL CONSIDERATIONS OF ANEMIA

CHAPTER FOUR

EFFECTS OF ANEMIA

On the basis of primary hematologic abnormalities or hematologic abnormalities resulting from other types of underlying disorders, many situations are found in which the blood has a decreased capacity to transport and deliver oxygen to body tissues. A number of signs and symptoms result from this decreased capacity of the blood to fulfill its primary function that are, to a large extent, seen irrespective of the disorder causing it. Consequently numerous general effects of anemia can be singled out that will be common to nearly all such situations. The development of symptoms in patients with anemia depends primarily upon (a) the degree of anemia present, (b) the changes in total blood volume, (c) the rapidity of the development of the anemia, (d) the status of the cardiovascular system, and (e) the causative disorder.

In acute blood loss (13) hemoglobin and plasma are reduced proportionately, and the immediate symptoms are mainly related to the decreased volume of circulating blood. Anemia (as indicated by grams of hemoglobin per 100 ml of blood, or hematocrit) does not develop until fluid enters the vascular tree to restore the plasma volume and concomitantly decrease the hemoglobin concentration. This begins rapidly but is complete only 48 to 72 hours after the hemorrhagic episode. Plasma proteins and then erythrocytes are regenerated. In man there are no stores of erythrocytes (comparable to the "splenic reservoir" of dogs), although there is evidence of shift of blood within the vascular tree (12), so replenishment of hemoglobin must await regeneration. The development of the decreased hemoglobin level in the circulating blood is delayed following acute hemorrhage and is indicative of compensatory adjustments.

If the development of anemia has been of an insidious nature, adjustments in the blood volume take place. In mild anemia the total blood volume is only slightly, if at all, reduced below normal (16, 18) because of a compensatory increase in plasma volume occasioned by the decrease in total hemoglobin-red-cell mass. Here the signs and symptoms are largely due to the decreased capacity of the blood to transport and deliver oxygen. In severe anemia, however, the total blood volume may be somewhat decreased—apparently as a means of maintaining a higher hemoglobin level in the circulating blood (45)—so that the additional signs and symptoms due to disproportion (actual or potential) between blood volume and vascular tree may be encountered.* It is in this latter situation that the status and responsiveness of the cardiovascular system plays an important role.

For brevity, the usual signs and symptoms encountered in anemia of whatever cause are given in outline form.

I. Integumentary
  A. Pallor: best and most reliably discerned in the mucous membranes, nail beds, and lines of the palm (usually pink until the hemoglobin concentration is less than 7 Gm per 100 ml) since skin color varies with vasoconstriction or vasodilatation, fluid content, and pigmentation
II. Respiratory (32, 38); cardiovascular (14, 21, 22, 26, 32, 39, 40, 41, 50, 51, 55); renal (8, 9, 19, 49)
  A. Exertional dyspnea, tachycardia, palpitation, angina of effort, claudication, night cramps, orthopnea, cough, air hunger in extreme anemia
  B. Increased arterial pulsation, capillary pulsation, bruits, cardiac enlargement, murmurs, ankle edema, urinary frequency
  C. Increased rate and depth of respiration
III. Neuromuscular (24, 27, 37, 42, 43, 46)
  A. Headache, vertigo, lightheadedness, faintness, tinnitus, roaring in ears
  B. Subjective sensitivity to cold, fatigability, lack of power of mental concentration
  C. Lesions in the optic fundus
IV. Gastrointestinal (30, 44, 56)
  A. Anorexia, nausea, flatulence, constipation, diarrhea
V. Genitourinary (8, 19, 49)
  A. Menstrual irregularity, cessation of flow, profuse flow
  B. Urinary frequency, nocturia, hyposthenuria
  C. Loss of libido and/or potency
VI. Metabolic
  A. Low-grade, sustained fever
  B. BMR increased 10 to 15 per cent above base line

In general, all these effects are the result of the blood's decreased ability to transport and deliver the oxygen required to meet the tissues' metabolic demands. If, as implied by the tissue dysfunction giving rise to the above signs and symptoms, the oxygen demands are not being met, one might expect a decreased total-body oxygen consumption. But this has not been demonstrated. Indeed, a 10 to 15 per cent increase in oxygen consumption has been reported by some investigators. Various compensatory mechanisms come into play, some of which have been adequately described.

If the supply of oxygen to tissues depended solely on the hemoglobin concentration, in severe anemia the oxygen requirement could not be met. Normally blood contains 15.6 Gm of hemoglobin per 100 ml. Since each gram of hemoglobin carries 1.36 ml of oxygen at complete saturation, arterial blood carries 21 ml of oxygen per 100 ml. Venous blood contains approximately 15 ml of oxygen per 100 ml, 6 ml of oxygen having been removed by the tissues. If the hemoglobin level of the circulating blood drops much below 5 Gm per 100 ml, less than 6 ml of oxygen per 100 ml of blood is available for tissue. The major adjustments are an increased rate of blood flow and deviation of blood from less to more vital areas.

The cardiac output remains constant until the hemoglobin level of the circu-

* Whyte (54) gives these figures: for each 10 per cent of deficiency of hemoglobin, the blood volume is decreased 4 per cent of the normal volume; for every 10 per cent fall in hemoglobin, the plasma volume increases by 2 per cent of the normal volume.

lating blood falls to about 7 or 8 Gm per 100 ml (10, 53). The output then increases proportionate to hemoglobin decrease and may reach four to five times the normal. The pulse rate,* stroke volume, and circulation rate increase; the viscosity of the blood and the peripheral resistance decrease (6, 7, 15, 20, 47). The result is that the work of the heart is only slightly increased. However, because of the peculiarities of the coronary circulation, the myocardium has only a borderline oxygen supply. As indicated by the extreme unsaturation of coronary sinus blood at rest (17), any increase in oxygen delivery must be effected by increased flow. Additional strain may overload the system, and angina, etc. result (3, 4, 17, 31, 57).

There is also an increase in the percentage of oxygen leaving hemoglobin and an increase in efficiency of carbon dioxide transport. Therefore, in moderate anemia (about 10 Gm of hemoglobin per 100 ml of blood), there may be little clinical evidence of circulatory changes at rest. Only with exertion do weakness, palpitations, dyspnea, etc. become evident.

Results obtained in recent work have indicated that in anemia a mild degree of arterial hypoxia is present. In severe anemia values of oxygen saturation in the high 80 per cent range are not unusual. This is due in part to a decreased diffusing capacity of the lung and a normal absolute, but relatively increased, venous admixture (33, 38). This degree of arterial unsaturation has been explained on the basis of a shift in the oxygen dissociation curve that has long been known to exist in many types of anemia (23, 36). This shift is to the right so that at arterial oxygen tensions (flat portion of the dissociation curve) only slight arterial unsaturation occurs, but at tissue oxygen tensions (steep portion of the dissociation curve) oxygen is more readily available to cells than normal. The displacement of

the dissociation curve is demonstrable by in vivo techniques in patients with hemoglobin levels less than 9 Gm per 100 ml of blood; it is moderate in those with levels 6.5 to 9 Gm per 100 ml, and more marked in those with levels less than 6.5 Gm per 100 ml. This shift in the dissociation curve is therefore beneficial in anemia since it facilitates the transport of oxygen from the lungs to the tissues, allowing an increase from 25 to 65 per cent in utilization of arterial oxygen (25). A relative intraerythrocyte acidity has been demonstrated in anemia but explains only part of the changes seen. Patients with various hemoglobinopathies might be expected to present a special situation (35). Oxygen dissociation studies made on dialyzed hemoglobin S show normal behavior of the pigment. The in vivo dissociation curve and the dissociation curve obtained using intact cells are shifted to the right. The shift in the dissociation curve is therefore not a result of the abnormal hemoglobin, but rather a result of the intracellular changes. However, in patients with sickle cell trait, a slight shift of the oxygen dissociation curve to the right has been demonstrated without any depression of the hemoglobin level of the circulating blood. It must be concluded that although several factors are known to influence the oxygen dissociation curve of red cells no explanations have been offered that satisfactorily and completely account for the changes observed in various situations.

The normal renal blood flow of 1,200 ml per minute may be reduced to 600 ml per minute in moderate anemia by mechanisms that direct blood to more vital areas (8, 9, 19). Even with this reduction in flow, an adequate supply of oxygen is brought to the kidneys. Because of the compensatory increase in plasma volume

---

* The mechanism by which the pulse rate is increased is unknown. The tissue(s) may have a plasma flow requirement that influences cardiac output by humoral or neural mechanisms.

when the red cell mass is reduced, the plasma flow per minute remains near normal, and clearance of blood urea nitrogen and other metabolites is usually unimpaired. However, there may be a specific tubular defect manifested by low specific gravity, albuminuria, and sodium chloride and water retention proportional to the hemoglobin deficit (49). Marked decreases in blood flow have also been observed in the skin and extremities (1, 2, 28) contributing to the preservation of the central circulation. Hepatic circulation is well maintained (30) and increases above normal as the cardiac output rises. Hepatic function is usually well maintained in severe anemia of acute (56) or slow (44) onset.

In general, the physiologic adjustments that take place when the hemoglobin concentration falls below a critical level of 7 Gm per 100 ml of blood are increased cardiac output, increased efficiency of carbon dioxide clearance, and deviation of blood to the most vital centers. But all are borderline adjustments and are easily overcome. Consequently patients are frequently comfortable and asymptomatic at rest in spite of significant hemoglobin deficit, but with exertion of almost any degree bothersome and noticeable defects become evident (5, 7, 48).

Bibliographic references for Chapter 4 begin on page 393.

CHAPTER FIVE

CLASSIFICATION OF THE ANEMIAS

TABLE 5.1.   Morphologic classification of the anemias

I. Macrocytic normochromic anemia (MCV 94 to 160 cu μ; MHC 32 to 36 Gm per 100 ml)

    A. Bone marrow shows abnormal ("megaloblastic") erythrocyte maturation (see Table 7.5)

        1. Pernicious anemia
        2. Sprue, idiopathic steatorrhea
        3. Megaloblastic anemia of pregnancy and puerperium
        4. Megaloblastic anemia of infancy
        5. *Diphyllobothrium latum* infestation
        6. Postgastrectomy: "surgical pernicious anemia" (occurring frequently after total gastrectomy, infrequently after subtotal gastrectomy)
        7. Intestinal abnormalities: diverticula, strictures, blind segments, terminal ileitis, resections
        8. Acute and chronic alcoholism and liver disease
        9. Dietary deficiency: vitamin B_{12} (extrinsic factor), folic acid, vitamin C (?)
      10. Refractory megaloblastic anemia
      11. Ingestion of anticonvulsant drugs or antifolic acid preparations (antimetabolites)

    B. Bone marrow does not show "megaloblastic" changes; usually shows "normoblastic" maturation

        1. Liver disease
        2. "Aplastic anemia," "hypoplastic anemia," refractory anemia of "chronic bone marrow failure"
        3. Associated with reticulocytosis
            a. Hemolytic with marrow response
            b. Posthemorrhagic with marrow response
        4. Scurvy (may be some element of maturation abnormality in bone marrow)
        5. Anemia secondary to multiple myeloma, myeloid metaplasia, uremia, myelophthisis, miliary tuberculosis (these anemias tend to become macrocytic when severe)

II. Normocytic normochromic anemia (MCV 80 to 94 cu μ; MHC 32 to 36 Gm per 100 ml)

    A. Sudden blood loss
    B. Hemolytic anemias
        1. Intracorpuscular defect (see Table 9.1)

TABLE 5.1   (*continued*)

        2. Extracorpuscular defect (see Table 9.1)
        3. Interaction of intra- and extracorpuscular abnormalities (see Table 9.1)
    C. Hemoglobin-red-cell mass deficit
        1. Chronic disease
           a. Infection: bacterial, viral, fungal
           b. Renal disease
           c. Malignancy
           d. Liver disease
           e. Rheumatoid arthritis
           f. Rheumatic fever
        2. Toxic agents
           a. Benzol
           b. Carbon tetrachloride
           c. Ionizing radiation
           d. Radiomimetic agents
           e. Antimitotic agents
           f. Antimetabolites
           g. Lead
        3. Malignancy
           a. Carcinoma
           b. Leukemia
           c. Lymphoma
           d. Multiple myeloma
           e. Myelosclerosis (myelofibrosis)
        4. Splenomegaly
          (See under Extracorpuscular abnormality, Table 9.1)
        5. Endocrine disorders
        6. Bone marrow failure (see Table 11.1)
           a. Aplastic (acquired or constitutional)
           b. Hypoplastic (acquired or constitutional)
    D. Hydremia associated with pregnancy
    E. Some compensated (or nearly compensated) hemolytic disorders
        1. Hemoglobinopathies (i.e., homozygous hemoglobin C disease; see Table 3.1)
        2. Hereditary spherocytosis $\leftarrow$ *Maybe ↑MCHC*
III. Microcytic normochromic anemia (MCV 60 to 80 cu μ; MCHC 32 to 36 Gm per 100 ml)   ↓   N
    A. Hemoglobin-red-cell mass deficit
        1. Chronic disease
           a. Infection: bacterial, viral, fungal
           b. Renal disease
           c. Malignancy
           d. Liver disease
           e. Rheumatoid arthritis
           f. Rheumatic fever
         2. Toxic agents
           a. Benzol
           b. Carbon tetrachloride
           c. Ionizing radiation
           d. Radiomimetic agents
           e. Antimitotic agents
           f. Antimetabolites
           g. Lead
        3. Malignancy
           a. Carcinoma
           b. Leukemia

TABLE 5.1 (*continued*)

      c. Lymphoma
      d. Multiple myeloma
      e. Myelosclerosis (myelofibrosis)
    4. Splenomegaly
      (See under Extracorpuscular abnormality, Table 9.1)
    5. Endocrine disorders

IV. Microcytic hypochromic anemia (MCV 60 to 80 cu μ; MCHC 20 to 30 Gm per 100 ml)
  A. Iron-lack anemia
    1. Chronic blood loss
    2. Outgrowth of supplies (in infants, adolescents)
    3. Excessive demand (in repeated pregnancies)
    4. Defective absorption
      a. Malabsorption syndrome
      b. Sprue, idiopathic steatorrhea, celiac disease, gastrectomy, etc.
    5. Copper deficiency: abnormal protein metabolism (very rare, only in infants)
  B. Chronic lead poisoning (mild hypochromicity)
  C. Thalassemia syndrome (see Table 3.1)
    1. Alone as trait or anemia
    2. Associated with hemoglobinopathy
  D. Vitamin B_6 (pyridoxine) abnormality (rare)
  E. "Crude liver factor" abnormality (rare)
  F. "Familial hypochromic microcytic anemia" (rare)
  G. "Sideroachrestic" anemia

TABLE 5.2. Physiologic classification of anemias caused by increased loss or destruction of hemoglobin-red-cell mass (with physiologically hyperactive bone marrow)

I. Anemia resulting from blood loss
  A. Acute
    1. External: building blocks (especially iron) not available for re-utilization
    2. Internal: building blocks (especially iron) subsequently available for reutilization
  B. Chronic
    1. External: building blocks (especially iron) not available
    2. Internal
      a. Lungs: iron not available for reutilization (idiopathic pulmonary hemosiderosis)
      b. Elsewhere: building blocks (especially iron) available for reutilization

II. Anemia resulting from excessive destruction of red cells (see Table 9.1)
  A. Owing to intracorpuscular defects
    1. Hereditary defect of red blood cell
      a. Hereditary spherocytosis
      b. Ovalocytosis
      c. Thalassemia
      d. Stomatocytosis
      e. Hereditary nonspherocytic disease
      f. Hemoglobinopathies (see Table 3.1)
        (1) Sickle cell anemia

Table 5.2   (*continued*)

          (2) Hemoglobin C disease
          (3) Other
          (4) Combinations with other defects
       g. Primaquine-sensitive hemolytic anemia (glucose-6-phosphate dehydrogenase deficiency); favism
       h. Erythropoietic porphyria
    2. Acquired defect of red blood cell
       a. Paroxysmal nocturnal hemoglobinuria
       b. Thermal injury
       c. Deficiency disease (vitamin B_{12}, folic acid, iron deficiency)
B. Owing to interaction of intra- and extracorpuscular abnormalities
    1. Primaquine-sensitive hemolytic anemia
    2. Favism
    3. Lead poisoning
    4. Vitamin B_{12} or folic acid deficiency
    5. Thermal injury
C. Owing to extracorpuscular abnormalities
    1. Immune mechanism: antibodies demonstrable
       a. Naturally occurring immunity
          (1) Anti-A and anti-B immunity (responsible for most hemolytic transfusion reactions)
       b. Acquired immunity
          (1) Rh factor immunity
          (2) Subgroup factor immunity
          (3) Cold agglutinin reaction
             (a) Paroxysmal cold hemoglobinuria
          (4) Cold hemolysin reaction (luetic, nonluetic)
             (a) Paroxysmal cold hemoglobinuria
          (5) "Autoimmunity"
             (a) Idiopathic acquired hemolytic anemia
             (b) Secondary or symptomatic acquired hemolytic anemia (secondary to leukemia, lymphoma, disseminated lupus)
             (c) Favism
             (d) Reaction to drugs (Fuadin, quinine, etc.)
             (e) Thrombotic thrombocytopenic purpura (rare)
    2. Nonimmune mechanism (no antibody demonstrable)
       a. Infectious agents
          (1) Red cell parasitism
             (a) Malaria
             (b) Oroya fever *Bartonella bacilliformis*
          (2) Bacterial toxins or hemolysins
             (a) *Cl. welchii*
             (b) Hemolytic streptococcus, bacterioides
       b. Chemicals toxic to normal cells
          (1) Arsine
          (2) Heavy metals: lead, etc.
          (3) Naphthalene
          (4) Phenylhydrazine
          (5) Oxidant compounds
          (6) Surface active compounds
          (7) Water (intravenous)
    3. Unknown mechanism
       a. Splenomegaly
          (1) Cirrhosis
          (2) Gaucher's disease
          (3) Splenic vein thrombosis

TABLE 5.2 (*continued*)

        (4) Myeloid metaplasia
        (5) Infection
    b. Acute and chronic infections
    c. Acute renal disease (hemolytic uremic syndrome)
    d. Chronic renal disease
    e. Malignancy
    f. Chronic inflammatory disorders
        (1) Rheumatic fever
    g. Infantile pyknocytosis
    h. Acanthocytosis

TABLE 5.3. Physiologic classification of anemias caused by decreased production of hemoglobin-red-cell mass (with physiologically hypoactive bone marrow)

I. Anemia resulting from specific deficiency (see Table 7.5)
  A. Vitamin B_{12} deficiency
    1. Defective diet (very rare)
    2. Deficiency of intrinsic factor
      a. Pernicious anemia
      b. Total, subtotal gastrectomy
    3. Defective absorption
      a. Sprue, regional enteritis, intestinal resection, blind loop syndrome
      b. Tapeworm (*Diphyllobothrium latum*) infestation
  B. Folic acid abnormality
    1. Defective diet
    2. Defective absorption
      a. Sprue
      b. Intestinal resection
    3. Defective utilization
      a. Scurvy; megaloblastic anemia of infancy
      b. Acute alcoholism and liver disease (?)
      c. Anticonvulsant drugs
    4. Increased requirement
      a. Pregnancy
      b. Hemolytic anemia
      c. Malignancy
    5. Etiology unknown
      a. Megaloblastic anemia of pregnancy
      b. Intestinal strictures, blind loop syndrome
  C. Vitamin C deficiency
    1. Induced deficiency of folic acid
    2. Pure dietary vitamin C deficiency (?)
  D. Iron lack
    1. Increased loss of iron
      a. Blood loss
    2. Increased requirements
      a. Pregnancy
      b. Growth
    3. Decreased intake
      a. Defective diet
      b. Malabsorption (chronic)
  E. Pyridoxine abnormality
  F. Crude liver factor abnormality

TABLE 5.3   (*continued*)

    G. Copper deficiency (?)

    H. Protein deficiency or abnormality

        1. Kwashiorkor

  II. Anemia resulting from endocrine abnormality

    A. Thyroid

    B. Pituitary

    C. Adrenal

    D. Erythropoietin (?)

 III. Anemia resulting from mechanical interference with marrow function

    A. Inadequate capacity (?)

        1. Newborn

        2. Premature

    B. Myelophthisis

        1. Malignancy

        2. Myelofibrosis

        3. Osteopetrosis

        4. Xanthomatosis (histiocytosis X)

        5. Miliary tuberculosis

 IV. Anemia resulting from relative marrow failure

    A. Infection

    B. Renal disease

    C. Malignancy

    D. Toxic agents

    E. Liver disease

    F. Rheumatic fever, rheumatoid arthritis

    G. Collagen diseases

    H. Endocrine disorders

  V. Anemia of bone marrow failure (aplastic or hypoplastic; see Table 11.1)

    A. Constitutional

    B. Acquired

        1. Toxic agents: antimetabolites, antimitotic agents, gold, arsenic, chloramphenicol, etc.

        2. Idiopathic

PART III] THE RED CELL: PRODUCTION

CHAPTER SIX

NORMAL RED CELL PRODUCTION*

The main function of the cells of the erythropoietic maturation series is to provide suitable vehicles for the synthesis, transport, and protection of hemoglobin molecules: to produce a respiratory pigment capable of accepting, transporting, and delivering oxygen and to provide an environment where the pigment can be maintained in its functional state.

Previous sections have dealt with the manufacture of heme and globin, and with the metabolism of iron, as these factors are involved in the biosynthesis of hemoglobin. Since *de novo* hemoglobin biosynthesis takes place within the immature cell, *effective* production can only be accomplished by the proper multiplication and maturation of erythropoietic precursors in the bone marrow and the escape therefrom by the more mature forms. A consideration will be made of normal (this chapter) and abnormal (next chapter) erythropoiesis from the point of view of the factors controlling multiplication, maturation, and release of erythrocytes and the alterations that result when controls are deranged or requisite factors lacking. It is evident that for the normal production of normal erythrocytes there are required multiplication and maturation of a most highly differentiated series of cells, the formation of unique enzyme systems and cytoplasmic constituents, and the precise si-

multaneous or sequential interaction of many factors over a considerable span of time. Table 6.1 shows the chemical composition of human erythrocytes and gives an indication of the multiplicity of factors known by animal, human, and natural experiment to be necessary for red cell production. Significant interference with, or abnormality of, the most critical of these factors usually results in a decrease in the number of adequately filled, properly functioning, normally surviving red cells delivered to the peripheral blood. Disease is thereby evidenced. Frequently the disease can be characterized by morphologic abnormalities of the red cells that are expressions of underlying biochemical defects. It is a great convenience of hematology that in many situations readily observable morphologic alterations can be accurately interpreted as indicators of specific biochemical alterations.

SITE AND SEQUENCE OF RED CELL PRODUCTION

Of the many theories that have been advanced concerning the ultimate progenitor(s) of the circulating cells, none can be supported by critical evidence capable of only one interpretation. Accordingly,

* General references and review articles: 8, 13, 17, 20, 25, 34, 35, 43, 48, 49, 55, 63, 70, 85, 88, 90, 93, 100, 101, 108, 110.

TABLE 6.1. Approximate chemical composition of human red blood corpuscles

	Gm/100 ml RBC
Hemoglobin	33.50
Methemoglobin	0.50
Nonhemoglobin protein	0.87
Lipids	0.48
Glucose	0.83
Minerals	0.67
Water	73.15

	mg/100 ml RBC
Stroma	
Proteins, total	500
Stromatin	300
Elinin	200
Blood group substances	
Enzymes	
Lipids, total	480
Phosphatides	
Cephalin	133
Lecithin	106
Sphingomyelin	73
Cholesterol (free)	130
Cholesterol esters	29
Neutral fats, cerebrosides	98
Glycolytic system, total	188
Glucose	74
Reducing substances calculated as glucose (2, 3-diphosphoglycerate, ATP, hexose-phosphates, DPN, TPN)	114
Water-soluble constituents other than proteins	
Glutathione	70
Ergothioneine	3.3
Elemental composition, total	767
Phosphorus	
Organic acid-soluble	55
Inorganic	3
ATP	10
Hexose mono- & diphosphate	15
2, 3-diphosphoglycerate	28
Sulfur	
Neutral	6
Inorganic sulfate	0.04
Ethereal sulfate	0.04
Copper	0.115
Zinc	1.44
Lead	0.057
Tin	0.026
Manganese	0.019
Aluminum	0.007
Silver	trace
K+	420
Na+	45
Ca++	
Mg++	3
Cl−	180

Table 6.1   (*continued*)

Vitamins and coenzymes

Thiamine	0.008
Cocarboxylase	0.01
Riboflavin	0.022
Flavine-adenine dinucleotide	0.075
Niacin	1.0
Diphosphopyridine nucleotide	10.0
Triphosphopyridine nucleotide	1.2
Pyridoxine	0.005
Pantothenic acid	0.025
Coenzyme A	0.144
Ascorbic acid	1.0
Adenosine (mono-, di-, triphosphate)	62

Compounds related to hemoglobin

Iron	115
Protoporphyrin (free)	0.031
Coproporphyrin (free)	0.002

Miscellaneous

Amino acids	30
Total NPN	44
Nucleotide-N	13
Amino acid-N	7.4
Urea	20
Creatine	2
Creatinine	8
Uric acid, uric acid riboside	

From Wintrobe, M. M., Clinical Hematology, ed. 5, p. 124, Lea & Febiger, Philadelphia, 1961.

vigorous proponents of the various monophyletic, dualistic, or polyphyletic accounts of hematopoiesis are at work. Unfortunately some have employed terms and assigned names disregarding usage by others, so that there is considerable duplication, overlap, and private definition, with much resulting confusion. No standard system of nomenclature or definition of cell types has been generally accepted, despite numerous reviews and "official" proposals. The following account makes use of terms and definitions that have been widely employed in investigation and teaching; however, this terminology necessarily cannot be supported any more convincingly than any other.

Bone Marrow

The adult red cell is produced by a process called normoblastic erythropoiesis. In normal bone marrow the formation of both granulocytes and erythrocytes takes place extravascularly, in the stroma of the marrow outside the sinusoids. Evidence for this has been at hand for some time from morphologic studies using light microscopy (17) and more recently electron microscopy (77, 107, 111). According to these observations the marrow is structured as follows. Leading into the marrow cavity through foramina in the bony cortex are the nutrient arteries. Inside the cortex these branch into distributing arterioles, which in turn give rise to an endosteal sinusoidal bed. From this sinusoidal bed penetrating sinusoids lead to a central vein: in cross section the marrow structure has been likened to a wheel with rim, spokes, and hubs. The marrow sinusoids are almost unique in their simplicity of structure: they are composed of a single layer of flattened littoral reticular cells (large mononuclear cells demonstrable with vital dyes). The walls are of variable thickness and are frequently discontinuous. The reticular cells are usually associated with a ground substance, but a basement membrane is not present unless the sinusoidal wall is adjacent to fat cells, in which instance a definite membrane with fibrillar structure is found. Blood is present within the sinusoids of the marrow, but for the most part erythroblasts and other hematopoietic and connective tissue elements are outside; no lymphatics are demonstrable. The reticular cells are unstable. If they become phagocytic or differentiate into other cell types, they leave their position in the sinusoid, making a gap in the wall. Perfusion with particulate matter (Thorotrast, etc.) reveals extremely rapid distribution in the intrasinusoidal and extrasinusoidal compartments.

The marrow is probably the most unstable tissue of the body and has been described as composed of "fugitive vessels, capable through the motility and multipotentiality of the reticular cell wall of changing the course, varying the completeness of the wall—even of forming and disappearing—in response to changing requirements for marrow functions of erythropoiesis, myelopoiesis, antibody formation, phagocytosis, lymphatic drainage, blood flow and delivery of cells to the circulation or sequestration of cells from the circulation" (107).

Having been formed outside the marrow sinusoids, the more adult red cells gain access to the intravascular compartment by diapedesis and probably not by forced entry brought about through pressure generated by a growing mass of cells as previously postulated (3, 95).

Erythrocyte Maturation Sequence

The most immature form of the red cell that can be identified as belonging to the erythrocyte series is the proerythroblast. Accurate identification can be made on the basis of both morphologic and biochemical criteria (radioiron uptake,

DNA, RNA). By processes of multiplication and maturation the proerythroblast produces adult red cells. Like all other blood cell progenitors, it is derived from a multipotential primitive cell, the stem cell. Curiously enough, even though calculations indicate that the stem cell must be present in significant numbers in the marrow, it has not yet been satisfactorily and acceptably identified by either morphologic or biochemical criteria. When the primitive stem cell undergoes division, one resultant cell is directed into a specific maturation sequence; the other cell remains undifferentiated and multipotential so that depletion of stem cells does not occur. The factor(s) that determines which daughter cell remains undifferentiated and which starts along a maturation sequence is unknown. A precise mechanism must exist, however, since even the most potent stimulus or urgent need for specific cells must not be allowed to deplete the stem cell pool.

During normoblastic erythropoiesis, maturation and mitotic divisions occur in a definite sequence that can now be roughly quantitated by various techniques (1, 2, 14, 56). For example, most of the iron destined for hemoglobin biosythesis is taken into the cell at the proerythroblast or early erythroblast stage. If radioactive iron is employed as an in vivo label, grain counts can be made by radioautography for the young cells and then similarly determined for the later stages (1, 2). Each mitotic division will result in halving the grain count of a labeled cell. It has been determined that approximately three mitotic divisions occur during the evolution of a proerythroblast into a normoblast (Figure 6.1). By timed studies it has been concluded that the intermitotic period is about 20 hours, and consequently the change from proerythroblast to normoblast takes approximately 2 days. At this time the nucleus has become pyknotic, the cell unable to carry out DNA synthesis (14) and con-

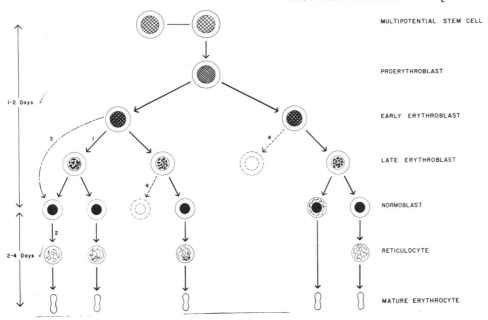

FIGURE 6.1.   Schema of erythropoiesis and possible mechanisms of action of erythro-poietin. Available evidence supports the conclusion that a main rate of erythropoietin stimulation is upon formation of proerythroblast from stem cells. Red cell production could also be increased by (1) shortening of intermitotic generation times, (2) accelera-tion of maturation during nonmitotic growth phase, (3) acceleration of maturation by omission of one or more intermediate mitotic divisions, and (4) diminution of death rate of red cell precursors (ineffective erythropoiesis). (Adapted from Erslev, A. J., Blood 14:386, 1959, and London, I. M., Harvey Lectures, series 56, p. 153, Academic Press, New York, 1961)

sequently incapable of further division. The nucleus then disappears from the cell, probably by extrusion (111). These direct observations agree very well with calculations based on marrow differential counts, mitotic indices, assumed time per mitosis, and known life span of the adult erythrocyte.

Following loss of the nucleus, the cell *usually* retains some of its RNA, account-ing for its polychromatophilic properties in Wright's stain and its reticulated char-acteristics in cresyl blue. The events of nuclear maturation, contraction, and ex-trusion are not always simultaneous with the cytoplasmic changes and hemoglobin formation. While some reticulocytes con-tain a pyknotic nucleus, most do not; orthochromatic normoblasts may be seen that develop into adult erythrocytes im-mediately after the nucleus is lost, with-

out the usual polychromatophilic or non-nucleated reticulocyte stage. Other perturbations come into the otherwise orderly maturation sequence (96, 97). Some 10 to 15 per cent of cells die at various stages of development according to pigment studies (see Ineffective Eryth-ropoiesis, page 139), and some few cells apparently skip mitotic division(s), since a small but definite proportion of heavily labeled reticulocytes is found by the ra-dioautographic grain-counting technique (1). However, it is evident that the vast majority of erythrocytes develop by im-perceptible gradations, through the or-derly controlled sequence arbitrarily divided into proerythroblast, early eryth-roblast, late erythroblast, normoblast, and reticulocyte, to mature red cells, with the usual number of mitoses (three) taking place in the proper time (4 days).

Very little is known concerning the mechanisms whereby cells are released from the marrow for delivery to the peripheral blood. Diapedesis of normoblasts and reticulocytes from their extravascular developmental site has been pictured in electron microscopy (3), and attention has been called to the mutual adhesiveness of the more primitive marrow cells. Reticulocytes are large and sticky and perhaps because of this are retained in the marrow (46) 2 to 4 days before release into the peripheral blood. If they prematurely escape into the peripheral blood, these large, sticky cells are filtered out by the spleen, in which they are probably held to full maturity (50).

DISTRIBUTION OF NUCLEATED, RETICULATED, AND ADULT ERYTHROCYTES IN BONE MARROW AND CIRCULATING BLOOD

The reticulocytes found in the marrow are larger, less mature, and contain more reticulum when stained supravitally than the reticulocytes of the peripheral blood. They are found outside the sinusoids in the "fixed tissue" of the marrow. Recent studies on humans indicate that all the non-nucleated and nonreticulated erythrocytes are in the circulating blood and that no adult red cells are present extravascularly in the normal marrow, which contains a "pool" of reticulocytes approximately equal in number to the nucleated erythrocytic cells. With appropriate hypoxic stimulation these marrow reticulocytes can be shifted to the peripheral blood; if total shift takes place the number of circulating reticulocytes is approximately doubled.

Reasonably accurate figures are now available for the number of cells present in the "fixed tissue," or stroma, of the marrow as well as in the circulating blood. These are given in Table 6.2 according to Finch and compiled from data presented by Donohue and Reiff (18, 19, 82).

THE ERYTHRON: CONCEPT AND CONTROL OF STEADY STATE

"Erythron" is a term employed by Castle and Minot (12) to indicate the combined mass of mature and immature red cells, the sum total of all cells in the erythrocyte series, extravascular as well as intravascular. The concept of the erythron is valuable since it emphasizes the functional unity of the red cells and their precursors whether in the peripheral blood or bone marrow. Since the erythron is maintained remarkably constant for prolonged periods of time but can change in orderly fashion in response to internal and external stimuli, regulating mechanisms must exist. Although the existence of these regulatory mechanisms had long been presumed, it is only recently that satisfactory experimental evidence has delineated something of their nature and mode of action. Realizing that the prime function of hemoglobin is to transport oxygen from air to tissue, Paul Bert in 1878 predicted that at high altitudes with low partial pressure of oxygen, physiologic adjustments would occur to compensate for the decrease in available oxygen so that by means of increase in the mass of circulating red cells and hemoglobin a normal amount of oxygen could be transported. His prediction was rapidly fulfilled by the demonstration of polycythemia in animals and individuals who resided at high altitudes. This remarkable insight implied the existence of regulatory mechanisms activated by tissue hypoxia and has evolved into the now generally accepted hypothesis that *the rate of red cell production* is related to tissue oxygen tension.

To maintain the erythron at a constant value a steady state is required in which the rate of cell production is precisely balanced by the rate of destruction. In the absence of disease, the life span of the red cell and consequently the rate of cell destruction is normal and con-

TABLE 6.2.   Distribution of nucleated, reticulated, and adult erythrocytes in bone marrow and circulating blood

Cell type	No. of cells per Kg body weight ($\times 10^9$)	Relative no. of cells	Estimated volume of cells (cu μ)	Total volume for 70–Kg subject ($\times 10^{12}$ cu μ)	
Nucleated red blood cells	5	1.5	250	88 ⎫	6% in
Marrow reticulocytes	5	1.5	120	44 ⎭	marrow
Circulating reticulocytes	3.3	1.0	100	23 ⎫	94% in peripheral blood
Adult erythrocytes	330	100	90	2,000 ⎭	eral blood

Adapted from Finch, C. A., Hematology Manual, p. 1, 1960 (privately printed).

stant. The steady state of the erythron is therefore controlled by changes in the rate of red cell production. The fundamental stimulus controlling erythropoiesis depends upon the relation between oxygen supply and metabolic requirements of tissues.

The net production of an article of given specifications can be speeded by increasing the rate of flow along an assembly line or, lacking this, by setting up a second assembly line. Theoretically red cell production could be controlled by alteration in the rate at which primitive cells are formed and differentiate into proerythroblasts (adding assembly lines) or by alteration in the rate at which the proerythroblasts multiply and mature (increasing the rate of flow). There is no evidence that in any situation the time required for a cell to pass from the first stage of differentiation to final maturation into a *normal erythrocyte* is shortened.[*] Consequently it has been concluded that as long as the metabolic environment is adequate the rate of red cell production[†] is determined solely by the rate of stem cell differentiation (the number of production lines set up). Red cell production depends upon alterations in the rate of erythropoiesis, which in turn are effected not by speeding the rate of maturation of the red cells but by increasing the number of stem cells and the number of red cell precursors formed therefrom.

PHYSIOLOGY OF TISSUE OXYGENATION

Oxygen is picked up in the lungs from inspired air, bound to the hemoglobin, and transported to the tissue capillaries. Here the oxygen must be at a pressure high enough to permit it to leave the capillary, diffuse through the tissue, and reach even the most distant cells. In highly vascular tissue a fairly low mean capillary oxygen pressure will be sufficient to ensure an adequate supply to all tissue cells, whereas a poorly vascularized tissue must depend on a high mean capillary oxygen tension. The mean capillary oxygen tension that determines the tissue perfusion pressure lies somewhere between the arterial and the venous oxygen tensions. Arterial oxygen tension is the same throughout the body and is determined by the oxygen tension in the atmosphere and the functional and ana-

[*] The rate of mitotic division and the intermitotic division time of individual nucleated red cells remains constant, as determined by radioautographic grain counting; the ratio of erythroblasts to normoblasts remains constant; and the metabolism of already formed nucleated cells is not altered despite widely varying conditions of anemia and anoxia (21).

[†] Under certain circumstances the time spent by the maturing cell in the bone marrow may be shortened by delivery to the peripheral blood at unusually early stages of development (nucleated red cells, reticulocytes). This is not really a change in the rate of maturation but rather a shift in the site at which the maturation takes place, i.e., from bone marrow to peripheral blood.

tomic integrity of the lungs. Venous oxygen tension varies from tissue to tissue and is determined by the amount of oxygen delivered, less that consumed. The amount delivered to a tissue depends on a number of factors: oxygen tension of inspired air, pulmonary function, hemoglobin concentration, cardiac output, and the vascular distribution of circulating blood among the individual tissues. From this amount of oxygen a certain fraction is extracted and consumed in the tissue. The oxygen tension in the capillary blood and in the venous blood leaving the tissue depends on the amount of oxygen left over and the shape of the oxygen dissociation curve. Consequently, many factors in addition to the hemoglobin concentration are involved in the establishment of the pressure gradient along which the oxygen moves. A change in any one will result in a change in the oxygen gradient, and the supply of oxygen will exceed or fall short of the demand. The resulting change in cellular metabolism will, in some way, mobilize compensatory mechanisms until the steady state is restored. In the individual tissue there may be an increase or decrease in the vascularity with a change in the distance between the cells and the nearest functioning capillary and a change in the amount of blood which perfuses the tissue. Furthermore, the mean capillary oxygen tension may be altered by appropriate changes in the oxygen dissociation curve, in the pulmonary vital capacity, in the cardiac output, and in the rate of red cell production. Of all these mechanisms, a change in the number of active tissue capillaries appears to be the most common compensatory response to minor local fluctuations in the degree of tissue oxygenation. However, an increase or a decrease in red cell production appears the preferred way by which tissues compensate for major and prolonged changes in tissue oxygenation. Since alterations in the red cell production only slowly effect a change in the oxygen-carrying capacity of blood, temporary pulmonary and cardiovascular adjustments protect the tissues until a new steady state has been restored. If the red cell mass decreases, the hemoglobin concentration and the oxygen-carrying capacity are diminished, and a greater fraction of the transported oxygen has to be extracted by the tissues to meet cellular demands. The arteriovenous oxygen difference increases, the mean capillary oxygen tension, or partial pressure, falls decreasing the pressure head required to facilitate adequate diffusion of oxygen, so that cells situated at a distance from capillaries become hypoxic. Conversely, increases in the red cell mass result in small arteriovenous differences, high pressure maintaining diffusion, and hyperoxia of cells. The evidence now available stands in strong support of the above-outlined presumption that the mechanisms controlling the erythron (cell production and circulating red cell mass) are triggered by changes in the tissue oxygen tension. Many clinical and experimental observations indicate that a decreased supply of oxygen to tissues (such as occurs at high altitudes, in pulmonary disorders, and in shunts carrying deoxygenated into oxygenated blood) results in increased erythropoiesis; an increased supply of oxygen to tissues (such as occurs when air with high oxygen tension is breathed, when polycythemia is induced by transfusions, or when the tissue demand for oxygen is decreased as in hypothyroidism, hypophysectomy, and starvation) results in decreased erythropoiesis.

It should not necessarily be presumed that an effect of tissue hyperoxia is inhibition of erythropoiesis but rather that the stimulus operative at normal oxygenation is to some extent diminished. Recent studies indicate that the erythropoietic tissue of hyperoxic subjects is very sensitive to stimuli (47) calling for increased red cell production.

FUNDAMENTAL STIMULUS TO ERYTHROPOIESIS

The fundamental stimulus to erythropoiesis and consequently to changes in size of the erythron is hypoxia (35). The sequence is as follows: the rate of red cell production determines the size of the hemoglobin mass, which determines the circulating hemoglobin concentration; the hemoglobin concentration determines the degree of tissue oxygenation, which determines the rate of cell production.*

DEFINITION OF ANEMIA

As will be discussed in Chapter 10, there is no general agreement upon the basis for the definition of anemia. Some maintain that anemia should be defined in terms of the *concentration* of hemoglobin in the peripheral blood. This position is taken because the oxygen supply to a tissue depends largely on the amount of functioning oxygen-containing hemoglobin that is perfusing the tissue, and the functional importance of the red cell mass is determined by the hemoglobin concentration it can maintain in the circulating blood. Others maintain that anemia should be defined in terms of the total hemoglobin-red-cell mass present in the body. This position is taken largely because of the physiology of polycythemia and situations that appear somewhat anomalous in terms of the former definition. For example, immediately following acute hemorrhage, the hemoglobin concentration temporarily remains the same as before hemorrhage; yet the subject obviously has a decreased hemoglobin-red-cell mass and compensatory mechanisms are immediately set in motion. Conversely, in the pregnant female, despite a decrease in hemoglobin concentration, there is an increase in absolute amount of hemoglobin: more hemoglobin than before the pregnancy, yet a lower hemoglobin concentration, and on that basis "anemia." Thus it would seem that the definition of anemia must be based upon the adequacy of oxygen supply to the tissue, which depends not only upon the concentration of functional hemoglobin but also on the rate of circulation and the adequacy of the functioning circulatory bed. This is most clearly illustrated by experimental "dilution anemia" induced by Dextran administration, where despite a drop in the concentration of the circulating hemoglobin and no change in the total hemoglobin-red-cell mass, the compensatory increases in cardiac output and capillary bed circulation result in better perfusion of the tissues and tissue hyperoxia so that erythropoiesis is reduced. However, a practical, workable definition of anemia taking into account all these conditions is patently impossible if only because tissue oxygen demands vary from tissue to tissue and from time to time. Therefore it would seem reasonable to define—arbitrarily—anemia on the basis of the concentration of the circulating hemoglobin. Abnormalities can then be readily identified by deviations from a normal range that has been determined by adequate statistical study.

Theoretically an equilibrium between oxygen supply and oxygen demand can be reached at almost any hemoglobin con-

* While the above hypothesis is reasonably derived from many observations and now is consistent with considerable experimental evidence, it must be acknowledged that other regulatory mechanisms may also exist. To account for the existence of a compensated hemolytic process (i.e., increased red cell production, increased red cell destruction, but normal hemoglobin level), it has been suggested that an inhibitor of erythropoiesis may develop in aging cells. If the inhibitor is prevented from forming or accumulating by premature red cell destruction, or if the inhibitor is removed (by bleeding, for example), then erythropoiesis will be allowed to increase beyond the normal level even in the presence of normal tissue oxygenation. There is no direct evidence in support of this position.

centration as long as pulmonary and cardiovascular adjustments are properly effected. In dogs, by measurement of oxygen consumption, arterial and venous oxygen concentrations, arterial pH, cardiac output, peripheral resistance, and maximum oxygen-transporting capacity at different hematocrit values but at maintained blood pressure, it was demonstrated that oxygen consumption *increased* as the hematocrit increased until the latter reached 42 per cent. At progressively higher hematocrit values, oxygen consumption decreased. By other calculations it was concluded that at a hematocrit of 42 per cent oxygen transport is maximal. Increasing the number of red cells of the blood increases the oxygen-carrying capacity but decreases the rate of flow by increasing the blood viscosity (Figure 10.1). An intermediate hematocrit value is therefore the one at which the oxygen-carrying and delivering capacity of flowing blood is the highest possible for a given perfusion pressure (16). Similar conclusions and values concern-

ing the normal, optimum, or "ideal" hematocrit have been reached from in vitro measurements of hematocrit, viscosity, and oxygen delivery in human blood (Figure 6.2). A general principle appears to operate in physiology that the average or normal is closely identified with, if not actually identical with, the optimal. (This obtains for physiologic, certainly not for intellectual, processes.)

SITE OF ACTION OF FUNDAMENTAL STIMULUS TO ERYTHROPOIESIS

Since erythropoiesis is stimulated under conditions in which oxygen delivery is insufficient to meet oxygen demand, and is restrained when the supply exceeds the demand, it was at one time assumed that a decrease in oxygen supply to the developing red cells themselves accelerated proliferative activity, while an excess of oxygen was suppressive. By this hypothesis, first proposed by Miescher in 1893 (69), hypoxia was thought to stimulate red cell production by acting directly on red cell precursors without intermedi-

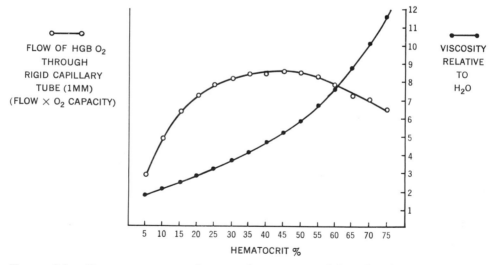

FIGURE 6.2.   Oxygen transport relative to hematocrit. Solid circles denote viscosity of whole blood relative to that of water at various hematocrits measured in Ostwald viscometer. Open circles denote flow of oxyhemoglobin through viscometer in arbitrary units at various blood hematocrits. (From Jandl, J. H., et al., *in* Page, L. B., and Culver, P. J. (ed.), Syllabus of Laboratory Examinations in Clinical Diagnosis, p. 100, Harvard University Press, Cambridge, Mass., 1960)

ary agents. Numerous studies designed to obtain direct evidence in support of this have not been fruitful.

Attempts by various workers to demonstrate marrow hypoxia by direct measurement of oxygen in aspirated samples or by polarography employing implanted electrodes in various types of anemia and following acute hemorrhage have yielded values not significantly different from normal (71). In vitro studies concerning the production of heme, the proliferative activity of the erythropoietic tissue, and the rate of hemoglobin synthesis show decreased function under hypoxic conditions and increased activity with increased oxygen tensions (65, 78). Because of the limitations of the techniques and short-time studies of necessity performed, these experiments do not form conclusive evidence against the theory that hypoxia stimulates marrow cells directly. However, since positive evidence for a factor in circulating blood has been forthcoming from other types of studies, attention has been directed to this line of investigation.

In 1950 Reissmann (83) found polycythemia and accelerated erythropoietic activity in the well-oxygenated partner of parabiotic rats when the other was exposed to low oxygen tensions. Since erythropoietic stimulation occurred despite demonstrably normal oxygenation, it was necessary to presume the existence of a factor in circulating blood derived from the anoxic rat. Since that observation patients have been studied with patent ductus arteriosus and reversed blood flow, a situation in which hypoxia (and cyanosis) is present in the lower half of the body while the upper half is normally oxygenated. Erythropoietic hyperplasia developed not only in the bone marrow of the hypoxic area but also in the normally oxygenated areas of the marrow. These studies made untenable the hypothesis that oxygen alone *directly* controls red cell production and caused a re-

evaluation of evidence supporting the theory that a circulating factor controls red cell production.

THE ERYTHROPOIETIC FACTOR (ERYTHROPOIETIN)

At the turn of the century Carnot and Déflandre (11) claimed that small amounts of serum obtained from anemic rabbits and infused into normal recipients doubled the red cell count in 3 days. Later workers showed that serum in the small amounts employed had no measurable activity and that this claimed rate of increase in red cell count did not occur under any physiologic circumstances. However, when plasma obtained from anemic (bled) rabbits was injected in *large quantities on successive days* to minimize dilution, reproducible results were obtained (37) in many different laboratories demonstrating erythropoietic stimulation and increases in reticulocyte count, hemoglobin level, hematocrit, and red cell count. Direct assessments of erythropoietic activity in such situations have been obtained by increases in (a) the number of nucleated red cells in the marrow, (b) the plasma clearance rate of radioactive iron, and (c) the red cell utilization of radioactive iron. The circulating factor responsible for stimulating erythropoiesis has been variously referred to as the erythropoietic factor, or erythropoietin, a name first suggested by Bonsdorff and Jalavisto in 1948 (6).

Physiology

Studies have also shown the erythropoiesis-stimulating factor to be present in increased amounts in the plasma of animals exposed to low oxygen tensions. Large amounts have been demonstrated in the plasma of animals in whom severe anemia had been induced by the hemolytic agent phenylhydrazine. Moreover, a proportional relation was demonstrable between the degree of induced hypoxia or anemia and the level of erythropoietic factor in the plasma (36). Increased amounts of erythropoietic factor appear within a few hours of induced hypoxia; the amounts increase gradually to a maximum at 12 to 24 hours and from 24 to 48 hours remain constant. With termination of hypoxia the level of circulating erythropoietic factor decreases rapidly over a 3- to 6-hour interval so that 50 per cent of the factor is cleared from plasma in 4 or 5 hours. However, if the bone marrow is damaged by x-ray or nitrogen mustard administration, the plasma level remains elevated for longer periods of time (60). The clearance of erythropoietin from plasma therefore depends in large part on bone marrow activity and presumably indicates utilization and degradation by erythropoietic cells during stimulation. When the imbalance of oxygen supply and demand is of minor degree, no excess erythropoietin is found in the plasma or urine: utilization equals production. But when a major, abrupt imbalance occurs, erythropoietin builds up in the plasma and urine because its supply exceeds the rate of utilization by the erythropoietic tissue.

Owing to limitations in the assay techniques mentioned below, it has not been possible to demonstrate conclusively in human beings that erythropoietic factor activity is decreased below normal with hyperoxia or induced polycythemia. Suggestive but indirect evidence is available.* The fact that it has not been possible to detect reliably normal or subnormal levels of erythropoietin has led some workers to propose that erythropoietin is produced only in response to significant stress hypoxia and is therefore a "panic mechanism" and not truly a regulator of physiologic erythropoiesis concerned with day-to-day fluctuations. However, within the limits of accuracy of the available methods the level of erythropoietic factor reflects in a general way the tissue oxygen tension. Since, in addition, its appearance in the peripheral blood seems to precede the increase in bone marrow erythropoietic activity, one requirement for a mediating "hormone" relaying information about the degree of tissue oxygenation to the bone marrow is satisfactorily fulfilled.

The ultimate test to certify the presence of erythropoietin must depend upon the demonstration of an increase in the number of cells stimulated to develop from the stem cell pool into the erythron or an increase in the size of the erythron: an enlargement of the total mass of red cell precursors and an unequivocal increase in the hemoglobin-red-cell mass. In actuality these criteria have seldom been met, and much confusion has resulted from lack of consideration of these basic principles. Most of the assay techniques—unfortunately almost of practical necessity—have substituted one or two readily obtainable measurements on the presumption that in the particular situation under study an accurate indication will be given of erythron augmentation. The measurements most often used are red blood count; hemoglobin concentration, hematocrit, and reticulocyte increase; alteration in bone marrow cellu-

---

* Animals made polycythemic by transfusion so that tissue hyperoxia is present show relatively greater response to the administration of known amounts of erythropoietic factor than do normal animals. Suggestively, the level of endogenously produced erythropoietic factor is lower in the hyperoxic than the normal. In addition, the observation demonstrates that hyperoxia does not inhibit erythropoiesis but rather that under these circumstances the activity is potentially responsive (47). Recent observations made employing hypertransfused rats and the appearance of radioiron in the red cells of the peripheral blood as indicators of erythropoietic activity show that the erythropoietic activity of normal rat serum is about 25 per cent of that of the serum of rats made acutely anoxic and *greater* than that of the serum of hypertransfused rats (81).

In this connection it may be pointed out that a thermostable factor in the plasma of animals with transfusion polycythemia has recently been described (54) that *inhibits* erythropoiesis. Confirmation of this work will be awaited with interest.

larity, both in vivo and in vitro (22, 68, 86); changes in the ratio of erythrocyte precursors to granulocyte precursors in the marrow; radioactive iron turnover; and red cell utilization of radioactive iron. Although in most instances the use of one or more of these measurements has been legitimate in that changes in the erythron are undoubtedly indicated, numerous exceptions have occurred, some of which will be pointed out below.

Moreover, it must be acknowledged that the presently available assay techniques—of necessity in vivo procedures—leave much to be desired in the way of sensitivity, standardization, and reproducibility. The most direct and convincing method of demonstrating the erythropoietic factor in plasma depends on the infusion of large volumes of plasma (20 to 30 per cent of the animal's blood volume daily for 2 to 3 weeks) into an adequate number of recipients of the same species and the observation of the erythropoietic effect in terms of reticulocyte response and subsequent hemoglobin and red cell changes. Normal plasma must be used as a control. Most of the basic information regarding erythropoietic factor obtained by means of this crude, laborious, and time-consuming technique is unquestionably sound. Even so, the responses obtained are not quantitatively equivalent to the changes observed subsequent to the animal's exposure to hypoxia even though the plasma infusions may be continued for prolonged periods.

Bioassay

Innumerable variations on this bioassay theme have been tried out—almost as many as the number of investigators working on the problem—but as yet no completely reliable method reproducible from one laboratory to the next has become accepted. These variations in the assay procedures make critical comparisons difficult (40, 52). No unit of erythropoietin has been adopted as standard,

although tentatively a unit has been defined as the amount that by standard assay procedure (52) effects a net incorporation of 20 per cent of injected radioiron into the red cells of a starved rat and several laboratories compare the induced response to that obtained following the administration of a known amount of cobaltous chloride (an effect equivalent to the increase of radioiron uptake induced by 5 μM of cobalt in a starved rat). No assay method yet tried is sensitive enough to demonstrate erythropoietin in normal human plasma or in plasma with slightly elevated levels without prior manipulation and concentration of the test plasmas. A number of attempts have been made to render the recipient animals more sensitive indicators. By and large these have been aimed at inducing a low base-line level of erythropoiesis and a decreased rate of red cell production so that, hopefully, small changes become more significant. Transfusion-induced polycythemia, increased oxygen tension of inspired air, hypophysectomy, starvation, sublethal irradiation, and nitrogen mustard administration are examples. Basically, all these methods, except possibly the latter two, depend upon modifying the organism so that the tissue oxygen supply is greater than the demand and consequently the marrow is more sensitive to stimulation by erythropoietin (39). Since the most acceptable method of evaluating erythropoietic response, outlined above, is so time consuming, tedious, and impossible to apply in small animals, many variations have been tried: reticulocyte count, 20-hour utilization of radioactive iron, plasma clearance of radioactive iron, etc. Attempts have been made to concentrate the active material for greater effect and to prepare plasma so that injection can be made from one species to another, preferably from large to small animals. Although not completely satisfactory, boiling plasma for short periods of time has been shown to result in an extract with little cross-species toxicity. However, since boiling also destroys a considerable proportion of the erythropoietic factor (92), careful concentration of the heat-stable supernatant must follow. By means of this technique, attempts have been made to isolate and identify the erythropoietic factor and to assess and define its role in human physiology.

Biochemical and Physical Properties

The factor is found in the muco-glyco-protein fraction which is electrophoretically located in the a_1- and a_2-globulin range (66, 67). It is relatively heat-stable, nondialyzable, and inactivated by proteases (89). Jacobson reports a product of 50,000-fold purification of the original plasma obtained from sheep's blood that is homogeneous at three different pH values by both electrophoresis and ultracentrifugation; it is also homogeneous by DEAE-cellulose chromatography. This substance, with a molecular weight of 40,000, has been further resolved into a large amount of inactive a–1–glycoprotein and a small amount of active hormone. It contains some 55 per cent protein, 11 per cent carbohydrate, 6 per cent sialic acid, and has some of the properties of an a–2–glycoprotein (108).

Mechanism of Action

Recently, the mouse with transfusion-induced polycythemia (39, 48, 231) has shown distinct advantages as an indicator of erythropoietin because endogenous erythropoiesis is virtually eliminated in a manner that does not exert any deleterious effect (at least none has been so far detected) on the animal's hematopoietic system (39). Animals so manipulated appear to be very sensitive responders to administered preparations of erythropoietin and, moreover, the results seem to be reproducible. Recent modifications by DeGowin et al. (17a) (injection of radioiron 2½ days after hormone

injection) have increased the sensitivity markedly and made it possible to demonstrate a sigmoidal curve describing the relation of log-dose of erythropoietin and response measured by erythrocyte radioiron incorporation. Of considerable interest here are the observations made by serial biopsies of spleens following injection of erythropoietin into the mice with transfusion-induced polycythemia (23). In the mouse the spleen is an active, important organ of hematopoiesis; following the induction of polycythemia, erythropoiesis in the spleen is virtually eliminated. After the injection of erythropoietin, proerythroblasts are evident at 24 hours, and by 72 hours maturation has progressed to normoblasts, early reticulocytes, and release of adult cells: a wave of erythropoiesis sweeps through the spleen beginning with the earliest recognizable cell of the erythrocyte series (derived from the stem cell) and progressing through the maturation series to the formation of adult red cells. These observations clearly support the above-outlined concept that differentiation of the multipotential stem cell into the red cell precursors is stimulated by erythropoietin and that normal maturation then follows if nutrition is adequate.

Increased Erythropoietin in Human Disease

Using one or the other of the assay variations mentioned above, it has been reported (38, 51, 57, 75, 75a, 79) that in the majority of patients with anemia, and in those with secondary polycythemia, the plasma is erythropoietically more active than normal: contains a higher-than-normal level of erythropoietic activity. The highest levels have been observed in the plasma of patients with the so-called aplastic anemias and Cooley's anemia. Substance with erythropoietic activity has also been isolated from urine of these patients (44, 45, 57, 109).

Increased amounts of erythropoietin

have also been demonstrated in the plasma of patients with pernicious anemia, iron-lack anemia, sickle cell anemia, erythroblastosis fetalis, leukemia, and various types of refractory anemias. In the latter instances it is probable that although the mechanism responsible for the production of erythropoietin is intact, inadequacy of the bone marrow prevents the appropriate response. The hope of possible therapeutic use of erythropoietin in these situations has not been sustained despite some early, apparently inaccurate, reports. In the anemias that accompany starvation, infection, chronic renal disease, and neoplasm no increase in plasma erythropoietin has been demonstrated.* However, these anemias do not respond to the administration of plasmas known to be rich in erythropoietin, so that a relative inadequacy of bone marrow responsiveness may be presumed.

It must once again be acknowledged that the findings have been inconsistent from one patient to another in any one laboratory and difficult to reproduce from one laboratory to the next. Nevertheless, enough sound work has been done on animals to sketch at least the outlines of the physiologic control of erythropoiesis, and there is sufficient evidence to conclude that the same principles obtain for human physiology.

Site of Production

There have been numerous attempts to locate the site at which erythropoietic factor is produced. The extirpation of spleen, the classic endocrine organs (thymus, gonads, thyroid, pituitary, adrenals, pancreas),† stomach, intestinal tract, or 90 per cent of the liver has not abolished red cell production. The administration of x-ray, nitrogen mustard, or thorium dioxide has not impaired the production or release of the erythropoietic factor. Removal of organs such as liver, heart, lungs, and central nervous

system has not been possible, and although extracts of these organs have not shown erythropoietic activity, they remain possible sites of production.

Because of the natural experiment available in the polycythemia associated with patent ductus arteriosus with reversed blood flow, described above, the site of production of erythropoietic factor in the human being can be located in the hypoxic, cyanotic areas of the body. It is usually stated that this means below the diaphragm, but it should be remembered that some of the arterial supply to the lung parenchyma arises from the aorta at the region of hypoxia so that on these grounds alone the lungs should not be excluded. Considerable attention has been given to the possible role of the kidneys because of the clinical observation of decreased erythropoietic activity in renal disease and the polycythemia sometimes associated with renal tumors and other renal abnormalities. Much evidence has been presented from several laboratories for (33, 72–74, 76, 84, 99) and against (20, 26, 27, 70) the proposition that the kidneys are the source of erythropoietic factor. Recent observations (87) employing parabiotic rats in which one partner could be subjected to either hypoxia alone or nephrectomy plus hypoxia indicate a slight increase in erythropoiesis when the nephrectomized partner was made hypoxic but much less increase than was demonstrable when one

---

* Technically, as pointed out above, it has not been possible to demonstrate normal or decreased levels in human beings.

† Although the influence of the endocrines upon erythropoiesis has not been here elucidated, they, of course, do play a very important role. Marked hematologic alterations are consistently seen in endocrine disorders (of pituitary, adrenals, thyroid, gonads). In general, however, although these glands do take part in the regulation of erythropoiesis, their effect appears to be exerted at second hand, through effects on metabolism and oxygen requirements, and not by direct effect upon the marrow or direct modification of the fundamental stimulus to hypoxia.

of an unoperated pair was subjected to hypoxia.

At present the site of erythropoietic factor production has not been conclusively established to the satisfaction of all, but it seems fair to conclude that although small amounts may be produced elsewhere in the body, the kidney is the main source of supply. Erythropoietic factor has been extracted from the kidney; natural experiments suggest the loop of Henle as a possible site of production (4); indirect evidence that the juxtaglomerular cell secretes erythropoietin has been obtained in experiments with rats (53a).

Summary

It is justified to conclude that under conditions of adequate nutrition the dynamic equilibrium of the erythron, which depends primarily upon the rate of red cell production, is controlled by a hormone, erythropoietin. An extraordinarily and exquisitely sensitive system is thereby set up that is based on a "feed-back" principle capable of monitoring and responding to even the normal day-to-day destruction of erythrocytes and, in addition, to changes induced by alterations in the external and internal environments.

ERYTHROPOIETIN VS. ERYTHROCYTOSIS-STIMULATING FACTOR

The above considerations of the control of erythropoiesis are based on the reasonable presumption that the stimulating factor of prime interest is the one involved in the normal physiology of the erythron: a factor vitally concerned with the moment-to-moment production of red cells to compensate exactly for red cell destruction and with the response to internal and external environmental alterations. The role of this factor is, then, the control of the size of the erythron by multiplication and differentiation of erythrocyte precursors in such a way that each of its component parts is increased but remains qualitatively normal. That is, the nucleated red cell precursors and the adult red cells must remain intrinsically normal and capable of normal life span. Were this otherwise, it would be obvious that the factor is not concerned with normal physiology. As defined in this way the erythropoietic factor has been chemically characterized as (a) relatively heat resistant, (b) nondialyzable, (c) subject to proteolytic destruction, and (d) not soluble in ether or lipid solvents and most likely an α–2–glycoprotein. The administration of the erythropoietic factor to suitable test subjects results initially in an increase in the stem cells and the most immature red cells of the marrow and later in generalized hyperplasia; reticulocytosis; increase in red cell count, hemoglobin concentration, and hematocrit value; and increase in the clearance of iron through the plasma and in the incorporation of iron into the hemoglobin of functionally competent red cells.

It is important to bring out these considerations again at this point because some workers have repeatedly demonstrated a factor, derived from plasma of animals made anemic by a variety of ways and from patients with different types of anemias, that is (a) stable to prolonged boiling and (b) ether-soluble and most likely a lipid (61). The administration of this factor to suitable test subjects results in increased numbers of nucleated red cells in the marrow, reticulocytosis, an increase in the red cell count, but *no* increase in hemoglobin concentration or hematocrit value and *no* enhancement of iron turnover or utilization. Erythrocytosis follows its administration owing to the formation of microcytes without associated hemoglobin response. Moreover, these microcytes are osmotically as well as morphologically abnormal and apparently do not long survive. This factor does not produce a response in the erythron such as occurs normally and consequently should not be termed erythropoietin. Those who have done the most critical work with it have been careful to term it the erythrocytosis-stimulating factor. It apparently functions by increasing the number of cellular divisions which the erythrocyte precursors undergo during maturation so that microspherocytes result but no net increase in hemoglobin production. As a lipid the factor is interesting since it has been known for some time that batyl alcohol $[CH_3(CH_2)_{17}\text{-}O\text{-}CH_2\text{-}CH(OH)\text{-}CH_2(OH)]$ induces the same unique change in animals (62). Accordingly it is thought that the erythrocytosis-stimulating factor may be identical with, or closely related to, batyl alcohol. However, to achieve results quantitatively comparable with plasma, amounts of this compound far in excess of physiologic values must be administered. Recent studies have indicated that with large doses of batyl alcohol all marrow elements are affected and that leukocytosis and thrombocytosis as well as erythrocytosis can be induced. This factor is of considerable interest because of its demonstrated role in cell multiplication and its relation to erythropoietin.

As might safely be predicted, other workers have found variations in responses to preparations of "erythropoietin" and differences in chemical or physical properties so that the occurrence of more than one erythropoiesis-stimulating factor has been proposed (8, 31, 103). Recent studies by Brecher and Stohlman (9) and Stohlman (95) indicate that when very large doses of an erythropoiesis-stimulating factor are employed, reticulocytes are produced at such an early time and of such large size that the most reasonable interpretation is that mitotic divisions have been skipped; the reticulocytes are so much larger than normal that it appears impossible that they could mature into normal-sized erythrocytes. Moreover, the life span is definitely decreased (97). In addition, Linman (64)

has reported that plasma from rabbits made anemic by phenylhydrazine-induced hemolysis contains two factors capable of influencing erythropoiesis: a relatively thermolabile substance that is orally inactive but capable upon parenteral administration of enhancing erythropoiesis by affecting the rate of erythrocyte differentiation from the stem cell, and a thermostable substance active upon oral administration and capable of enhancing erythropoiesis by influencing the number of mitoses the erythrocyte precursors undergo during maturation.

It may, then, well be that more than one factor is necessary to stimulate *normal* erythropoiesis and that an excess (or relative deficiency) of one or the other factor(s) results in skipped mitoses and short-lived macrocytes or, conversely, too many mitoses and short-lived microcytes.

ANDROGENS AND ERYTHROPOIESIS

The studies of hemoglobin and hematocrit values in relation to age and sex in human beings have long suggested that androgenic hormones are involved in erythropoiesis. Among children 2 to 14 years old, hemoglobin and hematocrit values increase with age with no significant sex difference. Between 14 and 20 years of age the values decrease in females and increase in males. These differences are present into the third decade, but following this there is a gradual fall in values for males whereas in females there is a tendency to a rise in values following menopause. The slight differences seen in the fifth and sixth decades persist until the ninth decade, at which time the values in males are lower. Although it is evident on the basis of extensive studies in animals and sparse observations in humans that the androgenic hormones are involved in these differences (53), the mechanism(s) whereby androgens bring about the changes is obscure. Clinical observations have indicated that androgens were effective as *replacement* therapy in the treatment of some types of anemia (hypogonadism, hypopituitarism, hypothyroidism). When testosterone was employed in "pharmacologic doses" in the treatment of carcinoma of the breast, elevations in the hemoglobin and hematocrit values in peripheral blood were noted. Recently androgenic preparations have been fairly extensively employed in various types of anemias (myeloid metaplasia, multiple myeloma, lymphatic leukemia, Hodgkin's disease, chronic bone marrow failure, etc.) not responsive to other agents (29). In a considerable number of adults significant elevations in hemoglobin and hematocrit values have been noted with a limited associated clinical improvement; in the aplastic anemia of childhood prolonged complete remissions have been induced. There is no physiologic or metabolic information to define the mechanism whereby pharmacologic doses of androgens produce their results, but the observed increased proliferation of erythrocyte precursors suggests that a primary effect is through the stem cell (29).

COBALT AND ERYTHROPOIESIS

One other element should be mentioned because of its biochemical and limited clinical interest. It has been known for a long time that the administration of cobalt (usually as cobaltous chloride) will induce polycythemia in animals. This is a true polycythemia with increases in hemoglobin and hematocrit values as well as in the red blood cell count. Studies have been made on the response of humans to the administration of cobalt over prolonged periods of time, and the substance has been demonstrated to have limited clinical utility in patients with refractory anemia associated with chronic infection or renal disease and in an occasional individual with idiopathic refractory anemia. Something of the mechanism whereby cobalt produces its effect has been elucidated by recent work dem-

onstrating an increased amount of erythropoietin in the plasma following administration of the element (10, 32). Since cobalt is known to interfere with certain enzymes concerned with the transport and utilization of oxygen (58), its administration may well result in a histotoxic hypoxia. Tissue hypoxia may then stimulate the production of erythropoietin, resulting in polycythemia. However, the identity of the erythropoietic factor stimulated by cobalt and that stimulated by bleeding or by phenylhydrazine-induced hemolytic anemia has, of course, not been established, and some difference in effects has been noted. Thus, cobalt is effective in increasing red cell production in animals with inflammation or renal disease, but these show a lack of response to bleeding and do not respond in a quantitatively appropriate way to administration of erythropoietin derived from bled animals (59). The problem cannot be resolved at present.

ERYTHROKINETICS

A steady state of the circulating hemoglobin-red-cell mass is maintained in the normal individual by the precise balance achieved between the amount removed from and the amount delivered to the peripheral blood per unit of time. Anemia results (a) when the amount of hemoglobin-red-cell mass delivered to the peripheral blood is decreased, (b) when the amount removed from the peripheral blood is increased and not balanced by a compensatory increase in delivery, or (c) when both occur together. This general statement forms the basis of the physiologic classification of the anemias given in Tables 5.2 and 5.3, which attempt to group hematopoietic disorders according to the physiologic competence of the bone marrow to respond in various situations, as "anemias caused by increased loss or destruction of hemoglobin-red-cell mass" and "anemias caused by decreased production of hemoglobin-red-cell mass";

some disorders appear under both headings. However, as investigations progressed it became evident that another aspect of bone marrow physiology was important but not necessarily implicit in that classification; namely, marrow could *apparently* be responding in terms of both morphologic evidence of increased erythropoietic activity and uptake of plasma iron and yet not be able to deliver the goods adequately to the peripheral blood. Here then is brought out the concept of *ineffective* as opposed to *effective* erythropoiesis. Ineffective erythropoiesis refers to the situations in which the marrow processes to a certain extent red cell and hemoglobin components as though it were engaged in the production of erythrocytes, but is unable to deliver the expected final product to the circulating blood. At some stage catabolic events nullify anabolic efforts, and the marrow is unable to produce viable cells. Even in the normal individual studies of hemoglobin production and destruction indicate that about 10 to 15 per cent of the total erythropoietic activity is associated with early pigment breakdown and not with the production of functionally competent cells. In certain anemias (Table 6.6) most of the erythropoietic activity is ineffective.

Accordingly, classifications have been attempted (25) wherein each component in the *total* erythrokinetic picture is evaluated: normal or increased destruction or loss of hemoglobin-red-cell mass, decreased stimulation of the marrow, decreased responsivity of marrow to stimulation, increased marrow response with effective erythropoiesis, increased marrow response with ineffective erythropoiesis. To define and quantitate these various facets of the total erythrokinetic picture, a series of measurements is available that can be separated into two main groups (7, 25, 30). The first series of measurements reflects the production of hemoglobin-red-cell mass; the second series reflects hemoglobin-red-cell mass breakdown. A balance between the two occurs when production equals destruction during the steady state achieved with an unchanging circulating hemoglobin-red-cell mass.

With the development of anemia* (a decrease in the circulating hemoglobin-red-cell mass) and the concomitant tissue hypoxia and increased output of erythropoietin, the marrow is stimulated to respond with augmented production. Production rates of about six times normal have been demonstrated by various workers, giving an indication of the range of capabilities of the marrow. In evaluating marrow response in the various anemias, comparison must be made between the erythropoietic response actually achieved and the optimum response of a normally reactive marrow to the same stimulus.

Quantitation of erythropoiesis is based upon the following considerations, measurements, and indices. In the normal individual, the total blood volume, hemoglobin-red-cell mass, and mean red cell life span (see Chapter 9) are established within the accuracies of the methods available. These values make it possible to draw up a balance sheet indicating the daily turnover of constituents of the hemoglobin-red-cell mass. These values, as given by Finch, are shown in Table 6.3. In preparing for the actual calculations the following measurements may be made.

A. Number of erythrocytic cells in the marrow. Since there is no practical way

---

* In an adequate nutritional setting no difference has been demonstrated in the magnitude of the marrow response to comparable degrees of anemia produced by blood loss or by hemolytic processes (24). Because possible inhibitory factors could not be satisfactorily assayed, this finding must be interpreted with caution as indicating "no difference has been demonstrated" and not taken as final evidence that differences in marrow response do not exist with reference to anemia produced by blood loss versus that caused by hemolysis.

TABLE 6.3.   Theoretical erythrokinetic data in normal (70–Kg) man

Assumptions	Calculated values	Daily turnover (0.83–1.0%)
Blood volume: 5,000 ml	Red cell mass: 2,000 ml	16.7–20.0 ml red cells
Venous hematocrit: 44.5%	Hemoglobin mass: 666 Gm	5.6–6.7 Gm hemoglobin
Mean body hematocrit: 40%	Circulating iron mass: 2,224 mg	18.5–22.3 mg iron
	Circulating pyrrole pigment: 22.5 Gm	193–234 mg urobilinogen

NORMAL CONVERSION CONSTANTS

Body hematocrit factor = 0.92 × venous hematocrit
Mean corpuscular hemoglobin concentration = 33 Gm/100 ml
Mean cell volume = 87 cu μ
Iron per gram hemoglobin = 3.38 mg
Daily red cell breakdown = 1/120 or 0.83%
Protoporphyrin molecular weight = 566
Stercobilinogen molecular weight = 580
Hemoglobin molecular weight = 66,000
Iron atomic weight = 56

From Giblett, E. R., et al., Blood 11:291, 1956.

of measuring total marrow mass, the evaluation is made by calculating the ratio of erythrocytic to myelocytic cells (E/M ratio) in a smear of marrow aspirate or section of marrow biopsy. Since this yields a ratio, the value is valid only if the myelocytic cells are normal and the marrow material is not contaminated by admixture with peripheral blood cells. The normal ratio is taken as 360 red cell precursors per 1,000 granulocytic cells, or 1:3. It is admittedly and obviously not very accurate or reproducible. The E/M ratio assays the *total erythropoietic activity* but does *not* give an indication of viable cell production or take into account increased production due to increase in total marrow mass, a phenomenon known to occur in many situations.

B. Plasma iron turnover. As discussed in the section on Ferrokinetics, in Chapter 2, the plasma iron turnover is calculated from the plasma iron level and the rate of clearance of the radioisotope from the plasma. The amount passing through the plasma may be calculated in milligrams by blood volume considerations. Since this is difficult and of limited practicality, the following formula has been applied to give the milligrams of iron per 100 ml of blood per day (assuming a normal blood volume):

$$\frac{\text{Plasma iron } (\mu g \text{ per 100 ml})}{\text{Radioiron clearance T/2 (min)}} \times \frac{\text{Plasmatocrit}}{100}$$

The normal value is taken as 0.6 mg per 100 ml of blood per day (range 0.4 to 0.8). However, not all the iron passing through the plasma is destined for incorporation into red cells: 0.15 mg per 100 ml per day is assumed to represent that not involved in erythrocyte turnover. The erythrocyte plasma iron turnover (EPIT) is 0.6 less 0.15, or 0.45 mg per 100 ml per day. This value is taken to indicate the *total erythropoietic activity,* since the plasma iron turnover, in general, correlates with total erythropoiesis as determined in a number of different situations.

C. Red cell utilization of iron. This measurement is derived from the plasma iron turnover and the percentage of injected radioactive material appearing in the circulating hemoglobin-red-cell mass 2 weeks after injection. The normal value is 0.45 mg per 100 ml of whole blood per day. In the absence of hemolysis (see section on Ferrokinetics), it reflects the new components of the hemoglobin-red-cell mass entering the circulation, or the *effective erythropoietic activity.*

D. Reticulocyte count. At the time of entry into the circulation most erythrocytes contain some RNA, precipitable as reticulum upon supravital staining. Accordingly an evaluation of the reticulocytes yields a figure indicative of the number of new cells delivered to the peripheral blood. By convention, the reticulocyte count is expressed as a percentage (number of reticulocytes per 100 red blood cells in the peripheral blood). To compensate for possible changes in the total erythrocyte count, which will of course influence the ratio, the reticulocytes may be expressed in terms of the number present per cubic millimeter of whole blood when the red blood cell count is known. If the red cell count is not determined, a similar modification of the reticulocyte percentage may be obtained by a "correction" employing the patient's hematocrit (or hemoglobin) value as compared with normal. A reticulocyte count of 36 per cent in a patient with a hematocrit of 15 per cent would therefore become a corrected value of 15/45 × 36, or a 12 per cent value.

As pointed out earlier in this section, there is in the marrow a reticulocyte pool approximately equal in size to that found in the peripheral blood. In various situations the pool may be shifted into the peripheral blood doubling the count there. However, the count is then no longer a reflection of daily erythrocyte production. Usually these marrow pool reticulocytes can be recognized by the increased amount of reticulum they contain and their association with nucleated red cells. Experience has shown that in such a situation dividing the reticulocyte count by two gives a better estimate of daily production.

Despite the errors and limitations inherent in attempts to bring the expression of the count into line with daily production, the reticulocyte count remains the most applicable and helpful method of assessing erythropoiesis in terms of marrow response to stimulation and delivery of hemoglobin-red-cell mass to the peripheral blood: the *effective erythropoietic activity.*

E. Red cell life span. This topic (and the following one) will be developed at length in Chapter 9. The methods ordinarily employed to determine red cell life span do not distinguish between loss from bleeding and from hemolysis, but they do yield a quantitation of the effective duration of the red cells in the peripheral circulation. When a steady state exists, determination of red cell life span therefore indicates the delivery rate per day of cells to the peripheral blood since the destruction rate per day is thereby balanced: *effective erythropoietic activity.*

F. Fecal urobilinogen. The amount of urobilinogen excreted in the feces gives an estimate of the total pyrrole pigment that is catabolized through the urobilinogen cycle. It measures not only the pigments broken down in the circulating blood but also the pigments in the marrow that for one reason or another do not reach the circulating blood. Accordingly, it is taken to indicate *total erythropoietic activity.* The numerous, important limitations of this procedure are outlined in a later section on hemoglobin catabolism (Chapter 9).

At this point it is desirable to give emphasis to the important concept behind this approach to erythropoiesis and types of bone marrow response. The total effort of the marrow to respond erythropoietically is indicated by (a) the E/M ratio and (b) the plasma iron turnover. In addition, by assessing, through the fecal urobilinogen determination, the catabolic products of the hemoglobin-red-cell mass, the rate of its destruction can be estimated and, accordingly, since production equals destruction in the steady state, the total erythropoietic effort thereby evaluated. But in some situations the marrow is not able to deliver the product of this total effort to the peripheral blood. The effective effort of the marrow can be indicated by (c) red cell utilization of iron and (d) reticulocyte count. Again, by assessing (e) the red cell survival in the peripheral blood, the rate of destruction of circulating cells can be determined and accordingly the effective effort evaluated. When the assessment of total erythropoietic effort does not balance with the assessment of effective erythropoietic effort, the difference can be ascribed to ineffective erythropoiesis. In short, *total erythropoiesis* is defined as total production of hemoglobin-red-cell mass regardless of whether entrance to the circulating blood is ever achieved. Effective erythropoiesis refers specifically to the portion of the hemoglobin-red-cell mass that enters into and remains in the circulating blood long enough to be measured. *Ineffective erythropoiesis* refers to that portion of the hemoglobin-red-cell mass not appearing in the circulation (Table 6.4).

In order to compare measurements between different individuals it is necessary to have standards of reference arbitrarily given in terms of 100 ml of whole blood. Table 6.5 shows the values given by Finch.

Values for these determinations and the E/M ratio as obtained from data on the patient are compared with normal values, and series of erythrokinetic indices results. These indices are then compared with the expected maximal responses of normal marrow at a comparable degree of anemia, and the responses of the patient's marrow are evaluated in terms of erythrokinetics. The term "proliferative anemia" is used for a maximal response of three to six times normal; "nonproliferative anemia" is used when the optimum response achieved is less than the maximal response of normal marrow.

The broad conceptual basis that underlies this erythrokinetic approach to evaluating bone marrow response and classifying the anemias is important, and the criticism which this approach directs at other methods of evaluation and classification is telling and profound. Moreover, the concepts that are threaded through the entire scheme leading up to quantitation and comparison with the normal are based on a dynamic and physiologic approach to the problems of erythropoiesis and will be repeated below in summary form for emphasis. It must be pointed out at this time that in the above account of the measurements required for quantitating erythrokinetics, qualifying limitations were kept at a minimum. It is very difficult to give an account of the actual measurements without adding one or more major and several minor qualifications for each and every assessment made. However, were these in-

TABLE 6.4.   Erythrokinetic measurements

Erythropoietic effort	Production	Destruction
Total	E/M ratio Plasma iron turnover	Fecal urobilinogen
Effective	Reticulocyte count Red cell utilization	Red cell survival

From Finch, C. A., and Noyes, W. D., J.A.M.A. 175:1163, 1961.

TABLE 6.5. Standard values for various erythrokinetic measurements

Measurements	Values per 100 ml whole blood per day
Erythrocytic plasma iron turnover	0.45 mg
Red cell utilization	0.45 mg
Reticulocyte count	6×10^9 cells
Fecal urobilinogen determination	3.3 mg
Life span measurement	0.42 ml RBC

Conversion of these measurements to this form of reference is for the most part apparent. In case of a Cr^{51} half-life survival time of 13 days in a patient with a hematocrit of 15, the calculation would be as follows:

$$\text{Destruction rate (ml RBC per 100 ml whole blood per day)} = \frac{120}{25} \times 0.42 \times \frac{15}{45} = 0.67$$

$$\text{Relative destruction rate} = \frac{0.67}{0.42} = 1.5 \times \text{normal}$$

where 25 is corrected life span, 120 is normal life span, 15 and 45 are hematocrit values of patient and normal individual. The one exception in the above calculation of the relative rate of production and destruction would be the E/M ratio of the marrow. Here, since the white blood cell reference may be assumed to adjust also to the individual's age, the ratio as obtained may be used.

From Finch, C. A., Hematology Manual, p. 38, 1960 (privately printed).

cluded here, the valuable considerations and contributions would be difficult to discern. The major limitations are set out in more detail in Chapter 2 (section on Ferrokinetics), Chapter 9, and earlier in this chapter. It would seem that by the very processes of attempting to compensate for the recognized limitations of the values, correcting them for variations, and comparing them with an arbitrary standard, the final figure is so transmogrified that it is almost surprising to find a reasonable index emerge. Not one of the individual assessments is truly acceptable on its own merits as more than a rough indicator of the general direction of change, but the aggregate of six appears in many situations to give information consistent with the physiologic concept underlying the process of erythropoiesis. The main criticisms emerging from the accounts of those who have worked with the determination and application of data have been that the methods now available for attempting quantitation are not consistently reliable enough to be used as arguments supporting the concepts (15, 42, 98, 102).

SUMMARY

The seemingly straightforward statement that anemia is the result of an imbalance between production and destruction can no longer suffice even though in itself it is not untrue. One must go further and state that anemia results when an imbalance *has occurred because.* . . . To complete the statement in a satisfactory manner complex considerations must be taken into account. Basic to this is that in terms of erythropoiesis the marrow responds according to the stimulation it receives from a circulating factor (erythropoietin) and according to its own inherent capacity to proliferate. In certain disorders (Table 6.6) there is a failure

TABLE 6.6.   Erythrokinetic classification of anemias

I. Nonproliferative anemias
   A. Decreased marrow stimulation
      1. Anemia of endocrine disorder
      2. Anemia of renal disease
      3. Anemia of infection
   B. Marrow failure
      1. Iron-lack anemia
      2. Anemia of marrow damage
      3. Idiopathic

II. Proliferative anemias
   A. Effective erythropoietic response
      1. Anemia of hemorrhage
      2. Hemolytic anemias
   B. Ineffective erythropoietic (dyspoietic) response
      1. Folic acid and vitamin B_{12} deficiency
      2. Thalassemia
      3. Pyridoxine-responsive anemia
      4. Idiopathic (refractory anemia with hyperplastic marrow)

From Finch, C. A., and Noyes, W. D., J.A.M.A. 175:1163, 1961.

in the production of the stimulating factor; in others the marrow fails to respond to an apparently adequately produced stimulating factor. If erythropoietic response does occur, it may be one of two types. An effective erythropoietic response delivers viable, functionally competent red cells to the peripheral circulation; an ineffective erythropoietic response occurs because the marrow is unable to deliver such red cells to the peripheral blood even though morphologically and biochemically it appears to be processing component parts as though it were going to do so. The total erythropoietic response is the summation of effective plus ineffective.

In addition to this, the capacity of the marrow to proliferate and produce must not be defined only in terms of its total erythropoietic and effective erythropoietic response, but the response must be compared with that of a normal individual at a comparable degree of stimulation. Some degree of failure is evidenced if erythropoiesis can be increased only threefold, when under comparable stimulation a normal response would be a sixfold increase. It must be realized that relative failure of the bone marrow occurs even when a marrow can increase its production to three times the normal output because under comparably increased stimulation normal marrow would increase its production six times normal.

Erythrokinetics considers the contributions to the disturbed balance of increased destruction or loss of hemoglobin-red-cell mass by indicating the effective duration of red cells in the peripheral circulation.

In continuing the statement "anemia results when an imbalance has occurred between production and destruction . . ." one might go on with "relative failure of bone marrow, ineffective erythropoiesis, and the delivery of abnormally short-lived erythrocytes to the peripheral blood." When possible, the etiology of these alterations would also be given, as, for example, "vitamin B_{12} deficiency."

A significant advance beyond the approach to the study of anemias represented by the morphologic classification given in Table 5.1 occurred with the physiologic approach, of which the classification in Tables 5.2 and 5.3 is perhaps a first approximation and the erythrokinetic classification (Table 6.6) a next approximation. The formalization of the erythrokinetic approach to the study of anemias (best regarded as a special treatment within the more general physiologic approach) has emphasized certain factors which, while not formerly excluded, were not necessarily implicit.

The erythrokinetic classification of disease has implicit in it concepts not necessarily brought out by prior classifications, and the erythrokinetic approach to the study of disease gives promise of greater potential for uncovering the unusual, different, or new and thereby adding to knowledge of disease processes, even though the techniques of measurement have not satisfactorily caught up with the concepts upon which the classification is based.

Bibliographic references for Chapter 6 begin on page 396.

CHAPTER SEVEN

PERNICIOUS ANEMIA
AND THE NON-ADDISONIAN
MEGALOBLASTIC ANEMIAS

ADDISONIAN PERNICIOUS ANEMIA[*]

Pernicious anemia results from a nutritional deficiency that usually occurs in later adult life and may make its presence known by systemic, gastrointestinal, neurologic, and hematologic manifestations. In recent years the presenting manifestations of the disease have changed considerably from those formerly seen. In the past the diagnosis could apparently be made with certainty on symptoms and signs; today in the majority of patients, no pathognomonic symptoms or signs are found.[†] This is undoubtedly due to the increased availability of medical care and a willingness of patients to seek medical attention earlier in the disease process. An accurately established diagnosis must now usually be based upon specific laboratory findings and the changes induced by appropriate therapy. Following the studies of Minot and Murphy (178) it has become evident that pernicious anemia no longer is a uniformly fatal illness but one treatable to such an extent that life expectancy is unshortened. It thus becomes of paramount importance to establish a correct diagnosis for each individual patient. There are several ap-

proaches to this and several ways to certify the diagnosis, all based upon knowledge of the pathophysiology of the disease.

Pernicious anemia occurs because of a *conditioned* nutritional deficiency of vitamin B_{12}. The abnormality that is basically responsible for the deficiency, or "conditions" it, is a failure of the gastric mucosa to secrete "intrinsic factor," a substance necessary for the normal absorption of vitamin B_{12}. The disease, therefore, is an example of a relatively pure deficiency of a single vitamin, something rarely seen in human nutrition. The evidence is now convincing that the gastric abnormality is genetically determined although usually not detectable until the second half of life. Those with the familial predisposition undergo a slowly progressive functional and anatomic degeneration of the gastric mucosa by which the ability to produce intrinsic factor is sufficiently cur-

[*] General references and review articles: 6, 9, 16, 36–39, 41, 53, 58, 60, 64, 68, 73, 75, 82, 89, 91, 92, 102, 117, 120, 132, 169, 179, 182, 203, 207, 234, 238, 248, 262, 263, 265, 267.

[†] "Disease is very old and nothing about it has changed. It is we who change as we learn to recognize what was formerly imperceptible." *J. M. Charcot.*

tailed to impair the absorption of vitamin B_{12}. Whether or not the picture of fully developed pernicious anemia appears in a given individual depends upon the severity and duration of the gastric lesion, the dietary intake of vitamin B_{12} and folic acid, and conditions which may alter the requirements for these vitamins.

To sum up, pernicious anemia is a body-wide deficiency of vitamin B_{12} brought on by a genetically determined failure of the stomach to secrete in adult life adequate amounts of intrinsic factor for the physiologic absorption of vitamin B_{12}. This defect in the absorption of physiologic amounts of vitamin B_{12} can be corrected by the administration of intrinsic factor even though the functional and anatomic degeneration of the gastric mucosa is irreversible.

Clinical Manifestations

Although seen chiefly in the white race, and in disproportionately high incidence among people of Scandinavian, English, and Irish extraction, the disease occurs in practically all peoples. It is very rare in Orientals but its formerly presumed low incidence in Negroes was evidently based on inadequate sampling. The occurrence in males and females is approximately equal. Instances of the disease in infancy and childhood have been documented with extreme rarity (144, 151, 237); few instances in adolescence and early adult life have been documented (180). A significant incidence appears in the fourth decade and increases slightly in each decade thereafter. The usual patient is an elderly individual who has not felt up to par for 6 months to a year. Several months ago, however, he noted a definite change for the worse and since then has felt himself going downhill at an increasingly rapid pace. Anorexia becomes very bothersome, with lack of energy and drive; he may have noted or had called to his attention in recent weeks a pallor or pale yellow complexion. Shortness of breath upon exertion, palpitations, and a sense of coldness and "poor circulation" in the extremities become very bothersome and limiting. Because of general malaise, lack of strength, pallor, and breathlessness upon exertion, he seeks medical advice. It should be noted that all these symptoms are nonspecific and could be indicative of decreased circulating hemoglobin concentration due to a large variety of causes. The physical examination may similarly reflect only the low hemoglobin levels. This is currently the usual picture presented. It is evident that a certain diagnosis can be achieved only by means of laboratory tests and/or therapeutic trials.

A more classic picture of the disease may occasionally be seen. The patient, formerly a pleasant individual, is now a cantankerous curmudgeon with prematurely gray hair, light complexion, blue eyes, large ears, broad cheekbones, lemon-yellow complexion with moderate scleral icterus, and vitiligo or melanotic pigmentation. He or she reports gastrointestinal upsets with episodic abdominal pain; alternating constipation and diarrhea; recurrent episodes of sore, painful red tongue; moderate weight loss; symmetrical numbness and tingling, with "pins-and-needles" sensations in the extremities; awkwardness while fastening buttons, lacing shoes, or sewing; difficulty in walking, maintaining balance, and knowing where the feet are, especially in the dark and while descending stairs. Often there is a family history of pernicious anemia (185). In such a situation a strong presumptive diagnosis of pernicious anemia *should* be made and will most likely be proved by the physical examination and laboratory procedures. Indeed the coexistence of signs and symptoms of anemia, symmetrical numbness and tingling of extremities, and gait abnormalities is sufficient to justify a presumptive diagnosis of pernicious anemia. When to these signs and symptoms are added lingual atrophy with or without painful irritation, splenomegaly, and additional manifestations of combined degeneration of the spinal cord (see below), the diagnosis becomes practically certain, lacking only crucial laboratory evidence and response to effective therapy to establish it unequivocally.

The central nervous system manifestations seen in association with pernicious anemia and etiologically related to the vitamin B_{12} deficiency are grouped under the term "subacute combined degeneration of the spinal cord and brain" (64, 130, 213, 218, 248, 269). Although this is an unsatisfactory term because the disease is usually chronic and not subacute and may involve only one and not combined systems, it is to be preferred to the older terms, "combined system disease," "subacute combined sclerosis," and "funicular degeneration of the cord." The disease is the result of diffuse but uneven degeneration of the white matter of the spinal cord and brain. In early cases only the posterior columns may be involved, with multiple foci of spongy degeneration. These lesions appear to spread up and down the cord as well as into the lateral columns. The pathologic changes are not limited to specific systems of fibers in the posterior and lateral columns but are irregularly scattered (Figure 7.1). When the dorsal and lateral columns of the spinal cord are involved, the classic symptoms of ataxia, variable degrees of spasticity, and weakness are present, progressing to severe paraplegia and flexion deformities if unchecked by appropriate therapy. In far-advanced, long-standing vitamin B_{12} deficiency the *spinothalamic* tract may be involved, and patients who have similar lesions in the white matter of the brain show mental symptoms (5). Although there is no general agreement among the occasional studies that have

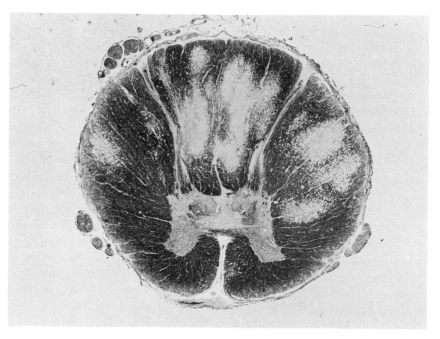

FIGURE 7.1.   Subacute combined degeneration of spinal cord. Areas of spongy degeneration indicating active, advancing lesions are seen here to involve mainly the dorsal and lateral columns. Nevertheless, lesions are not limited to specific fiber tracts but are somewhat irregularly scattered and overlap into other areas

been done, it is probable that associated peripheral neuropathy may be present to account for some of the symptoms.

Mental signs are frequent—irritability, apathy, somnolence, suspiciousness, and emotional instability (69, 85). In the day-to-day management of the patient this must be recognized as part of the disease, for not infrequently a quite different personality emerges following effective therapy. So-called "megaloblastic madness" (232) may be manifested by marked confusional or depressive psychoses: intellectual deterioration and disorientation. Olfactory involvement and perversion of taste are reported frequently if specifically asked about; visual impairment is rare and takes the form of centrocecal scotoma (154) with occasional optic atrophy (71, 111). Recent evidence indicates that some toxic amblyopias (from tobacco, alcohol, etc.) may be specifically caused by vitamin B_{12} deficiency (114).

In the development of subacute combined degeneration patients first notice general weakness and paresthesias: "pins-and-needles" numbness, stiffness, deadness, tightness, feelings of heat or cold, formication, shooting pains. These symptoms are usually constant and steadily progress; they are invariably symmetrical and involve distal parts first. The weakness and stiffness progress (especially notable in the legs), and along with them the defect in postural sensation produces a weak, unsteady gait and awkwardness of the limbs. Early in the course there may be no objective signs. Involvement of the posterior column results in loss of vibratory sense (probably the most constant and common of all neurologic findings) most pronounced in the distal portions of feet and hands and less frequently found in the arms and hands than in the lower limbs. It may, however, become extensive enough to involve the trunk. Position sense is somewhat less frequently involved. The motor system shows loss of strength, spasticity, changes

in tendon reflexes (absent or hyperactive), clonus, extensor plantar responses. The abnormalities are governed by the relative involvement of posterior and lateral columns, and the gait may be ataxic or spastic or both.

The lesions of the posterior columns (ascending fibers) account for the paresthesias, impairment of vibratory and position sense, ataxia and the Romberg sign, and perhaps the loss of tendon reflexes. Involvement of the lateral columns (pyramidal tracts, descending fibers) accounts for the weakness, spasticity, increased tendon reflexes, and Babinski's sign.

Having described at some length the manifestations of far-advanced pernicious anemia, it must immediately be pointed out that for one to expect to find these manifestations is more likely to hinder than to help early diagnosis. A survey (58, 59) contrasting the characteristics presented by patients with the disease in 1908–1923 and in 1944–1956 produced the following comparisons: fever, formerly noted in 79 per cent of patients, occurred in only 22 per cent in recent years; the incidence of glossitis was found to have dropped from 40 to 5 per cent; of atrophic glossitis, from 94 to 64 per cent; of splenomegaly, from 27 to 8 per cent; of spinal cord damage, from 11 to 7 per cent. Jaundice, formerly present in most cases, was uncommon in the recent group.* It is evident that because the early stages of the disease, rather than the classic picture, are usually seen, one must be alert to minimal changes that are by and large not pathognomonic and be ready to rely on laboratory findings and physiologic tests to establish the diagnosis. One other point must be made and emphasized at this time (although somewhat out of place): the neurologic ab-

* This incidence is based on criteria which would ordinarily be taken as advanced involvement: paresthesias were not an acceptable criterion, and loss of vibratory sense had to involve the trunk.

normalities may be seen without the usual peripheral blood changes and anemia. From the survey mentioned above it is obvious that most patients have anemia and no combined degeneration of the cord and brain. The inverse of this must also be expected, and fortunately today the physiologic tests and assay methods are available to establish vitamin B_{12} deficiency as the cause of the neurologic manifestations (19, 140, 248). The importance of instituting appropriate therapy as early as possible cannot be too strongly stressed, since the longer the vitamin B_{12} deficiency exists the more extensive and crippling the neurologic manifestations may become and the less readily they may be reversed to normal to rehabilitate the patient. Today the complication most to be feared in pernicious anemia is the development of irreversible crippling neurologic manifestations because of tardy or inadequate vitamin B_{12} therapy.

Peripheral Blood Findings

The peripheral blood findings typically include abnormalities in all formed elements of the blood: red cells, white cells, and platelets. The red cells are macrocytic in well-established anemia: mean corpuscular volume may be 110 to 150 cu μ. They are normochromic unless the unusual complication of iron lack coexists, in which situation the mean corpuscular hemoglobin concentration is below the normal limits of 32 to 34 Gm per 100 ml. Since the cells are predominantly macrocytic, disproportionate lowering of the red cell count compared with the hemoglobin concentration is seen; less than 2 million red cells per cubic millimeter is not unusual with a hemoglobin concentration of 8 Gm per 100 ml. Examination of the stained blood film shows extreme variation in the size of the cells, so that the moderate numbers of microcytes (4 μ in diameter) may be readily contrasted with the large, well-filled oval macrocytes that may measure 14 μ or more at greatest diameter. All gradations are seen, but the dominant cell is large, oval, bulky, well filled with hemoglobin, and usually does not have a central pale zone. Numerous intermediate-sized bizarre forms are seen. Reticulocytes are few in number, especially if calculated in absolute terms, both because of the red blood count depression and the low percentage seen. Definite leukopenia is so frequent that its absence should raise serious doubts about the validity of the diagnosis of pernicious anemia, provided complications such as infection can be adequately excluded, since it is well established that patients with pernicious anemia are capable of appropriate leukocytic responses. A commonly occurring abnormality is polymorphonuclear neutrophilic leukocytes with unusually large numbers of lobes or nuclear segments: hypersegmented polys or macropolycytes with six to ten nuclear segments. Formerly thought to represent older-than-normal cells (shift to the right), these multilobed polys more likely represent the product of the abnormal nuclear divisions that occur during mitosis of myelocytic cells. Calculated in absolute terms there is a neutropenia. The differential shows relative lymphocytosis. The platelets are consistently reduced in number but only unusually into the range associated with hemorrhagic manifestations.

In general, the more severe the anemia the more gross are the above changes: in profound anemia the macrocytosis is extreme. However, it is important to note that significant morphologic changes may be seen even in the absence of anemia. Various observers have emphasized that early in the "preanemic" stage of vitamin B_{12} deficiency typical well-filled oval macrocytes and hypersegmented polys are found; therefore, these constitute extremely sensitive diagnostic indicators.

Bone Marrow Findings

Profound and highly characteristic changes are found in the bone marrow (53, 68, 135, 156, 170, 207, 250). The volume of the marrow is increased by replacement of fat, extension along marrow cavities, and increased cell concentration. Striking morphologic alterations are seen in the precursors of all three formed elements. Instead of the usual E/M (erythrocyte to myelocyte) ratio of approximately 1:4 or 1:3, the red cell hyperplasia may shift the ratio to 1:1. Moreover, the red cells show characteristic morphologic alterations and abnormal maturation. Instead of the usual normoblastic proliferation, so-called megaloblastic proliferation occurs. In the light of inconclusive evidence megaloblastic proliferation is probably most accurately regarded as the route of erythrocyte production available to vitamin B_{12}–deficient red cell precursors: a deficient but not a new or different maturation series. The normal proerythroblast in the deficient state takes on abnormal characteristics. Moreover, in this situation the abnormalities are readily perceived at each level as the cell passes through the maturation series on its way to becoming an oval, well-filled macrocyte ("megalocyte"). The abnormal proerythroblast* is a cell that usually covers a larger area on the stained blood film than its normal counterpart. It should be noted that this is not necessarily the same as saying that it is larger in size than is the normal proerythroblast. It usually covers a larger area but appears thin in contrast to the normal proerythroblast, which seems to rise up with definite "focal-plane thickness" from the cover slip. An abundant, intensely dark-blue cytoplasm is present and lacks granules. Its periphery is frequently irregular, with one or several "dog-ear" projections. The nucleus is centrally located and occupies a large area of the cell. The most important feature of the cell is the extremely fine, delicate nuclear chromatin, which is uniformly dispersed so that it is punctate in appearance rather than strand-like or condensed. One or more large blue nucleoli may be present. As maturation proceeds there is dyssynchrony of nuclear and cytoplasmic development. At an unusually early age, as judged by nuclear maturation, the cytoplasm begins to take on an acidophilic hue, reflecting hemoglobin development. The nucleus persists in occupying a large area of the cell even though the nucleoli disappear and the chromatin gathers into knots and clumps. It thereby remains open with large clear spaces between the chromatin. Sometimes hemoglobin production progresses in the cytoplasm to orthochromatic proportions while the nucleus remains large and fairly open. Ultimately, however, considerable condensation and pyknosis occur, followed presumably by extrusion, leaving the large oval macrocyte. The number of mitotic figures is increased in megaloblastic proliferation, and diploid and tetraploid forms may be identified. Although all stages of the red cell maturation series corresponding to the various arbitrary steps of normoblastic proliferation may be singled out, the majority of the cells are primitive—analogous to the proerythroblast or early erythroblast. Very few cells analogous to normoblasts are present. This has given rise to the concept of "maturation arrest" with the implication that development proceeds to a certain phase and

* Because it has been used differently by so many different workers, the term megaloblast has become difficult to deal with in any satisfactory fashion. Some authors equate the megaloblast with the abnormal proerythroblast, some with the abnormal normoblast. It would seem most consistent (although undeniably cumbersome) to reserve the word to designate a type of abnormal maturation, *megaloblastic proliferation,* and employ the nomenclature used for the normal maturation series (proerythroblast, early and late erythroblast, normoblast, etc.). For example, one would speak of an early erythroblast of megaloblastic proliferation.

then stops. In a limited sense this is probably true, but the "arrest" is partial at best, for as described above abnormal maturation does proceed to macrocyte production.

Morphologic alterations in the leukocyte and megakaryocyte series, while very evident, are usually not as vividly portrayed as the erythrocyte abnormalities. Giant myelocytes, metamyelocytes, and multilobed megakaryocytes (polykaryocytes) are present.

For grossly abnormal megaloblastic proliferation to be present, evidence indicates that two factors are necessary in varying degree of balance: (a) vitamin B_{12} deficiency (of prime importance) and (b) tissue hypoxia with resultant stress on erythropoiesis. Observations have shown that if a patient with untreated pernicious anemia and marrow showing abnormal maturation and abnormal proerythroblasts is transfused to a normal hemoglobin level with washed red cells (thereby relieving hypoxia without administering therapeutically effective amounts of vitamin B_{12} or folic acid), a decrease in number of abnormal proerythroblasts takes place, but evidence of abnormal maturation persists without reticulocyte response (56, 172). A reasonable explanation would seem to be that relief of tissue hypoxia decreases erythropoietin formation; a decrease in this factor relieves the stimulus for proliferation from stem cells (setting up several production lines) but the other maturation abnormality persists unchanged. In fact, patients are seen with tissue (glossal, neural) evidence of vitamin B_{12} deficiency, but without anemia, who have typical maturation abnormalities in the marrow and as mentioned above a few macrocytes and hypersegmented polys in the peripheral blood.

Although specific tests (some of which will be mentioned below) indicate profound disturbances of many metabolic systems, the usual screening tests relative to blood chemistry yield unremarkable results. One or more liver function tests may be abnormal, but no consistent pattern of hepatic dysfunction has been found. The bilirubin concentration is usually within normal limits, but the value is increased above that expected for the low concentration of circulating hemoglobin. Aside from a lack of ability to concentrate, urine findings are unremarkable. In the presence of combined degeneration of the spinal cord the spinal fluid may show moderate increases in protein but is otherwise normal. Amino-aciduria has been noted (82, 137) especially in the presence of combined degeneration of the spinal cord (245).

Gastric Findings

In the vast majority of patients with pernicious anemia tests of gastric secretory ability show a histamine-refractory achylia and achlorhydria, and examination of the gastric mucosa by gross or histologic techniques shows a marked atrophic gastritis of the fundal portions or a severe gastric atrophy involving all coats of the stomach wall (168, 169, 238, 261, 266). Notable exceptions to this are the *few* patients with authenticated pernicious anemia in infancy, adolescence, and early adult life (180, 237). Otherwise, the rule is so well followed that for practical purposes *if histamine-fast achylia and achlorhydria do not exist the patient cannot have pernicious anemia.* In a normal individual 1 hour following histamine stimulation between 100 and 200 ml of clear gastric juice can be readily aspirated which has a pH of 1 to 2 and 50 to 100 titratable units of "free hydrochloric acid." The same procedure performed on a patient with pernicious anemia yields 10 to 20 ml of cloudy, grumous material, aspirated with some difficulty, which has a pH of 6 to 8 and no "free hydrochloric acid." The achylia is as important to note as the achlorhydria, since the latter occurs in an increasing proportion of otherwise normal individuals apparently as a concomitant of the aging process. Histamine-fast achlorhydria* is present in approximately 3 per cent of subjects aged 20 to 29; 4 per cent of subjects aged 30 to 39; 14 per cent of subjects 40 to 49; 16 per cent of subjects 50 to 59; 25 per cent of subjects 60 to 69; and 28 per cent of subjects over 70 years old. Therefore, it must be remembered that achlorhydria need not be evidence *for* a diagnosis of pernicious anemia, but that the presence of "free hydrochloric acid" for practical purposes *excludes* the diagnosis. However, although no extensive studies are available, it is generally acknowledged that achlorhydria *plus* true achylia as described above must be taken as strong evidence in favor of pernicious anemia.

In connection with this discussion of atrophic gastritis, achylia, and achlorhydria, it is important to point out that the incidence of gastric carcinoma is increased in pernicious anemia. Various extensive surveys (17, 126, 136, 185, 195, 272) indicate the increase to be from three to ten times that found in comparable age groups.† The incidence of gastric polyps is also increased, and transition from apparently benign polyps to malignant neoplasms has been observed. Because of this each patient must undergo *repeated* careful searches for gastrointestinal abnormalities. As the patient is being followed under treatment, careful investigation must be done at the slightest provocation (G.I. series, gastric cytology, fecal guaiac test, etc.). Some of the studies on gastric carcinoma in pernicious anemia indicate that the majority of the lesions occur in the fundus, a region only difficultly examinable with accuracy by usual roentgenographic techniques, so that special procedures are called for.

Criteria for Diagnosis

We have here developed the criteria by which a *presumptive diagnosis* of per-

nicious anemia may be made. The symptoms and physical findings are today usually nonspecific and at best constitute suggestive evidence *unless* central nervous system manifestations are present. Lacking these, however, the evidence must come from the laboratory in the form of (a) typical peripheral blood findings, (b) typical bone marrow alterations, and (c) histamine-fast achlorhydria and achylia. With these criteria fulfilled, a *presumptive diagnosis* of pernicious anemia may be made. The fourth and most important criterion for the diagnosis is a typical orderly clinical and hematologic response (Figure 7.2) to the administration of a therapeutic agent of known potency in physiologic amounts (now almost invariably vitamin B_{12}). With the fulfillment of these four criteria, the diagnosis is for practical purposes assured, and the chance of an inaccurate diagnosis very slight. Nevertheless, it must be pointed out that none of the above criteria is necessarily based upon the defect that is fundamental to and causal of pernicious anemia, namely, the genetically determined tendency toward degeneration of the gastric mucosa that leads to inability to produce intrinsic factor. When Minot empirically established the efficacy of liver administration in the treatment of pernicious anemia, it became evident (130) that it was possible to reverse completely or halt the progression of all clinical and laboratory manifestations except one: the gastric defect,

---

* Recent studies by various workers on patients formerly classified as having achlorhydria by the usual histamine test show that some 60 per cent had normal acid secretion by the augmented histamine test—unfortunately something of an ordeal for the patient. Patients with pernicious anemia do not so respond to the augmented histamine test: there is no increase in the volume of juice secreted, and in over 90 per cent the juice actually becomes more alkaline (34, 257).

† A notable exception to these findings is the experience of Wilkinson (259), who reports no increased incidence in a series of 1,820 patients personally observed for many years.

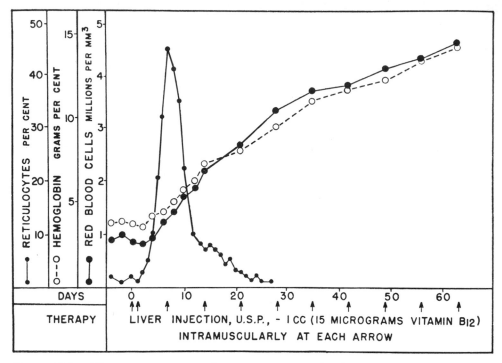

FIGURE 7.2.   Characteristic maximal response to specific therapy by severely anemic patient with pernicious anemia. (From Castle, W. B., *in* Cecil, R. L., and Loeb, R. F. (ed.), A Textbook of Medicine, p. 1131, Saunders, Philadelphia, 1959)

or, expressed in later physiologic terms, the inability of the patient to secrete adequate quantities of intrinsic factor. As defined above, the manifestations of pernicious anemia are the consequence of a lack of intrinsic factor. Therefore, establishment of an unequivocal diagnosis demands the demonstration of this ultimate causal defect. In actual practice, as pointed out above, this is seldom necessary, even though at present it can fairly readily be done by the appropriate combination of modern radioactive techniques and long-established physiologic principles.

Pathology and Pathophysiology: Basic Observations

In 1855 Addison gave a rather vague description of a disease now acknowledged to be pernicious anemia and frequently referred to as Addisonian pernicious anemia. In view of the amazing

physiologic and anatomic complexity of the disease known today, it is astonishing that shortly thereafter the anatomic expression of the primary cause of the disease came under suspicion. Atrophy of the glandular portion of the stomach was noted on autopsy examination, and Austin Flint wrote: "I suspect that in these cases there exists degenerative disease of the glandular tubuli of the stomach. . . . Fatal anaemia must follow an amount of degenerative disease reducing the amount of gastric juice so far that assimilation of food is rendered wholly inadequate to the wants of the body."[*]

The first experimental approach to this theory came from the observations of Fenwick in 1870 when he demonstrated that the acidified scrapings of gastric

[*] One hundred years later it is curious to note that the quotation ends: "I shall be ready to claim the merit of this idea when the difficult and laborious researches of someone have shown it to be correct."

mucosa obtained post mortem from a patient with pernicious anemia failed to diminish the weight of a cube of hard-boiled egg white. He concluded that "the progressive atrophy of the stomach had prevented the digestion of the albuminous materials of the food." No studies of significance along these lines followed until the unsuccessful attempts of Peabody to overcome the digestive inadequacy of pernicious anemia by forced feeding. These studies were given needed direction and selectivity by Whipple's experiments with dogs, outlined in Chapter 3, which demonstrated the hemoglobin-producing capacities of various foods, of which liver was found especially efficacious. Based upon these observations, Minot and Murphy (178) convincingly demonstrated the therapeutic effectiveness of the systematic daily feeding of half-pound quantities of raw or lightly cooked liver and established beyond question that the disease was the result of a nutritional deficiency and that the absorptive defect could be overcome by selective forced feeding. This therapeutic triumph by Minot and Murphy served to emphasize the crucial role of the gastric abnormality, since this alone was irreversible among the various manifestations of the disease. This fact prompted Castle (39) to initiate studies into the *physiologic* nature of the gastric defect, since by that time gastric atrophy and lack of hydrochloric acid in the gastric contents had been shown to be universally present.

It was well established that the administration of large quantities of meat to patients with pernicious anemia did not induce a clinical or hematologic remission. Castle first obtained clinical and hematologic remission by employing meat that had been predigested by temporary residence in a *normal* stomach immediately prior to its administration to patients with pernicious anemia. By observations made sequentially *in the same patient*, he then demonstrated by hematologic evaluation that (a) although patients with pernicious anemia were unable to derive a required nutritional factor from the ingestion of beef alone, (b) if the meat had been predigested by exposure to normal human gastric juice within a normal alimentary tract, patients could then obtain from it the indispensable factor. In essence, Castle had substituted the products of gastric digestion of beef successfully effected by the normal human stomach for those of the defective digestion of pernicious anemia, and by the correction of the hematologic derangement had shown that pernicious anemia resulted not from a simple nutritional deficiency but from a *conditioned* deficiency. Even though the requisite nutrient factor is present in ingested food, the patient is deprived of it because of a specific lesion that prohibits utilization. Subsequent observations demonstrated that therapeutic results were obtained from the daily administration of mixtures of 200 Gm of beef muscle and 150 ml of normal human gastric juice. Using this technique it was concluded that the development of erythropoietic activity resulted from contact within the alimentary tract of a thermostable food substance (extrinsic factor) with a thermolabile compound in gastric juice (intrinsic factor).

Extensive use was made in these early studies and many subsequent ones of a technique known as the serial reticulocyte response (double reticulocyte response) by which the erythropoietic activity of various substances can be assessed and compared (179). To a patient with untreated pernicious anemia maintained on a base-line diet, a daily uniform amount of a given substance is administered for a 10-day period of observation and its erythropoietic effectiveness assessed by daily quantitation of the reticulocytes. During a second similar and contiguous period, the erythropoietic activity of a second substance may be assessed by the reticulocyte response which, when present, indicates the second substance to be more potent than the first (Figure 7.3). A positive response in the second period must be obtained to permit a conclusion; failure to increase the reticulocyte count in the second period could mean that (a) an inactive substance was being administered or one less active than that given in the first period, or (b) the initial response had been maximal.

In Castle's most rigorous test of his hypothesis and observations, during a first 10-day observation period the daily administration of beef and normal human gastric juice produced *no* reticulocytosis (had no erythropoietic activity) when the substances were given *separated by a 12-hour interval;* however, when in a second, contiguous 10-day interval the substances were administered *simultaneously,* reticulocytosis occurred, indicating the development of significant erythropoietic activity when in the gastrointestinal tract an interaction was possible between extrinsic and intrinsic factors.* These perdurable observations, which have withstood the test of time and become "obstinate facts" of clinical experimentation, have formed the basis for the great majority of the studies concerned with pathophysiology that have subsequently been done. From this point may be traced two distinct but interconnected stories, the one concerned with the nature and mode of action of intrinsic factor and the other with the nature and mode of action of extrinsic factor. And it is upon the physiologic principles established by the obstinate facts that present-day radioactive diagnostic tests are based.

Intrinsic Factor

To consider the nature and mode of action of intrinsic factor it will first be necessary to present briefly evidence concerning some properties of extrinsic fac-

tor. The classic source of extrinsic factor was, of course, beef muscle, but in addition early experiments demonstrated that casein, eggs, and 70 per cent alcoholic extracts of beef muscle possess extrinsic factor activity. Extraction and substitution procedures demonstrated that none of the then-known vitamins, including folic acid, possessed extrinsic factor activity singly or in combination. Extrinsic factor was not isolated as such from the classic sources, but its identity became known by comparison of its activity with that of the antipernicious anemia factor isolated from liver extracts. Very early it was demonstrated that the erythropoietic activity of crude liver extracts was enhanced by the simultaneous oral administration of normal human gastric juice. Consequently crude liver possessed extrinsic factor activity. Meanwhile the "chemical dissection of liver" was pursued until extracts were available that contained none of the known vitamins but were therapeutically effective against pernicious anemia when administered parenterally in amounts of 1 ml per month. In 1948 it was found that the erythropoietic activity of orally administered purified liver extracts was also potentiated by gastric juice. During this same year Merck Laboratories in the United States announced the isolation of a red crystalline substance that they called vitamin B_{12}. A few weeks later

---

* The double reticulocyte response is a most valuable tool in hematology and is only now being supplemented or replaced in certain situations by radioactive techniques. As pointed out by Castle, in single patients it was possible to determine the comparative erythropoietic activity of two or more experimental liver fractions or various iron compounds. Later the existence of distinct clinical deficiency of folic acid and quite recently pyridoxine abnormality were so established. "Double deficiencies" of thyroid hormone and vitamin B_{12}, of thyroid hormone and iron, of vitamin B_{12} and iron, of folic acid and vitamin C were clearly documented. Moreover, the inhibitory effect of intercurrent infection, toxic chemicals, and hyperoxia, or the stimulating action of hypoxia, on erythropoietic function were clearly established in man.

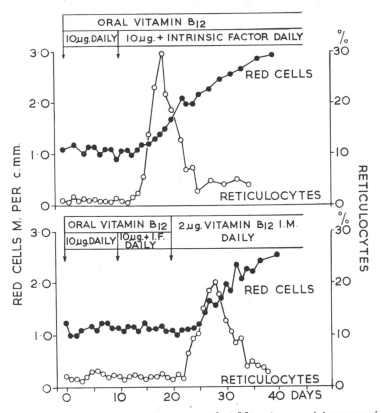

FIGURE 7.3.   Hematologic response of patient with Addisonian pernicious anemia (upper figure) and of patient with intestinal malabsorption syndrome (lower figure) to treatment with small daily oral dose of vitamin B₁₂ given alone, and then with potent source of intrinsic factor. Patient with intestinal malabsorption syndrome subsequently received small daily injections of the vitamin. (From Mollin, D. L., *in* University of London, British Postgraduate Medical Federation, Lectures on the Scientific Basis of Medicine, vol. 7, p. 94, Athlone Press, London, 1957)

independent isolation of the same substance was announced by the Glaxo Laboratories in England. This vitamin, injected parenterally, was found to be highly effective in the treatment of pernicious anemia. And still in 1948 it was found that although 5 μg of vitamin B₁₂ was erythropoietically inert when given daily by mouth to patients with pernicious anemia, erythropoietic and clinical response promptly followed the daily simultaneous administration of 5 μg of vitamin B₁₂ and normal human gastric juice. Although separated by 20 years from Castle's original observation, the experimental design and the techniques employed to demonstrate this were the

same, except that instead of 200 Gm of beef muscle, 5 μg of vitamin B₁₂ was given with the normal human gastric juice to the patient. Only after the active principle of liver extract had been found to be vitamin B₁₂ did it finally become apparent that vitamin B₁₂ is identical with the so-called extrinsic factor. The chemistry of vitamin B₁₂ as antipernicious anemia principle and something of its function will be dealt with later. At present a consideration will be made of the nature and mode of action of intrinsic factor, referring to vitamin B₁₂, or extrinsic factor, when appropriate.

PROPERTIES. In 1937 it was shown that intrinsic factor activity of normal human gastric juice required that the mixture of beef muscle and gastric juice be given to the patient at a pH of not less than 5.* The activity of such a mixture was destroyed at once by boiling or by 70 per cent alcohol. Intrinsic factor was shown unable to pass through an ultrafilter or dialysis membrane, and at least part of it was precipitated by half saturation with ammonium sulfate. These properties suggested a large molecule, presumably a protein or an enzyme. It could not be identified with pepsin, lysozyme, polypeptides, and other gastric enzymes.

As little as 10 ml of gastric juice could potentiate the erythropoietic activity of 1 μg of vitamin B_{12} when the two were given daily simultaneously by mouth. However, intrinsic factor failed to augment the activity of vitamin B_{12} when both were given simultaneously by intravenous injection, daily, and subsequent to sterile incubation. It appeared that the essential activity of instrinsic factor was to enhance the gastrointestinal absorption of vitamin B_{12}. In 1952 radioactive vitamin B_{12} became available by the incorporation of Co^{60} into the molecule. The first studies relative to intrinsic factor activity employed the estimation of radioactivity in the feces for a few days after the oral administration of a tracer dose of the labeled vitamin. The amount of radioactivity excreted by patients with pernicious anemia was consistently and significantly greater than the amount excreted by normal persons. When intrinsic factor and the labeled vitamin were given simultaneously, the patients' fecal radioactivity decreased. These studies, strictly speaking, did not demonstrate the absorption of vitamin B_{12} but rather the changes in excretion of Co^{60} *presumed* to be in the intact vitamin B_{12} molecule. Under comparable situations it was possible to demonstrate the accumulation of radioactivity in the region of the liver by directional external radioactive counting. Less radioactivity accumulated in the liver region in patients with pernicious anemia than in normal individuals, but again the amount could be augmented by the simultaneous administration of a source of intrinsic factor.

THE SCHILLING TEST. The most conclusive studies relative to absorption of the vitamin B_{12} molecule were accomplished by Schilling employing (a) measurement of the radioactivity appearing in the urine following oral administration of labeled vitamin B_{12}, (b) measurement of the increase in urinary excretion of radioactivity when intrinsic factor was also given, and (c) demonstration that the urinary radioactivity was due to the presence of intact labeled vitamin B_{12}. In this technique, now referred to as the Schilling test (90, 221, 264), a tracer dose of labeled vitamin B_{12} is given orally to a patient who has fasted overnight; following this, the urine is collected for 24 hours (some workers employ 48- to 72-hour collections). Because under ordinary circumstances an undetectable amount of radioactivity appears in the urine even in the normal person, 1,000 μg of *unlabeled* vitamin B_{12} is administered *parenterally* 2 hours after the oral dose to serve as a "flushing dose" that in some way (saturation of binding sites, carrier action in exceeding renal clearance, etc.) allows the excretion of labeled vitamin B_{12} into the urine in readily detectable amounts (4). Both by chemical procedures and by microbiologic assay the radioactive label appears to be due to the presence of intact vitamin B_{12}.

When the Schilling test is performed in patients with pernicious anemia, very small amounts of radioactive vitamin B_{12} are excreted in the urine: 0 to 3 per cent of the administered dose. In normal individuals the excretion is in the range of 5 to 40 per cent. If to the patient with

---

* This pH dependence of intrinsic factor activity has been confirmed in the recent in vitro studies to be described later (124).

pernicious anemia a source of instrinsic factor is administered simultaneously with the radioactive vitamin B_{12}, the excretion of the vitamin in the urine is significantly enhanced into the normal range. The Schilling test convincingly demonstrates the absorption of vitamin B_{12} from the gastrointestinal tract, its entrance into the circulation, and its excretion by the kidneys. By utilizing the simultaneous oral administration of intrinsic factor, the enhanced excretion (dependent upon absorption) of vitamin B_{12} may also be demonstrated.

Probably the most direct demonstration that intrinsic factor plays a necessary role facilitating the absorption of vitamin B_{12} are studies in which radioactive vitamin B_{12} was added to preparations of intrinsic factor in amounts to saturate available binding sites. This preparation was given orally to a patient with pernicious anemia, and at the moment before administration nonlabeled vitamin B_{12} was added to the mixture. The reverse procedure was also done: nonlabeled vitamin B_{12} was bound to the intrinsic factor preparation with radioactive vitamin added just before oral administration. In both situations it was found by fecal and urinary assay that the vitamin

B_{12} bound to the intrinsic factor preparation was the one preferentially absorbed.

Three types of studies—fecal excretion, hepatic accumulation, and urinary excretion of labeled vitamin B_{12}—are being extensively employed in the investigation of pernicious anemia. Simultaneous measurements in groups of normal individuals and patients have shown the three tests to give results comparable and consistent with one another (199; Table 7.1). Recently whole-body counting has been used to measure the absorption of cobalt-labeled vitamin B_{12} (211).

It should be noted that, unlike assays employing the double reticulocyte response, these tests may be performed even on treated patients whose hematologic symptoms are in remission. This is based upon the observation that the gastric lesion is not corrected by treatment. They are therefore extremely valuable diagnostic tools (19, 140, 181, 201). Because of the equipment involved and the ease of sample collection, the Schilling test is the most widely employed. A word of caution must be sounded, however: the excretion of labeled vitamin B_{12} depends on reasonably intact renal function, an adequate urinary output, and an accurate urine collection; this test

TABLE 7.1.   Absorption of radioactive vitamin B_{12} by normal individuals and patients with pernicious anemia, as determined by various tests

Method	Normal values[a]	Values in pernicious anemia[a]
Schilling test		
0.5 μg dose	15–40%/24 hr	0–7.5%/24 hr
1.0 μg dose	5–40%/24 hr	0–3.0%/24 hr
2.0 μg dose	5–20%/24 hr	0–2.5%/24 hr
Fecal excretion		
0.5 μg dose	3–67% excreted	70–100% excreted
1.0 μg dose	13–74% excreted	72–100% excreted
Hepatic uptake		
0.5–1.0 μg dose	300–7,300 cpm/μc B_{12} Co^{60} given	0–100 cpm/μc B_{12} Co^{60} given
Plasma increment		
1.0 μg dose	Peak activity 3–12 $\mu\mu$g B_{12}/ml	Peak activity 0–1 $\mu\mu$g B_{12}/ml

[a] These figures are intended as examples rather than standard values.

From Grasbeck, R., Advances Clin. Chem. 3:299, 1960.

cannot be employed in patients with significant renal disease (206).

MODE OF ACTION. These observations provide evidence concerning the mechanism of action of intrinsic factor. Previous analyses of the problem hypothesized the following possibilities: (a) *enhanced absorption* of the vitamin by action of intrinsic factor; (b) *protection* of the vitamin from destruction or utilization (bacterial) in the gastrointestinal tract so that lacking intrinsic factor there is insufficient opportunity for adequate absorption; and (c) *interaction*, presuming activation or alteration of the vitamin B_{12} molecule so that it becomes hematopoietically more potent. As yet there appears no conclusive evidence to exclude any one of these possibilities, but the available evidence most convincingly supports enhanced absorption of unaltered vitamin B_{12} as the mode of action of intrinsic factor. The basic abnormality, then, in pernicious anemia is defective production of intrinsic factor, which in turn is responsible for the faulty absorption of vitamin B_{12} and the consequent body-wide deficiency. Castle has stated that "pernicious anemia would not develop if the patient could effect daily the transfer of one-millionth gram of vitamin B_{12} the distance of a small fraction of a millimetre across the intestinal mucosa and into the blood stream."

Intrinsic factor is produced in the stomach, and one phase of its action may well begin in this region (48). Experimentally, normal human gastric juice can competitively remove from foods the vitamin B_{12} naturally bound to proteins or polypeptides (beef, pork, casein) or added radioactive vitamin B_{12}. The vitamin B_{12} then bound by intrinsic factor is not dialyzable. This competitive removal and preferential binding is favored by an acid medium. The first step in intrinsic factor action may then be to bind the vitamin B_{12} released from food by the acid environment of the stomach.

Evidence has recently been obtained that the principal site of absorption of vitamin B_{12} in man is the distal half of the ileum (7, 11, 22, 44, 81). If labeled vitamin B_{12} is administered orally prior to laparotomy, measurement of the location of the vitamin by direct scanning of the loops of bowel with scintillation detectors shows that 3 hours after administration the radioactivity is entirely in the distal half of the ileum. Since this occurs at the time when the plasma level of radioactive vitamin B_{12} is beginning to increase, a selective retention in the distal ileum is indicated. Confirmatory evidence that the distal ileum is the major site of vitamin B_{12} absorption comes from documented deficiency in patients with diseases of the ileum or following major surgical resections (7).

There have been many investigations into the mechanisms whereby intrinsic factor brings about the transmucosal passage of vitamin B_{12}. Although substances without intrinsic factor activity may bind vitamin B_{12}, all preparations known to possess intrinsic factor activity have the capacity to bind vitamin B_{12} and alter its electrophoretic mobility, dialysis characteristics, availability to microorganisms, etc. (212). The evidence now indicates that the binding is of a specific nature, since intrinsic factor preparations will not bind in comparable fashion analogues of vitamin B_{12} or degradation products (30, 31). Alterations in either the nucleotide or planar part of the molecule (Figure 7.4) prevent or weaken the attachment to intrinsic factor. This probably can only be explained by linkage between the two molecules at two, three, or more sites.

It has been suggested that the principal action of intrinsic factor is to bind vitamin B_{12} and thereby render it unavailable to microorganisms of the intestinal tract. This hypothesis was based on the results of microbiologic assay techniques in which it was shown that preparations containing intrinsic factor activity did not support the multiplication of vitamin B_{12}–dependent organisms. This effect could be abolished by heating, a procedure known to destroy intrinsic factor activity. The theory was made somewhat attractive by reports of bacterial flora present in the gastrointestinal tract of patients with pernicious anemia in greater-than-normal numbers and at sites ordinarily relatively free of bacteria in the normal person. However, a number of proteins and substances are capable of tightly binding vitamin B_{12} and preventing its microbial utilization but do not possess intrinsic factor activity, and from the evidence discussed below this does not appear to be the physiologically significant role of intrinsic factor governing the absorption of vitamin B_{12}. Nevertheless, it may indeed be a partial explanation of the vitamin B_{12} deficiency seen in association with the broad tapeworm, *Diphyllobothrium latum* (24, 104, 189, 251). Approximately 20 per cent of the population in Finland harbors the tapeworm, but only 1 in 3,000 becomes anemic. The deciding factor appears to be the level of attachment of the worm: when it is present high in the gastrointestinal tract, it contains considerable quantities of vitamin B_{12}, which it apparently preferentially takes up at the host's expense.*

It was mentioned previously that when the administration of intrinsic factor is separated by 12 hours from the administration of vitamin B_{12}, no evidence is obtained for potentiation of the latter or for interaction between the two factors. When the time between administrations is reduced, a point is reached at which interaction does take place. It is then possible to show that intrinsic factor preparation given *prior* to the vitamin B_{12} has a more potent hematopoietic effect than the reverse sequence. This suggests an important interaction between the intrinsic factor and the intestinal mucosa, in which the latter is presumably modi-

fied so that it can accept the vitamin and more readily transfer it through the gut wall. This concept has received some intriguing support by in vitro studies concerning the mechanisms whereby vitamin B_{12} is bound to intestinal mucosa (everted sacs or homogenates) or liver slices (118, 119, 121, 124, 177). When isotopically labeled vitamin B_{12} is employed, the amount adsorbed to intestinal mucosa in the presence of intrinsic factor may be quantitated. It has been repeatedly demonstrated that prior exposure of the tissue to intrinsic factor increases quite significantly its ability to take up vitamin B_{12}. Following exposure to intrinsic factor the tissue may be repeatedly washed without removing the factor that augments vitamin B_{12} uptake. However, if the initial step is done in the presence of a chelating agent (EDTA), enhancement of uptake does not occur. This effect of EDTA may be overcome by the presence of calcium ions. From this it has been concluded that intrinsic factor attaches to receptor sites on mucosal cells by a specific binding action requiring calcium ions. Vitamin B_{12} is attached to the intrinsic factor and from there is transported into the cell.† This proposed mechanism of action provides a ready explanation for the observation that there is an optimum ratio for the amounts of

---

* Tests on these patients also show that intrinsic factor is destroyed or inhibited to some extent. The development of vitamin B_{12} deficiency is accordingly the result of defective intrinsic factor activity, decreased dietary intake of vitamin B_{12}, and preferential uptake of vitamin B_{12} by the worm when located high in the intestinal tract (251).

† Suggestive support for the concept that this is the mode of action in humans is derived from the observation that the defective absorption of vitamin B_{12} sometimes seen in steatorrhea may be improved by the administration of calcium ions. Presumably in these patients the calcium is otherwise bound by intestinal fatty acids in the form of soaps. In tropical sprue, however, similar studies showed that the impaired absorption of vitamin B_{12} was not improved by either calcium lactate or intrinsic factor (214).

vitamin B_{12} and intrinsic factor present for maximal absorption of the vitamin to occur. If excess intrinsic factor is present, the absorption of vitamin B_{12} is progressively decreased. In this situation it is visualized that in addition to the molecules of intrinsic factor saturating the mucosal cell receptor sites, some of the excess intrinsic factor becomes bound to vitamin B_{12}, thereby blocking its absorption, since the receptor sites are occupied by intrinsic factor alone.

SPECIES SPECIFICITY. At this point it must be mentioned that there is evidence for some degree of species specificity relative to source of intrinsic factor. In the human being, gastric juice or mucosal extract of hog, monkey, and rat is effective, but dog's gastric juice is not. In the rat, rat intrinsic factor is effective but human gastric juice and intrinsic factor from hog stomach preparations are ineffective or even inhibitory (188, 253). This idea of species specificity has become important in recent times in the care of patients. There are available and in wide use preparations for the treatment of pernicious anemia composed of vitamin B_{12} and intrinsic factor. At first blush this appears reasonable: the deficiency in gastric secretion is corrected by intrinsic factor and the vitamin B_{12} is readily absorbed. In point of fact these preparations *are* potent and effective hematopoietic agents. Since, initially at least, the human being is, with respect to vitamin B_{12} absorption, not very discriminative about the source of intrinsic factor, a partially purified preparation derived from the hog's stomach has been widely used. But in several series of patients maintained on these preparations for prolonged periods of time, somewhere between 20 and 30 per cent have experienced clinical and hematologic relapse (18, 139, 196, 223, 241). Testing by the Schilling procedure demonstrated that in these patients the particular hog intrinsic factor preparation employed for therapy was no longer effective for enhancing the absorption of vitamin B_{12} (224–226). The patients had become refractory to the specific preparation and had indeed developed a circulating blood factor that could inactivate intrinsic factor activity (132a, 161, 241, 242). If serum from a refractory patient was administered along with an intrinsic factor preparation in the Schilling test, the expected enhancement of radioactive vitamin B_{12} excretion did not occur, and the inhibition of intrinsic factor activity varied with antibody titer as assayed by a hemagglutinin technique. This refractoriness and inhibition was species specific: enhanced vitamin B_{12} absorption could still be promoted by normal human gastric juice. The inhibitor was demonstrated (132a) to be in the γ-globulin fraction and to react in vivo with intrinsic factor–Co^{60}–vitamin B_{12} complex and alter its electrophoretic migration. It is assumed that the patients had developed a circulating antibody to a molecule that was, in part at least, altered or foreign and consequently antigenic. The point of great practical importance is that this type of preparation is unsuitable for the treatment of pernicious anemia.

Vitamin B_{12} adsorbed to intestinal mucosa by the intrinsic factor mechanism is there held by firm bonding (118–121). Apparently a specific mechanism is required to start it on its transmucosal migration (48). By in vitro studies it was shown that an aqueous extract of rat intestine was capable of releasing vitamin B_{12} from its bond to rat intrinsic factor. The rat extract released vitamin B_{12} from rat intrinsic factor much more readily than from human intrinsic factor. Moreover, the rat extract was not effective against hog intrinsic factor. There is therefore a striking species specificity in action of the aqueous extracts. In addition, the calcium-dependent bond holding the rat intrinsic factor–vitamin B_{12} complex to rat intestinal mucosa became unsusceptible to EDTA inhibition more quickly than it did when human intrinsic factor–vitamin B_{12} complex was employed. This led to the hypothesis that at or within the intestinal cell there occurs a species-dependent release of vitamin B_{12} from intrinsic factor. Experiments only incompletely reported indicate that not only is rat intestinal extract capable of releasing vitamin B_{12} *preferentially* from rat intrinsic factor, but human intestinal extract is capable of releasing vitamin B_{12} *preferentially* from human intrinsic factor.

It may be that the species dependence of intrinsic factor plays a role neither in the binding of vitamin B_{12} to intrinsic factor nor in the attachment of intrinsic factor to the intestinal mucosa but rather in the stage concerned with *release* of vitamin B_{12} from intrinsic factor by a presumed enzyme in the ileal mucosa. The unusual cases of specific malabsorption recently described in adults and children may be the result of reduction or absence of small intestinal receptors for intrinsic factor or reduction in the vitamin B_{12}-"releasing" enzyme or factor (45, 46).

CHEMISTRY. The list of substances thought at one time to be intrinsic factor or to contain intrinsic factor activity, and subsequently proved not to, is long and need not be itemized here. In 1952 it was suggested that intrinsic factor might be a soluble mucoprotein originating from the gastric glands. Analyses of such preparations by various workers (70, 146, 147) using different physical and chemical means indicate that the active principle is a neutral mucoprotein of molecular weight 70,000, an acid mucoprotein of molecular weight 40,000 or 15,000, or a mucopolypeptide of molecular weight 5,000. In an additional preparation all the vitamin B_{12}–binding capacity of hog glan-dular mucoprotein resided in a fraction that contained neutral polysaccharides coupled to a protein moiety. It seems possible that the "native" substance, as secreted, has a high molecular weight but that it is degraded to subunits of several sizes retaining clinical activity, or alternatively that a prosthetic group active as intrinsic factor is secreted separately from various carriers and combines subsequently. Two teams of workers have detected at least fifteen amino acids and also hexosamine, mannose, galactose, and a fucose (40) in the hydrolysate of "purified" preparations.

Taylor et al. (243) have described the finding of intrinsic factor activity derived from *human* gastric mucosa in two forms: in a particle-free fraction and in association with mitochondria. The fraction associated with mitochondria is of constant composition by ultrafiltration and electrophoresis but at pH 5 splits into two components, one having intrinsic factor activity and the second, inhibitory action.

SITE OF PRODUCTION. Early clinical observations employing the double reticulocyte response had shown intrinsic factor to be secreted throughout the fundus and cardia of the human stomach. Radioautography of sections of rat stomach labeled with radioactive vitamin B_{12}, on the assumption that the vitamin may be bound at sites of intrinsic factor secretion, indicates the chief (pepsinogen) secreting cells at the base of the gastric glands as its source. These cells have the characteristics of *protein*-secreting cells, not those of *mucus*-secreting cells (138).

PATTERN OF INHERITANCE OF DEFECTIVE PRODUCTION. Since the defective production of intrinsic factor conditions the development of vitamin B_{12} deficiency and the clinical picture of pernicious anemia, studies concerning the genetic factors *predisposing* to pernicious anemia have been based upon the ability of relatives of patients to absorb vitamin B_{12} as assayed by the Schilling test (33, 173). The most extensive studies report measurements on 136 relatives of 34 patients and 97 healthy control subjects. A significantly greater proportion of the family members than of the controls had low test results. Moreover, the number of family members with low vitamin B_{12} absorption increased with age, while no such variation was noted in the control group. The data indicate that the predisposition to pernicious anemia is most probably inherited as a single dominant autosomal factor.

SUMMARY. In summary, the absorption of physiologic amounts of vitamin B_{12} appears to take place at the terminal ileum through an intrinsic factor–dependent mechanism.* The substance possessing intrinsic factor and vitamin B_{12}–binding activity is found in association with mucoprotein or mucopolypeptides and is secreted mainly in the fundus of the stomach. In the stomach the vitamin B_{12} present in animal protein is freed from its loose binding by the acid environment. Intrinsic factor then firmly binds the free vitamin. The vitamin B_{12}–intrinsic factor complex is then adsorbed to the mucosal cells of the ileum at specific receptor or acceptor sites through a pH- and calcium-dependent bond. By a species-dependent intestinal mucosal factor the calcium-dependent bonding of the intrinsic factor–vitamin B_{12} complex is altered so that quick release of vitamin B_{12} and penetration into the intestinal wall takes place. It has been suggested that this is effected by "pinocytosis" at a molecular level by contractile receptor proteins at the surface of the cell (2). Recent studies indicate that vitamin B_{12} is transferred directly to the blood stream and does not enter by the lymphatics (210).

Extrinsic Factor (Vitamin B_{12})

In order to pursue the intrinsic factor story, it was pointed out that when vitamin B_{12} was crystallized from liver, it was very shortly thereafter identified as extrinsic factor. Part of the proof of this identity was provided by a study showing that when a suitably prepared extract of beef muscle (classic extrinsic factor source) was administered parenterally and without contact with gastric intrinsic factor to patients with untreated pernicious anemia, it had potent antipernicious anemia activity as judged by reticulocyte, clinical, and hemoglobin responses. By microbiologic assay and by clinical assay using the double reticulocyte response it was demonstrated that the hematopoietic activity of such beef

* Granting the terms of the experiments, there has been no serious questioning of the accuracy of either the observations or the interpretations of the findings concerning Castle's gastric intrinsic factor hypothesis as initially demonstrated and subsequently elucidated by a most remarkable series of perspicuous investigations (37, 39). Recently, however, the *physiologic relevance* of Castle's gastric intrinsic factor as the critical conditioning factor in the development of the vitamin B_{12} deficiency of pernicious anemia has been challenged; the accuracy of the observations has not been questioned, but they are considered interesting epiphenomena of no pathophysiologic import in the metabolism of vitamin B_{12}.

Work has been reported concerning the absorption of liver-bound radioactive vitamin B_{12} (190, 209) in which, without exposure to added intrinsic factor, greater absorption of radioactivity took place from a preparation containing labeled vitamin B_{12} in a bound, or conjugated, form derived from liver than from crystalline radioactive vitamin B_{12}. It has also been reported (183, 184) that patients with pernicious anemia can be treated with and maintained on vitamin B_{12} administered orally (without contact with added intrinsic factor) if the vitamin is in the form of a peptide complex derived from fermentation.

Since neither the naturally occurring "food forms" of vitamin B_{12} nor the coenzyme forms was available for testing, the possibility was raised that gastric intrinsic factor might not be required for the absorption of the naturally occurring forms or complexes of vitamin B_{12}. An alternate function of intrinsic factor was studied, and it was shown that the hepatic uptake of vitamin B_{12} was enhanced by the *parenteral* administration of intrinsic factor (192, 193, 247). Perhaps then the true role of intrinsic factor was not in the intestinal absorptive phase of the natural forms of vitamin B_{12} but in enhancing

muscle extracts and purified liver extracts could be accounted for *in toto* by their vitamin B_{12} content. Vitamin B_{12} was thus identified as both extrinsic factor and the antipernicious anemia principle. With this double role in mind, a consideration will be made of the chemistry and metabolism of vitamin B_{12} and the consequences of its deficiency.

CHEMISTRY. Vitamin B_{12} and related compounds are unique among the vitamins in that they are synthesized exclusively by microorganisms; all other organisms are directly or indirectly dependent upon this source. The vitamin B_{12} found in higher plants is due to contaminating or symbiotic organisms. It is a joy to the pharmaceutical houses involved in the industrial production of vitamin B_{12} that *Streptomyces griseus* and *S. aureofaciens* produce the vitamin as well as the antibiotics streptomycin and chlortetracycline, so that vitamin B_{12} may be obtained as a by-product from streptomycin "slops" (155). Vitamin B_{12} crystals are dark red and readily soluble in water in concentrations of biologic interest. The structure of vitamin B_{12} (Figure 7.4) was announced in 1955 after a 7-year study employing chemical synthesis and degradation, x-ray crystallographic analysis, and electronic computation involving some 10 million calculations. Early in the studies cobalt was found to be a component, and the element was thereby added to the list of essential nutrients for man. The vitamin B_{12} molecule is divided into two main portions: (a) a "planar group," a ring structure surrounding the cobalt, that resembles the porphyrin ring of heme except for a bond linking two pyrrole rings directly together instead of through a bridging carbon atom (a corrinoid ring); and (b) a "nucleotide group" containing a base, 5, 6-dimethylbenzimidazole, and phosphorylated ribose esterified with 1-amino, 2-propanal. Finally a cyanide group is carried by the trivalent cobalt

atom, which is also linked to the benzimidazole base. Under certain conditions the cyanide group dissociates from the molecule and can be replaced by hydroxide, aquo, and nitro groups. These compounds are now referred to as the cobalamines. Prefixes are employed to denote the group attached to the cobalt: cyanocobalamine (vitamin B_{12}); hydroxocobalamine (vitamin B_{12a}); aquocobalamine (vitamin B_{12b}); nitrito- (or nitro-) cobalamine (vitamin B_{12c}), etc. All these compounds have about the same biologic activity. A number of derivatives have been produced by removing and/or substituting component parts.

---

the liver uptake in the vitamin's postabsorptive phase. It should be pointed out again that the observations and interpretations drawn from the experiments with gastric juice, beef meat, liver extract, and cyanocobalamine cannot be questioned, but that their physiologic relevance was challenged. They were considered perhaps a series of accurate, interesting observations, irrelevant in that they had nothing to do with the pathophysiology of pernicious anemia and the metabolism of naturally occurring vitamin B_{12}.

The observations employing the vitamin B_{12}–peptide complex (HHP/1) have lacked suitable controls with respect to both the amounts of vitamin B_{12} employed (see reference 72 for remissions in pernicious anemia induced by small oral doses of purified vitamin B_{12}) and prior studies in the same patients concerning responsiveness to the doses employed. They have obtained independent support from a study on normal subjects and patients with partial gastrectomy (176). Recent studies employing the vitamin B_{12} peptide "in identical dosage and test methods" (231) have shown it to be similar in clinical and hematologic effects to crystalline vitamin B_{12}, although serum levels showed a comparatively greater rise at the low dosage. Studies employing a cobamide coenzyme show that intrinsic factor is required for its absorption as for cyanocobalamine (150, 268). The absorption of hydroxocobalamine, now thought to be an important form in which vitamin B_{12} occurs naturally in the liver (246), is enhanced by intrinsic factor. Thus, although the critical studies have not been done concerning the naturally occurring form(s) of vitamin B_{12}, there is no need to be diffident in stating that it must still be considered firmly established that the role of intrinsic factor in facilitating the absorption of physiologic amounts of vitamin B_{12} is central in the pathophysiology of pernicious anemia.

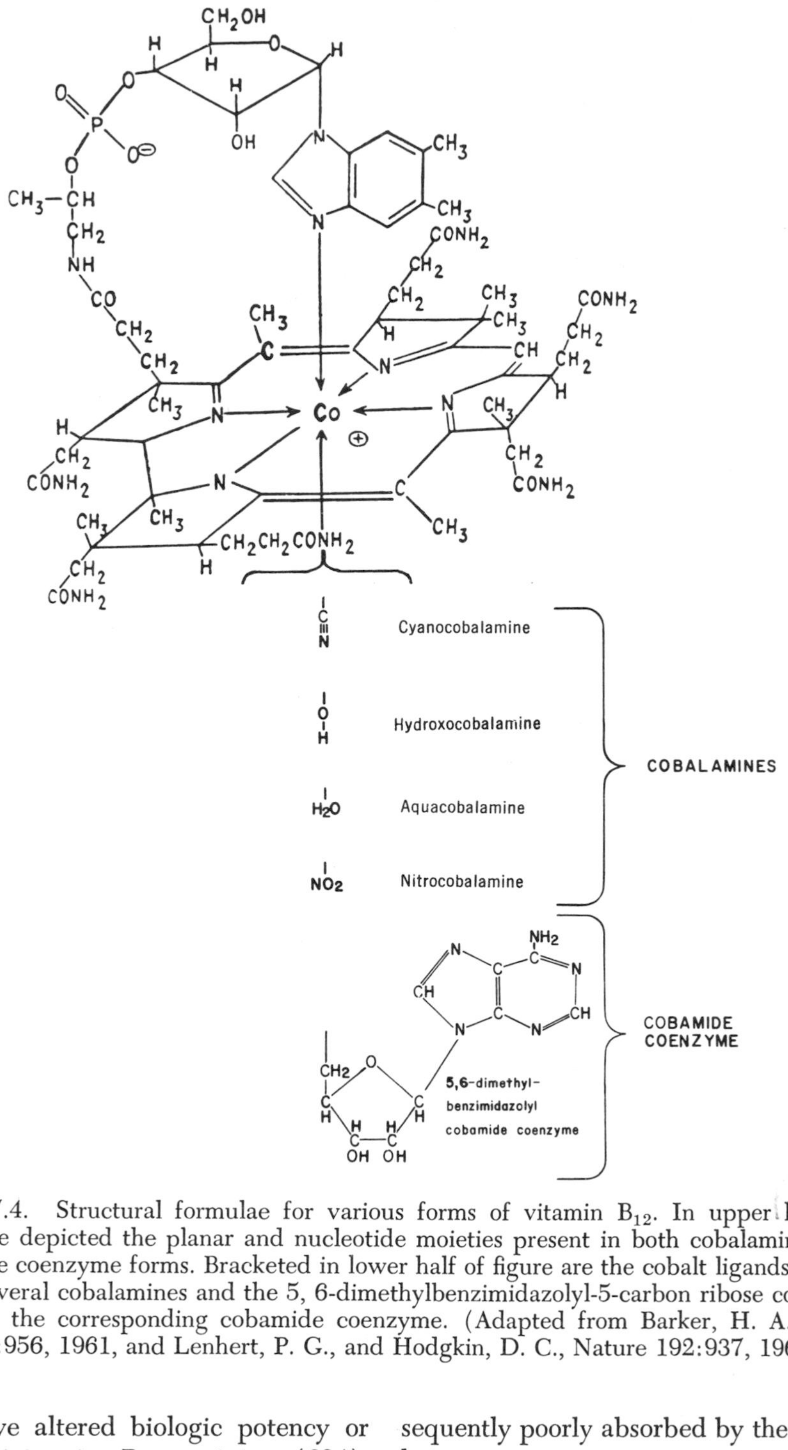

FIGURE 7.4. Structural formulae for various forms of vitamin B_{12}. In upper half of figure are depicted the planar and nucleotide moieties present in both cobalamine and cobamide coenzyme forms. Bracketed in lower half of figure are the cobalt ligands found in the several cobalamines and the 5, 6-dimethylbenzimidazolyl-5-carbon ribose complex found in the corresponding cobamide coenzyme. (Adapted from Barker, H. A., Fed. Proc. 20:956, 1961, and Lenhert, P. G., and Hodgkin, D. C., Nature 192:937, 1961)

Some have altered biologic potency or even antivitamin B_{12} activity (234). When adenine is subsituted for the benzimidazole base, a compound designated pseudovitamin B_{12} results, which is only weakly bound by intrinsic factor and con-sequently poorly absorbed by the human being.

NATURAL FORM. In nature vitamin B_{12} occurs complexed with a protein or an eighty-amino-acid polypeptide chain of known composition (115, 116) to which it is probably linked at several points, one of which is the cobalt atom. Moreover, recent work indicates that the naturally occurring compounds are chemically different from the originally isolated (vitamin B_{12}, or cyanocobalamine) molecule and that perhaps only in the naturally occurring forms is biologic activity present. These biologically active compounds are now termed the "cobamide coenzymes."* Three of the cobamide coenzymes have been isolated and characterized in detail, and one has been crystallized. In general, the base may be substituted for by an adenine base (or other heterocyclic base); no cyanide radicle is present; the cobalt is trivalent and linked to an additional adenine base through a ribose (153; Figure 7.4). These compounds are unstable. That the classic cyanocobalamine and hydroxocobalamine compounds are readily formed by exposure to cyanide, light, or pH changes and are mainly artifacts induced by the isolation procedure accounts for the fact that the coenzyme forms had previously been overlooked (246). There is evidence that a number of cobamide coenzyme forms exist. The three most extensively studied are (a) adenyl cobamide (AC), which contains one cobalt, one phosphorus, and two adenine groups; (b) benzimidazolyl cobamide (BC), which contains one cobalt, one phosphorus, one benzimidazole, and one adenine group; and (c) dimethylbenzimidazolyl cobamide (DBC), which contains one cobalt, one phosphorus, one 5, 6-dimethylbenzimidazole, and one adenine group. As indicated in Table 7.4, specific enzymatic reactions are controlled by these cobamide coenzymes.

Nutritionally, physiologically, and biochemically the coenzyme form is the one of primary interest, since it alone is natually occurring and biologically active. Practically all the studies on pernicious anemia have been done employing cy-anocobalamine because this is the chemically stable, available form. It remains to be demonstrated whether or not the observations made and the principles established for cyanocobalamine obtain for the coenzyme form. Recent studies concerning the hepatic uptake of 5, 6-dimethylbenzimidazolyl cobamide following oral administration demonstrate that it cannot be absorbed without intrinsic factor, that it forms a stronger attachment to the intestinal mucosa prior to absorption than does vitamin B_{12}, and that when orally administered with intrinsic factor less DBC than labeled vitamin B_{12} is deposited in the liver of patients with pernicious anemia (150). Similarly, employing the Schilling test (268), negligible amounts are excreted in the urine of patients with pernicious anemia unless intrinsic factor is administered simultaneously. Although its excretion is thereby enhanced, the increase is not of the same magnitude as is seen with vitamin B_{12} under similar circumstances.

ASSAY. The assay of vitamin B_{12} is accomplished mainly by microbiologic techniques employing organisms that are unable to synthesize the vitamin and whose growth is therefore strictly dependent upon the vitamin B_{12} content of the media. Various strains of lactobacilli, *Escherichia coli* mutants, and *Euglena gracilis* have been used; the latter is probably the most reliable and sensitive (215, 216). By and large, colorimetric or chemical methods cannot be employed because the amounts to be assayed are so minute: normal serum values range from 100 to 900 $\mu\mu$g per milliliter. However, a recent isotope-dilution technique based upon known properties of the intrinsic factor–vitamin B_{12} complex yielded similar values (217). The results of such assays indicate severe deficiency of the vitamin in

* The original term "vitamin B_{12} coenzyme" has been dropped since it implies a chemical structure and composition not actually present in the coenzyme.

the blood, urine, and tissue of patients with untreated pernicious anemia. These findings are consistent with earlier studies that demonstrated the lack of antipernicious anemia principle in extracts from the livers of patients who were untreated at the time of death. As a result of microbiologic, physicochemical, and hematopoietic assays on human material, there is no question that in pernicious anemia a profound deficiency of vitamin B_{12} exists and that the importance of the metabolism of vitamin B_{12} is secondary only to that of intrinsic factor (140, 148, 149, 249).

DIETARY SOURCES AND ABSORPTION. The average American diet is said to contain some 5 μg of vitamin B_{12} per day. Since, as mentioned above, higher plants do not contain the vitamin, it must be derived almost exclusively from foods of animal origin. Liver and mollusks are such sources, and adequate amounts are usually present in milk, meat, sausage, cheese, fish, and eggs. Consequently it was to be expected, and in point of fact was demonstrated, that "Vegans," a sect that completely abstains from all animal foods and foods derived from animals, would become deficient. Vegetarians on the other hand usually allow the consumption of milk and eggs even though derived from animals and thereby gain a significant degree of protection. Vitamin B_{12} deficiency resulting from defective intake (pure extrinsic factor deficiency) is seldom seen in the United States and has rarely been demonstrated in adequate fashion (112, 200). The fact that it does occur indicates that the human being cannot utilize the significant amounts of vitamin B_{12} synthesized by his gastrointestinal flora but is dependent upon exogenous supplies. Ironically enough, even the patient with untreated pernicious anemia excretes daily an amount of vitamin B_{12} that would constitute adequate therapy could he but utilize it. Therefore, practically all instances of abnormal vitamin B_{12} metabolism are caused by defective intestinal absorption, and a consideration of naturally occurring deficiency should be related to the *physiologic* absorption of vitamin B_{12} from ordinary food. This is unfortunately not yet possible. The early studies were made by feeding crude preparations, but of recent years crystalline preparations have been widely employed, most frequently with an incorporated radioactive label (54). As pointed out above this is not a physiologic compound and more needs to be known about the absorption of, for example, the newly discovered coenzyme forms.*

TWO MECHANISMS OF ABSORPTION. It must be emphasized that in studies of this nature physiologic amounts (amounts not greater than those found in a normal diet) must be employed. There are at least two mechanisms of absorption (65). In the mechanism discussed above, mediated by the action of intrinsic factor, microgram quantities of vitamin B_{12} are involved which are certainly in the physiologic range. The percentage of radioactive vitamin B_{12} absorbed decreases rapidly with increasing doses (94). A maximal normal absorption of about 1.5 μg per dose, certainly less than 5 μg, is generally accepted (2, 32, 239). Moreover, radioactivity does not appear in the plasma for 4 hours, after which it rapidly reaches a maximum in 8 to 12 hours. This delay probably indicates the specific and complicated mechanism of absorption discussed above.

Contrariwise, when milligram quantities of labeled vitamin B_{12} are administered, a small percentage is absorbed (even in patients with pernicious anemia); absorption takes place without delay: radioactivity is immediately detectable in the plasma and the amount ab-

* The situation may well be analogous to iron metabolism, where a disparity is seen between the metabolism of organic food complexes and inorganic, nonphysiologic iron preparations.

TABLE 7.2.   Values for serum vitamin B_{12} concentration obtained in clinical studies

Type of person	No. of persons	Serum vitamin B_{12} concentration	
		Range ($\mu\mu g/ml$)	Mean ($\mu\mu g/ml$)
Normal individuals	223	100–900	356±12.3
Pernicious anemia patients	320	<10–110	<38± 1.1
Total gastrectomy patients	12	25–130	66±10.7
Partial gastrectomy patients	22	35–160	87± 7.7
"Vegans"	14	30–110	75± 5.9

From Grasbeck, R., Advances Clin. Chem. 3:299, 1960.

sorbed is proportional to the dose given. This is due to a supraphysiolgic or "pharmacologic" mechanism, probably involving mass action. Since the absorption of very large amounts of vitamin B_{12} may thus be induced, this method has been successfully used in the treatment of pernicious anemia (26, 174). In these instances enormous doses of vitamin B_{12} (1,000 μg per day) have been employed.

PLASMA TRANSPORT. Transport of vitamin B_{12} across the mucosa under the influence of intrinsic factor has been detailed above. The step involving the specific adsorption of intrinsic factor and the binding of vitamin B_{12} apparently is a "passive" physical phenomenon, since it occurs in hypothermia and in poisoned rats. However, the mucosal intake of the vitamin is probably dependent upon energy-requiring metabolic processes and pinocytosis. It is not known whether intrinsic factor is also absorbed. In the plasma the vitamin circulates at a concentration that has now been well established by the microbiologic tests mentioned above. It is obvious that determination of the concentration may be of considerable help in differential diagnosis and in nutritional and physiologic investigations. The serum vitamin B_{12} concentration has been shown to be a very sensitive indicator of the status of vitamin B_{12} stores and metabolism (Table 7.2).

A proportion of vitamin B_{12} circulates in the plasma in a "free," or unbound, state,* by which is meant it is directly available to microorganisms. About 80 to 85 per cent is carried in bound form, attached to a protein carrier designated "erythroglobulin," which has a molecular weight of 50,000 and migrates as an α-globulin (254). When so bound, the vitamin is not available for microorganisms. Accordingly, in estimating total vitamin B_{12} concentration the serum or test substance must be heated or digested to free the vitamin. The concentration is usually reported as free, bound, and total vitamin B_{12} values. Despite the fact that some is "free," plasma is able to bind added vitamin B_{12}; apparently other globulins (α_2, β, and γ) are available for this.

Vitamin B_{12} deficiency may thus be diagnosed even in the absence of typical clinical signs and the usual laboratory alterations. The determination of serum vitamin B_{12} concentration has been extremely valuable in the investigation of combined degeneration of the spinal cord and in estimating the efficacy of treatment in replacing vitamin B_{12} stores. Vitamin B_{12} assays have been done in a large number of diverse conditions. Extremely high concentrations have been found in myeloid leukemia (27) and some related conditions (175), where the

---

* It is most probably loosely bound to the β-globulins.

binding capacity of the plasma is greatly increased. High concentrations have also been demonstrated in acute and chronic liver disease, where the phenomenon is thought due to release of the vitamin by hepatocellular lesions comparable to that seen in experimental carbon tetrachloride poisoning. These are most probably secondary phenomena and not due to alterations in primary metabolism of vitamin B_{12}.

The main point to be emphasized here is that in normal subjects and patients with "pure" vitamin B_{12} deficiency, the serum vitamin B_{12} concentration provides a reliable measure of the magnitude of the vitamin B_{12} stores in the body. Limited studies on simultaneous assay of liver biopsy material and serum have shown good agreement.

The dynamic aspects of vitamin B_{12} transport have been assessed by the use of radioactive preparations with high specific activity (27, 74, 106, 255). Here a word of caution must be introduced. Since the values for plasma concentration are so minute, the amounts of vitamin B_{12} employed in studies become critical, for if the normal, physiologic values are exceeded the substance employed cannot be considered a true tracer substance, necessarily capable of yielding the desired information. The early studies on plasma clearance rates involved the injection of 1.5 μg of vitamin B_{12} so that significantly detectable amounts of radioactivity would be available. However, this amount was more than double the vitamin B_{12} content of all the circulating plasma and could hardly be termed a tracer amount.

When small amounts of radioactive vitamin B_{12} are given orally to normal subjects, or together with a source of intrinsic factor to patients with pernicious anemia, radioactivity appears in the plasma only after about 4 hours, reaches a peak at 8 to 12 hours, and then declines slowly so that detectable amounts are present as late as 7 days (65–67). At the peak levels only about 2 per cent of the oral dose is present in the plasma. When small doses of radioactive vitamin B_{12} with high specific activity are injected parenterally, 50 to 70 per cent of the dose disappears in 5 minutes, and by 15 minutes only 10 to 30 per cent remains. Following this the decline is much slower. The plasma clearance in patients with myeloid leukemia and pernicious anemia is somewhat lower, perhaps in association with the increased binding capacity (107, 175).

DISTRIBUTION AND CONCENTRATION IN BODY TISSUES. Clearance from plasma is effected by transfer to tissues; in human beings the liver appears to be the main site of storage. When small, physiologic doses are given orally or parenterally, only minute fractions of the administered dose are lost from the body.

When supraphysiologic doses of cyanocobalamine (500 to 1,000 μg) are administered intramuscularly, large amounts (60 to 69 per cent by 72 hours) are lost through the kidney. Since it has been demonstrated that the blood levels reached after parenteral injection are not proportional to the amounts retained in the body, it seems likely that the vitamin is adsorbed to tissue receptor sites or converted to an inactive form (3). When supraphysiologic doses of hydroxocobalamine (500 to 1,000 μg) are administered intramuscularly, higher serum levels are immediately obtained than for comparable doses of cyanocobalamine. The levels persist for longer periods of time (2 to 4 weeks) and smaller amounts of the vitamin are lost through the kidneys (16 to 27 per cent by 72 hours); as with cyanocobalamine, the hydroxo compound eventually becomes located in the liver (97, 98, 141). Because of these findings it may well be that hydroxocobalamine will prove to be the superior in the maintenance treatment of patients with pernicious anemia.

Studies in the human being concerning

the body distribution of vitamin B_{12} are, of course, restricted almost exclusively to external directional counting, and these are limited by the fact that the unabsorbed amounts retained for a considerable time in the gastrointestinal tract following oral administration obscure the directional counting for 2 to 3 days. However, the evidence indicates that when absorbed by the intrinsic factor mechanism, nearly all the vitamin is taken up by the liver. Following parenteral administration of physiologic amounts, radioactivity is at first found in many organs and tissues (muscle, kidney, liver, etc.) but then is slowly fed back to the liver, where it is found present again in almost the same amount as originally administered. In the liver at least 50 to 70 per cent of the vitamin appears to be in the recently described coenzyme forms (15, 246). Studies prior to the identification of the coenzyme indicated that the vitamin B_{12} was "bound"* probably by a peptide complex through cobalt to a β-globulin. Within the liver cell differential centrifugation shows the vitamin to be located in the mitochondrial, nuclear, and supernatant fractions.

As Table 7.3 shows, the concentration of vitamin B_{12} in human and animal organs has been assayed by a number of authors with fair agreement in results (50, 198, 240). The average total-body content of vitamin B_{12} is about 4 mg (range 0.8 to 11.1 mg), of which about 1 mg is present in the liver. Observations by

means of tracer studies indicate that the biologic half life of the radioactivity in the liver is about 1 year (222). Evidence indicates that the radioactivity is still in the form of vitamin B_{12} and not of degradation products and that this stored form is resistant to removal, for example, by flushing doses of nonradioactive vitamin B_{12} (96).

It is of interest to note that studies concerning the body-wide distribution of vitamin B_{12} in pernicious anemia indicate that the levels are diminished proportionately in all organs and tissues, usually to one-tenth to one-twentieth of the normal amounts (109).

EXCRETION. To complete our understanding of the nutritional cycle of vitamin B_{12} the excretion pattern must be known. For some time this has been obscured by the large amount synthesized in the gut and excreted in the feces, which, as pointed out above, is not available to the individual. The information needed is, of course, the amount of endogenous vitamin B_{12} lost daily from the body. Confirmation of the very small amount excreted by the kidney (0 to 270 mμg per day), as determined by microbiologic testing and by radioactive studies, precludes the excretion of large amounts of degradation products. It is, therefore, unlikely that extensive breakdown of endogenous vitamin B_{12} takes place. Gastric juice and pancreatic juice contain small amounts of vitamin B_{12}, but since normally these secretions are produced in large amounts, they play a significant role in total metabolism. It has recently been established that a considerable amount of vitamin B_{12} is eliminated in the bile (two to three times as much per day as the fecal loss), but most of this is reabsorbed (enterohepatic circulation), probably by

TABLE 7.3. Concentration of vitamin B_{12} in various organs, based on experiments by different workers

Organ	Range (μg/Gm wet weight)	Average (μg/Gm wet weight)
Liver	0.4 –2.6	1.1
Kidney	0.04–0.39	0.21
Spleen	0.01–0.17	0.08
Adrenals	0.11–0.53	0.25
Muscle	0.01–0.21	0.09

* The vitamin B_{12} may be liberated from tissue (except serum and bone marrow) by minor manipulations. Heating and digestion are not required for it to become available to microorganisms.

the intrinsic factor mechanism (125, 191, 193, 208). However, even following bile duct ligation some radioactivity continues to be excreted in the feces as vitamin B_{12}; this is presumably due to the vitamin content of rapidly desquamating mucosal cells (101).

The biologic half life of radioactive vitamin B_{12} in the liver is approximately 365 days (222). In comparable studies supplemented by total-body counting 0.2 to 0.3 per cent of the total radioactivity is lost per day. The average daily loss of endogenous vitamin B_{12} in a normal subject is thus about 8 μg. (Preliminary studies on cobamide coenzymes indicate similar orders of magnitude.)

The essential points in this cycle may well be brought together here. The average daily intake of vitamin B_{12} in food is approximately 5 μg. Of this, approximately 1 to 4 μg may be absorbed by intrinsic factor transport; the remaining amount is lost in the feces. The total-body content of vitamin B_{12} is calculated to be 4 mg (4,000 μg). There is evidence to indicate that little, if any, of this is degraded. The daily excretion of vitamin B_{12} amounts to 0.2 per cent of that present in the body, or an endogenous loss of 8 μg per day for the average individual. When the body stores have been depleted to one-tenth to one-twentieth of the normal, as in typical pernicious anemia, the excretion is reduced to 0.8 to 0.4 μg per day.

It is evident that at this stage the nutritional balance studies concerning vitamin B_{12} are imprecise; the orders of magnitude are indicated, but little else. Nevertheless, starting with normal stores and utilizing the known metabolism of vitamin B_{12}, from the above figures it has been calculated that with cessation of intake, as would occur following total gastrectomy (i.e., "surgical pernicious anemia" due to removal of intrinsic factor) some 400 days would be required for the development of a severe deficiency. (The calculations are as follows: 4 mg of vitamin B_{12} equals 4,000 μg; when the deficiency state has been reached, the store is reduced to one-twentieth of the original, or to 200 μg—3,800 μg less than normal. At a loss of 8 μg of vitamin B_{12} per day, this would take some 425 days. With decrease in stores, the amount lost per day would be decreased; 425 days is, therefore, probably a minimum value.) This is in good agreement with clinical observations on the development of vitamin B_{12}–deficiency anemia in a large series of patients followed after gastrectomy or after cessation of treatment of Addisonian pernicious anemia (55). It usually takes between 1 to 3 years for a macrocytic, megaloblastic anemia to develop that is responsive to vitamin B_{12} alone. Moreover, maximal hematopoietic responses are achieved in pernicious anemia by the administration of 1 μg of vitamin B_{12} intramuscularly per day, and this dose also assures maintenance of adequate hematopoiesis. This amount would sufficiently balance the daily loss at the time of deficiency (0.4 to 0.8 μg). With this degree of clinical confirmation, one can fairly confidently presume the major outlines of the metabolic scheme to be correct, even though the final word is not available.

BIOCHEMICAL ROLE OF VITAMIN B_{12} AND THE COBAMIDE COENZYMES. What then are the biochemical, pathophysiologic, and clinical changes resulting from deficiency and/or alterations in the metabolism of vitamin B_{12}? It has not yet been possible to pinpoint a specific biochemical function of vitamin B_{12} in terms of human metabolism. Several roles are provocatively suggested by studies on patients with pernicious anemia and on vitamin B_{12}–deficient microorganisms, and recently specific roles have been assigned the cobamide coenzymes in important enzymatic reactions. All these will be briefly described, but it is well to acknowledge from the outset that none provides a final picture of the mechanism of action of vitamin B_{12}, and the roles of the cobamide coenzymes have thus far been clearly delineated only in microorganisms.

Vitamin B_{12} has been observed to have an effect on the reduction of some sulfhydryl-containing compounds from the (S-S) to the (SH) state in in vitro enzyme systems and this has been correlated with in vivo studies on levels of reduced and oxidized glutathione and levels of oxidized and reduced vitamin C in patients with pernicious anemia. Because methionine has the capacity to substitute for vitamin B_{12} in some microbiologic systems and because vitamin B_{12} can exert a methionine-sparing action in chicks by promoting the methylation of homocysteine to methionine, vitamin B_{12} has been implicated in one-carbon transfers. But until very recently these activities have been inextricably enmeshed with those of folic acid. It now seems clear from studies on the "folic acid cycle" that one form of vitamin B_{12} is necessary for the folic acid–mediated methyl transfer that occurs in this reaction (see section on Response to Folic Acid).

From the beginning it was generally taken almost for granted that vitamin B_{12} was involved in the synthesis of the desoxyribonucleic acids, the ribonucleic acids, and proteins in general. However, here again no specific sites or modes of action have been elucidated and confirmed. Some systems are known in which ribosides and/or ribotides are directly reduced to the desoxyribosyl compounds without molecular cleavage at the glycosidic bond. The conversion of small amounts of purine and pyrimidine ribonucleotides to desoxyribonucleotides has been demonstrated by enzymatic action. Although vitamin B_{12} is presumed to be involved, the systems have not been sufficiently purified to evaluate the exact vitamin B_{12} requirement in satisfactory fashion. However, several lines of evidence provocatively point to these and have

been recently summarized (16). The obligatory requirement of *Lactobacillus leichmannii* for vitamin B_{12} can be bypassed by the addition of desoxyribosides (not free desoxyribose or ribosides); isotope studies indicate a poor conversion of ribosyl groups to DNA desoxyribose in the absence of vitamin B_{12}; there is a large and abrupt increase of desoxyribotides and DNA after the addition of vitamin B_{12} to deficient cultures; and vitamin B_{12} starvation of *L. leichmannii* produces an "imbalanced" growth (impaired DNA synthesis, unimpaired RNA and protein synthesis) resulting in inability to divide and long filamentous organisms. Consequently it is proposed that vitamin B_{12} participates in the synthesis of the desoxyribosyl groups, specifically the conversion of appropriate components of RNA to DNA.

With the discovery of the coenzyme forms of vitamin B_{12}, it has become evident that the cobamide coenzymes are in the main the biologically active forms of the vitamin (15). Several specific steps and sites of action in enzymatic processes have been demonstrated to be under their influence or control (1, 13, 14, 152, 202, 234). Their general function is to facilitate within a given compound the transfer of hydrogens from one carbon to an adjacent carbon. Specifically, they have been shown to take part in isomerization of several important compounds and in intramolecular oxidation-reduction reactions (Table 7.4).

It was originally reported that the cobamide coenzymes facilitated the exchange of carbon dioxide with the carboxyl groupings in pyruvate (205). Recent work by Peel (197) indicates that under anaerobic conditions the carbon dioxide–pyruvate exchange reaction proceeds without the cobamide coenzyme and that under aerobic conditions the coenzyme is not specific for the reaction but rather functions with mercaptoethanol to protect the required enzyme from oxygen.

TABLE 7.4.   Known functions of the cobamide coenzymes

Reaction	Coenzyme
Glutamate$\rightleftarrows\beta$-methylaspartate$\rightleftarrows$mesaconate	AC BC
Methylmalonxyl-CoA$\rightleftarrows$succinyl-CoA	BC DBC
1, 2-propanediol$\rightarrow$propionaldehyde Ethylene glycol$\rightarrow$acetaldehyde	AC BC DBC

AC, adenyl cobamide; BC, benzimidazolyl cobamide; DBC, dimethylbenzimidazolyl cobamide.

If this turns out to be a general function of vitamin B_{12} or its derivatives, the vitamin may prove to be an indirect participant in many enzyme systems.

The exact role of the coenzyme(s) in human vitamin B_{12} deficiency has not yet been determined in terms of organ dysfunction or pathophysiologic changes. Nevertheless, the assignment of specific functions to the biologically active form of vitamin B_{12} should more rapidly lead to a clearer understanding of alterations that follow the development of deficiency.

In summary it may then be stated with certainty that vitamin B_{12} (a) participates with folic acid in methionine synthesis from homocysteine, (b) participates in glutamate-isomerase reactions, (c) participates in methylmalonyl-CoA-isomerase reactions, and (d) participates in the conversion of diols to desoxyaldehydes. With less certainty it is presumed to participate in the synthesis of desoxyribosyl derivatives in the transformation of RNA to DNA. However, it must be stressed again that these reactions have so far been demonstrated to occur only in microorganisms.

Morphologic Changes Associated with Vitamin B_{12} Deficiency

During the development of vitamin B_{12} deficiency, depletion apparently occurs proportionately in almost all tissues and the deficiency actually is body-wide. Confirmation of this is found in the morphologic abnormalities that have been demonstrated in epithelial cells (20, 225) recovered from skin and tongue and from buccal (76), gastric, small intestinal, rectal, bladder, and vaginal linings (75). Without going into individual characterization of the noted changes, it may be said in general that they are somewhat analogous to the morphologic changes seen in marrow cells and are promptly reversed by the administration of vitamin B_{12}. The abnormalities are especially notable in cells that have a rapid turnover rate and consequently an increased nucleoprotein synthesis. Most of the studies concerning the biochemical alterations accompanying vitamin B_{12} deficiency have been made on bone marrow obtained from patients with untreated pernicious anemia, and special attention has been focused on the red cell series.

Microspectrophotometry with ultraviolet light has demonstrated that during *normal* red cell maturation cytoplasmic RNA concentration diminishes rapidly and has almost disappeared at the time hemoglobin appears (Figure 3.1). In pernicious anemia (99), several observers have noted, the RNA disappears much more slowly and persists into the stages at which hemoglobinization is well advanced (258). In both normal and deficient cells the diameter of the nucleus progressively decreases, and there is gradual disappearance of DNA. Analytic procedures on individual cells and whole marrow from untreated patients have shown that, unlike the normal, greater amounts of RNA in proportion to DNA are present. DNA differs from RNA in that it contains desoxyribose instead of ribose, and thymine instead of uracil. In the marrow of patients with untreated pernicious anemia the ratio of uracil (RNA) to thymine (DNA) is increased and decreases rapidly to normal following specific therapy (186). The suggested interpretation has been that the biosynthesis of DNA is catalyzed by vitamin B_{12} in the methylation of uracil to thymine (which is 5-methyl uracil). In the deficient state the biosynthesis of DNA would be impeded and the ratio shifted from the normal to that observed. However, since other studies have demonstrated similar changes in primitive but otherwise normal cells, the described changes were probably due to the immaturity of the marrow cells rather than to their deficiency. In addition, the increased absolute amounts of DNA and the still greater increases in RNA that have been demonstrated in pernicious anemia suggest the possibility of other mechanisms.

Bone marrow may be cultured in vitro by well-standardized techniques, and the morphologic appearance of the cells is well preserved for a sufficient number of days to permit study of megaloblastic-normoblastic maturation. Most observers agree that the abnormal proerythroblasts of pernicious anemia grown in serum obtained from untreated patients will mature along megaloblastic lines and will be replaced by normoblastic cells only following the addition of liver extract. Although conflicting results have been reported, the addition of vitamin B_{12} to similar preparations also induces a change to normoblastic maturation.

By incorporation of C^{14} formate into the thymine of DNA its rate of synthesis

has been measured in deficient cells suspended in pernicious anemia serum (244). A significant increase in the rate of synthesis was noted after the addition of vitamin B_{12}. Most observers have agreed that intrinsic factor from gastric sources is not necessary for this action of vitamin B_{12}.

Some observers have claimed the production of morphologically abnormal cells in normoblastic marrow grown in pernicious anemia serum. Contrary to the original interpretation that this was the result of a toxic or "inhibitory" factor in the serum, it is probably due to the development of cellular vitamin B_{12} deficiency caused by binding action and can be corrected by the addition of minute amounts of vitamin B_{12}. From what has been said previously about the biologic activity of vitamin B_{12} and the cobamide coenzymes, it is evident that for greater clarity these studies should be repeated employing the coenzyme. Nevertheless, some in vivo confirmation of these culture studies has been obtained by Horrigan et al. (127), who demonstrated that the instillation of vitamin B_{12} directly into the marrow cavity (without contact with gastric intrinsic factor) could induce local transformation from megaloblastic to normoblastic proliferation without inducing changes in distant marrow (opposite iliac crest). This indicates local fixation of the vitamin B_{12}, probably conversion to the coenzyme form, and local correction of the deficiency.

The chief distinguishing characteristics of megaloblastic proliferation are the finely dispersed chromatin of the nucleus and the delayed disappearance of RNA from the cytoplasm. Reisner (207) has proposed that megaloblastic proliferation results from prolonged resting phases between mitoses (allowing more complete dispersion of chromatin throughout the nucleus). The prolonged resting phases between mitoses are a consequence of the inability of deficient cells to synthesize in the usual time the extra amounts of DNA required for mitosis. Since a principal source of the extra DNA is cytoplasmic RNA, the deficient cell also shows a persistence of RNA.

Numerous studies have documented by means of serial aspiration the remarkably rapid changes that occur in bone marrow following specific therapy (57). Within a matter of 4 to 6 hours observable changes are present in the form of decreased numbers of abnormal and increased numbers of normal proerythroblasts. Progressive alteration to near normal composition takes place in about 2 days, and a predominantly normoblastic marrow is present by 4 days or earlier, at which time reticulocytes begin to enter the peripheral blood in increasing numbers. It is unlikely that the abnormal cells are transformed into normal ones following therapy. Rather, the abnormal proerythroblasts continue their megaloblastic-type maturation through early and late erythroblasts and normoblasts to megalocytes, but no *new* abnormal proerythroblasts are formed, so normoblastic maturation proceeds from the stem cell. In this connection it is important to note that for the most accurate interpretation of the marrow picture, the specimen must be obtained *before* specific therapy is begun lest the main characteristics be rapidly obscured.

Although the marrow of untreated pernicious anemia has been characterized as primitive, with long intermitotic periods and "maturation arrest," it is by no means inactive as far as iron and pigment metabolism are concerned.

Pathophysiology: Observations from Tracer Studies

INEFFECTIVE ERYTHROPOIESIS. In 1922 Whipple suggested that the greatly increased output of substances derived from hemoglobin catabolism in untreated pernicious anemia was partly the result of rapid destruction of *circulating* red cells, but on a quantitative basis concluded that there must be additional sources of the pigments.

Various sources considered possible at one time or other have been (a) erythrocytes of extremely short life span, (b) "stillborn" erythrocytes destroyed in the marrow cavity before delivery to the peripheral blood, (c) direct synthesis of bilirubin by unknown pathway, or (d) an extracellular turnover of pigments in the marrow (131). In view of present knowledge of heme biosynthesis this latter now seems definitely excluded.

The use of N^{15}-labeled glycine (158, 159) in studying untreated pernicious anemia has not only demonstrated a decreased red cell life span but also established that some 40 per cent of the products of hemoglobin breakdown are derived from sources other than the hemoglobin of the circulating erythrocyte (Figure 7.5). Labeled urobilinogen was excreted by the patients within a few days after N^{15}-glycine administration in such quantities that it could not have been derived from the tagged hemoglobin of the circulating erythrocytes, which at that time showed no augmented destruction. These studies, combined with observations on iron metabolism to be outlined next, indicate pigment synthesis in the marrow but failure of the marrow to deliver the pigment to the peripheral blood as properly packaged hemoglobin (i.e., viable red cells), a process designated *ineffective erythropoiesis*.

It must be remembered that there is a definite hemolytic component to pernicious anemia. Numerous studies have demonstrated that the life span of the erythrocytes of untreated patients is significantly decreased (110). Since the life span of erythrocytes from such patients is shortened whether tested in the patient or in a normal subject, an intrinsic cellular defect is present that is corrected only with adequate specific therapy. In addi-

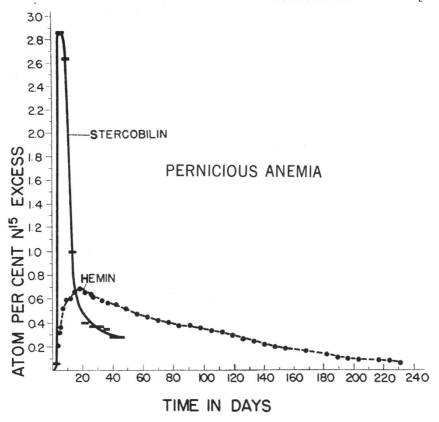

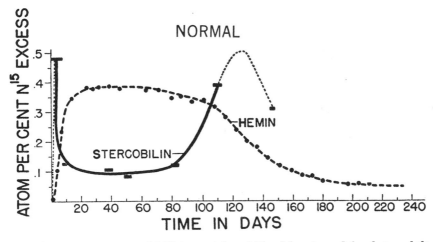

FIGURE 7.5. Concentration of N[15] in peripheral blood hemin and fecal stercobilin after feeding N[15]-labeled glycine for 2 days. (Adapted from London, I. M., et al., J. Biol. Chem. 184:351, 359, 1950)

tion, the survival of normal erythrocytes in untreated patients is significantly shortened. A hemolytic factor is present extrinsic to the erythrocyte that again is corrected by specific therapy. This situa-

tion exemplifies a combined extra- and intracorpuscular hemolytic mechanism: in the untreated patient an intrinsically defective cell is circulating in a deleterious environment. There is thus clear-cut evidence that a significant hemolytic component is present in pernicious anemia.

FERROKINETICS. In untreated pernicious anemia the concentration of iron in the circulating blood is typically elevated above normal, and the concentration of iron-binding protein is slightly subnormal. Increased iron stores are consistently seen in pernicious anemia (hepatic siderosis and marrow siderosis) mainly owing to diversion of the large amount of iron normally present in the circulating hemoglobin to the tissues with the development of anemia. But additional metabolic abnormalities are present since, unlike uncomplicated iron overload, the turnover of radioactive iron through the plasma is very rapid (Figure 7.6). This iron, when followed by external tracking techniques (Figure 7.7), accumulates with abnormal rapidity in the bone marrow. However, after retention there, it is gradually released, most of the iron moving to the liver rather than into the circulating erythrocytes. Indeed, determination of the percentage incorporation into the peripheral erythrocytes (Figure 7.8) yields markedly subnormal values (trace to 40 per cent instead of nearly 100 per cent). Therefore, despite a very large turnover in absolute values of iron through the plasma, only a subnormal amount is successfully incorporated into erythrocytes and delivered to the peripheral blood. A significant amount is delayed in the marrow for a time and then moved on to the liver.

ERYTHROKINETICS. Absolute values of the various measurements of ferrokinetics and erythrokinetics vary considerably from individual to individual owing to difference in size and variation in blood volume. To avoid these factors Finch et al. have expressed such data according to certain standards and then compared the results with similar data for normal individuals (77). A series of "erythrokinetic indices" is thereby obtained indicating total erythropoiesis, effective erythropoiesis, and destruction. The activity of the marrow is evaluated by (a) E/M ratio, (b) plasma iron turnover, (c) urobilinogen excretion, (d) red cell utilization of iron, (e) peripheral erythrocyte survival, and (f) reticulocyte count. Of these, the first three measure total heme turnover ("total erythropoiesis"); the remainder measure actual delivery of cells to the circulating red cell mass ("effective erythropoiesis"). Studies have indicated that in untreated pernicious anemia the *total* marrow erythropoiesis is about three times normal, but the *effective* red cell production is no more than normal. Since the erythrocytes that are delivered to the peripheral blood do not long survive, an equilibrium is reached at a significantly anemic level. This is comparable to the changes seen in thalassemia major. *Total* erythropoiesis is somewhat less, and *effective* erythropoiesis considerably less, than would be *expected* of a normal marrow under *comparable sustained hypoxic stimulus*. Thus, in addition to the hemolytic component, relative bone marrow insufficiency also occurs in untreated pernicious anemia.

An enormous number of studies have been done concerning the pathophysiology of every organ system in the body and the biochemical changes present in untreated pernicious anemia. It is safe to say that in most, significant derangements have been found many of which have relevance to other disease processes. Throughout the years pernicious anemia has engendered interest that might appear disproportionate to the incidence of the disease, and the investigative interest continues despite the fact that it is a disease for which a satisfactory treatment has long been available. This has been most fortunate since the knowledge and insight gained through these studies have been valuable in terms of physiology and biochemistry, both in general and in relation to other diseases.

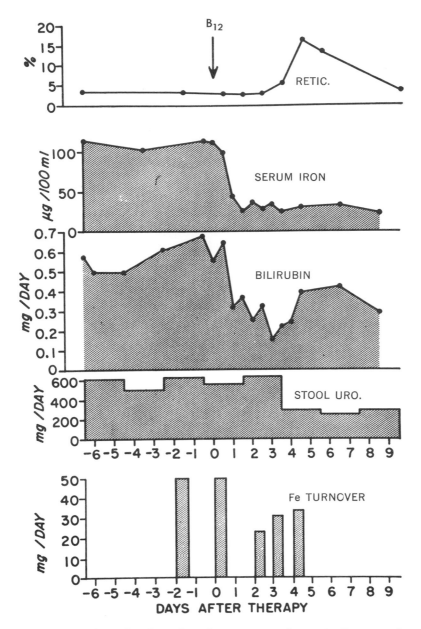

FIGURE 7.6.   Changes brought about by administration of vitamin B_{12} to patient with pernicious anemia. In relation to reticulocyte response are seen rapid changes in serum iron and bilirubin levels, slower decrease in output of fecal urobilinogen, and marked decrease in plasma iron turnover. These occur as the marrow progressively shifts from ineffective to effective erythropoiesis. (From Finch, C. A., et al., Blood 11:807, 1956)

Response to Folic Acid

So far pernicious anemia has been considered as a discrete, almost uncomplicated problem: a disease that results from a nearly pure deficiency of vitamin B_{12} and which responds specifically to the administration of vitamin B_{12}. This is, of course, true. However, in the course of

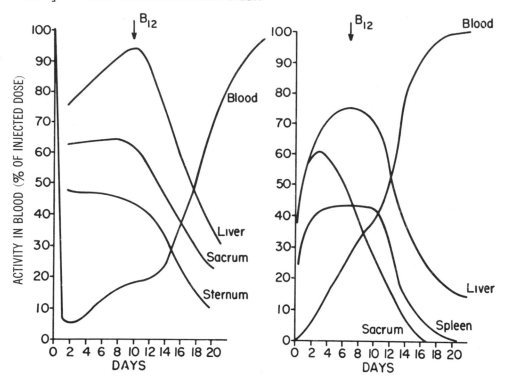

FIGURE 7.7.   Shifts in distribution of radioactive iron in response to vitamin B_{12} therapy in two patients with pernicious anemia. Ordinate refers only to blood counting, where 100 per cent represents the maximum utilization of radioiron in the red cell mass during the period of study. Counts over body surface in relation to designated organs are expressed as they relate to one another and do not have significance as absolute values. Before treatment there is decreased red cell utilization of radioiron and accumulation of activity in liver, spleen, and marrow; following therapy the iron is rapidly drained from tissues and appears in the circulating red cell mass. (Adapted from Finch, C. A., et al., Blood 11:807, 1956)

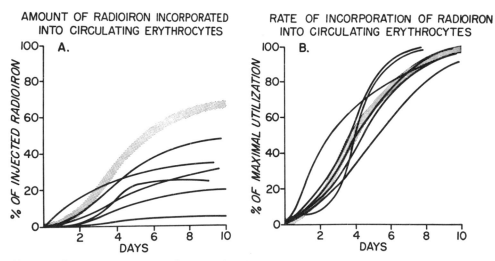

FIGURE. 7.8.   Percentage and rate of radioactive iron incorporation into circulating erythrocytes in six patients with untreated pernicious anemia. Shaded areas represent normal ranges for this method. (From Finch, C. A., et al., Blood 11:807, 1956)

studies searching for the antipernicious anemia principle of crude liver extract a compound was isolated that was later designated folic acid. When this was administered orally to patients with untreated pernicious anemia in amounts of 5 mg per day, a clinical and hematologic response occurred. But this compound was not found in refined liver extract to which pernicious anemia also responded. Therefore, the existence of a *second* hematopoietic factor *distinct* from the active principle of refined liver extract subsequently identified as vitamin B_{12} was established. However, it was soon demonstrated that although the administration of folic acid could initiate satisfactory clinical and hematologic response, the drug was *not* satisfactory for maintenance therapy. Very early it was found that despite adequate hematologic status the signs and symptoms of combined degeneration of the spinal cord and brain might appear and progress during the continued administration of the drug (47); more recently this has been observed to occur in conjunction with the administration of multivitamin preparations containing small doses of folic acid (12). Indeed, if the administration of folic acid is persisted in long enough, hema-

tologic relapse also ensues. It was evident, therefore, that folic acid did not constitute adequate replacement therapy, as did refined liver extract (vitamin B_{12}), for pernicious anemia (227). The most decisive and best controlled observations concerning this problem have been published by Vilter's group (260). In these studies a number of patients with pernicious anemia but without evidence of combined degeneration of the cord were given maintenance doses of folic acid and followed with frequent careful hematologic and clinical evaluation. A significant number developed neurologic, hematologic, and glossal symptoms (Figure 7.9). These relapses responded adequately to the administration of greater amounts of folic acid but in all instances again occurred after a variable interval of time, usually with a more severe degree of abnormality than before. Adequate response to vitamin B_{12} was always seen except in patients maintained for very long periods of time on folic acid; these developed an anemia associated with marrow that morphologically appeared relatively aplastic. Prolonged vitamin B_{12} administration was then required, and the response was slow, suboptimum, and atypical. Because of these decisive studies and many other

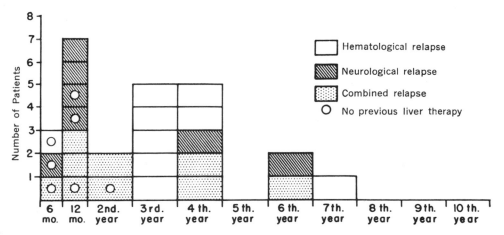

FIGURE 7.9. Number of hematologic, neurologic, and combined relapses which occurred over a 10-year period in thirty-six patients with pernicious anemia who were taking only folic acid. (From Will, J. J., et al., J. Lab. & Clin. Med. 53:22, 1959)

clinical observations, there is no question but that folic acid *should not* be used in the treatment of pernicious anemia.

A completely satisfactory explanation based on suitable evidence for the hematologic response to folic acid seen in pernicious anemia has not been advanced. Studies do not indicate that folic acid enhances the intestinal absorption of vitamin B_{12}; there are no studies concerning its influence on the permeability of cells to vitamin B_{12}. The administration of folic acid to patients with pernicious anemia probably does not mobilize vitamin B_{12} since the serum concentration remains low and often even decreases (21, 149). Measurements indicate that while the serum and tissue content of vitamin B_{12} is one-tenth to one-twentieth of normal in untreated pernicious anemia, its concentration in the bone marrow cells and peripheral blood cells is decreased only to one-half of normal. It has been suggested that by the administration of folic acid erythropoiesis is forced through by perhaps a mass action effect. Since the content of vitamin B_{12} in the bone marrow and peripheral blood cells remains relatively higher than in other tissues, with the induced hematopoietic response the other tissues are further drained of their vitamin B_{12} and made even more deficient. Hence, the appearance of neurologic symptoms, which are the incontrovertible sign of vitamin B_{12} depletion. In this connection it is of interest that to produce a hematologic response in uncomplicated pernicious anemia, folic acid must be given in pharmacologic doses of 5 to 15 mg per day. Physiologic doses in the range of 25 to 400 μg daily are usually ineffective, although they *are* effective in other nutritional megaloblastic anemias secondary to folic acid deficiency (171, 230). This finding is consistent with the concept that a hematologic response in pernicious anemia may be brought about by a mass action effect of pharmacologic (supraphysiologic) doses of folic acid.

Some workers have interpreted the available findings to indicate that a *folic acid* abnormality is basic to megaloblastic maturation and that the abnormality in folic acid metabolism is secondary to the vitamin B_{12} deficiency (51, 249). Without an adequate amount of vitamin B_{12}, folic acid coenzymes cannot take part in their critical roles in nucleic acid synthesis and cell division. Other workers believe that the vitamin B_{12} (or a coenzyme form) is per se essential to prevent megaloblastic maturation, and consequently they place this vitamin, rather than folic acid, in the central and critical role.

The recent work (79), mentioned briefly above, concerning vitamin B_{12} as a necessary cofactor in the folic acid cycle by which methionine is formed from homocysteine through transmethylation (145, 220) would appear to support the concept that folic acid (or derivative) may be the actual operational compound and that for it to function (to be derived from a precursor or transformed into a biologically active compound) vitamin B_{12} is required. In this cycle, which was worked out in *Escherichia coli* mutants, a new folic acid derivative, N5-methyltetrahydrofolic acid (N5-methyl-THF) (Figure 7.11) was found to be the key link connecting enzyme reactions involving a "B_{12} enzyme."[*] N5, 10-methylene-THF plus DPNH react under enzyme control to form N5-methyl-THF. This latter compound donates its methyl group to homocysteine to produce methionine and THF under the influence of the B_{12} enzyme and four cofactors.[†] THF picks up formaldehyde to re-form the original starting compound, N5, 10-methylene-THF, and the cycle is completed. With a deficiency of vitamin B_{12}, the B_{12} enzyme would be present in insufficient

[*] The form of this "B_{12} enzyme" is unknown. It is not cyanocobalamine or one of the cobamide coenzymes.

[†] Cofactors are DPNH, a flavine adenine nucleotide (FAD), ATP, and magnesium cations.

supply to allow the transformation of N5-methyl-THF to THF; the former would be expected to accumulate and the latter to be decreased. THF is pictured as essential to the production of purines (29) and pyrimidines of nucleic acids from their precursors (79).

With respect to the possible accumulation of N5-methyl-THF, it is of considerable interest that Waters and Mollin (252) have recently reported the blood folic activity in untreated pernicious anemia to be increased above normal as assayed by *Lactobacillus casei,* an organism known to respond to N5-methyl-THF. Moreover, the blood levels of folic activity decreased to normal following the administration of vitamin B_{12}.

It should be emphasized that the folic acid cycle described above has as yet been demonstrated only in microorganisms. However, N5-methyl-THF is an important folic acid derivative known to occur in human liver and blood (125a). On the basis of the above findings a short supply of THF (because of its role in formation of purines and pyrimidines from nucleic acid precursors) would be the proximate and basic lack in megaloblastic proliferation. A short supply of THF could be brought about by a folic acid deficiency (see below) or by a deficiency of vitamin B_{12} blocking the transformation of N5-methyl-THF to THF.

Summary

Pernicious anemia results from a genetically determined defect in intrinsic factor production that is nearly always associated with gastric atrophy, achylia, and achlorhydria. As a result of the defective production of intrinsic factor, the nutritional balance of vitamin B_{12} (cobamide coenzymes) is altered, and a body-wide deficiency results. The balance is upset because of the impaired absorption of vitamin B_{12} that results from insufficient production of intrinsic factor. In pernicious anemia the impaired absorption can be corrected by the administration of intrinsic factor. The pathophysiologic consequences of the deficiency are classically reflected by changes in the central nervous system, hematopoietic system, and gastrointestinal system, but numerous other changes in other organ systems are seen. In association with morphologic alterations, hematopoiesis is abnormal in all cell series (erythrocytic, leukocytic, megakaryocytic). Erythropoiesis is ineffective and relatively insufficient, and combined extra- and intracorpuscular hemolytic mechanisms exist with pigment abnormalities. Except for the defective production of intrinsic factor, gastric atrophy, achylia, and achlorhydria, the abnormalities may be reverted to normal by correcting the vitamin B_{12} deficiency: the progression of central nervous system lesions will be halted and reversion of the lesions may take place, the extent depending largely on the prior duration of the vitamin B_{12} deficiency. The administration of physiologic doses of folic acid will not effect a clinical or hematologic remission; the administration of pharmacologic doses of folic acid will effect a *temporary* clinical and hematologic remission, but the remission may not long persist and irreversible neurologic damage may occur. The establishment of a diagnosis of pernicious anemia should be based on the following criteria: (a) typical peripheral blood changes; (b) typical bone marrow changes; (c) perhaps combined degeneration of the spinal cord; (d) histamine-refractory achylia, atrophic gastritis, and achlorhydria; (e) deficiency of vitamin B_{12}; (f) typical response to the administration of vitamin B_{12}; (g) defective absorption of vitamin B_{12} because of insufficient production of intrinsic factor as result of a genetic abnormality; and (h) correction of the metabolic derangements of vitamin B_{12} by the administration of intrinsic factor. As mentioned previously, in practice it is seldom necessary to fulfill all these criteria.

TABLE 7.5.   Classification of vitamin B_{12} and folic acid abnormalities

VITAMIN B_{12} ABNORMALITY (DEFICIENCY)

I. Inadequate intake (extrinsic factor defect)

II. Defective absorption
    A. Defective production of intrinsic factor
        1. Genetic: pernicious anemia
        2. Surgical: total or subtotal gastrectomy
        3. Chemical or radiation: destruction of mucosa
    B. Malabsorption syndromes
    C. Lack of availability of ingested vitamin B_{12}
        1. Fish tapeworm competition (*Diphyllobothrium latum*)
        2. Bacterial competition (blind loop, diverticulae, etc.)

FOLIC ACID ABNORMALITY (DEFICIENCY OR ALTERED UTILIZATION)

I. Inadequate intake
    A. Megaloblastic anemia of infancy
    B. Megaloblastic anemia of pregnancy
    C. Nutritional megaloblastic anemia
    D. Liver disease associated with alcoholism

II. Defective absorption
    A. Malabsorption syndromes
    B. Lack of availability of ingested folic acid because of bacterial competition (blind loop, etc.)

III. Inadequate utilization or increased requirement
    A. Folic acid antagonists
    B. Vitamin C deficiency
    C. Administration of anticonvulsants
    D. Preferential uptake by fetus or neoplastic tissue
    E. Hemolytic anemia (?)
    F. Liver disease (?)

NON-ADDISONIAN MEGALOBLASTIC ANEMIAS

It can be appreciated from the above consideration that pernicious anemia is a discrete entity in which the changes are unusually well documented. As such it may serve as a prototype for the other so-called megaloblastic anemias. With extremely few satisfactorily documented exceptions, the megaloblastic anemias are due to varying degrees of abnormality in the metabolism of vitamin B_{12} or folic acid or both together.* Accordingly they may be classified as shown in Table 7.5.

Vitamin B_{12} Abnormality

Many of the clinical entities indicated by the above classification will not be dealt with here. Obviously they all have in common bone marrow morphology indis-

tinguishable from that seen in pernicious anemia. If the abnormality is due to vitamin B_{12} deficiency, many or all of the criteria outlined above for pernicious anemia will be fulfilled. Some exceptions may be briefly noted. Inevitably following total gastrectomy (9, 108, 166, 194, 256), probably frequently following extensive resection of the jejunum and ileum (7, 35), and infrequently following

* "Non-Addisonian megaloblastic anemia" has been described in tropical and nontropical sprue, nutritional macrocytic anemia, megaloblastic anemia of pregnancy, megaloblastic anemia of infancy, various intestinal disorders (blind loops, fistulae, diverticulosis, ileitis), corrosive and neoplastic lesions of the stomach, acute and chronic liver disease, carcinomatosis of bone marrow, extensive neoplastic growth; following total or subtotal gastrectomy, administration of anticonvulsant and antileukemic drugs; in vitamin C deficiency, in parasitic infestations, associated with excretion of orotic acid (129), and in refractory anemia (87).

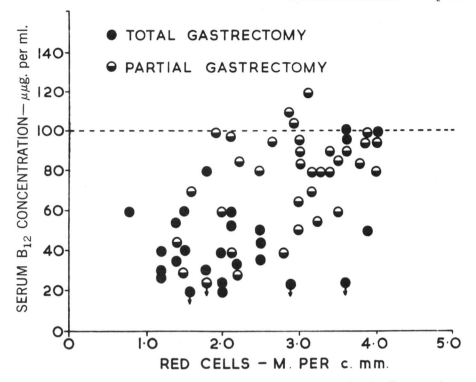

FIGURE 7.10.   Pretreatment serum vitamin B_{12} concentration and red cell count of group of patients with megaloblastic anemia due to total or partial gastrectomy. Interrupted line represents lower level of range found in control subjects. (From Mollin, D. L., *in* University of London, British Postgraduate Medical Federation, Lectures on the Scientific Basis of Medicine, vol. 7, p. 94, Athlone Press, London, 1957)

subtotal gastrectomy (25, 62, 63, 157, 160, 165, 167), vitamin B_{12} deficiency develops (Figure 7.10). Because of the surgically induced lack of intrinsic factor in the postgastrectomy syndrome, vitamin B_{12} absorption is impaired but is corrected by the administration of intrinsic factor (61).* Following extensive resection of the small bowel, the impairment in vitamin B_{12} absorption is due not to lack of intrinsic factor but to the absence of the specific receptor sites of the vitamin–intrinsic factor complex. In the so-called malabsorption syndrome vitamin B_{12} deficiency may develop, again owing to impaired absorption of the vitamin, but here the absorptive defect is *not* corrected by the administration of intrinsic factor, since the basic abnormality appears to reside in the intestinal wall

rather than in the production of intrinsic factor (86, 89, 182; Figure 7.3). Contrariwise, the deficiency developing because of inadequate intake of vitamin B_{12}, as would be expected, shows no impairment of vitamin B_{12} absorption,† and exogenous intrinsic factor is not needed (200). When the deficiency is due to lack of availability of the vitamin to the host because of preferential uptake by the parasite (tapeworm, blind loop bacteria,

* In some patients with *partial* gastrectomy, the absorption of vitamin B_{12} is increased if the pure vitamin is given *with* a meal rather than in the fasting state. This is not true for *total* gastrectomy or Addisonian pernicious anemia (61).

† It is reported that with long-standing exogenous vitamin B_{12} deficiency atrophy of gastric mucosa may become so severe that the production of intrinsic factor is decreased. There are no satisfactory studies concerning the reversibility of these lesions.

etc.), vitamin B_{12} absorption is impaired, is not corrected by the administration of intrinsic factor, but is corrected by appropriate chemotherapy or surgery (10, 23, 88). Today these abnormalities of vitamin B_{12} metabolism are readily detected by radioactive techniques (Schilling test, hepatic uptake test; 81). The results of these techniques confirm those previously found by clinical assay and by determination of the double reticulocyte response. As in pernicious anemia, a hematologic response may be obtained following the administration of pharmacologic doses of folic acid; combined degeneration of the spinal cord may also follow the prolonged administration of folic acid.

Folic Acid Abnormality

Referring again to the classification shown in Table 7.5, if the abnormality is due to alteration in folic acid metabolism, then except for the bone marrow changes and to some extent the peripheral blood changes, entirely different criteria must be used to establish a diagnosis. "Pure" folic acid deficiency or abnormality is seldom seen, for the clinical picture is usually complicated by other nutritional deficiencies superimposed on gastrointestinal malfunction and obvious dietary inadequacies or excesses. It is, therefore, usual for such patients to show considerable weight loss on initial examination. Glossitis is frequently present or has occurred some time in the past. But, as with pernicious anemia, in this country the initial complaints and signs may be nonspecific. Unless the folic acid abnormality is complicated by vitamin B_{12} deficiency, the neurologic manifestations are irritability and peripheral neuropathy. As mentioned above, the maturation abnormalities seen in the bone marrow are indistinguishable from those of pernicious anemia. The changes in the peripheral blood are also very similar; however, macrocytosis and anisocytosis are usually not as extreme, and leukopenia is only an inconstant finding. The blood and bone marrow picture is more frequently distorted by complicating factors such as infection and concomitant iron lack. Where suitable observations have been made in uncomplicated subjects, the pathophysiology appears to approximate very closely that of pernicious anemia with respect to pigment metabolism, iron metabolism, red cell defect, individual organ dysfunction, and biochemical changes.

Folic Acid

While studying megaloblastic anemias seen in Hindu women, Wills demonstrated hematologic responses to an autolyzed yeast preparation, Marmite, and to crude liver extracts; however, responses were not obtained with purified liver extract. The condition now termed "nutritional megaloblastic anemia" was accordingly differentiated from pernicious anemia, and the existence of a hematopoietic agent separate from that found effective in pernicious anemia (vitamin B_{12}) was demonstrated. A similar anemia could be produced in monkeys, and it was later found that this could also be relieved by crude liver and autolyzed yeast; the active factor was named vitamin M. Microbiologic studies demonstrated that diverse organisms required for growth a factor present in yeast and crude liver. It was shortly thereafter found that the yeast or crude liver could be replaced by pteroylglutamic acid (folic acid) or related substances. To complete the cycle, it is now known that patients, apparently similar in every way to those originally studied by Wills, respond adequately to the administration of pteroylglutamic acid, as do also the nutritionally deficient monkeys.

CHEMISTRY. As might be expected this hematopoietically active substance accumulated many names in the time before it was chemically identified as pteroylglutamic acid (PGA); it has been called vitamins M, B_c, B_c conjugate, B_{10}, B_{11}, R,

S, and U, and *Lactobacillus casei* factor. It has now been synthesized and consists of a pteridine grouping linked through *p*-aminobenzoic acid to a single glutamic acid residue (Figure 7.11). It is now conventionally referred to as folic acid, folacin, pteroylglutamic acid, or PGA. It is found in nature in conjugated forms in which varying numbers of glutamic acid residues are attached by peptide linkages to the glutamic acid radicle of PGA. Some of these conjugates have been syn-

thesized. In yeast it occurs mainly as pteroylheptaglutamic acid.

It was demonstrated that to become biologically active pteroylglutamic acid had to be converted to another form. A triphosphopyridine nucleotide–dependent enzyme found present in many tissues was required for this transformation, which could be greatly facilitated by ascorbic acid through stabilization of the product. That this was pertinent to man was demonstrated by a markedly in-

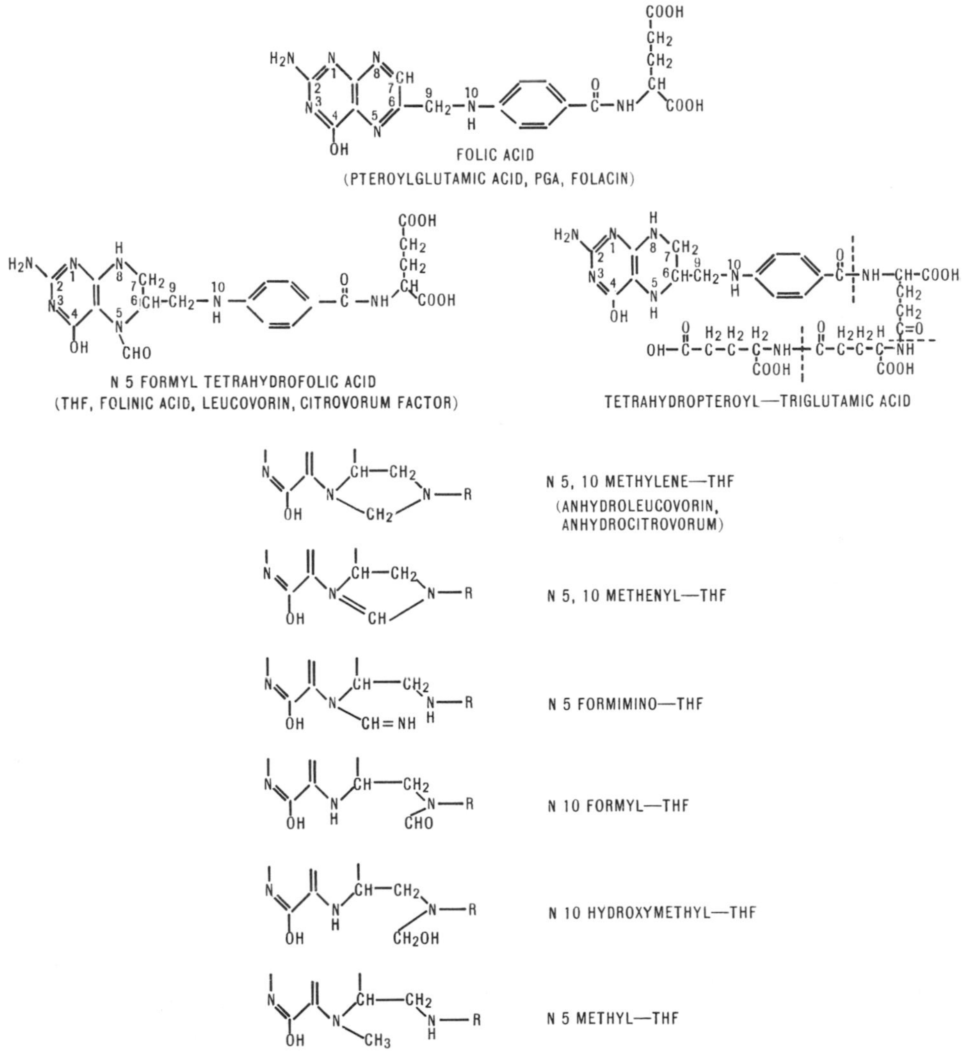

FIGURE 7.11. Chemical structures of folic acid and various conjugates and derivates of folic acid. The metabolic pathways in which they participate are indicated in Table 7.4

creased urinary excretion of the altered folic acid following the administration of vitamin C. The altered form was found to be 5-formyl-tetrahydropteroylglutamic acid (Figure 7.11). Since the factor was found necessary for the growth of a microorganism, *Leuconostoc citrovorum*,* the name citrovorum factor was assigned. It is also designated folinic acid and leucovorin, has now been synthesized, and has been shown to be hematopoietically effective in the treatment of megaloblastic anemias.

Various other reduced coenzyme forms of folic acid are illustrated in Figure 7.11 and will be mentioned later in association with the enzyme reactions in which they are known to participate.

DIETARY SOURCES, ABSORPTION, AND BODY DISTRIBUTION. Folic acid (in free and conjugated forms), folinic acid, and related forms are widely found in foods: yeast, leafy vegetables, liver, fruits, grains, nuts, eggs, milk, etc. The figures usually given for human requirement are at best rough estimates and range from 100 to 1,000 μg per day. The average diet in the United States (even after cooking) supplies much in excess of this when assayed for "total folic activity"; diets supplying less than 1,000 μg per day must be grossly abnormal. Moreover, a considerable amount of folic acid and allied substances is produced by bacteria in the gastrointestinal tract, so that the amount excreted exceeds the daily intake. Pteroylglutamic acid appears to be taken in through the jejunum by passive absorption; the conjugated polyglutamates are absorbed less efficiently but nothing is known about the details of the absorptive mechanism. Intrinsic factor is not implicated. Except in instances of severe malabsorption, folic acid (and allied compounds) appears to be absorbed very readily and is as effective upon oral as on parenteral administration. The amounts of endogenous folic acid and allied com-

pounds that are lost per day are unknown.

Folic acid activity has been found in all body tissues analyzed. The total-body content is estimated at 6 to 10 mg; 4 to 6 mg is present in the normal liver. Unlike the situation with regard to pernicious anemia and vitamin B_{12}, there are few studies concerning the level of folic activity in tissues and cells of patients presumed deficient (198).

ASSAY METHODS AND SERUM LEVELS. Many microbiologic methods have been available for folic acid assay but until recently have not had the required sensitivity to detect reliably the amounts circulating in the blood. The growth response of a microorganism to compounds of the folic acid group (folates) may vary according to the number of glutamic acid residues present in the compound as well as to the various reduced coenzyme forms. Of the three organisms in general use, *L. citrovorum* responds to the monoglutamate, N5, 10-methylene-THF, and citrovorum factor; *S. fecalis* does not respond to polyglutamates or N5-methyl-THF; while *L. casei* responds to all forms, whether mono- or polyglutamate, oxidized or reduced. Since evidence now indicates that the monoglutamate, N5-methyl-THF, is a most important component of blood and tissue folic activity in man (125a), much important information concerning the physiology of folic acid in normal and abnormal situations is being revealed by employing *L. casei*, which alone detects it.

Employing modifications introduced by Herbert (123) to increase the sensitivity of the *L. casei* method and prevent inactivation or deterioration of folic activity in the sample to be assayed, several groups of workers have independently

* It is curious to note that owing to an error the organism originally thought to be *L. citrovorum* was actually *Pediococcus cerevisiae*. Mercifully the name has not been changed accordingly.

concurred in establishing the normal serum level and agree that a clear separation can be made between normal and abnormal (43, 49, 104a, 122, 123, 252) although the lower limit of normal cannot be precisely defined. Waters and Mollin (252) find that serum folic activity is composed of a stable and a labile* component. In the normal individual 65 to 94 per cent of the total activity is labile, and this is the component most useful as an index of folic acid metabolism. In normal subjects the serum level is given as 5.9 to 21.0 mμg per milliliter (9.9 $\pm$ 0.3); in patients with megaloblastic anemia requiring folic acid for therapy, less than 4.0 mμg per milliliter; in patients with pernicious anemia, 6.0 to 27.0 mμg per milliliter (16.6 $\pm$ 1.1), and in patients with pernicious anemia with combined degeneration of the spinal cord, 14.4 to 36.8 mμg per milliliter (24.8 $\pm$ 2.4). As mentioned above, the lower limit of normal cannot be precisely defined, but there is general agreement that the assay is reliable at levels greater than 2.5 mμg per milliliter, and a clear separation between normal and abnormal is made by a level of 3 to 4 mμg per milliliter.

Assay of whole blood for folic activity (104a) indicates considerable amounts present in normal red cells but almost complete depletion in the red cells of folic-deficient patients. Consequently determinations of whole blood folic activity may prove to be more reliable than serum levels in differentiating normal from abnormal.

The application of these techniques should be helpful in defining the various clinical situations in which folic acid abnormalities and deficiencies have been suspected or implicated. It will also, most probably, largely replace the investigations into folic acid metabolism (because only insensitive assay techniques were previously available) made by measuring (a) urinary output following parenteral and oral administration of folic acid, (b) rise in serum level of folic acid activity after a test dose, and (c) clearance from the blood following injections. Because of technical difficulties and interpretational pitfalls,† none of these manipulations has been generally adopted.

Use has also been made of known biochemical actions of folic acid in attempts to obtain indirect indicators of deficiency. In the metabolism of histidine a derivative of folic acid (tetrahydropteroylglutamic acid) is necessary for transformation of the histidine to glutamic acid that is then excreted in the urine. Histidine is normally metabolized to formiminoglutamic acid (FIGLU), which in turn yields its formimino group to tetrahydropteroylglutamic acid, resulting in citrovorum factor (5-formyl-tetrahydropteroylglutamic acid) and glutamic acid. In the absence of folic acid, FIGLU accumulates and appears in the urine, where it can be assayed (28, 142, 143, 163). When the test is performed on patients, loading doses of histidine are given to increase its sensitivity (162). However, although the results are as might be expected in the majority of instances (increased FIGLU excretion in patients with nutritional megaloblastic anemia, in those receiving folic acid antagonists as antileukemic therapy, in those with megaloblastic anemia of pregnancy, etc.), notable exceptions have occurred (increased excretion in some 50 per cent of patients with pernicious anemia whose serum levels of folic acid activity are not below normal and who do not respond to physio-

* The activity is lost to autoclaving or storage, even at $-20°C$; the change is prevented by vitamin C in phosphate buffer with certain time limits; the lost activity may be restored to serum by the addition of vitamin C.

† For example, urinary output is measured as an index of enteral absorption, but if the body stores are depleted excretion will be down because of retention after absorption. Prior priming or saturating doses have improved the test sufficiently to warrant its use in clinical investigation.

logic doses of folic acid, in rats and chickens deficient in vitamin B_{12}, in some patients with iron-lack anemia and some with hereditary spherocytosis (43a), etc.). Moreover, some folic acid–deficient animals do not excrete excess FIGLU. Consequently FIGLU may be excreted in vitamin B_{12} deficiency and *not* be excreted in folic acid deficiency.

Interpretation of the results of this test is also made difficult by the demonstration that in certain animals dietary methionine influences the amount of FIGLU excreted in the urine (83, 84). Nevertheless, some workers feel that the excretion of abnormal amounts of this compound may be a more sensitive indicator of folic acid abnormality than are serum levels (103) and that in pernicious anemia, for example, FIGLU abnormalities are attributable to folic acid abnormalities mediated through the folic acid cycle and the deficiency of vitamin B_{12}.

A most promising tool has recently become available in the form of tritium-labeled folic acid (8, 133, 134). It was expected that by this means the amount of folic acid absorbed from an oral dose could be assayed by determining the fecal and/or urinary excretion of radioactivity. Although there was some overlap in values, control subjects excreted less radioactivity in the *feces* than patients with megaloblastic anemia associated with the malabsorption syndrome. Patients with megaloblastic anemia not associated with malabsorption (pernicious anemia, heritable or surgical) excreted normal amounts in the feces. Control subjects and patients with malabsorption excreted similar amounts of radioactivity in the *urine* after small doses; when large doses were employed, the urinary execretion of the control subjects was three times that of the patients with malabsorption. The injection of 15 mg of nonlabeled folic acid did not interfere with the absorption of tritium-labeled folic acid but did enhance the urinary excretion of patients and controls.

This, in conjunction with the low serum levels now demonstrated, is apparently the best evidence available indicating the defective absorption of folic acid in some patients with malabsorption syndrome and the depletion of tissue folic acid in these conditions.

When tritiated folic acid is administered intravenously to normal individuals at a dose of 1 μg per kilogram of body weight, 60 per cent is cleared from the plasma in one circulation time; 90 to 95 per cent is removed in 3 minutes. In the plasma about 64 per cent is bound to protein. The rapid clearance suggests a selective uptake and specific binding at or in cells. At low doses most of the radioactivity is retained in the tissues; the small amounts found in the urine are mainly associated with folic acid activity, although some of the label is associated with citrovorum factor activity. At the higher doses (30 μg per kilogram of body weight) the fraction taken up by the tissues is lower and more appears in the urine, 90 per cent as unchanged folic acid. Up to 3 days after the initial injection, the tissue-bound radioactivity can be displaced by a flushing dose of folic acid; thereafter, the amount displaced decreases with time. This suggests that after its initial uptake, the folic acid becomes more firmly bound, tranferred to a "deeper" location, or changed in form.

On the whole it is obvious that only a very preliminary account can be given of the intake, absorption, transport, storage, and excretion of folic acid in normal and abnormal conditions.

BIOCHEMICAL ROLE OF FOLIC ACID AND COENZYME FORMS. Concerning biochemical functions, there is evidence that in the body folic acid exists in active forms that have coenzyme-like functions in cell metabolism in a number of reactions in which *single carbon atoms are transferred*

to or built into intermediates (203, 204).
The various metabolic systems dependent on the folic acid coenzymes are listed
in Table 7.6, which also gives the coenzyme form and the chemical moiety implicated in the one-carbon transfer units.
Figure 7.11 shows the chemical structures
and relations of the various coenzyme
forms. The reported isolation of folic acid
and citrovorum factor from natural materials rather than the other tetrahydropteroylglutamic acid derivatives is a reflection of the chemical lability of the
latter, and stability of the former, compounds, rather than a true indication of
the forms present. As with vitamin B_{12},
practically all the clinical studies and until very recently the in vitro studies have
been done employing the chemically stable, readily available forms, folic acid and
citrovorum factor, and not the biologically active coenzyme forms. Moreover,
the microbiologic and biologic activities
depend also on the number of glutamic
acid residues present in the compound.
The reported isolation of monoglutamates rather than polyglutamates is probably also a reflection of the instability of
the latter rather than an indication of the
actual presence of the monoglutamate in

tissue. Enzymatically active polyglutamates recently isolated and characterized
from natural materials with appropriate
precautions appear to have three or seven
glutamic acid residues.

There is evidence (a) that the enzymatic systems for synthesizing polyglutamates from monoglutamates occur in
man, (b) that conjugase in human blood
can split the higher polyglutamates to
triglutamates, and (c) that enzymes are
present in many tissues capable of converting folic acid to the various *reduced*
tetrahydrofolic (THF) forms (123).
Nevertheless, recent evidence indicates
(125a) that in human tissues folic acid
activity is due to a monoglutamate, N5-
methyl-tetrahydrofolic acid, the newly
described intermediate that depends
upon vitamin B_{12} for its activity in the
folic acid cycle described above.

A great deal of evidence concerning
nucleic acid anabolism has been assembled during the last decade. Two anabolic pathways have been demonstrated:
(a) construction of the nucleotides from
simple precursors; and (b) assimilation
of larger prefabricated bases, nucleosides, and nucleotides (the phosphori-

TABLE 7.6.   Metabolic systems dependent on folic acid coenzymes

System	Coenzyme form and chemical moiety implicated		
Serine ⟷ glycine Methionine biosynthesis, Thymine biosynthesis	N5, 10–methylene–THF	–CH₃	methyl
Serine ⟷ glycine Thymine biosynthesis	N10–hydroxymethyl–THFᵃ	–CH₂OH	hydroxymethyl
Purine biosynthesis	N5, 10–methenyl–THF	–CHO	formyl methenyl (formic acid)
Purine degradation, Histidine degradation	N5–formimino–THF	–CH=NH	formimino
Methionine biosynthesis	N5–methyl–THF	–CH₃	methyl
Purine biosynthesis	N10–formyl–THF	–CHO	formyl

ᵃ N10–hydroxymethyl–THF exists chiefly and perhaps exclusively in the anhydro derivative N5, 10–methylene–THF.

bosides of nucleosides). The pathways and steps involved in the biosynthesis of purines and pyrimidines are outlined in Figure 7.12. Although the exact sites of action in human metabolism have not been established for the vitamin B_{12} and folic acid coenzymes in these anabolic pathways, the folic acid coenzymes have been shown to participate in several critical steps involving formyl donation (29). In addition to the different sugars, DNA and RNA are chemically distinguished by the pyrimidine bases they contain; both contain the purines adenine and guanine plus the pyrimidine cytosine. RNA in addition contains the pyrimidine uracil, while DNA contains the pyrimidine thymine. It is therefore of considerable biochemical interest that various megaloblastic anemias have been shown to respond to the administration of some of the immediate precursors of RNA and DNA (249). Certain pyrimidine precursors (Figure 7.12) have been therapeutically effective: uracil (15 to 30 Gm daily, orally) and thymine (10 to 15 Gm daily, orally). Although there is one report of positive response to the administration of thymidine in pernicious anemia, other workers have consistently obtained negative results (236). A mixture of cytidylic and uridylic acid has produced positive results. The administration of orotic acid (3 to 6 Gm daily) has produced suboptimum and unsustained responses (218). In this regard it is of considerable interest that a child with megaloblastic anemia, who excreted enormous amounts of orotic acid in the urine, has been described as refractory to vitamin B_{12} and folic acid. A block was demonstrated in the conversion of orotic acid to the later pyrimidine precursors (235). Hematologic response followed the administration of a mixture of uridylic and cytidylic acids, presumably by bypassing the block (128, 129).

In addition to the cytochemical and analytic evidence cited in association with the megaloblastic changes in vitamin B_{12} deficiency, there is considerable evidence that abnormalities in RNA and DNA synthesis exist and that clinical and hematologic responses can be obtained by the administration of RNA and DNA precursors. Although the lack of response to thymidine is inexplicable at present, available evidence indicates that vitamin B_{12} deficiency and folic acid abnormality result in megaloblastic anemias and bodywide changes because of defects in RNA and DNA biosynthesis. The resultant changes consequently are most evident in cells that normally multiply rapidly.

No attempt will be made here to deal with the complicated clinical pictures presented by the entities listed in the classification in Table 7.5. Although response to folic acid administration is almost invariably adequate, the complete picture is seldom due to pure folic acid deficiency or abnormality; complicating factors are not unusual. In the megaloblastic anemias of infancy and pregnancy vitamin C deficiencies have been sometimes implicated.* In severe malabsorption syndromes (late sprue, steatorrhea, etc.) deficiencies of iron, vitamin B_{12}, and vitamin C may be concomitants. In a study relating the serum vitamin B_{12} level and the dose of folic acid to the hematopoietic responsiveness of patients with the megaloblastic anemia of sprue, Sheehy et al. (228–230) found that the lower the vitamin B_{12} level, the larger the dose of folic acid had to be to elicit a response. In some instances inhibitors of folic acid metabolism have been either definitely implicated (antileukemic agents such as Aminopterin and Amethopterin; anticonvulsant agents (42, 78, 105, 113, 164), in

---

* Severe macrocytic anemia with megaloblastic proliferation in the marrow is sometimes seen in scurvy. It is not clear from the few reported controlled observations whether vitamin C alone is implicated as a hematopoietic agent, whether folic acid deficiency is implicated, or whether (in some patients) both are interrelated and implicated (52, 270).

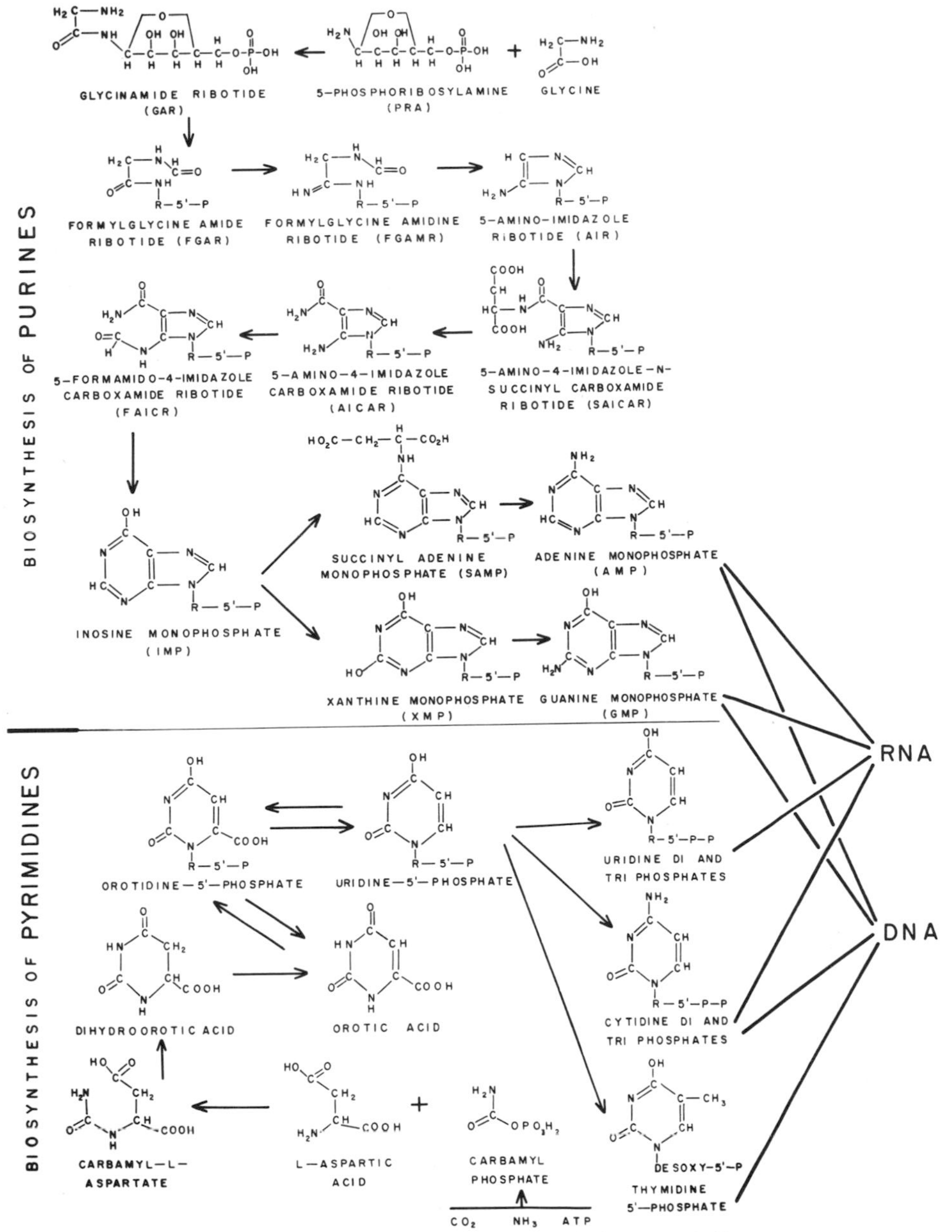

FIGURE 7.12. Main steps and some important intermediate compounds in biosynthesis of RNA and DNA

particular the hydantoin derivatives) or suggested (liver disease and alcoholism). As might be predicted from these brief notes, the management of these patients may present complicated problems in initial replacement and maintenance therapy. The presence of vitamin B_{12} deficiency is almost certain when megalo-blastic anemia is associated with combined degeneration of the cord and is most probable when gastric secretion is deficient in volume and acidity. From what has been pointed out above, these patients must *not* be treated with folic acid in the amounts usually employed for therapy, namely 5 to 15 mg per day. Since (practically) all patients with megaloblastic anemia (whether the abnormality relates primarily to vitamin B_{12} or folic acid) will respond to this dose, no differentiation can be made at that level. However it has been shown in several series of patients that the oral or parenteral administration of physiologic amounts of folic acid (25 to 400 μg per day) will produce adequate hematopoietic response in persons with folic acid abnormality but *not* in those with pernicious anemia (171). Conversely, in patients with folic acid deficiency, the administration of large doses of vitamin B_{12} (500 μg daily, intramuscularly) may induce hematologic responses perhaps by increased mobilization and/or utilization of folic acid. Small daily doses (1 to 5 μg intramuscularly) will induce hematologic responses only in patients with vitamin B_{12} deficiencies (271). Use of physiologic doses, therefore, may permit identification of the abnormalities as due to one or the other of the two vitamins at a clinical level without the aid of the more elaborate biochemical, radioactivity, or microbiologic measurements.

So.

Treatment	PA	Folic acid def.
High folic acid	o	+
Low B_{12}	+	o
Dmt:		
Low folic acid	+	+
High B_{12}	+	+

Bibliographic references for Chapter 7 begin on page 402.

PART IV] THE RED CELL: METABOLISM

CHAPTER EIGHT

RED CELL METABOLISM
AND METHEMOGLOBINEMIA

NORMAL RED CELL METABOLISM[*]
Function of the Red Cell

For many years the anatomy and main purpose of the adult erythrocyte have been accurately evaluated: it is a non-nucleated, biconcave, disc-shaped cell, containing hemoglobin in high concentration and so organized that during its 120-day life span and 175 miles of travel an effective means is provided for feeding oxygen to all tissues. However, because of a naïve belief in its simplicity, the red cell until very recently has been grossly underestimated. It has come into its own only through the deserved appreciation of its complex ultrastructure and the dynamic mechanisms that operate to maintain it as a properly structured and functioning unit. The *developing red cell* (as discussed in Chapters 1, 2, and 3) is organized for the biosynthesis of some 400 million molecules of hemoglobin that ultimately make up 95 per cent of its dry weight; the *adult red cell* is so organized that this hemoglobin may most effectively fulfill its oxygen-transporting function. The great change in attitude toward the adult erythrocyte has come about because of a forced recognition that for this transport to take place there is required

not only a mechanical contrivance or conveyance but also a "dynamo of activity." The adult erythrocyte retains, after having lost its nucleus and subcellular particles (mitochondria, RNA granules, etc.), a most impressive array of enzymes, proteins, carbohydrates, lipids, anions, and cations, many of which have been demonstrated to be in active metabolic flux.

This job of supplying oxygen to all tissues is indeed a prodigious one. In the average individual in a basal state about 250 ml of oxygen *per minute* is inspired, picked up by the red cells, transported and delivered to tissues; this value is, of course, much increased by activity. For a turnover of this magnitude, extremely rapid and nearly complete oxygenation of hemoglobin must occur in the lungs and comparably rapid deoxygenation in the tissues. Some concept of the effectiveness and rapidity of the actual reactions may be gained from the calculations of Roughton, who concluded that the average time a blood cell spends in a pulmonary capillary is 780 milliseconds and that very nearly complete oxygenation takes place

[*] General references and review articles: 2, 4, 10, 16, 17, 26, 35, 38, 42, 44, 47, 51, 53, 56, 59, 62, 63, 67, 71, 89, 90, 115, 116, 120, 121, 126, 154, 167, 171–173, 180, 181, 188, 220, 221, 228.

within the first third of that transit time (62, 193). For this to occur, the total surface area of the circulating erythrocytes exceeds 1,500 times the body surface, and there exist very precise and delicate facilitating mechanisms within each cell. It is pertinent here to point out that were hemoglobin not appropriately divided into corpuscular units, the resulting hemoglobin solution of approximately 15 Gm per 100 ml would be too viscous for effective circulation, the osmotic pressure of the plasma would be increased to some five times that of the plasma proteins, and the rate of oxygen uptake from capillaries would be less than one-third that for a suspension of intact red cells (195). The turbulent mixing that is imparted to the cells by circulation mechanics greatly enhances the capacity of a limited amount of hemoglobin to take on or give up oxygen. Thus, in addition to removing hemoglobin from the general metabolic pool

and turnover (the half life of hemoglobin circulating free in the plasma is 200 minutes (110) as opposed to 120 days for intracellular hemoglobin) and providing a locus in which enzyme systems can effectively function to maintain hemoglobin in the chemical state required for oxygen transport, important mechanical requirements are satisfactorily fulfilled by the packaging of hemoglobin into cellular units.

Anatomy of the Red Cell

Classically, the red cell was thought to be composed of two main parts: a retaining membrane and a highly concentrated solution of hemoglobin. However, the biconcave, discoidal form of itself indicates some definite structural arrangement (Figure 8.1). Geometric analysis indicates that the surface area of the cell is larger than the minimal area required to enclose its actual volume, as would be

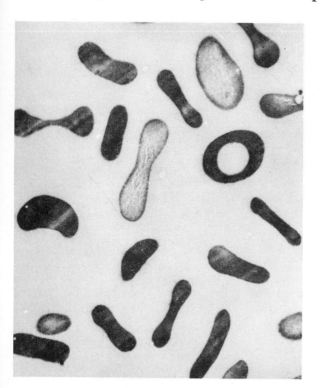

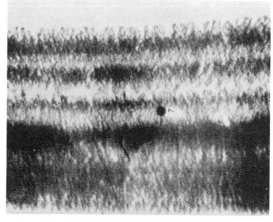

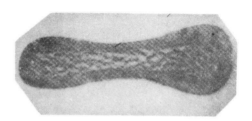

FIGURE 8.1.   Electron microscopic studies of thin sections of normal red cells at different magnifications. (From Ponder, E., Protoplasmalogia 10:1, 1955)

the situation for a simple spherical form. Therefore, some constituent molecules are constrained to take up preferred positions, and a definite ultrastructure to the cell is required.

The findings of Nakao et al. (160) relative to the isolation from red cells of a protein analagous to that found in muscle and variations in the shape of the cell according to its adenine nucleotide content suggest the possibility that the biconcave, discoidal configuration is partly maintained by an ATP-dependent contractile protein.

Osmotic stress or lytic agents can induce leakage of the hemoglobin, leaving a "posthemolytic residue" (otherwise termed ghost, stroma, envelope, red cell membrane, etc.). Since the posthemolytic residue can, under suitable conditions, reassume the configuration (biconcave disc) of the intact erythrocyte even though leached nearly free of hemoglobin, it is evident that the stroma comprises the main framework, or underlying architectural structure, of the cell (76). Nevertheless, it is now becoming more and more apparent that a sharp differentiation of stroma and hemoglobin cannot be made at all times, but rather that hemoglobin probably is an essential structural component (a coacervate) of the functioning cell and that the membrane in turn, by means of the ultrastructure, to some extent determines the ordering and functioning of hemoglobin.

The average red cell is 8.4 μ in diameter, 2.4 μ thick at the periphery and 1 μ thick at its narrowest portion in its native state. It is composed (172) of some 71 per cent water, 28 per cent hemoglobin, 7 per cent lipid such as cholesterol, lecithin, etc. (154, 168), and 3 per cent sugars, salts, enzyme protein, etc. (131). The stroma itself has been shown to be birefringent, or doubly refractive, indicating a patterned molecular structure (154). It is made up of a lipoprotein complex in which the lipids have an intrinsic radial

birefringence and the proteins a birefringence indicating a parallel arrangement at right angles to the lipids. Electron microscopy shows the surface of the human red cell to be covered by a layer of circular, plaque-like structures approximately 100 by 500 by 30 Å (74). The interstices of the plaques are thought to represent the channels, or pores, that allow for the ingress and egress of water, electrolytes, etc. The lipids of the plaques are oriented so that the hydrophobic acid groups project outward and impart a strong negative charge to the surface of the cell. This charge has never been satisfactorily measured in terms of an isoelectric point but is probably so strong that intercellular repelling forces are enough to prevent cells from touching each other. Beneath the plaques are proteins arranged in long fibrillar elements (elinin), positioned side by side and parallel to the surface, so that they in effect wrap around the cell in layers (167, 172, 173). Measurements on elinins extracted from the membrane by certain methods indicate that they are approximately 2,500 to 10,000 Å long and 125 Å wide. They are probably linked together laterally by the ether-extractable lipids to form the framework (stromin). The ABO and CDE antigens are associated with the elinin fractions. Other less accurately defined proteins, such as S protein, antisphering substance (30, 171), etc., are also presumed to be located here. The structure is highly oriented at the surface and contains little hemoglobin; it is less ordered toward the center and contains progressively more and more hemoglobin. From surface to center the protein and lipid concentrations progressively decrease while the hemoglobin concentration increases, so that no absolute dividing lines can be drawn. The individual molecules of hemoglobin are fairly ordered at the surface, while the orientation progressively decreases toward the center. Nevertheless, some ordering of the hemoglobin molecules persists throughout the cell, since low-angle x-ray scattering shows that the molecules can individually move freely but only within their own limited spaces, packing being such that only 10 Å separates one from another (9).

Numerous studies have been made concerning the thickness·of the membrane (162, 167, 172). By chemical analysis and by calculations of molecular size and arrangement, values of 100 to 500 Å have been obtained, values that check reasonably well with direct measurements made on ghosts. However, electron microscopic examination of intact cells—either by estimating the depth of pits produced by heating or by direct measurement of thinly sliced cells—yields values of 500 to 1,000 Å. This range is too great to be accounted for by the mass of the stromal components alone and indicates that hemoglobin is an integral part of the membrane. Originally it was thought that a small fraction of the hemoglobin (2 to 6 per cent) was "anchored" in, and very difficultly separable from, the ghost, since even repeated washing of ghosts still left a small residuum of hemoglobin (5). However, by radioactive tracer techniques, Hoffman et al. have shown complete mixing of unlabeled intracellular hemoglobin with labeled extracellular hemoglobin at the time of osmotic lysis, so that there would not appear to be any structurally, or irreversibly, fixed hemoglobin (77).

It must be acknowledged that there are major inconsistencies in this simplified presentation of erythrocyte structure; many points could be amplified, disputed, or refuted. In electron microscopy it is difficult to separate artifact from true object, to distinguish changes induced by preparative techniques from inherent structure, and to determine whether size is truly representative or altered by the state of hydration. The results of many analyses of intact red cells and stroma have been shown to vary significantly with the methods of preparation, the anticoagulant used, the method of lysis, and even the number of washings during which the cell is ostensibly freed of plasma contamination. It has been shown, for example, that repeated washing may result in significant loss of lipid and protein although hemolysis is negligible. Ponder has demonstrated that unwashed erythrocytes may be readily broken into smaller particles by mechanical disruption, while cells thrice washed in isotonic saline are disrupted only with difficulty. Another fact which apparently has to be learned over and over again is that the cellular composition, in terms of lipid, water, protein, ion, and enzyme content and specific gravity, varies considerably with the *age* of the cell. It is obvious that to make accurate meaningful comparisons, similarly aged populations of cells must be employed.

Structure and Functions of Hemoglobin

Studies on the anatomy of the hemoglobin molecule* reveal four iron atoms in the centers of four protoporphyrin rings. Analysis of x-ray diffraction pictures (86) shows that these four heme groups are located in shallow depressions of the surface of the globin moiety (Figure 8.2), each heme group in association with one of the four polypeptide chains (168). The iron in each porphyrin ring is hexacovalent, i.e., it can bind six atoms or atom groups. In the plane of the porphyrin ring it links with the four nitrogen atoms of the pyrrole rings. When the fifth bond is attached to the proper site (probably the imidazole moiety of a histidine residue) in the globin peptide chain and the heme is properly positioned in relation to the polypeptide chain (probably by means of carboxyl bonding of its propionic side chains to arginine residues),

---

* The studies by Perutz were made employing horse hemoglobin, but there is reason to think that the results may be applied to human hemoglobin.

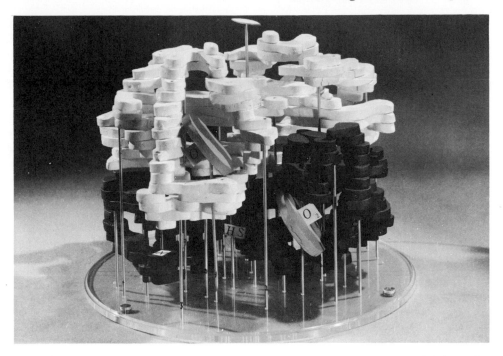

FIGURE 8.2.   Perutz's model of horse hemoglobin molecule calculated at 5.5 Å resolution. The two kinds of polypeptide chains are indicated: two white and two black chains; the heme groups are indicated by gray disks. (From Perutz, M. F., et al., Nature 185:416, 1960)

the remaining covalent bond can attach reversibly to oxygen (50, 101). Evidence also indicates that the heme groups lie near sulfhydryl groups. Whatever the actual positions of the heme groups in relation to the polypeptide chains, they confer on the iron atoms the remarkable and difficultly imitable property of reversible oxygenation: the ability to take on and give up oxygen without a change in valency. Magnetic studies of ferrous hemoglobin indicate that the iron has four unpaired electrons in the third (outer) shell (29). Oxygen is known to possess two unpaired electrons. Upon combination of oxygen with ferrous hemoglobin, a change in the magnetic susceptibility takes place indicating that all the unpaired electrons of the iron and oxygen have paired. In this form oxygen cannot accept an electron in transfer and hence cannot act as an oxidizing agent.

OXYGEN ASSOCIATION AND DISSOCIATION.

The situation with respect to oxygen uptake and transport by hemoglobin is enormously complicated by the presence of four heme groups per hemoglobin molecule and the consequent fact that each ferrous hemoglobin molecule may exist binding none, one, two, three, or four molecules of oxygen (53, 88). But this complexity also confers an enormous physiologic advantage upon hemoglobin. When one heme group takes on oxygen, a change in the affinity for oxygen is induced in the remaining heme groups so that they can much more readily bind to oxygen; when the second heme group is oxygenated, the affinity of the remaining two heme groups is again changed; etc. The combination of the oxygen ligands with hemoglobin takes place in four separate steps, and this occurs in such a way that the oxygenation of one heme group facilitates the oxygenation of the others. Presumably because of their association with similar polypeptide chains, the interactions in human hemoglobin occur in pairs: the first and third ligands are loosely bound and the second and fourth are tightly bound. The mechanism whereby this heme-heme interaction takes place is not known. Present models indicate that the heme groups are too widely separated for the oxygenation of one of them to affect the oxygen affinity of its neighbor directly (168). As discussed in the section on the sickling phenomenon, there is evidence for a gross rearrangement of the polypeptide chains with respect to each other upon oxygenation and deoxygenation; such a reorganization of the molecule would be expected to alter the affinity of the heme groups because of environmental changes local to them.

The physiologic consequences and advantages of this heme-heme interaction are most important. When the percentage of hemoglobin saturated with oxygen is determined experimentally with respect to the partial pressure of oxygen in standardized and equilibrated suspensions of erythrocytes, the curve so obtained—called the oxygen dissociation curve of hemoglobin—is found to be sigmoidal in shape, as indicated in Figure 8.3. The position and shape of this oxygen dissociation curve may be altered by changes in the pH, ionic strength, or temperature of the hemoglobin environment (188, 189). A lowering of the pH, for example, shifts the curve to the right so that more oxygen is given up by the hemoglobin at a given oxygen tension (or less taken up) than under standard conditions.

The physiologic relevance of these observations is evident from the following considerations. Normally, the partial pressure of oxygen varies between 30 and 100 mm Hg. With reference to the oxygen dissociation curve of hemoglobin, this means that one is usually dealing with the steeply ascending part of the curve and the less rapidly ascending top

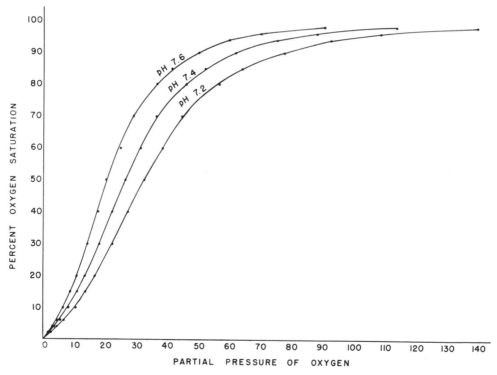

FIGURE 8.3.   Oxygen dissociation curves of human hemoglobin at various pH values

portion. Therefore, minor changes in the partial pressure of oxygen, in the region of 30 mm Hg, bring about the association or dissociation of large amounts of oxygen from the hemoglobin. Full oxygenation is effected only by proportionately greater changes in oxygen tension. Nevertheless, conditions are such that in the lungs *almost* complete saturation of the hemoglobin with oxygen is achieved. Full oxygenation is achieved only by oxygen tensions found under artificial laboratory conditions. Thus, the heme-heme interaction provides an excellent mechanism for loading or unloading large amounts of oxygen stimulated by relatively minor physiologic changes in the partial pressure. Moreover, as mentioned above, the position of the curve is altered by pH and temperature changes, and in such a fashion that at the lower pH value and increased temperature expected in rapidly metabolizing tissues producing carbon dioxide, oxygen is all the more readily dissociated from the hemoglobin.

Hemoglobin has a function, in addition to oxygen transport, important to total-body economy; namely, aiding in the transport of carbon dioxide from tissues to lungs for expiration. In doing this hemoglobin also exerts its considerable buffering effect (0.7 mole of carbonic acid, as bicarbonate ion, per mole of oxygen exchanged, or about 70 per cent of the total carbon dioxide without any pH alteration).

OXYGEN AND CARBON DIOXIDE TRANSPORT. In the tissues CO_2 is produced by diverse metabolic processes and exists there at a high partial pressure. Accordingly, it moves along pressure gradients into the circulating plasma and cells. In the plasma a small portion is transported in simple physical solution, but in the main CO_2 and H_2O react *slowly* to form H_2CO_3, which in turn dissociates into H^+ and HCO_3^-. At pH 7.4, according to the Henderson-Hasselbalch equation, the ratio of HCO_3^- to H_2CO_3 will be 20:1. A considerable amount of H^+ is taken up by the plasma proteins. The major portion of the CO_2 produced by the tissues diffuses into the erythrocytes, where it is handled by two different mechanisms: (a) some of the CO_2 combines directly with the amino acid residues in the reduced hemoglobin to form carbaminohemoglobin—$HHgbNH_2 + CO_2 \leftrightarrows H$-$HgbNHCOOH$; (b) the major portion of the CO_2 is hydrated *rapidly* to H_2CO_3 facilitated by the erythrocytes' carbonic anhydrase. Then the H_2CO_3 dissociates to H^+ and HCO_3^-.[*] Coeval with this the O_2, under a pressure gradient, dissociates from the Fe and diffuses to the tissues. The deoxygenated hemoglobin can accept the H^+ (the reverse of the oxygenation effect described below) and by this buffering action help to preserve the pH stability of the cell, plasma, and body. This has been termed the "isohydric cycle." The HCO_3^- now diffuses out of the cell into the plasma because of its concentration gradient, thereby leaving an excess of cations in the erythrocyte. The major positively charged ion in the erythrocyte is of course K^+. But the efflux of this ion is *relatively* slow due to the low permeability of the membrane to it. However, the membrane is *highly* permeable to Cl^-, and Cl^- accordingly enters the cell to maintain electrostatic balance. This phenomenon has been called the "chloride shift." Although the entrance of Cl^- maintains electrical equilibrium, it also upsets the osmotic equilibrium so that H_2O enters with a consequent increase in cell size. The entire sequence is referred to as the "Hamburger shift."

When blood comes to the lungs, O_2 enters the red cell because of the pressure gradient and adds to the sixth coordination link of Fe, displacing the H_2O associated there in the reduced hemoglobin

[*] The CO_2 is transported in 5 per cent simple physical solution, 20 per cent carbaminohemoglobin, 75 per cent bicarbonate ion.

form. The addition of O_2 causes the resonating electrons of the porphyrin group to shift toward the O_2 and brings about the dissociation of a proton (H^+) from the imidazole ring of histidine in a peptide chain of globin (67).* The H^+ combines with HCO_3^- to form H_2CO_3. The intracellular conversion of H_2CO_3 to H_2O and CO_2 is rapidly effected by the carbonic anhydrase of the cell, and the CO_2 released diffuses along pressure gradients out of the cell, through the plasma, capillaries, and alveolar walls, into the alveolar spaces. Thus the reverse of the isohydric cycle and chloride shift occurs with oxygenation.

Precise measurements recently made by Roughton (194, 195) have for the first time made it possible to calculate the dissociation constants for each of the four heme moieties. Roughton has stated: "We now know enough about the kinetics of the reactions of gasses with hemoglobin to deal with the physiological problems of oxygen transport in the circulation— further work is being undertaken in order to find out more about the reactions for their own sake."

INFLUENCE OF CELL MEMBRANE AND CELL SHAPE ON OXYGEN TRANSPORT. It is interesting to note that the red cell membrane plays a significant role in oxygen transport. Various kinetic studies show that the *rate* of oxygen uptake is some twenty times slower in red cell suspensions than in hemoglobin solutions (61, 62, 223). This is due in the main to the resistance of the membrane to oxygen passage. In addition to this, as the first molecules of oxygen enter the cell and combine with the outermost layer of hemoglobin, they form a barrier that progressively slows down the entrance of additional oxygen. At a concentration of 30 Gm of hemoglobin per 100 ml of solution and by reason of the relatively fixed positions of the hemoglobin molecules because of the cell's ultrastructure, the translatory motion, or diffusion, of the

hemoglobin molecules is nil, thus impeding oxygen entrance to the interior of the cell for complete saturation. An ever-increasing barrier to oxygen is built up.† There is reason to believe that the differences in the over-all kinetics of hemoglobin reactions in red cells and in solutions are due to diffusion factors, and that the purely chemical kinetics are the same. Despite these diffusion disadvantages imparted largely by the cell membrane, the packaging of hemoglobin into discrete units confers an overwhelming advantage on the total organism in terms of oxygen transport.

The biconcave form of the erythrocyte has been thought to allow optimum diffusion of gases by permitting a more uniform proximity of the surface membrane and the internal hemoglobin than would be possible in the spherical form. Moreover, recent studies indicate that a 40 per cent decrease in surface area takes place during the formation of microspherocytes. This decrease in surface area and the unavailability of central hemoglobin molecules should by calculation give a 20 per cent advantage to the biconcave, discoidal form over the spherical form in terms of the kinetics of oxygen transport (236). Exact measurements made by Carlsen and Comroe employing the stopped-flow technique show that disc-to-sphere transformations (induced by heat or hypotonic solutions) are not accompanied by measurable changes in the rate of gas uptake (33, 34). That the method has the required sensitivity to detect such a change is illustrated by the

---

* This effect—hemoglobin becoming more acidic on oxygenation—is called the "Bohr effect."

† Evidence by Hemmingsen and Scholander indicates that this barrier effect is much less than previously estimated (73, 203). By a presumed "bucket-brigade mechanism," oxygen is readily passed from one hemoglobin molecule to the next; hemoglobin solutions allow the passage of oxygen more rapidly than would be predicted on the basis of other kinetic studies (39).

observation that cells dehydrated by hypertonic solutions so that the mean corpuscular hemoglobin concentration (MCHC) increased 50 per cent do show a significant decrease in the rate of gas uptake. Although for technical reasons these studies were made with carbon monoxide and nitrogen monoxide, there is reason to believe that the finding can be applied to the kinetics of oxygen transport.

INFLUENCE OF DIFFERENT FORMS OF HEMOGLOBIN ON OXYGEN DISSOCIATION. It has been mentioned that the position and shape of the all-important oxygen dissociation curve of hemoglobin can be altered by pH, temperature, and ionic environment. The position can also be shifted by changes (a) in the heme-to-protein attachment, as in the abnormal hemoglobin M and variants (56); (b) in the ligand attached to iron, as in carboxyhemoglobin; and (c) in the valency of the iron, as in methemoglobin in which the iron is oxidized to the trivalent state because of defective cell enzymes (41). By and large, the minor abnormalities in the oxygen dissociation curves determined on suspensions of red cells containing abnormal hemoglobins such as S and C appear to be due to intracellular alterations, since solutions of these abnormal hemoglobins yield normal curves (188). This also appears to be the situation for fetal hemoglobin; however, in this latter instance the oxygen dissociation curve determined for cell suspensions is markedly shifted from the normal to a position physiologically more advantageous to the fetus (238). As can be seen from Figure 8.3, a position of the curve to the left of normal indicates that larger amounts of oxygen can be picked up by the cells at the partial pressure of oxygen in maternal arterial blood in the placenta than would be possible by normal cells. Because of the steepness of the curve, oxygen unloading to fetal tissues takes place effectively under oxygen and carbon dioxide partial pressures of fetal tissues.

Carboxyhemoglobin (carbonmonoxyhemoglobin, HgbCO) is produced by the combination of carbon monoxide with the iron of the heme radicle. Although carbon monoxide combines more slowly with hemoglobin than does oxygen, it is bound some 210 times more firmly and is consequently only difficultly dissociable. Carboxyhemoglobin is therefore unavailable for hemoglobin's essential role of oxygen transport. The toxic effects of the inhalation of carbon monoxide are due solely to tissue hypoxia from the decreased oxygen transport. The decrease in transport comes about not only because carbon monoxide renders the hemoglobin unavailable, but also because the presence of carboxyhemoglobin, even in small percentages, shifts the dissociation curve of the otherwise normal hemoglobin so that it less readily gives up its oxygen. Carboxyhemoglobin is a bright cherry-red pigment, and when clinically suspected because of exposure or signs of hypoxia without cyanosis, its presence can be determined by spectral absorption curves or by a simple dilution procedure. Dilute solutions of oxyhemoglobin appear yellowish-red to the unaided eye; carboxyhemoglobin appears pink or bluish-red.

Methemoglobin is a derivative of hemoglobin in which the iron of the heme complex has been oxidized to the ferric form by electron transfer to oxygen. Oxygen that is linked to hemoglobin in this fashion is not dissociable by changes in the partial pressure of oxygen; the pigment is consequently of no value for respiration. The iron can be reduced to its normal form by various reducing agents or by enzymatic action; the hemoglobin then returns to its functional state. Reduced hemoglobin (Hgb) is susceptible to *oxidation* by molecular oxygen to form methemoglobin (MHgb) during the normal process of *reversible oxygenation* with molecular oxygen to form oxyhemoglobin ($HgbO_2$). Quantitatively the oxidation reaction is hardly significant. However, even the small amount of oxidation estimated to occur per day (3 per cent) would in the long run represent a serious physiologic problem, since nonfunctioning methemoglobin would gradually increase with time. In the normal erythrocyte methemoglobin is continuously being formed; it is also continuously being reduced by specific mechanisms so that the concentration at any given time is very small, less than 1 to 2 per cent of the total pigment (49, 107). In addition to its presence owing to an abnormal globin (hemoglobin M), abnormal quantities of methemoglobin appear in the blood (a) when the rate of *reduction* of the methemoglobin is altered (hereditary methemoglobinemia) or (b) when the rate of *production* of methemoglobin exceeds the rate at which the reducing mechanisms can function (acquired methemoglobinemia due to various oxidant compounds).

To maintain hemoglobin in the reduced form in which it can be reversibly oxygenated and deoxygenated requires the continual production of energy in the erythrocyte through glycolysis and the regeneration of reduced pyridine nucleotides.

Metabolic Capabilities of the Red Cell

The developing nucleated red cell contains all the necessary subcellular components and enzyme systems for replication, maturation, and differentiation (Table 8.1). It is capable of synthesizing many different types of compounds (proteins, lipids, carbohydrates) and can therefore add to its structural materials and enzyme components. The production of heme and globin is, of course, the cell's major effort. To meet its energy requirements, it has available to it the tricarboxylic acid cycle, the Embden-Meyerhof cycle, and the pentose phosphate pathway (16, 17, 228). By the time the developing red cell has reached the normoblast stage, it has lost its ability to synthesize DNA and can therefore no longer reproduce itself by mitotic division. It is therefore probably accurate to state that senescence of the erythrocyte begins at or slightly before its normoblast stage of development (23, 108).

The young red cell, or reticulocyte (36, 126), although it has lost its nucleus and the ability to multiply and divide (125), still retains the capacity (albeit in mi-

TABLE 8.1. Metabolic characteristics of red cell at various stages of its development

	Nucleated cell	Reticu- locyte	Adult cell
Replication	+	0	0
DNA synthesis	+	0	0
RNA synthesis	+	0	0
RNA present	+	+	0
Lipid synthesis	+	+	0
Heme synthesis	+	+	0
Protein synthesis	+	+	0
Cytochrome and electron transfer system	+	+	0
Carbohydrate metabolism			
Krebs' tricarboxylic acid cycle	+	+	0
Embden-Meyerhof pathway	+	+	+
Pentose phosphate pathway	+	+	+
Maturation and/or senescence	+	+	+

nute quantities) to synthesize protein (mainly globin) and heme, to take aboard iron and incorporate it into hemoglobin. It also contains the enzymes necessary for the *de novo* production of compounds containing considerable potential energy for cell metabolism, the purine and pyridine nucleotides. Both the Embden-Meyerhof cycle and the pentose phosphate shunt are active, and at this stage of development the cytochrome system and the tricarboxylic acid, or Krebs', cycle are intact and to some extent functional for electron transport (47). There is evidence that lipids can be synthesized at this stage (141) and that the red cell and plasma are in a dynamic state of exchange with respect to lipids and phospholipids (96, 119, 124, 143, 144, 184).

The nonreticulated mature erythrocyte has lost its RNA and its ability to form heme and synthesize proteins; very probably it cannot synthesize lipids (31, 141). The tricarboxylic acid cycle is no longer functional although a few of its enzymes persist. However, the entire set of enzymes necessary to carry carbohydrate metabolism through the Embden-Meyerhof and pentose phosphate pathways still persists and functions (6, 7). From this metabolism of glucose various compounds of high potential energy and/or reductive capacity are produced that become available for translation into the actual work that must be performed to keep the erythrocyte in a properly functioning state. To direct the utilization of the potential energy and reductive capacities of these compounds the mature red cell retains a remarkable array of enzyme systems (4, 37); the channeling mechanisms and ultimate utilization are discussed on pages 211ff. In addition to enzymes with known functions (maintenance of hemoglobin in a form capable of reversible oxygenation and protection from degradation, for example), many enzymes are present whose functions are

presently obscure, such as acetyl cholinesterase, which suggestively is associated with the lipoprotein components on the outside surface of the stroma (200).

Although it is not known whether the mature erythrocyte can synthesize glutathione *de novo* from the component parts (glycine, glutamic acid, and cysteine), studies employing labeled glycine indicate that the red cell is capable of incorporating (or exchanging) the amino acid into glutathione.

A most important problem with respect to the adult erythrocyte concerns its ability to synthesize or renew its critical compounds containing high potential energy and/or high reductive capacity. It is known that rabbit reticulocytes can synthesize *de novo* the purine nucleotides (adenosine and guanosine triphosphate) but that the adult erythrocytes do not have the complete pathway for *de novo* purine formation. They are, however, able to complete the final steps of *nucleotide synthesis* and utilize ribosyl derivatives for nucleoside triphosphate formation—the so-called salvage pathway for incorporation of purines into nucleotides (128–130). Mature human red cells can utilize preformed purines for nucleotide synthesis but are deficient in their capacity to convert inosinic acid to adenylic acid (121). It has been demonstrated that mature human erythrocytes can synthesize DPN from nicotinic acid (182) and also incorporate nicotinic acid into the pyridine nucleotides TPN and DPN (94, 182).

It is of interest that the erythrocyte is unique among biologic units in that the cell itself does no work in fulfilling its primary functions of oxygen and carbon dioxide transport. Because of the peculiar properties of hemoglobin, these are passive functions not requiring the expenditure of energy produced by the cell. Energy expended by the cell is directed at maintaining the cell in a functional state so that these passive activities can go on. Although not established, it is conceivable that the red cell also serves as a transport device for lipids, carbohydrates, proteins, nonhemoglobin iron, various ions, hormones, and vitamins. If any of these possibilities turn out to be so—for example, if there is a net delivery of lipids (21) to a specific site—then it is likely that actual work is accomplished by the red cell. But at present the evidence indicates that the energy produced and made available by erythrocyte metabolism is expended in maintaining the cell so that its passive functions may properly proceed.

Aging of the Red Cell

The studies detailed in Chapter 9 document that the erythrocyte has a finite life span and that normally the erythrocyte is removed from circulation *after* it has lived out its 120-day span. During any given period of time a certain number of cells are destroyed; the evidence indicates that the ones destroyed are those that have reached their full age. It is reasonable to suppose that the biochemical and biophysical changes concerned with aging ultimately determine the cell's removal from circulation and destruction. Consequently considerable investigative activity has been directed toward defining the changes that occur with age in (a) the structural components, (b) the chemical composition, (c) the energy sources, and (d) the critical functional components of the erythrocyte.

An ordinary peripheral blood sample contains a mixture of cells of all ages. Some technique is necessary for identifying and separating the cells into appropriate age groups. It has been known for a long time that when blood is sedimented, the reticulocytes are preferentially distributed at the top of the red cell column. Since the reticulocyte is a *young* cell, this position is indicative of a cell newly formed and released. This slower sedimentation is due to the greater water content and consequent lower density of the reticulocyte (75). After centrifugation (24) and ultracentrifugation (187) also the young cells are found in the top layers, from which they can be obtained for various analytic procedures, leaving behind in the column cells whose age is greater than the mean of the original population.

By means of radioactive iron a limited population of cells can be labeled and followed as an identifiable phalanx through their life span. When this is combined with centrifugation at various time intervals after administration of the radioiron, it has been shown that the radioactivity first appears in the top layer and then progressively descends the column of cells.

It has been noted that the young cells from the top of the column are more resistant to osmotic lysis than those at the bottom (138). Employing cells labeled with radioactive iron, the amount of radioactive hemoglobin liberated by cell lysis during the osmotic fragility test indicates the age of the cells destroyed at any given tonicity. Serial studies by this technique confirm the observation that cells become progressively more susceptible to osmotic lysis during their life span (75). These conclusions are confirmed by a technique employing a graded decrease in ionic strength of the media to induce osmotic lysis (40). Samples may be obtained for characterization of the erythrocytes at any point during the progressive changes induced.

The cells most resistant to osmotic stress (younger cells) may be recovered for study or the products of the lysed (older) cells subjected to study. Analyses employing various combinations and modifications of these techniques have yielded information concerning aging.

Changes in the structural components of the red cell can be directly indicated by a decrease in surface area and by chemical analyses that show, for example, less lipid in old cells as compared with young; structural changes may also be inferred from the different ionic composition and from behavior in mechanical and osmotic fragility tests (decreased potassium content and decreased mechanical and osmotic resistance in old cells; 75). Considerable evidence is now available concerning the alterations in cell energetics (14): oxygen utilization is, of course, high at the nucleated stage, falls off sharply following extrusion of the nucleus and loss of subcellular particles to reach its low point, and then rises slightly with increasing age. The rate of glucose disappearance and Embden-Meyerhof glycolysis decreases progressively (14). Observations on the cation steady state indicate a low level of active transport in the older cells.

The many studies concerning changes in the levels and activities of various enzymes in health and disease (2, 137, 139, 140, 163, 177, 178, 180, 235), particularly those involved in glucose utilization (14; Table 8.2), have demonstrated significant decreases in many instances, but it has not been unequivocally established that they fall below a rate-limiting range during normal life span (36a, 137, 139, 140, 202). Because of a decrease in cellular ATP and an increase in ADP (117) and the correlation of decreased survival of ATP-deficient cells as they age in vivo and in vitro, this seems likely but has not been demonstrated.

Some workers have reported an increased concentration of methemoglobin in older cells (28, 239), the increase being appreciable at about 50 days of age and mounting steadily thereafter. This finding, admittedly disputed by some workers (18), would be consistent with a progressive inability of the cell to protect its hemoglobin from deleterious changes that can lead to its oxidation, denaturation, and destruction (186).

A number of studies have demonstrated that the ability to reduce methemoglobin to hemoglobin is a function of cell age: the reticulocyte has the greatest capacity (142); the capacity of the old erythrocyte is less than the young or mature cell (12, 100). Jalavisto and Solantera (95) conclude that the same decay curve is found for the methemoglobin reduction rate as for the erythrocyte survival. No studies have shown a striking change in the enzymes (methemoglobin reductases) as a cause of the cell's decreased capacity: some of the fall-off in methemoglobin reduction capacity can be explained by diminished glucose utilization and a resultant decrease in the generation of reduced pyridine nucleotides required for enzyme function.

In the section on Primaquine-sensitive Hemolytic Anemia in Chapter 9 evidence will be noted to link the protection of hemoglobin to the equilibrium between reduced and oxidized glutathione (35), which, as has been pointed out, is dependent upon glucose metabolism and the pyridine nucleotides (43). It is of interest that increased amounts of hemoglobin A_3 (147) have been described in older cells since this component is made up of an altered denatured hemoglobin derived from hemoglobin A. Differences in the oxygen saturation of old and young cells have been described that are due to macromolecular changes within the cell and very probably represent alterations in the structure of the hemoglobin molecule that progress with age (46). Accordingly the proposition has been advanced that if through aging and the consequent loss of metabolic capabilities the red cell is unable to protect its critical functional component, hemoglobin, from changes that lead to its degradation, the same or similar changes may allow alterations in the cell membrane that lead to destruction of the cell (11). The recent observations that animal and human erythrocytes become progessively more susceptible to hemolysis by immune antibodies and complement may also be

TABLE 8.2. Chemical changes recorded in old and young red cells

ENZYME CHANGES	
Glucose–6–phosphate dehydrogenase	Increased activity in young cells
6–phosphogluconic dehydrogenase	Increased activity in young cells
Phosphohexose isomerase	Increased activity in young cells
Triose phosphate dehydrogenase	Increased activity in young cells
Aldolase	Increased activity in young cells
Lactic dehydrogenase	Little or no difference
Methemoglobin reductase	Increased activity in young cells
Purine nucleoside phosphorylase	Little or no difference
Cholinesterase	Increased activity in young cells
Catalase	Increased activity in young cells
Glyoxalase	Increased activity in young cells
METABOLIC CHANGES	
Glycolysis	Increased in young cells
Oxygen utilization	Decreased in young cells
Nucleoside utilization	Increased in young cells
CONSTITUENT CHANGES	
Phosphate esters	No difference
	Doubtful fall in easily hydrolyzable phosphate (mainly ATP) and 2, 3–phosphoglyceric acid
Glutathione	No difference
Total–SH	Increased in young cells
Lipids	Increased in young cells (but not per unit surface area)
Electrolytes:	
Potassium	Increased in young cells
Sodium	{ Increased in young cells (Joyce, 99) { Decreased in young cells (Bernstein, 14)
K^{42} exchange	Decreased in young cells
Water	Increased in young cells
Methemoglobin	Increased in old cells
Oxygen dissociation	Decreased in old cells
STORAGE CHANGES	
Phosphate esters	Decreased breakdown of ATP and 2, 3–phosphoglyceric acid in young cells
Electrolytes	Decreased loss of potassium from young cells

Adapted from Prankerd, T. A. J., The Red Cell, Blackwell, Oxford, 1961.

taken as evidence of an age-dependent susceptibility to destruction (68, 121).

In addition, there may be an accumulation of metabolites noxious to the metabolic activity of the cell. Although it is clear that during its sojourn in the circulation the normal erythrocyte undergoes a process of aging, and it seems most probable that its final destruction is the result of this aging process, there is no direct evidence to establish this as fact. It may well be that the changes noted so far are mechanisms designed to hold off final destruction as long as possible or are merely incidental, concomitant alterations and not the changes directly responsible for the vulnerability of age. The critical reaction(s) that actually determines the life span of the erythrocyte is not known.

Cellular Energetics

PRODUCTION OF COMPOUNDS OF HIGH POTENTIAL ENERGY. Although it has been known for some time that the adult eryth-

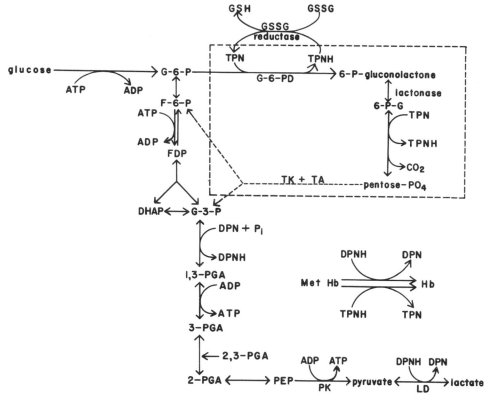

FIGURE 8.4.   Glucose catabolism in human erythrocytes. GSH, reduced glutathione; GSSH, oxidized glutathione; G–6–P, glucose–6–phosphate; F–6–P, fructose–6–phosphate; FDP, fructose–1–6–diphosphate; DHAP, dihydroxacetone phosphate; G–3–P, glyceraldehyde–3–phosphate; LD, lactic dehydrogenase; TPN, oxidized triphosphopyridine nucleotide; TPNH, reduced triphosphopyridine nucleotide; DPN, oxidized diphosphopyridine nucleotide; DPNH, reduced diphosphopyridine nucleotide; 6–P–G, 6–phosphogluconate; G–6–PD, glucose–6–phosphate dehydrogenase; TK, transketolase; TA, transaldolase; Pi, inorganic phosphate; ADP, adenosine diphosphate; ATP, adenosine triphosphate; PEP, phosphoenolpyruvate; PK, pyruvic kinase; 1, 3–PGA, 1, 3–phosphoglyceric acid; 3–PGA, 3–phosphoglyceric acid; 2–PGA, 2–phosphoglyceric acid; 2, 3–PGA, 2, 3–diphosphoglyceric acid; Met Hb, methemoglobin; Hb, reduced hemoglobin

rocyte metabolizes glucose and utilizes a small amount of oxygen, the details and mechanisms of cellular energetics have until recently not been analyzed. By identification of intermediates (7) and studies of specific enzymatic activities, it has been shown that the Embden-Meyerhof pathway* is present and functional, metabolizing glucose to lactic acid, with the production of potential energy in the form of ATP. Similarly, it has now been demonstrated that the pentose phosphate pathway† is operational, utilizing glucose to

produce carbon dioxide and a source of potential energy and high reductive capacity, TPNH. These two pathways can be linked together in at least one point. As illustrated in Figure 8.4, studies have shown that the ribose phosphate of the pentose phosphate pathway enters pools of the Embden-Meyerhof pathway and is there further metabolized to lactic acid,

* Also called the glycolytic pathway.
† Also called the phosphogluconic acid pathway and the hexose monophosphate pathway or shunt.

with the production of ATP as a source of high-energy phosphate bonds as potential energy.

It had usually been considered that the amount of glucose metabolized by way of the pentose phosphate pathway was negligibly small. Accordingly, the energy possibly made available by this pathway, and the oxygen consumption of the erythrocyte, were of necessity regarded as nugatory. However, recent studies by Murphy (156, 157) have indicated that the relative amounts of glucose metabolized by either pathway vary significantly with pH and partial pressure of oxygen. Szeinberg and Marks (226) have similarly shown an increased rate of glucose catabolism by the pentose phosphate pathway *without* increased rate of glucose utilization or lactic acid formation by the addition of the physiologic components (cysteine, ascorbic acid, pyruvate) and chemical agents (primaquine, phenylhydrazine, nitrofurantoin, etc.). Under circumstances simulating in vivo conditions as closely as presently possible, it has been estimated (157) that some 11 per cent of the total glucose metabolized passes through the pentose phosphate pathway. These calculations were made employing glucose labeled with C^{14}. Since carbon dioxide is produced only by metabolism through the pentose phosphate pathway, and not through the Embden-Meyerhof pathway, the recovery of labeled carbon dioxide indicates that the pentose phosphate pathway *is* functional. By employing glucose labeled either uniformly or in various positions, the contribution of the different metabolic pathways can be assessed. It has been found that glucose labeled with C^{14} in the one position results in a good yield of labeled carbon dioxide; glucose labeled with C^{14} in the six position does not result in a comparable yield of labeled carbon dioxide. Figure 8.4 indicates that this occurs because in

the pentose phosphate pathway the C^{14}-labeled carbon dioxide is produced only from the one carbon of glucose. Similarly, the recovery of C^{14}-labeled oxygen from uniformly labeled glucose in amounts greater than that recovered from glucose labeled only in the one position may be taken as evidence for recombination and recycling of fragments. Additional evidence for this comes from the observations that ribose phosphate has been shown to undergo cleavage and recombination to form a hexose labeled in the one position. This hexose returning to the pentose phosphate pathway, results in production of C^{14}-labeled oxygen. Moreover, the data indicate that pyruvate is transformed only to lactate because the labeled carboxyl position of pyruvate contributes only a very minute amount of C^{14} to carbon dioxide. Because of this recycling of metabolic fragments taking place above pyruvate, uniformly labeled glucose can and must be used to assess the total contribution of the pentose phosphate pathway in the metabolism of glucose.

With these pathways an established background, calculations were made by Murphy (157) of the relative amounts of potential energy derived from each. For each mole of glucose metabolized through the pentose phosphate pathway, 2 moles of TPN is converted to TPNH. When glucose is metabolized through the Embden-Meyerhof pathway, the reaction must be first primed by the utilization of 2 moles of ATP. Each hexose is split into two trioses, and for each triose continuing through the pathway 2 moles of ATP is formed. The net production is, therefore, two high-energy phosphate bonds, as ATP, for each glucose molecule metabolized through the Embden-Meyerhof pathway. In addition to this, consideration must be made of the intermediates of the pentose phosphate pathway which are further metabolized by crossing to and continuing through the Embden-Meyerhof pathway, for these also result in the production of ATP.

As indicated in Table 8.3, 11 per cent of the glucose is metabolized through the pentose phosphate pathway; this contributes, in the form of TPNH, 25 per cent of the available energy. The remaining 75 per cent of the total available energy is in the form of ATP and is contributed from the 89 per cent of the total glucose that is metabolized through the Embden-Meyerhof pathway.

From these calculations it is apparent that the potential energy contribution of the pentose phosphate shunt is considerable and not the insignificant amount formerly proposed. In general these two forms of potential energy are *not* interchangeable. The adult red cell does *not* have a mechanism for converting the energy of TPNH to high-energy phosphate bonds such as occurs in oxidative phosphorylation. Consequently TPNH serves primarily in glutathione reduction and in protecting the cell against various

oxidant compounds. In the normal red cell the concentration of TPNH may be slightly higher than TPN (16.0×10^{-6} moles per liter of whole blood as opposed to 11.6×10^{-6} moles per liter of whole blood). DPNH is also formed but is probably mainly utilized in the transformation of pyruvate to lactic acid. In the normal red cell (as in other tissues) the concentration of DPN exceeds that of DPNH (33.0×10^{-6} moles per liter of whole blood as opposed to 4.6×10^{-6} moles per liter of whole blood; 118).

In addition to ATP other phosphate compounds are generated, but the exact roles and contributions of these compounds to the total picture of the energetics of the erythrocyte are largely unknown. The erythrocyte, for example, contains unusually large amounts of 2, 3-phosphoglyceric acid, and in most situations the concentration rises and falls as does ATP. This compound may therefore serve as a store of energy held in reserve and utilized only when the metabolism of glucose is inadequate. As such it would

TABLE 8.3. Potential energy from glucose metabolism in the erythrocyte

Calculation	Relative amount	
	TPNH	ATP
Average percentage of over-all glucose metabolism	11	89
Units of TPNH produced (PP × 2)	22	
Units of ATP from glucose not metabolized by PP (net EM × 2)		178
Units of ATP from pentose of PP further metabolized by EM (11 × 1.66)		18
Total units of TPNH and ATP	22	196
Equivalent units of potential energy[a] (1 TPNH = 3 high-energy PO_4)	66	196
Percentage of total potential energy	25	75

PP, pentose phosphate pathway; EM, Embden-Meyerhof pathway.

[a] It should be noted that in the adult red cell there is no mechanism available for converting TPNH to high-energy phosphate bonds. These calculations are of theoretic interest only.

Adapted from Murphy, J. R., J. Lab. & Clin. Med. 55: 286, 1960.

be somewhat comparable to the muscle stores of glycogen, a compound not found in normal erythrocytes. It has been shown recently that 2, 3-phosphoglyceric acid has considerable buffering capacity, so that in combination with glutathione and other phosphorylatable compounds the buffering effect of hemoglobin may be equaled in the cell. Because of this, it is hypothesized that this buffering ability may form a pH link with the red cell metabolic processes.

UTILIZATION OF THE POTENTIAL ENERGY. To what purposes and works are these sources of potential energy directed? The energy requirements of certain erythrocyte functions are fairly well delineated; some are poorly adumbrated; some are completely obscure. It is evident that at present the uses to which a considerable proportion of the total available energy is put remain unknown. In the adult erythrocyte the *demonstrated* uses to which the available energy is channeled are (a) maintaining various transmembrane gradients and running the sodium and potassium pump or ferry, (b) maintaining hemoglobin in a functional state capable of reversible deoxygenation, (c) maintaining the normal equilibrium of oxidized and reduced glutathione, (d) maintaining the considerable lipid turnover,* (e) priming the Embden-Meyerhof pathway, and (f) synthesizing DPN and TPN and completing (by the salvage pathway) purine nucleotides. Beyond this only speculation is possible at present relative to such terms as "integrity of the membrane," "metabolic viability," etc. The possibility that some of the energy is utilized for the synthesis of lipids is under active investigation and debate at this time (122–124). There is no direct evidence *for* the synthesis of lipids by the mature erythrocyte, and the available evidence is against this (31, 96, 140, 184, 196, 197).

As discussed in Chapters 1 and 2, specific receptor sites are maintained on the surface of the developing red cell for iron uptake from the plasma transport system. Glucose is required to maintain these sites and for the subsequent transfer of iron into the cell. Only remnants of these functions can be demonstrated in adult erythrocytes.

Beyond the observations that the high-energy terminal phosphates of ATP are in rapid turnover and that ATP functions as a specific coenzyme for many metabolic reactions, a mediator of energy transfer, and a precursor of some coenzymes, there are only a few preliminary observations concerning the metabolism of ATP itself. As measured in rabbits by experiments using labeled adenine (127), labeled ATP declines exponentially and reaches a low value in 55 days, but it is not known whether the decline is due to dilution with unlabeled ATP from (a) exchange with plasma sources (none found), (b) *de novo* synthesis of adenine (none demonstrated), (c) exchange of adenine or (d) adenosine (each can be utilized), or (e) utilization of intermediate compounds leading to adenosine. Studies by Lowy and coworkers (129, 130) have demonstrated that rabbit reticulocytes can synthesize *de novo* the purine nucleotides (adenosine and guanosine triphosphate) but that the adult erythrocytes do not have the complete

---

* The transport of various carbohydrates across the cell membrane is dependent upon specific structural, or steric, arrangements of the sugar molecules; only those with a specific molecular configuration are admitted. Competitive interference has been demonstrated so that evidently only specific loci of the membrane will admit the molecules. This has been referred to as "facilitated diffusion." The result is the same as for simple diffusion, but the mechanism and kinetics are those of a carrier-linked system. Under physiologic conditions, penetration of the red cell by glucose is rapid and as though by simple diffusion, so that energy is not expended. For lipid turnover (184) as with chloride anion penetration and the passive movements of sodium and potassium cations, it can be argued that expenditure of energy must be taking place to maintain the membrane in the proper condition, molecular configuration, or electrochemical state to allow this (109, 109a, 112–115, 166).

pathway for *de novo* purine formation. Adult rabbit erythrocytes can complete the final steps of *nucleotide synthesis* and utilize purines and ribosyl derivatives for nucleoside triphosphate formation. Mature human red cells can utilize preformed purines for nucleotide synthesis but are deficient in their capacity to convert inosinic acid to adenylic acid (121). Löhr et al. (117) have presented some evidence that with aging there is a decline in the concentration of ATP and a concomitant rise in the concentration of ADP, so that a loss of ability to phosphorylate ADP has been attributed to effete red cells.

Sodium and Potassium Transport in Red Cells

There is no question but that energy derived from glucose metabolism is required to drive the sodium and potassium pump (134, 135). The background and evidence for this statement are as follows. Erythrocytes are highly permeable to anions such as Cl^- and HCO_3^- and to H_2O (164). Cl^-, for example, has been shown to cross the cell membrane very rapidly (a half-time exchange of 0.24 second) and to be probably at all times at concentration and thermodynamic equilibrium across the membrane (230). The behavior of cations is, however, extremely different (133). To start with, the concentration of K^+ within the human red cell is 143 mM per liter of cell H_2O as opposed to 5 mM per liter of plasma H_2O; the intracellular concentration of Na^+ is 13.9 mM per liter of cell H_2O as opposed to 154 mM per liter of plasma H_2O. Thus, the total cation concentrations inside and outside the cell are at approximate equality, and with the high concentration of intracellular hemoglobin there are no osmotic pressure differences across the cell membrane. The evident large concentration gradients for Na^+ and K^+ must be maintained by some metabolically active process, since the calculated electrical potential across the cell membrane (no direct measurements have as yet been technically possible, as in muscle fibers or axons) is far too small to account for the observed asymmetric distribution, and evidence is *against* specific ion binding in the cell interior.

Studies employing radioactive tracers of Na^+ and K^+ indicate that both ions are in a constant state of flux across the membrane. It is known that for each ion the transmembrane migration is of two types: (a) active transport across the membrane requiring the expenditure of energy and involving a required exergonic chemical process, and (b) passive movement of diffusion during which the ion follows electrochemical concentration gradients. In general the following description obtains for the mechanism of the Na^+ and K^+ movements. For K^+, *entrance into the cell* involves transport up an electrochemical potential gradient, an active process dependent upon a chemical reaction and the expenditure of energy; *movement out of the cell* (leakage) is by passive diffusion. For Na^+, *transport out of the cell* (*extrusion*) involves transport up an electrochemical potential gradient and is effected by an active process requiring a chemical reaction and the expenditure of energy; *movement into the cell* is by passive diffusion. In addition, it has been demonstrated that the active components of K^+ influx and Na^+ extrusion are linked together and are interdependent (174). Under these circumstances, unlimited increase in intracellular K^+ and unlimited decrease in Na^+ are prevented by passive leakage, which, of course, occurs in both directions. The net movements are *out* for K^+ and *in* for Na^+, and a steady state is reached when the passive components just balance the active movements. Evidence for these statements has been derived from the following observations.

GLUCOSE METABOLISM AND ION TRANSPORT. It was noted that cells stored in the cold in the absence of glucose became progressively depleted of K^+, while the intracellular Na^+ content increased concomitantly. If these altered cells were then incubated at body temperature but still without glucose, no significant change in ionic constitution took place.* However, if the cells were then incubated with glucose, restitution toward a normal ionic composition followed: K^+ was pumped into the cell; Na^+ was pumped out. When altered cells were followed after infusion into a normal recipient similar restitution was found to occur in vivo (64). These ionic shifts were elegantly confirmed by radioactive tracer techniques, and the long-taught principle of the impermeability of red cells to cations had to be abandoned. Moreover, the radioactive techniques showed that the transport against a gradient requiring metabolism of glucose is being constantly effected so that K^+ is moved into and out of the red cell at an estimated hourly rate of 1.6 to 2.1 mM per liter of red blood cells at 37°C and Na^+ at an hourly rate of 3.0 mM per liter of red cells, a half-time exchange of 31 hours. This is a 5×10^5-fold difference from the half-time exchange of the freely permeable Cl^- (230). Thus the movement of Cl^- across the red cell membrane is nearly one million times faster than the movement of Na^+ and K^+ (231).

To determine which stage of glucose metabolism provided the energy to drive the so-called transmembrane pump, various substitution and inhibition studies have been made. Glucose, mannose, and fructose supported the extrusion of Na^+ and the accumulation of K^+ during the incubation of previously cold-stored and depleted red cells; galactose, arabinose, pyruvate, lactate, and disaccharides were not effective. Sodium fluoride and iodoacetic acid inhibited glycolysis, K^+ influx, and Na^+ extrusion, and increased the rate of diffusion of K^+ and Na^+ across the membrane. Metabolic poisons that did not inhibit glycolysis failed to affect the net reaccumulation of K^+ and extrusion of Na^+ (NaCN, 2, 4-dinitrophenol, NaN_3, and CO). Methylene blue (which increases the O_2 consumption of the red blood cells), sulfanilamide, fluoroacetate, and malonate were without net effect on cation transport. Since, as these studies showed, active transport was dependent on glycolysis (Embden-Meyerhof metabolism of glucose), the next question concerned whether the energy is made available as ATP or whether the transport mechanism is tied up with a particular reaction in the Embden-Meyerhof glycolytic sequence. Under various experimental conditions a parallel decline in ATP content and rate of K^+ accumulation was demonstrable (242).

In general, human erythrocytes in which the K^+ concentration was experimentally being increased, maintained, or decreased showed normal, stable, or falling concentrations of ATP, respectively. But variations in other components of the metabolic sequence also occurred (of which 2, 3-diphosphoglyceric acid is of particular interest), so that the evidence was compatible with, but not definitive for, ATP's being the source of potential energy. A similar position had been reached with respect to ionic transport across the membranes of nerves and muscles, where the problem was susceptible of solution because it was technically feasible to inject ATP into an axon or fiber and demonstrate that the quantity of Na^+ extruded was roughly proportional to the amount of ATP injected. This technique was not feasible in erythrocyte study (red blood cells are impermeable, or very slightly permeable, to ATP), but use was made of the previously observed phenomenon of reversible hemolysis (78).

As mentioned above, if cells are he-

---

* For complete accuracy it should be stated that the cells pick up small quantities of K^+ until the existing glucose intermediates capable of yielding energy are depleted.

molyzed by osmotic stress in the presence of radioactive labeled hemoglobin, the radioactive hemoglobin distributes itself freely throughout the cell at the moment of lysis (77). If the tonicity of the surrounding medium is then returned to isotonic values, a functional red blood cell is reconstituted containing labeled hemoglobin. Similarly, if cells depleted of ATP and K^+ are lysed in a cold 10 per cent solution of ATP and then reconstituted by restoration of isotonicity, the cells contain some 4 mg of ATP per milliliter and are then able to accumulate K^+ actively without further substrate. Recent studies report that any reaction that will generate ATP will run the membrane pump: ADP (a phosphate acceptor), PEP (phosphoenolpyruvate), inosine. The accumulated evidence indicates that ATP is the source of potential energy and that upon hydrolysis of ATP energy is liberated and converted to the work of active transport.

MECHANISM OF ION TRANSPORT. That the actual active mechanism of ion transport is mediated by a chemical reaction is made probable by the demonstration of saturation kinetics, a high temperature coefficient of activation, and competition among various ions. Two other observed facts are pertinent here. The active transport of Na^+ and K^+ occurs only at a fixed ratio over a wide range of rates and intra- or extracellular ionic concentrations. Two atoms of K^+ are transported inward for every two Na^+ atoms extruded.* These active transports are then considered to be parts of a single tightly linked system (174). On the basis of studies made on excretory glands, it has been proposed that the carrier substance is phosphatidic acid (79, 80). Although the actual chemical carrier in the red cell membrane is unknown, several means are available to dissociate carrier activity from glycolysis. Various organic solvents (*n*-butanol) can induce the loss of the erythrocytes' capacity to retain K^+ and

exclude Na^+ (84). Lead, which has been shown to attach to lipid-soluble acceptor sites on the red cell membrane, also induces a net loss of ions. Strophanthin and digitonin are known to block active transport with little effect on glucose metabolism (201). These substances probably act directly on the pump, perhaps by displacing K^+ from the carrier sites. Perhaps by steric dislocation of the carrier mechanism from the energizing source, the sickling phenomenon converts a cell behaving normally with respect to ionic equilibrium to one that rapidly changes its ionic composition. Mercury becomes principally bound to sulfhydryl groups of cell stroma and hemoglobin and inhibits the uptake of glucose and induces a loss of K^+ and decrease in osmotic fragility (241).

There is additional evidence from work employing more specific inhibitors that membrane sulfhydryl groups are involved in ion transport, erythrocyte shape and viability (88a, 212). Employing *n*-ethylmaleimide (NEM), a sulfhydryl inhibitor *freely permeable* throughout the cell, it was shown that the agent combined with intracellular glutathione stifled glycolysis, disrupted the cation gradient across the membrane, with a loss of K^+ and gain of Na^+ and H_2O that ultimately led to swelling of the cells, spherocytosis, and hemolysis. Although glycolysis was inhibited and ATP levels must have declined, the rate of K^+ loss indicated a membrane effect over and above the effect on glucose metabolism. Employing *p*-mercuribenzoate (PCB), a *nonpermeable* sulfhydryl inhibitor, the cation gradients were similarly disrupted by a loss of K^+ and gain of Na^+ and H_2O that ultimately led to swelling of the cells, spherocytosis, and hemolysis. In this instance, however, these effects were produced without changes in intracellular

---

* Various ratios are reported by different workers. The variations appear to be due to differences of experimental conditions: pH, partial pressure of oxygen, etc.

glutathione or glycolysis. The mechanism whereby membrane sulfhydryl inhibition impairs cation gradients is unknown.

Recently Post et al. have prepared an (thirty-one-fold purified) insoluble ATP-cleaving enzyme system from human red cells that they propose as a *participant* in the transmembrane movement of Na^+ and K^+ (175, 176). Considerable support for this proposal comes from an unusual constellation of characteristics common to it and the transport system: (a) the ATP-ase is located in the membrane, (b) it uses ATP in contrast to ITP (inosine triphosphate), (c) it requires Na^+ and K^+ together for activation, (d) the concentration for half-maximum activation by K^+ in the presence of Na^+ is 3 mM for the enzyme and 2.1 mM for the transport, (e) the concentration for half-maximum activation by Na^+ in the presence of K^+ is 24 mM for the enzyme and 20 mM for the transport, (f) there is competitive inhibition of K^+ activation by high concentration of Na^+, (g) the concentration for half-maximum inhibition by ouabain in the presence of Na^+ and K^+ is 10^{-7} M for the enzyme and 3 to 7 $\times$ 10^{-8} M for the transport, (h) ammonium ions substitute for K^+ but not for Na^+, (i) concentration for half-maximum activation by ammonium in presence of Na^+ is 8 mM for the enzyme and 7 to 16 mM for the transport.

In addition to providing evidence for the participation of the ATP-cleaving enzyme in the transmembrane movement of Na^+ and K^+, a further implication is that Na^+ and K^+ are more than simple co-factors. As substrates for transport they should be moved from one part of the system to another at a rate dependent upon dephosphorylation of ATP. The reciprocal competitive inhibition between Na^+ and K^+ means that on each side of the membrane the linked transport system must free itself of one transported substance before it can take on the other for transport.

MEMBRANE PORES. Aside from the observations made by electron microscopy, the evidence for the existence of membrane pores connecting the interior with the exterior of the cell is almost entirely inferential. Measurements made on the rate of entry of H_2O into erythrocytes under different circumstances* indicate the likely existence of H_2O-filled channels and provide a means for calculating the pore size (65, 219–221). For human erythrocytes, the pores are estimated to have a radius of 3.5 Å. It is of interest that the values for the radii of hydrated Na^+, K^+, and Cl^- are smaller than this (2.56 Å, 1.98 Å, and 1.93 Å, respectively) so that passage through the pores is possible but tight. The existence of a low-density assemblage of positive charges within the channel would provide a potent barrier to the passage of Na^+ and K^+ as demanded by the experimental data. Since the electrophoretic mobility of Cl^- equals that of Na^+ or K^+, and the erythrocyte membrane is very nearly freely permeable to Cl^-, a barrier must exist by which the movement of Na^+ into and K^+ out of the cell is impeded. This could most readily be effected by the existence of positive charges within the channel. Solomon believes that Ca^{++} within the membrane may be the responsible cation.

A 10 per cent increase in cell volume induced by osmotic swelling decreases the rate of H_2O diffusion by some 28 per cent. Presumably the alterations in the hydration of the membrane result in membrane swelling and compression of the pores. But there is only a very small effect on the rate of K^+ exchange. This dissociation of effects probably indicates that the pores responsible for the transport of H_2O are different from those used for K^+.

* Employing rabbit erythrocytes, Olmstead (165) has shown that in hypertonic and hypotonic solutions equidistant from intracellular osmolarity, the influx of H_2O exceeds the efflux and that alterations can be induced by changes in temperature, pH, and O_2 uptake of the cell.

According to present thinking the anatomic routes whereby H_2O and K^+ and Na^+ move across the cell membrane are pores or channels penetrating the membranes. These are about 3.5 Å in radius; some are filled with H_2O and others contain a certain assemblage of positive charges that form a barrier to passage of K^+ and Na^+. K^+ enters by a different route than does H_2O and exits by a pathway different from its entrance.

SUMMARY. Thus the red cell membrane is constructed in such a fashion that K^+ efflux and Na^+ influx occur along an electrochemical gradient by relatively slow passive diffusion through aqueous pores containing a high concentration of fixed positive charges. The membrane allows the rapid passage of Cl^-, HCO_3^-, and other small anions nearly one million times as rapidly as the cation diffusion. K^+ influx and Na^+ efflux are mediated almost entirely by a specific chemical reaction and carrier, or pump, that is driven by the energy liberated through the hydrolysis of ATP. In terms of the total energetics of the cell, thermodynamic calculations indicate that to run the pump responsible for the cation fluxes only 7 per cent (218) to 30 per cent (13) of the energy released by hydrolysis of available ATP is required. Considerable potential energy in the form of ATP remains available to the cell for other use.

Preservation of Red Cells

The erythrocyte's osmotic fragility and to some extent its mechanical fragility are dependent upon the ionic composition of the cell. Although the exact relation between these in vitro measurements and the cell's ability to survive in vivo is unknown, there is some correlation between observed abnormalities of osmotic and mechanical fragility and shortened survival time. For these and other more general reasons the question of the relation between the in vivo survival ability of an erythrocyte and its metabolism—specifically glucose metabolism—has been extensively investigated. The prime mover of the studies has actually been the need for methods of blood preservation that allow optimal survival after transfusion of the stored erythrocytes.

On empiric grounds it was long ago determined that ACD solution* employed as an anticoagulant and preservative resulted in an in vivo erythrocyte survival time significantly better than or equal to that obtained with other anticoagulants or preservatives tested (8). Since the cells were stored at 4°C, on the basis of the above-described metabolic changes, ionic shifts involving loss of potassium and increase of sodium would be predicted and were found to occur. There also occurred significant changes in osmotic and mechanical fragility, decreased incorporation of labeled acetate into stroma (3), decreased ability to utilize glucose, a shift in the oxygen dissociation curve, and a decreased post-transfusion survival ability correlated with duration of storage (214). Two approaches then seemed possible in the field of blood preservation.

The first was to arrest cell metabolism by freezing and preservation at very low temperatures. This has indeed turned out to be feasible, and cell preservation at −80°C or below can be carried out for prolonged periods (months or even years) without evidence of deterioration or decreased post-transfusion survival time (153, 224, 225). However, the processing of the blood and its reconstitution for use is presently a formidable undertaking. The high cost of the equipment needed makes the process impractical in all but the few research centers where it is currently employed.

The second approach was to attempt control of the metabolic changes that occur at 4°C in the ACD solution or to correct any induced deleterious alterations

* Acid citrate, sodium citrate, and dextrose.

(52). The original studies indicated that the metabolic changes were not primarily due to factors external to the erythrocyte (composition of ACD; use of fresh, aged, or dialyzed plasma; condition of leukocytes, platelets, stroma; gas phase; etc.) but were due to an intrinsic derangement. Measurements of the phosphate partition indicated marked decline in organic phosphate and increase in inorganic phosphate, with total phosphate somewhat decreased. This induced "storage lesion" could be partially repaired by transfusion. As the cell circulates in the normal environment, its ability to utilize glucose is improved, the phosphate partition returns to normal, its osmotic and mechanical fragility return toward normal, and its oxygen dissociation curve returns to normal.

Although circumstantial, the accumulated evidence indicates beyond reasonable doubt that the post-transfusion viability of the normal human red cell is dependent upon its continual metabolism of glucose during storage at above-freezing temperatures. Consequently the *intrinsic* derangement is in the main secondary to alterations in glucose metabolism. At 4 to 5°C the cellular utilization of glucose is greatly reduced but usually sufficient to exhaust unaugmented blood glucose in about a week. At this time cell viability falls precipitously. A major advance was made in blood preservation when it was found that the addition of glucose would extend the cell's life. It was also found that storage at pH of about 7.1 resulted in better survival than storage at higher pH. The ACD preparation presently used supports a minimum red cell survival of 85 per cent after 2 weeks, and 70 per cent after 3 weeks, of storage at 4°C. After this period of storage the post-transfusion survival is so limited that the blood is largely unsuitable for clinical use. A striking feature of red cell chemistry during storage after the optimum period is the rapid and extensive breakdown of the phosphorylated intermediates ordinarily replenished by glucose metabolism; most of the organic phosphate is converted to inorganic phosphate.

By various studies it was determined that the in vitro addition of purine nucleosides (52, 159), such as adenosine, inosine, guanosine, could return the phosphate pattern to normal and extend the preservation of red cells stored in ACD solution (from 21 to 28 days). It was originally thought that the nucleoside phosphorylase, known to be present on the surface of erythrocytes, released a phosphorylated ribose that, penetrating the cell, was used as enzyme substrate (Figure 8.4). Especially remarkable was the finding that after a period of storage in ACD when almost all the water-soluble organic phosphate had disappeared, the addition of a nucleoside followed by incubation at 37°C led to a large resynthesis of organic phosphates (210, 211). Because it was the least toxic of the nucleosides, inosine had been selected for extensive study. However, after the initial studies, marked inconsistencies in the post-transfusion viability results raised questions concerning variability in the composition of the inosine preparations employed and other possible effects of the purine nucleosides. Some workers (159) reported that a combination of adenine and inosine at the beginning of storage resulted in better red cell shape, osmotic resistance, ATP content, and post-transfusion viability than with either alone or none. These inconsistencies and peculiarities made it evident that the original hypothesis concerning release and utilization of phosorylated ribose was inadequate. Subsequent observations demonstrated a net synthesis of adenine nucleotide after incubation of nucleotide-depleted cells with adenosine or with inosine (244). Shafer and Bartlett (211a) have demonstrated that after 6 weeks of ACD storage inosine is capable of regenerating ATP. However, after 18 weeks of ACD storage inosine will not regenerate ATP, but either adenine plus inosine or adenosine alone will allow ATP regeneration.

Recent studies by Simon (215) have demonstrated that supplementation of the ACD preservative with small amounts of adenine alone results in slightly higher intracellular ATP levels, better glycolytic capacity, and viability of greater than 70 per cent of human cells after storage for 5 weeks. While it is known that human red cells can incorporate adenine into adenine nucleotides (244), it is not known whether this mechanism is the one responsible for the effects observed.

Although the effects of adenine on viability were considerably greater than on ATP, from these studies it would appear that cell deterioration begins at the time the ATP fall-off exceeds production. At this point glucose utilization also decreases and an even more rapid decrease in ATP results. At the present time it has not proved feasible to make practical use of these interesting findings in blood-banking and blood-preservation programs. But again the implications of the relations between the ability of the cell to maintain "normal concentrations" of compounds possessing potential energy and the maintenance of viability and cellular integrity are most intriguing and suggestive.

However, it should be pointed out that the storage lesion is basically different from the alterations associated with in vivo aging. The changes of in vitro aging are apparently due to exhaustion of substrates and accumulation of metabolic products; the changes of in vivo aging are apparently due to the instability of certain proteins that are necessary for critical enzymatic reactions.

METHEMOGLOBINEMIA

Another area of erythrocyte metabolism in which glucose utilization is demon-strably involved concerns the mechanisms required to maintain hemoglobin in its normal functional state: specifically, the reduction of methemoglobin to a hemoglobin capable of reversible oxygenation. Methemoglobin (containing ferric protoporphyrin 9) is continuously being formed in the erythrocyte and as such cannot take part in oxygen transport and delivery. As stated previously, the prime function of the erythrocyte is to feed oxygen to all tissues. For this to occur, very precise and delicate mechanisms are set up and maintained in the red cell, so that (a) the formation of methemoglobin is kept at a minimum and (b) any that is formed is reduced to the functional state required for reversible oxygenation (191). Oxidant compounds capable of changing hemoglobin to the oxidized, or met-, form (especially hydrogen peroxide) may be destroyed by glutathione peroxidase and catalase;[*] various reducing substances such as ascorbic acid, glutathione, and other sulfhydryl compounds are present in the cell for direct action on oxidants but probably only function with failure of enzyme systems (150, 151); mechanisms are normally present that are capable of reducing methemoglobin as it is formed by means of methemoglobin reductase(s). Of the above mechanisms the most important are dependent upon glucose metabolism for the supply of DPNH or TPNH. Abnormalities in these systems either through heritable defects (hereditary methemoglobinemia) resulting from an intraerythrocyte enzymatic defect or an abnormal hemoglobin (hemoglobin M), or induced by chemical agents (acquired methemoglobinemia), may result in symptomatic and sometimes fatal disease.

[*] However, since individuals with hypocatalasemia and acatalasemia do not have increased amounts of methemoglobin and the activity of glutathione peroxidase does not appear very great, these mechanisms are of questionable importance (227).

Hereditary Methemoglobinemia

Hereditary methemoglobinemia* is a rare condition of which approximately one hundred cases have been reported in the literature. It is characterized by cyanosis, a variable amount of hemoglobin (usually about 30 per cent) in the oxidized form, typically a compensatory polycythemia, and no other pathologic findings. The condition is present at birth and persists for life. In only approximately fifteen families have multiple members been shown to have the disease; however, in some of these families the condition has been demonstrated in three or more generations. The incidence is slightly greater in males than females. Available evidence indicates that the condition is inherited according to the pattern of a recessive trait, with homozygosity required for full expression. Symptoms are usually mild and at most consist of moderate fatigability, vertigo, headache, cramps or discomfort in major muscle groups, slight exertional dyspnea, and reduced tolerance of exercise. Clubbing of the fingers is *not* present. Life expectancy is apparently normal. However, biochemical evidence for a physiologic disadvantage is the elevated lactate levels following exercise.

This disorder is another example of an inborn error of metabolism. The defect is located in the patient's red cells, an intracorpuscular abnormality (45, 51). If cells from a patient are incubated in normal plasma for 24 hours and normal cells are similarly incubated in the patient's plasma, methemoglobin is not significantly reduced in the patient's cells or produced in the normal cells. If normal erythrocytes are transfused into a patient, methemoglobin does not appear in appreciable amounts in these cells. If a patient is suitably treated (see below) to convert nearly all the hemoglobin from oxidized to reduced form, and his cells are then infused into a normal recipient,

it can be shown that methemoglobin accumulates in the abnormal cells at the rate of approximately 3 per cent per day. Methemoglobin does not appear in the recipient's normal cells in abnormal amounts. The transformation of hemoglobin to methemoglobin at the rate of 3 per cent per day in the normal recipient is the same as the reappearance rate of methemoglobin in the patient following treatment. It is, therefore, most improbable that any abnormal factors external to the red cell influence the formation of methemoglobin. An instrinsic cellular defect is responsible for the disease.

It has long been known that a *solution* of hemoglobin obtained by lysing normal red cells shows a progressive increase in methemoglobin concentration until at 5 days or more (depending on pH, temperature, etc.) all the hemoglobin has been converted to the oxidized form. *Intact* red cells possess a mechanism which prevents this from occurring and maintains the hemoglobin in the reduced state. If sodium nitrite is added to the normal cells as an oxidizing agent, methemoglobin is formed and then progressively reduced to normal in the following 12 hours. Cells from a patient with hereditary methemoglobinemia have no ability to reconvert methemoglobin to normal. In the in vivo counterpart of this experiment sodium nitrite was administered intravenously to a normal individual and a patient (45). In both, approximately the same amount of methemoglobin was formed. In the normal person the methemoglobin was reduced; there was no reduction in the patient. These findings indicate that the intrinsi-

* This is, of course, a misnomer: "hemoglobinemia" is used to indicate the presence of extracellular hemoglobin circulating in the plasma, and methemoglobinemia should accordingly indicate the presence of extracorpuscular pigment. In the disease referred to here, the hemoglobin remains intracorpuscular while in the oxidized form. Familial methemoglobinemia, idiopathic methemoglobinemia, congenital methemoglobinemia, Codounis' disease, and hereditary methemoglobinemic cyanosis are synonyms.

cally abnormal cell of hereditary methemoglobinemia is incapable of reducing methemoglobin back to its properly functioning state.

Ascorbic acid and glutathione are substances present in erythrocytes and plasma capable of reducing methemoglobin. In vitro studies show that sufficient quantities of ascorbic acid can effectively reduce the methemoglobin of patients' cells. Similarly the administration of vitamin C in large doses reduces, temporarily, the percentage of methemoglobin in vivo in patients. Assay of cells and plasma from patients indicates low values for, but not depletion of, these compounds.* They probably function only as a second line of defense during failure of the normal reduction system.

As mentioned above, if normal intact cells are incubated in suitable media, there is no change in the (normal) low methemoglobin content of the cells. However, if the cells are incubated in a media devoid of glucose, abnormal quantities of methemoglobin are formed after the intracellular supply of glucose has been exhausted. If the glucose is replenished, normal cells are again capable of converting the previously formed methemoglobin back to reduced hemoglobin; glucose is utilized and lactate appears. This effect can be inhibited with iodoacetate.

It is evident that the methemoglobin reduction system depends on the metabolism of glucose for proper function. Various studies, many repeated in different laboratories, have been unable to show any defect in glucose metabolism of cells from patients with hereditary methemoglobinemia. These studies involved, among other things, measurements of oxygen consumption, glucose utilization, lactate production, phosphorylation, phosphate partitions, hydrolyzable phosphate as a measure of ATP content, and direct assay of the activity of various intermediates involved in the sequences of glucose metabolism in both the Embden-Meyer-

hof and the pentose phosphate pathways (93). Since hydrogen peroxide, a potent oxidizing agent in biologic systems, may be produced intracellularly and then decomposed by catalase, it was thought that a deficiency in catalase might be responsible for excessive formation of methemoglobin. However, catalase content is normal in the abnormal cells.

It is evident then that in the cells of a patient with hereditary methemoglobinemia an essential link is defective that in the normal joins glucose metabolism with the reduction of methemoglobin. Since this type of reduction (ferric to ferrous) must involve electron transfer, the intracellular abnormality is resolved into one of defective electron transport from a source of potential energy produced through glucose metabolism to methemoglobin.

Methylene blue is a compound known to act as an electron-transporting substance in various redox systems. It has been demonstrated that the addition of methylene blue causes an approximately tenfold increase in erythrocyte oxygen consumption (240). Such an increase also occurs in cells from a patient with hereditary methemoglobinemia but does not occur in either normal or abnormal cells in the absence of glucose. Methylene blue oxidizes the TPNH produced by the pentose phosphate pathway. This increase in TPNH oxidation results in increased metabolism through the pentose phosphate pathway (five- to ninefold increase). This is effected by an increase in total glucose utilization and an enhancement of recycling of intermediates (25).

When blood from a patient with methemoglobinemia is treated with methylene blue in the presence of glucose, complete reconversion of the methemoglobin to active hemoglobin rapidly occurs. The action of methylene blue is most likely due

* However, see p. 225 for a type of methemoglobinemia associated with defective synthesis of glutathione and reduced content.

to a combination of enhanced glucose utilization (oxygen consumption) and a coupling of the cell's potential energy source with methemoglobin by substituting for the defective link in electron transport (25).

There has been much interest in the nature of the defective compound and the source of energy. These points at present are not settled and confirmed. Recently two different "methemoglobin reductases" have been described with different properties, one optimally dependent upon TPNH for enzymatic function, the other more specifically dependent upon DPNH (Figure 8.5).

METHEMOGLOBIN REDUCTASE—TPNH DEPENDENT. The methemoglobin reductase described by Huennekens et al. (82, 83) is a red heme-containing pigment (of molecular weight 185,000) that can be

oxidized, reduced, or oxygenated. It is apparently similar to a TPNH-dependent methemoglobin reductase that had been isolated and characterized by Kiese et al. (103, 106). Huennekens found that the purified enzyme is specific for TPNH; only 20 per cent as much activity is observed with DPNH. As terminal electron acceptors either oxygen, methylene blue, or cytochrome C can be used. This substance requires methylene blue or an unknown obligate intermediary when functioning as methemoglobin reductase. Therefore, in this system the naturally occurring cofactor substituted for by methylene blue is known.

METHEMOGLOBIN REDUCTASE—DPNH DEPENDENT. In 1947 and 1949 Gibson et al. (27, 58–60) proposed that hereditary methemoglobinemia resulted from a deficiency of diaphorase I. No direct evi-

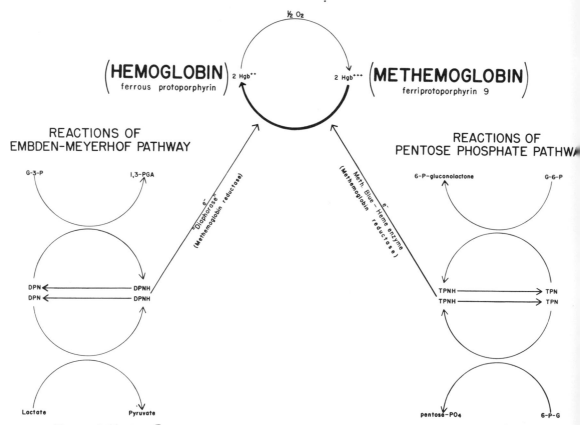

FIGURE 8.5.   Mechanisms available in the red cell for effecting reduction of methemoglobin to hemoglobin. Abbreviations for the various compounds are same as in Figure 8.4

dence for this was available until the recent work by Scott et al. (204–208), who have isolated a diaphorase-like enzyme from normal cells that catalyzes the reduction of methemoglobin by DPNH. Methylene blue is *not* required for its activity. This erythrocyte diaphorase is lacking in the red cells of patients with hereditary methemoglobinemia. Parents of methemoglobinemic children have less diaphorase activity than normal, and the inheritance of methemoglobinemia is consistent with a recessive pattern, with homozygosity required for full expression. Scott's studies have apparently been confined to hereditary methemoglobinemia in Eskimos of Alaska, in whom there is an unusually high incidence and in whom the disease takes some unusual forms. The incidence is to all appearances disproportionately high in the children as opposed to adults, and the amount of methemoglobin appears to decrease with age. These observed peculiarities might be due to dietary influences, but other possibilities cannot be excluded. It has been reported (102, 145, 146, 190) that the erythrocytes of neonates* are unusually susceptible to the formation of methemoglobin, there is a gradual decrease in the *susceptibility* of erythrocytes to the induction of methemoglobin by sodium nitrite solutions during childhood, and there is a rapid increase in resistance at puberty.

DEFICIENT GLUTATHIONE SYNTHESIS. Townes and Lovell (233) have recently reported a new variant of methemoglobinemia exhibiting dominant inheritance, decreased capacity of the cells to reduce methemoglobin, but *no* deficiency of either the TPNH- or DPNH-dependent methemoglobin reductase. The significant biochemical abnormality of the various enzymes and metabolic functions tested (234) appeared to be a decreased glutathione content. The primary abnormality is postulated as a defect in glutathione synthesis. This deficiency is thought to

result in impaired triose phosphate dehydrogenase activity and inadequate formation of the DPNH required for the methemoglobin reductase.

Determination of the oxygen dissociation curve in various patients with methemoglobinemia has yielded normal results in some and abnormal results in others. When abnormal, the curve is shifted to the region where impaired delivery of oxygen is expected (41). Moreover, appropriate treatment (see below) is reported in most patients to return the abnormal absorption curve to normal, but in others there is apparently no shift.

Clinical management of patients with hereditary methemoglobinemia is effected by oral administration of methylene blue or high doses of ascorbic acid (22, 51). Since treatment is usually given for cosmetic purposes but also for the relief of the minor complaints previously mentioned, it should be borne in mind that methylene blue is not innocuous and may produce a hemolytic anemia if improperly administered (66). The inconstantly seen mild compensatory polycythemia disappears with continued adequate therapy.

A positive diagnosis of hereditary methemoglobinemia can now be made only by identification of the compound by spectrophotometry (49, 56). It has a characteristic spectrum with a prominent absorption band at 630 mμ. This absorption band is abolished by cyanide, a phenomenon that certifies the identity of the compound and differentiates it from sulfhemoglobin. The necessity for this biochemical identification of the compound is made evident from the following considerations.

Cyanosis may be due to many different causes; the presence of 4 to 5 Gm of reduced hemoglobin per 100 ml of blood is required to produce a clinically recog-

---

* This is due in part to the presence of fetal hemoglobin which is more easily oxidized than adult hemoglobin (111).

nizable degree of cyanosis. Since this amount is most frequently seen in patients with congenital or acquired heart defects or pulmonary disorders, it is not unusual for patients whose cyanosis results from a pigment abnormality to have been followed under mistaken diagnosis for many years.* Methemoglobin in a concentration of 1.5 Gm per 100 ml results in evident cyanosis. Since patients frequently have 30 per cent of their total pigment in this form, it is not unusual for them to have 5 Gm or more of methemoglobin per 100 ml of blood and present a startling and alarming clinical cyanosis. Sulfhemoglobin in concentrations of less than 0.5 Gm per 100 ml results in obvious cyanosis. A concentration of 30 per cent of the total hemoglobin as hemoglobin M is reported to be associated with dramatic cyanosis so it seems likely that much less than that amount is clinically detectable.

Hemoglobin M Disease

In 1948 Hörlein and Weber (81) demonstrated the presence of a methemoglobin with unusual spectral characteristics in the blood of a family showing dominant transmission of a cyanotic condition. By splitting the hemoglobin into its heme and globin components and recombining them with complementary derivatives of normal blood, it was demonstrated that the anomalous spectral behavior was attributable to an abnormality of the globin. Combination of normal heme with abnormal globin resulted in a compound with spectral properties comparable to the original hemolysate from the patient. A normal spectral curve was obtained from the compound obtained from the reciprocal interchanges. This finding, made about a year before Pauling's publication of the abnormal electrophoretic pattern of sickle hemoglobin, was actually the first demonstration that a disease resulted from a hemoglobin of an abnormal molecular species.

Localization of the abnormality in the globin is consistent with current opinion regarding the biochemical defect in abnormal hemoglobins. It has more recently been reported that the abnormal pigment can be demonstrated by electrophoresis. The red cells of patients with the abnormality contain a mixture of normal adult hemoglobin (70 per cent) and hemoglobin M (30 per cent). By means of the "fingerprint" technique, comparison of trypsin-digested fragments indicates the presence of amino acid alterations in at least one fragment. It has been hypothesized that the mutation represented by one type of hemoglobin M (there is evidence of a multiplicity of M types†) results in the substitution of a tyrosine residue for the amino acid occurring at this point in the normal sequence (57). Abnormal properties of the hemoglobin molecule with respect to oxygen need not therefore result solely from changes in the heme group as formerly presumed but may be attributable to an abnormal amino acid sequence in the globin. It is thought that the abnormal amino acid residue in the globin may be responsible for the formation of an active group in the globin portion of the molecule which

* A patient has been reported with intense but asymptomatic cyanosis associated with a hemoglobin characterized by a reduced affinity for oxygen and an altered (probably absent) heme-heme facilitation (185). The lack of symptoms is attributable to the observation that the same 35 per cent of the hemoglobin's oxygen capacity as in the normal was given up to the tissues, which had the usual partial pressure of oxygen of 35 mm Hg. (Normal oxygen saturation drops from 95 to 60 per cent; in the patient the saturation dropped from 60 to 25 per cent.) The hemoglobin was shown to have an abnormal electrophoretic migration and abnormal spectra as alkaline and acid methemoglobin. It may therefore belong to the hemoglobin abnormalities designated hemoglobin M (185).

† The Boston type, hemoglobin M_B, has peaks of absorption at 605 and 495; the Milwaukee type, hemoglobin M_M, has peaks at 625 and 495 and cyanide removes the 625 peak; the Saskatoon type, hemoglobin M_S, has different intensities of maximal absorption at 605 and 495 than M_B. By similar criteria $M_{Chicago}$, $M_{Leipzig}$, and M_{Iwate} have also been characterized (19, 54–56, 98, 170).

forms an internal complex with the ferric iron. It must be recognized that these patients do not have "normal methemoglobin" in their blood, that the usual test for methemoglobin, abolition of the 630 mμ absorption peak with cyanide, may be negative, and that only a partial reduction at best is effected by either in vitro or in vivo treatment with ascorbic acid or methylene blue.

It is of interest to note that a normal methemoglobin-reducing system has been demonstrated in the red cells of these patients by the induction of "normal methemoglobin" and subsequent reappearance of reduced hemoglobin. Apparently the abnormally reactive heme groups cannot be reduced to the ferrous state by the normal methemoglobin reductase system(s). Consistent with present knowledge of genetic mechanisms and the anatomy of the hemoglobin molecule, it would be expected that only two of the four polypeptide chains would be abnormal and consequently not all the heme groups would be abnormally reactive. By means of the spectral changes following the reaction of the methemoglobin of hemoglobin M with cyanide, the presence of normally reactive heme groups is demonstrable in addition to the abnormally reactive heme groups of the same molecule.*

The red cell of a patient with hemoglobin M disease contains therefore normal and abnormal hemoglobins. The normal methemoglobin-reducing system is present, as evidenced by the fact that the normal hemoglobin is in the reduced, functional state. In the hemoglobin M, some of the heme groups are normally reactive while some are abnormally reactive, and in these latter the iron is maintained in the trivalent state because of the altered polypeptide chain.

Acquired Methemoglobinemia

Acquired, or secondary, methemoglobinemia results when the rate of formation of methemoglobin exceeds the rate of reduction because of the action of certain chemical agents (Table 8.4). Nitrites, sulfonamides, and aniline derivatives have been the most frequently incriminated drugs.

Through an unknown chemical interaction, nitrites produce methemoglobin at a rapid rate in a nearly stoichiometric reaction. Although usually absorbed from the gastrointestinal tract (nitrates may be reduced by bacterial action), nitrites may be inhaled by chemical workers, arc welders, cardiac patients receiving amyl nitrite, etc. Numerous instances and some fatalities (infants) have been reported from the ingestion of well water high in nitrates (32), use of bismuth subnitrate as an antidiarrheal agent, and the intake of food high in nitrates (192). Some of the sulfonamide drugs formerly employed (sulfanilamide, Prontosil, sulfathiazole, and sulfapyridine) frequently produced both methemoglobin and sulfhemoglobin. Aniline derivatives are probably the most potent formers of methemoglobin; inhalation of fumes or dust, oral ingestion or dermal absorption of any of the aromatic nitro- or amino-compounds may result in profound pigment changes. They probably work through the formation of breakdown products. Kiese and Waller (104) noted, for example, that nitrosobenzene must be reduced to phenylhydroxylamine by TPNH and methemoglobin reductase before the compound can oxidize hemoglobin to methemoglobin. Although most frequently seen because of industrial accidents or misuse, instances have also been described as caused by exposure to diaper labels or freshly dyed blankets or

---

* A group of cyanotic patients has been described who had no abnormal amounts of oxidized pigment in the circulating blood. After in vitro oxidation, however, a fraction of the methemoglobin was found to have an abnormal spectral absorption curve with characteristics similar to those of hemoglobin M (213). It was assumed that some of the hemoglobin was incapable of reversible oxygenation and was designated hemoglobin M_1.

Table 8.4.   Compounds capable of producing methemo-globinemia

Direct oxidants	Indirect oxidants

Nitrites
  Preserved meat
  Therapeutic uses
	Aryl-, amino-, and nitro-
	  compounds

Nitrates (reduced to nitrite
  by bacteria in gut)
  Well water
  Bismuth subnitrate
  Ammonium nitrate
	Aniline
	Acetanilid
	Acetophenetidin
	Nitrobenzene
	Nitrotoluenes

Chlorates Therapeutic uses	Sulfonamides
Quinones Naphthaquinones	
Methylene blue High dose	
Hydrogen peroxide In absence of catalase	

From Prankerd, T. A. J., The Red Cell, Blackwell, Oxford, 1961.

shoes, or ingestion of colored crayons. Acetophenetidin and acetanilid are two of the most commonly used compounds that may produce methemoglobinemia.

The rapidity with which a drug induces methemoglobin and the persistence of methemoglobin are, of course, dependent upon the drug's metabolism and excretion. These are most important considerations in relation to treatment (22). The symptoms may vary from pure alarm at having noted cyanosis, to headache, gastrointestinal disturbances, coma, and death. In general, patients with methemoglobin values less than 30 per cent of total pigment *and not rising* do not need treatment except discontinuance of the causative agent. The normal intraerythrocytic reducing mechanism will return the hemoglobin to its functional state within 5 to 12 hours. Patients with methemoglobinemia above 30 per cent of total pigment should be carefully followed, and repeated methemoglobin determinations should be made as indicated by the nature of the intoxicating material and clinical evaluation. The intravenous administration of dextrose is advocated by some. Most experienced workers agree that the use of methylene blue is not justified unless demanded by clinical status, type of intoxicating agent, or extremely high values of methemoglobinemia (i.e., over 60 per cent). Except under unusual circumstances reconversion by normal mechanisms takes place by 15 to 20 hours. Ascorbic acid is not of value in secondary methemoglobinemia because of the slow reconversion action. In extreme circumstances, exchange transfusions have been employed in conjunction with methylene blue administration (22, 132, 136, 158).

Sulfhemoglobinemia

Sulfhemoglobinemia is of importance mainly in that it must be ruled in or out when pigmentary causes of cyanosis are considered (51, 60, 148, 149, 214). The chemical nature of the compound is not known with certainty; the sulfur may substitute for one of the nitrogen atoms in the pyrrole ring or between the iron and its polypeptide bond (148). It is identified by an absorption band at 618 mμ, which is unaffected by cyanide but dispersed with hydrogen peroxide. In the red cell there is no mechanism for converting this compound to normal hemoglobin; it persists for the life of the erythrocyte (97), which may be somewhat shortened (86). Clinically it is seen in association with the habitual ingestion of an oxidizing drug (Bromo Seltzer, acetanilid, acetopheditin, etc.) and not infrequently is accompanied by chronic constipation (26).

Methemoglobin and Red Cell Destruction

It is pertinent here to point out that many drugs implicated in the induction of methemoglobinemia and sulfhemoglobinemia, and the methylene blue employed in the treatment of methemoglobinemia, may induce red cell damage of variable degrees (20). Some drugs, nitrites for example, produce methemoglobin almost exclusively, although Heinz bodies have been noted; phenylhydrazine acts in vivo to produce mainly red cell destruction. Some, such as potassium chlorate and arsine, produce massive hemolysis *and* methemoglobinemia. Some drugs which in most patients produce only methemo-globinemia will, on occasion, produce extensive cell destruction (48). In Chapter 9, in the section dealing with drug-induced hemolytic anemia, it is pointed out that cell destruction may be effected by several different mechanisms: oxidant compounds that produce abnormal osmotic fragility and some degree of methemoglobinemia; drug-antibody-complement mechanisms that produce alterations in osmotic fragility but no methemoglobinemia; agents that usually produce hemolysis with no change in osmotic fragility or methemoglobinemia in patients with enzyme-defective red cells (primaquine-sensitive type); and similar agents that may on occasion produce hemolytic anemia, methemoglobinemia, and alterations in osmotic fragility in patients with otherwise demonstrably normal red cells. The available evidence indicates that the presence of methemoglobin (or sulfhemoglobin) is not *necessarily* accompanied by changes in osmotic fragility or shortening of the erythrocyte life span (85; Figure 8.6). A normal erythrocyte survival time for the method employed has been demonstrated for the cells of patients with hereditary methemoglobinemia whether the cells are circulating in the patient or a normal recipient. It is of considerable in-

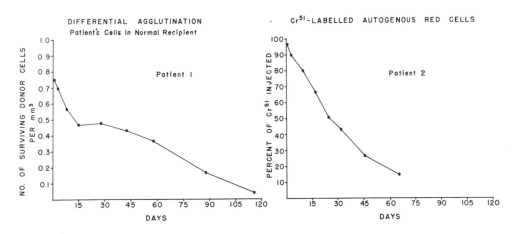

FIGURE 8.6. Survival of erythrocytes of patients with hereditary methemoglobinemia. (Drawn from data supplied by R. W. Weisman, Jr.)

terest that all these reactions are, under some conditions, demonstrably associated with glucose metabolism and cellular energetics: (a) normal osmotic fragility is dependent upon preservation of ionic equilibrium and/or preservation of the "integrity of cell membrane," (b) maintenance of hemoglobin in the functional state by reduction from methemoglobin, and (c) maintenance of the normal equilibrium of glutathione between the oxidized and reduced form by an enzyme dependent upon TPNH. (This equilibrium and its significance will be considered in Chapter 9.) The interrelations are obscure, but it appears evident that for the preservation of normal erythrocyte function, integrity, and survival, production of the potential energy of the cell through glucose metabolism and the conversion of that energy into actual work must proceed without aberration.

Bibliographic references for Chapter 8 begin on page 415.

PART V] THE RED CELL: DESTRUCTION

CHAPTER NINE

RED CELL DESTRUCTION AND THE HEMOLYTIC DISORDERS*

RED CELL DESTRUCTION

The essential abnormality common to all hemolytic disorders is a reduction of the erythrocyte survival time. For one reason or another the red cell cannot live out its normal life span and is prematurely destroyed in the body. The life span, or survival time (T), of the normal erythrocyte is now accurately known. Many different methods have been employed to determine the normal red cell survival time (20); † all yield essentially the same result, 100 to 130 days, but 120 days is the figure usually given (19, 87, 106). Frequently it is more convenient to speak in terms of the erythrocyte half life (T/2). This value is usually given as 50 to 65 days. From the nature of the methods employed and the analytic procedures required to calculate results, it is inevitable that some variations will exist in the final derived figures. But by and large the variations between methods are not great enough to affect the *clinical interpretation* of the results. For clinical purposes it matters little if one method of analyzing the data yields an average, or mean, life span of 20 days and a second method indicates 30 days. The survival time in either instance is significantly shortened.

In most hemolytic disorders the average survival time is in the range of 10 to 60 days.

Definition of Hemolytic Disease

Hemolytic disease exists in any situation in which the red cell life span is shorter than normal. If the increased rate of destruction is of such degree that augmented red cell production can compensate for the loss, no anemia develops. This is a *compensated hemolytic process* which is seen infrequently in some of the hemoglobinopathies but is seen often in hereditary spherocytosis. It is an abnormal situation in that the mass of erythropoietic tissue is increased above normal

* General references and review articles: 4, 11, 20, 23, 24, 37, 38, 43, 69, 70, 72, 80, 81, 99, 117, 129, 145, 152, 156, 158, 164, 173, 180, 218, 232, 234, 251, 278, 283, 285, 312, 332, 333, 335, 336, 348, 356.

† Indirect calculations have been made from marrow composition and intermitotic times, DNA turnover, pigment excretion, carbon monoxide production, iron turnover, etc.; more direct assessment has been made using identifiable labels occurring as cell characteristics or induced by various manipulations: the techniques of Ashby agglutination and differential hemolysis depend on blood type, sulfhemoglobin, elliptocytosis, N^{15}, deuterium, radioiron, Cr^{51} (87), DFP^{32} (88, 100, 106, 143), C^{14}, selenium, *p*-iodophenylhydroxylamine. Some of these techniques will be described presently.

and there may be a partial shift of reticulocytes from the marrow to the peripheral blood. When the shortening of the erythrocyte life span is of such magnitude that a normal hemoglobin level of the circulating blood cannot be maintained even by hyperactive erythropoiesis, anemia results. Stated quantitatively, the maximum effective erythropoietic effort of normal uninhibited marrow cannot compensate for a chronic hemolytic process in which the erythrocyte survival is less than 15 to 20 days (one-sixth to one-eighth of normal). Or, in other terms, normal marrow can increase its effective output of hemoglobin some six or eight times normal, but this is its maximum, and when the rate of destruction cannot be matched by increase in production, *hemolytic anemia results* (63).

Determination of Red Cell Survival Time

REQUISITE CONDITIONS. If the conditions under which erythrocyte survival time may be accurately determined are analyzed, it is found, as might be expected, that the requirements are seldom, if ever, fully met. Nevertheless, data that are suitable for clinical and pathophysiologic interpretation are obtainable in most situations. For the determination of erythrocyte survival time, the red cell (and only the red cell) should have a readily detectable label that either forms a part of the cell or is irreversibly bound to it. If the label is designed for incorporation into the cell during its production, it must be available for only a short period of time and undergo no metabolic cycling or recycling prior to incorporation; if the label is to be irreversibly bound to circulating cells, it must distribute itself uniformly among all cells without preference relative to age or other characteristic. The label must not of itself modify the survival of the cell. It must not be reutilized for new cell formation at the termination of the erythrocyte's survival but rather should be completely de-

graded and/or excreted. The label should be detectable by techniques that can accurately measure it in a convenient volume of blood. (This has recently been obviated by *whole-body* radioactive counting techniques.) Moreover, the subject or patient should be in a hematologically stable state (production balancing destruction) with no change in total red cell mass during the period of observation and no escape of intact labeled cells from the intravascular compartment by either external or internal hemorrhage. The loss of labeled cells to the exterior affects the results so that a false, shortened survival time is obtained. If a hematologically stable state does not exist, the red cell population will be shifted so that there is a predominance of young or old cells. If there is a predominance of old cells present at the time the label is added, the results will falsely indicate a short survival time; if there is a predominance of young cells, the results will falsely indicate a long survival. The method employed should be such that the survival of the red cell can be determined in its natural habitat, namely, the patient. Despite these formidable limitations, determination of an erythrocyte survival time is frequently undertaken in clinical and investigational studies and does yield valuable, interpretable, reproducible data.

THE CROSS-TRANSFUSION TECHNIQUE. Red cell survival in health and disease was originally studied in man by means of the Ashby technique of differential agglutination. From these studies came the present-day classification of hemolytic diseases according to whether the abnormality mainly responsible for red cell destruction is intrinsic or extrinsic to the red cell: whether the abnormality is built into, resides in, is part and parcel of the red cell (intrinsic, or intracorpuscular, as in sickle cell disease) or resides in the plasma or body tissues external to the red cell (extrinsic, or extracorpuscular, as in an acquired hemolytic disease due to a circulating cold hemolysin).

In the Ashby "cross-transfusion" technique, red cells, compatible but serologically distinguishable, are transfused into a recipient. In samples of blood obtained at intervals from the recipient postinfusion, the number of transfused red cells can be counted after agglutinating out the recipient's cells. Thus, type O cells may be transfused into a compatible type A recipient. Blood subsequently obtained from the recipient contains a mixture of O and A erythrocytes. By means of a potent anti-A serum, the recipient's A cells can be agglutinated, leaving the unagglutinated type O cells free for enumeration. The obvious disadvantages of the system are: (a) the techniques are laborious and exacting and ultimately depend on a red blood cell count with all its inherent error, (b) the donor and recipient red cells must differ in antigenic constitution but not be incompatible for transfusion,* (c) a large volume of blood must be transfused to obtain sufficient cells for counting, and (d) the life span of the subject's own red cells cannot be measured in his own circulation. Nevertheless, by this technique it was clearly established that the hemolytic disorders could be divided into two main classes: those in which the bone marrow produces faulty cells incapable of normal survival (intracorpuscular, or intrinsic, defect); and those in which essentially normal cells are produced by the marrow but their survival is cut short by abnormal plasma or tissue factors (extracorpuscular, or extrinsic, defect). By and large, the nature of the erythrocyte defects and the mechanisms responsible for erythrocyte destruction can be held accountable for the clinical signs and symptoms and the pathophysiologic changes that characterize and distinguish the diseases or syndromes of these two main divisions.

Normal results. When the percentage of normal donor cells surviving in a nor-

mal recipient is plotted against time on an arithmetic scale (Figure 9.1), the points fall on a straight line intersecting the time axis at about 120 days. This straight-line fall-off would be expected if each red cell had a total life span of 120 days and left the circulation at that time: if a constant proportion of the *original* number became obsolete each day because of senescence. Actually, of course, each cell does not live exactly 120 days. It has been estimated that the coefficient of variation in normal subjects is in the order of 5 per cent. Therefore the figure 120 days represents the *mean, or average, life span.*

Results characteristic of intracorpuscular defect. When cells from a patient with an intracorpuscular defect are transfused into a normal recipient, their survival time is shortened even though the cell environment is now normal. This finding certifies that the cellular abnormality is truly intrinsic and responsible for premature destruction of the erythrocyte. Curve I of Figure 9.2 shows the survival of red cells from a patient with paroxysmal nocturnal hemoglobinuria (PNH) after transfusion to a normal recipient. The initial part of the curve is linear and shows markedly accelerated destruction, but after a certain proportion of the cells (here 60 per cent) have been removed from circulation, the slope becomes less steep. The shape changes and alterations in slope of the survival curve indicate two populations of cells, one with a severe defect and consequent short life and the other with minor defects and nearly normal survival. There is thus considerably more spread of the red cell life span than in the normal, and estimation of the mean life span for the *entire* red cell population becomes a complex mathematical analy-

---

* In practice, cross transfusions are largely limited to giving type O blood to an A recipient or NN blood to an MM or MN recipient because of the lack of suitable potent antisera to other groups.

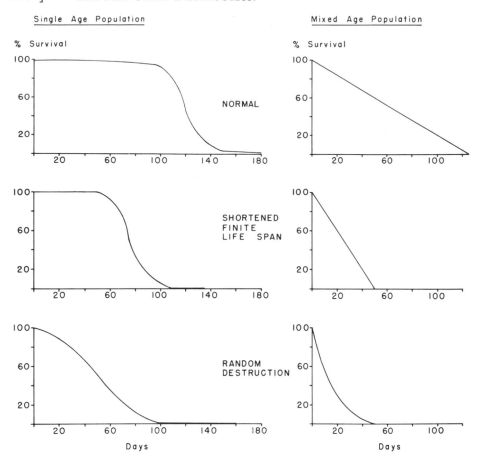

FIGURE 9.1.   Red cell survival times in various circumstances. Curves on left show results of in vivo labeling, as with N^{15}-tagged glycine; curves on right show results of
cross-transfusion technique, of in vitro labeling with Cr^{51} (corrected for elution), or of
in vivo or in vitro labeling with DFP^{32}. (Adapted from figure devised by A. G. Motulsky
in Finch, C. A., Hematology Manual, 1960. Privately printed)

sis and calculation. The mean life span of
the short-lived cells is estimated by extrapolation of the original slope to the
axis (here 6 days). (See discussion of
pathophysiology of PNH.) If red cells
from a normal donor are transfused into a
recipient whose red cells have an intracorpuscular abnormality, the normal cells
have a normal survival time, attesting to
the fact that the critical defect resides
solely in the recipient's red cell and is
nontransferable, and that the environment is normal.

*Results characteristic of extracorpuscu-
lar defect.* Curve E of Figure 9.2 shows

the survival time of normal red cells in
the circulation of a patient with an extracorpuscular defect. The life span of
the normal cells is short. Moreover, the
curve has an exponential form indicating
the destruction of a constant percentage
of the cells present on any given day.
Since the slope of the survival curve is
constantly changing throughout, the average life span cannot be estimated by the
extrapolation method. However, it has
been shown that the time taken for survival
to fall to 33 per cent of the original zero
time value represents the average life
span (219). When red cells from a pa-

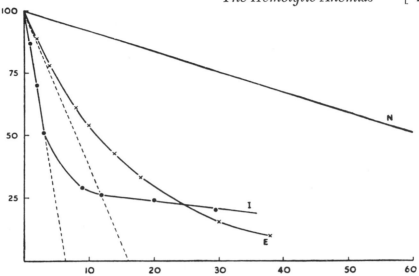

FIGURE 9.2. Red cell survival time determined by cross-transfusion technique. Abscissae, days after transfusion; ordinates, percentage survival of transfused red cells; curve N, survival of normal red cells in normal recipient; curve E, survival of normal red cells in subject with extrinsic hemolytic mechanism (idiopathic acquired hemolytic anemia); curve I, survival of red cells from patient with intrinsic red cell defect (paroxysmal nocturnal hemoglobinuria) (from Dacie and Mollison, 1949); dotted lines represent extrapolation of tangents to curves at zero time. (From Mollison, P. L., Brit. M. Bull. 15:59, 1959)

tient with an extracorpuscular defect* are transfused into a normal recipient, the donor cells survive normally, attesting to the fact that it is the environment in which they were circulating that was responsible for premature destruction and not a fault in the cell itself.

Interaction of intra- and extracorpuscular defects. Utilizing the cross-transfusion technique it is possible to localize the defect responsible for abnormal red cell destruction and thereby gain considerable insight into the pathophysiology of the hemolytic process. However, it should be noted that the classification of hemolytic disorders is not as exact and mutually exclusive as has so far been implied. The hemolytic anemia associated with ingestion of fava beans depends not only upon the presence of a red cell with an intrinsic chemical abnormality but also upon the presence of a factor in the circulating blood presumably produced through a hypersensitivity phenomenon. In associa-

tion with thermal burns (126, 252, 254) and lead poisoning an obviously extracorpuscular abnormality may induce a largely irreversible intracorpuscular abnormality so that the cells can no longer normally survive even in a normal environment.

THE RADIOACTIVE CHROMIUM TECHNIQUE. In many circumstances the information sought concerning red cell survival is precisely that which cannot be obtained by the Ashby technique: the behavior of the patient's red cell in his own circulation. Because of this and because of the technical difficulties in the Ashby procedure, mentioned above, the determination of red cell survival is today usually done by means of labeling with radioactive chromium (87, 108, 168, 220, 328).

* If a critical degree of *irreversible* damage has been inflicted on the red cell due to the effects of the extracorpuscular abnormality, it will, of course, have a shortened life-span even when transfused into a normal recipient.

When the red cells of a normal subject are labeled with Cr^{51} and returned to the donor (autosurvival) or infused into another normal recipient, the points plotted from the data obtained by serially sampling and assaying the peripheral blood radioactivity do not fall on a straight line as do the points derived from an Ashby test. The Cr^{51} survival time* is the resultant of the loss of red cells by aging and the loss or elution of Cr^{51} from the red cells. By comparison with other survival-determining techniques, the rate of Cr^{51} elution has been shown to be approximately 1 per cent per day in the normal (87). At present there is no generally accepted method to correct for elution, and it has become customary to present the uncorrected results. Moreover, there are no good data to settle the constantly recurring question whether or not Cr^{51} is eluted from cells involved in extra- or intracorpuscular hemolytic processes at a rate comparable to that determined for normal cells. Nevertheless, the information derived from survival studies using Cr^{51} is so valuable and the technique so satisfactory and widely applicable that the method is deservedly popular. In addition, because over 90 per cent of the Cr^{51} is bound to the hemoglobin, the label may be used to detect (and quantitate) gastrointestinal blood loss and to determine by external directional measurement of radioactivity the sites in which red cells are sequestered and destroyed (152, 162, 193, 219, 283, 350). The presently available data indicate that the labeling chromium enters the cell, changes valency, and is firmly bound to hemoglobin; the data are conflicting about whether it is bound to the α- (52) or β- (136, 247) chains of hemoglobin. The small amount of chromium that does elute from the cells and the chromium freed by cell destruction are excreted in the urine and do not relabel cells to an appreciable extent.

For convenience in recording, in comparative studies concerning erythrocyte life span it is customary to give the half life (T/2) of the cells, i.e., the time in days at which 50 per cent of the labeled cells have been removed from the peripheral blood. For Cr^{51} studies uncorrected for elution the normal half life is usually 28 to 38 days.† Values below this range are considered abnormal although it is at once evident that the shape of the curve should be known for more complete information. However, except for special studies and precise determinations, the single half-life figure yields the essential information most frequently desired concerning red cell life span.

SUMMARY. Employing the additional information that becomes available by means of the Cr^{51} labeling techniques (Figure 9.3), the criteria for the classification of hemolytic disorders may be restated briefly as follows.

In hemolytic disease due to an intracorpuscular abnormality the red cell is intrinsically defective and the defect is nontransferable. The patient's cells have a shortened survival time in himself or in a normal subject. Normal cells survive normally in the patient.

In hemolytic disease due to an extracorpuscular abnormality the environment of the red cell is abnormal. Both normal cells and the patient's cells have a shortened survival time in the patient, whereas the patient's red cells survive normally in a normal subject.

In hemolytic disease due to combined intrinsic and extrinsic defects normal cells are destroyed in the patient at an abnormally fast rate but usually not as fast as the patient's own defective cells. The

---

* Strictly speaking this is a chromium survival time and not a *radioactive* chromium survival time, since the technique corrects for the radioactive decay. This decay must not be confused with the elution of the Cr^{51} from the red cells.

† This normal range must be determined in each laboratory for the particular method and modifications that are employed.

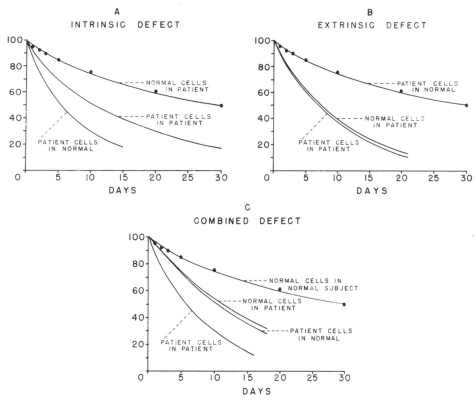

FIGURE 9.3. Red cell survival time determined by radioactive chromium technique (not corrected for chromium elution). (Adapted from Finch, C.A., Hematology Manual, 1960. Privately printed)

same patient's red cells are destroyed at a slower rate in a normal subject than in himself but, even so, at a more rapid rate than normal.

The ultimate criterion for a definitive diagnosis of a hemolytic disorder is, then, a shortened erythrocyte life span. However, it is obviously not always practical, desirable, or possible to start a red cell survival study and wait the required number of days or weeks to define the curve.

The biochemical and morphologic changes that result from increased red cell destruction are many and usually provide adequate evidence for the existence of a hemolytic process. These changes are usually readily and rapidly detected and quantitated, many of the procedures employed falling into the class of so-called screening tests. They follow as a direct consequence of the shortened erythrocyte survival time.

Mechanisms of Red Cell Destruction

Before describing the biochemical and morphologic changes that go along with increased red cell destruction, it might be well to acknowledge that upon close analysis it is not possible to give a satisfactory accounting of the final steps in the mechanism of erythrocyte destruction—just what happens to the cell at this point of its dissolution, or moment of truth.

In 1923 Rous (278) wrote: "Somewhere there must exist in the body, if only for a moment, morphologic evidence of the disintegration of every red cell." It is somewhat frustrating to realize that despite a destruction rate of some three million cells per second the evidence has by and large eluded investigative efforts to the present day. In a number of instances it is possible to give an accounting of the mechanisms required to bring the erythrocyte to the brink of destruction, but beyond that, for any given process, little information of in vivo relevance can be offered. The main routes of cell destruction proposed have been (a) osmotic lysis; (b) chemical, bacterial, or complement-antibody lysis; (c) mechanical trauma; (d) phagocytosis; (e) degradation or inhibition of enzymes necessary for "cell integrity"; and (f) other. Each of these will be further discussed in conjunction with a disease or syndrome best suited to illustrate the mechanism or demonstrate its unreasonableness or shortcoming.

Even the events occurring at the time of in vitro disruption or dissolution of red cells are poorly understood.

In 1929 Comandon and DeFonbrune (58) described the occurrence of large tears or rents in the erythrocyte membrane as it was subjected to gross osmotic stress to induce lysis. The hemoglobin was pictured as escaping through the membrane opening. For years this was accepted as the mechanism by which hemolysis took place. However, Bessis (22) was unable to confirm these findings and employing electron microscopy could not locate any break or point of rupture in the membrane of most red cells after osmotic lysis had occurred.

Employing high-speed microcinematography, Parpart (244) in 1954 described a general oozing of hemoglobin that occurred all over the cell surface during lysis by osmosis and by immune antibodies, not rupture at one point with escape of contents through an opening. It appeared that rather than a break occurring in a retaining surface, restraining or stabilizing forces holding the individual hemoglobin molecules in place were overcome, and the hemoglobin was then free to escape.

In some manner the cell is altered so that its macromolecular contents escape the confines of the membrane. Studies concerning altered permeability of erythrocytes and tumor cells during the process of lysis by immune antibodies (118) show that in suspensions of low protein content potassium ions, amino acids, and ribonucleotides are lost; the cell becomes permeable to sodium, swells, and then macromolecules (hemoglobin or RNA) escape. In suspensions of higher protein content (enough to balance the colloid osmotic pressure of the cells), the sodium and potassium distribution is altered; amino acids escape but no swelling or loss of macromolecules takes place. The conclusion was drawn that "functional holes" are induced in the membrane by complement-antibody action which lead to redistribution of small molecules, increase in cellular osmotic pressure, influx of water, and stretching of the membrane so that macromolecules are permitted to escape.

It should be pointed out that previous and subsequent workers have described *no* cellular swelling or spherocytosis during lysis in complement-antibody systems. However, studies employing the nonpermeable agent *p*-mercuribenzoate to block membrane sulfhydryl groups by Jacob and Jandl (148a) (see section on Mechanism of Ion Transport in Chapter 8) have demonstrated the disruption of the cation gradients across the cell membrane with loss of potassium cations and a gain of sodium cations and water. The water moves into the cell to compensate for the oncotic activity of hemoglobin and other macromolecules and leads to swelling of the cell, distention of the membrane, and distortion of the "pores." This allows a loss of macromolecules and eventually leakage of hemoglobin, i.e., hemolysis. The changes induced by osmotic imbalance in the above sequence can be prevented by balancing the intracellular oncotic activity by extracellular oncotically active material (albumin) or nonpenetrating osmotically active material (sucrose). It is suggested (148a) that in complement-immune lysis, more direct and extensive alterations in the cell membrane are induced than with sulfhydryl inhibitors, resulting in relatively large holes so that hemoglobin leakage can occur with little prior osmotic swelling of the cell.

"Intra-" and "Extravascular" Hemolysis

With respect to in vivo hemolysis, disruption or dissolution of cells may take place *within* the general circulation, so that the cellular components are for a restricted time free in the plasma ("intravascular hemolysis"), or after trapping and sequestration in certain regions of the circulation (spleen, liver, bone marrow), so that the cellular hemoglobin is for the most part degraded *in situ* ("extravascular hemolysis"). In the latter situation— by far the most common—trapping or sequestration is effected either (a) by surface adherence of the cells to the endothelium or reticuloendothelium by chemical or electrostatic forces or (b) by filtration brought on by physical means. It is not unlikely that both together occur in some situations. At any event, in addition to the above, Jandl et al. (152) have pointed out that phagocytosis is inescapably a process secondary to filtration and/or surface adherence and, moreover, is usually a posthemolytic event in vivo.

Radioactive techniques, especially labeling of erythrocytes with Cr^{51}, have made possible observations on the fate of normal, damaged, and diseased erythrocytes with respect to body site of destruction. As will be detailed later, it has been demonstrated that in certain situations cells may be destroyed in the spleen, the liver, both, or elsewhere. The attempt will be made, in the appropriate sections, to develop the reasons why sequestration occurs in one area in preference to another, but in general it seems likely, on the basis of cells injured by heat, chemicals, antibodies, or metabolic derangement, that the site of destruction depends on the degree of injury rather than on the exact type of injury and that the spleen is the primary organ for the removal of damaged or altered cells from the circulation (148, 148a, 331a).

Biochemical and Morphologic Changes Resulting from Increased Red Cell Destruction

BIOCHEMICAL CHANGES ASSOCIATED WITH COMPENSATED HEMOLYTIC DISEASE. As mentioned above, in a *compensated hemolytic process* characterized by a moderately shortened red cell life span, a depression of the hemoglobin level of the circulating blood below normal limits may not occur. This is accomplished largely by an increase in the total mass of erythropoietic tissue—the red cell precursors. There are no readily available means for assaying total functional erythropoietic tissue, but autopsy findings and bone marrow biopsies show an increase in the numbers of red cell precursors that is absolute as well as proportional to leukocyte precursors. The active red marrow extends into the normally yellow marrow areas and the proportion of fat cells is decreased. The proportionate change is also seen in bone marrow aspirates and is indicated by a larger percentage of erythrocyte precursors (usually referred to as normoblastic hyperplasia) and an increase above the normal E/M ratio (erythrocytic to myelocytic cells) of 1:3. Under these circumstances, the percentage of reticulocytes present in the circulating blood is minimally elevated, sometimes inconstantly so. The other biochemical and morphologic changes resulting from the decreased red cell survival to be enumerated below are minimal (or at least not detectable by present techniques, probably because of the limitations of accuracy).

BIOCHEMICAL CHANGES ASSOCIATED WITH HEMOLYTIC ANEMIA. In an *overt hemolytic process* (red cell life span shortened to less than one-seventh of normal; 63) the following changes can confidently be predicted. Directly consequent upon the increased rate of red cell destruction, pigment metabolism will be altered due to augmented hemoglobin breakdown. When hemoglobin is liberated from the red cell, its immediate fate depends to some extent upon the site and mechanism of erythrocyte destruction—extravascular or intravascular. Assuming for the moment the apparently more usual route, extravascular destruction, the heme is separated from the globin, catabolized through the bilirubin-urobilinogen cycle, and practically all of it is excreted. Various intermediates in this catabolic sequence can be qualitatively or quantitatively analyzed and the results interpreted to indicate the presence and magnitude of the hemolytic process.

Extravascular destruction and hemoglobin catabolism. The conversion of hemoglobin to bilirubin probably takes place in the entire reticuloendothelial system, but the extent of participation by various organs (spleen, liver, bone marrow, etc.) is unknown (64, 117, 180, 285, 335, 336). With reference to Figure 9.4, outlining hemoglobin catabolism, it is not certain whether (a) in the first step the iron-porphyrin complex is split from the globin to form hematin (a hydroxide of the trivalent iron derivative of heme) and the porphyrin ring then opened and the iron lost to form the straight-chain bilirubin compounds or (b) the oxidation of hemoglobin at the initial step opens the porphyrin ring to yield choleglobin, a green bile pigment iron-globin complex. Upon subsequent loss of the iron and globin the bilirubin compound is formed.

By either route the opening of the porphyrin ring occurs at one of the α-methene bridges, and 1 mole of carbon monoxide is formed. Measurement of carbon monoxide production has been used as an indication of hemoglobin breakdown (94, 233).

The transformation to hematin has been demonstrated in vitro, but circulating hematin has not been detected under physiologic conditions in vivo. In certain hemolytic disorders hematin is detected in the circulating plasma (as methemalbumin), and it is likely that normally it is catabolized only in the reticuloendothelial cells. The transformation to choleglobin has been demonstrated in vitro, but methodologic difficulties make suspect its detection in other situations. In either instance, the iron ultimately liberated is tenaciously retained in the body and reutilized mainly for new hemoglobin synthesis; the globin is degraded and returned to the general amino acid pool. Freed of globin and iron, the straight chain resulting from the cleavage of the porphyrin ring is converted to biliverdin and then reduced to bilirubin.*

Bilirubin is transported in the plasma to the liver. It is virtually insoluble in water but has strong avidity for albumin, with which it is transported. At the liver the bilirubin must be transported *to* the parenchymal cells, across the membrane *into* the cell and *to* the surface or interior of the microsomes, for in conjunction with the liver microsomes, the bilirubin is conjugated with glucuronide by enzymatic processes. In these processes the diglucuronide is mainly formed; some bilirubin exists as monoglucuronide, and a

---

* It should be noted again that the available evidence indicates that the bilirubin-urobilinogen compounds are derived from the heme ring and *not* from the heme precursors. There is no evidence that coproporphyrin, for example, gives rise to bilirubin-urobilinogen complexes. Consequently the heme precursors represent an anabolic process, the bilirubin-urobilinogen compounds a catabolic process, with reference to heme.

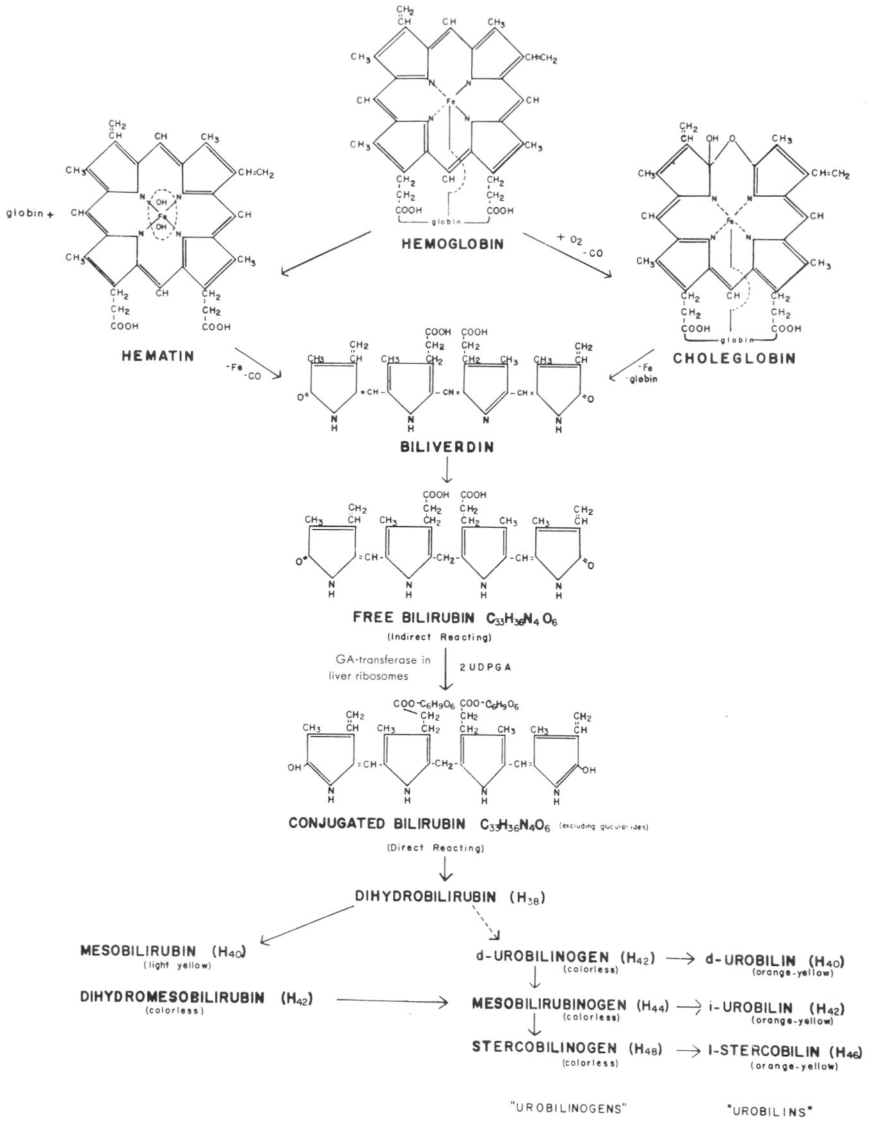

FIGURE 9.4. Hemoglobin breakdown through bilirubin-urobilinogen pathway. It is not known whether the in vivo pathway proceeds through hematin, choleglobin, or both, in the initial steps

small proportion as sulfates. The conjugated form (bilirubin glucuronide) is then excreted into the bile. At any one of these steps malfunction may occur and result in retention of bilirubin. Several such malfunctions have now been found to account for some of the nonhemolytic hyperbilirubinemias seen in human diseases. The glucuronides are highly polar compounds that confer water solubility upon the otherwise insoluble unconjugated bilirubin. As water-soluble compounds the conjugated bilirubin participates in a color reaction with Ehrlich's diazo reagent in the van den Bergh test. The *immediate* development of color upon addition of Ehrlich's reagent to aqueous solutions is called a direct reaction and indicates the presence of conjugated bilirubin (formerly called immediate, or direct-reacting, bilirubin). The free, un-conjugated water-insoluble bilirubin does not participate in the color reaction until alcohol is added to the mixture to solubilize the bilirubin or catalyze the color reaction.* That portion of the color developing after the addition of alcohol to the mixture in the van den Bergh test is due to the free, unconjugated bilirubin (formerly called indirect-reacting bilirubin).

In the normal individual most of the bilirubin glucuronide is excreted into the bile, but some escapes back into the circulating plasma giving rise to detectable levels, and some is probably absorbed from the gastrointestinal tract (191, 238). In a large series of normals the range for the van den Bergh partition test has been established as 0.11 ± 0.05 mg of conjugated bilirubin per 100 ml of plasma, and 0.62 ± 0.25 mg of *total* bilirubin per 100 ml of plasma (334, 357). Because of a skewed distribution curve, the upper limits of normal are difficult to establish but are accepted to be for conjugated bilirubin 0.25 mg per 100 ml, and for total bilirubin slightly less than 1.5 mg per 100 ml; most values for total bilirubin fall between 0.3 and 1.0 mg per 100 ml.

With increased catabolism of hemoglobin due to augmented red cell destruction, the various steps leading to conjugation may be overloaded and levels of unconjugated bilirubin may increase in the circulating plasma. Presumably because of its water insolubility, the unconjugated bilirubin is not excreted by the kidney, despite levels high enough to produce clinical icterus, and the classic acholuric jaundice of hemolytic anemia is seen.

Bilirubin is the principal bile pigment formed and excreted into the gut. A small but unknown proportion of the bilirubin may be excreted as mono- or dipyrroles, but these have been technically difficult to detect and quantitate. In the gut the bilirubin is progressively reduced by bacterial action into the members of the urobilin-urobilinogen groups. This degradation of bilirubin by bacterial action is so effectively done that only extremely small quantities of bilirubin have been detected in feces with radioactive labeling techniques. As indicated in Figure 9.4, the members of the urobilin and urobilinogen groups are chiefly defined by their optical activity and numbers of hydrogen atoms: d-urobilin (H_{40}), i-urobilin (H_{42}), l-stercobilin (H_{46}), and their corresponding colorless "-ogen" compounds.

The "-ogen" compounds are colorless but yield red complexes with Ehrlich's aldehyde reagent; the urobilins show intense green fluorescence with Schlesinger's solution (zinc acetate in alcohol). Both series of compounds are conventionally known collectively as urobilinogens. Their production is much depressed and the proportions altered by the administration of broad-spectrum antibiotics; they are not found in germ-free animals (122), and can be re-established by infection with a specific strain of coliform organism, so there is no longer doubt about the concept of their enterogenous formation.

The greater proportion of the urobilin group of compounds passes out in the feces, some is absorbed from the gut and transported back to the liver for re-excretion (the enterohepatic circulation). With an adequately functioning liver, the compounds are so effectively cleared from the blood that minimal elevations in the systemic circulation and urine occur even in the face of greatly increased production (297). If there is incidental or associated liver damage, effective clearance does not take place and an abnormally increased amount is detected in the urine. In any event, the amount excreted by the kidney is usually minor in propor-

---

* Probably due to urea and to solubilizing agents, a *small* proportion of the unconjugated bilirubin is "direct reacting," accounting in large measure for the increases in "direct-reacting" bilirubin levels seen in hemolytic jaundice (324).

tion to that eliminated in the feces. The composition of the urobilinogen group in the urine, bile, and feces varies with the efficiency of bacterial reduction, the degree and site of absorption, and the mobility and filling of the colon. When tested for in the urine or feces, they are usually grouped together and collectively quantitated as representing an equivalent number of milligrams of urobilinogen. Consequently, the excretion of bile pigments is usually given in milligrams of urobilinogen per day.

Since bile pigments may be derived from any heme chromogen, it is evident that contributions are made by multiple metabolic sources: myoglobin, catalase, cytochromes, peroxidase. The quantities of these compounds present in the body are small but their turnover times are unknown. Nevertheless, it is quite clear that in the normal person the most important source of bile pigments is the circulating hemoglobin. Consequently an elevation of unconjugated bilirubin in the peripheral blood constitutes strong presumptive evidence for the existence of a hemolytic process and an elevation in fecal urobilinogen constitutes virtually definitive evidence for the existence of a hemolytic process.

A quantitative estimation of daily urobilinogen excretion can be arrived at by the following calculations based on the figures provided in Table 6.3. A normal 70-Kg man with a blood volume of 5,000 ml and a mean body hematocrit of 40 per cent (mean hemoglobin concentration of 13.3 Gm per 100 ml) has a total hemoglobin mass of 666 Gm. The daily breakdown is 0.83 per cent per day, or 5.6 to 6.7 Gm of hemoglobin. On a molecular weight basis (hemoglobin, 66,000; four molecules of urobilinogen, 2,320), each gram of hemoglobin can yield 35 mg of urobilinogen. Therefore, the excretion of urobilinogen should theoretically be 193 to 234 mg per day.

To arrive at the total circulating hemoglobin mass, the blood volume has to be determined, estimated, or guessed—usually with considerable error and especially so in the presence of anemia. Consequently only gross deviations from normal values of urobilinogen excretion may be accepted as adequate evidence. However, the fact that the amount of bilirubin and urobilinogen derived from hemoglobin obviously depends on the total hemoglobin mass means that the values for each should be interpreted only after taking into account the circulating hemoglobin level. In attempts to meet this requirement certain "hemolytic indices" have been set up relating hemoglobin levels to urobilinogen excretion.

Another discrepancy must be mentioned. Observations made with N^{15}-tagged glycine have demonstrated the excretion of labeled urobilinogen at such an early time following administration of the label that it could not have been derived from the hemoglobin of circulating erythrocytes (Figure 7.5; 199). In the normal this amounts to 10 to 20 per cent of the total urobilinogen excreted; in some anemias with ineffective erythropoiesis it amounts to as much as 60 per cent of the daily excretion. The source of this pigment is unknown, but it is thought perhaps to be erythrocytes destroyed in the marrow before release to the peripheral circulation (stillborn cells) or heme groups not incorporated into hemoglobin (the so-called marrow shunt of ineffective, as opposed to *effective*, erythropoiesis). The catabolism of myoglobin and other heme-containing pigments are other possible sources. Whatever the true source, it is a variable that at present makes strict interpretation of urobilinogen excretion difficult.

In a few instances (excluding those in which pigment excretion is suppressed by antibiotic administration) apparently accurately determined urobilinogen excretion simply does not seem to reflect the red cell turnover. The excretion values may be normal or low in the presence of a documented hemolytic process. This has given rise to the suspicion that hemoglobin may also be degraded through a different and as yet unknown metabolic cycle. Consequently, while values for urobilinogen excretion can be interpreted as indicating red cell destruction, this must be done with the realization that about 70 per cent is derived from mature circulating erythrocytes and undetermined amounts of hemoglobin may be degraded through other pathways.

The case against determination of fecal and total urobilinogen excretion has probably been somewhat overstated above. The method has yielded considerable valuable information in some hands. Nevertheless, it would be fatuous not to acknowledge that the real reason more determinations and studies have not been made is the necessity for accurate, prolonged collection of feces and the unpleasant nature of the technical procedure itself.

Intravascular destruction and hemoglobin catabolism. If intravascular hemolysis is the predominant mechanism by which the cells are destroyed, hemoglobin is liberated directly into the circulating plasma (48, 127) and a somewhat different metabolic pathway is followed. There exists in the plasma a protein which will specifically bind and transport extracorpuscular hemoglobin quantitatively. This is an a_2-globulin called haptoglobin, that can bind two molecules of hemoglobin and form a complex of molecular weight 310,000 (1, 2, 14, 35, 111, 137, 161, 183–185, 306, 343, 345). Several haptoglobins are now known by their different electrophoretic migration patterns, and it is now established that the type(s) of haptoglobin(s) possessed by any given individual is genetically determined (14). All types apparently have equal hemoglobin-binding capacities. Normally, sufficient haptoglobin is present to bind 100 to 140 mg of hemoglobin per 100 ml of plasma. The haptoglobin-hemoglobin complex has a molecular weight of such magnitude that it is not excreted by the kidney. It is, however, taken up by the reticuloendothelial system and degraded in such a fashion that the heme is turned over to the bilirubin-urobilinogen cycle outlined above (226, 232, 234, 239). Extracorpuscular hemoglobin may therefore be present in amounts up to 100 to 140 mg per 100 ml of plasma without spilling into the urine to produce hemoglobinuria.

The hemoglobin-haptoglobin complex is cleared from the plasma at a rate of approximately 15 mg hgb. / 100 ml / hr; with respect to time, the fall-off follows a straight-line disappearance (100a).

In many situations haptoglobin may be used up in the extracorpuscular hemoglobin transport and metabolized faster than it can be synthesized or delivered to the blood so that the concentration falls to immeasurable levels. A depressed haptoglobin level provides evidence for abnormal utilization and probably constitutes a sensitive indicator of the presence of abnormal erythrocyte destruction (239). Recently considerable work has been done verifying this general conclusion but also demonstrating variations in haptoglobin levels in association with other factors: genetic, infection, liver disease, malignancy, etc. (232, 234, 240). When haptoglobin is absent or the binding capacity of the circulating haptoglobin is exceeded, hemoglobin, unbound by the protein, circulates in the blood. Unbound hemoglobin (molecular weight 66,000) is filtered by the glomerulus and passed on to the tubular system. Hemoglobinuria results after the resorptive capacity of the proximal renal tubules is also exceeded (183–185, 201). Some of the extracorpuscular hemoglobin may be split into heme and globin fractions before being otherwise metabolized or excreted. The heme, oxidized to the trivalent iron hematin, is bound to albumin (1, 2, 100, 195, 275), forming a substance, methemalbumin, that has a characteristic absorptive band and behavior. Employing the Schumm test, the presence of this substance in the peripheral blood is taken as evidence for a *recent* intravascular hemolytic episode, since it is rapidly cleared from the circulation and demonstrated in no other situation. The fate of this compound is not accurately known, but it is probably taken up by the reticuloendothelial system for processing through the bilirubin-urobilinogen cycle. Neither protein-bound hemoglobin nor methemalbumin appears in the urine during hemoglobinuria.

The iron-containing pigments (chiefly hemoglobin) that reach the renal tubules are apparently degraded *in situ*, and in an attempt at conservation, the iron is incorporated into apoferritin to form ferritin and hemosiderin. It is assumed that a portion of this is reabsorbed and reutilized for hemoglobin production. However, with continued build-up of hemosiderin in the tubular cells, some iron is apparently excreted into the urine. Most of the iron appearing in the urine is apparently derived from cells containing hemosiderin that have been desquamated and disrupted (183–185). Hemosiderin is not found in the urine at the onset of an intravascular hemolytic episode (even with hemoglobinuria) but does appear in a few days after the onset. Hemosiderinuria is, in fact, a fairly reliable sign of chronic intravascular hemolysis (62). (It is also seen on occasion in patients with iron overload and hemochromatosis.)

From what has been briefly described here, it might be concluded that a rather clear separation can be made between intravascular and extravascular hemolysis and support found for that separation in measurements of haptoglobin levels, methemalbumin, etc. In general, such a con-

clusion would probably be correct, but critical evidence does not establish a clear separation between intravascular and extravascular hemolysis. It is possible that methemalbumin can form to some extent in extravascular sites and diffuse into the plasma or that extravascular hemoglobin or hematin can diffuse into the plasma and there form methemalbumin (186). With regard to haptoglobin, any chronic hemolytic anemia of significant severity, apparently regardless of the mechanism of cell destruction, is usually associated with a lack or diminished level of haptoglobin. Again the possibility exists that extravascular hemoglobin may diffuse into the plasma, there complex with haptoglobin and depress its circulating level by increased utilization. It must be acknowledge that the line dividing intravascular from extravascular hemolysis is difficult to draw and that the changes seen may depend upon the rate and quantity of red cell destruction as well as upon the mechanism of destruction.

Reticulocyte response. Of the two major changes seen in hemolytic disorders that follow directly from the shortened erythrocyte life span, we have first considered the alterations in the various pigments seen in the different stages of hemoglobin catabolism. The other major change results from alterations in red cell production that follow the attempt made by the bone marrow to compensate for the abnormal destruction. Increases in total erythropoietic mass and in the erythrocytic/myelocytic ratio occur early in the process, and delivery of new red cells to the peripheral blood is hastened, in accordance with the physiologic controls of erythropoiesis previously described. The result is that more cells are delivered to the peripheral blood and as young cells they are identified as reticulocytes.

In the normal the reticuloctye count is usually between 0.5 and 1.5 per 100 erythrocytes,* or in absolute numbers 25,000 to 75,000 per cubic millimeter of blood. In hemolytic anemia the proportion is frequently 10 to 20 per cent, rarely 80 per cent or more. Although there is no precise correlation between the rate of cell destruction and degree of reticulocytosis, in general the highest reticulocyte counts are observed in the most brisk hemolytic anemias. Continuing reticulocytosis is good evidence of a hemolytic process, and although exceptions do occur, augmented red cell destruction is most frequently accompanied by a reticulocyte response.

Since the younger cells—most readily identified as reticulocytes—are larger than mature erythrocytes due mainly to an increased water content, significant reticulocytosis is accompanied by an increase in mean cell volume in the red cell indices and a macrocytic-appearing smear. In general, for every 10 per cent increase in reticulocytes, there is an increase of about 10 cu μ in the mean cell volume. Most of the severe hemolytic anemias are therefore somewhat macrocytic by erythrocyte indices and in appearance.

The number of normoblasts may be slightly increased in the peripheral blood of patients with hemolytic anemia, usually less than 1 per 200 white blood cells. With severe anemia, hypoxia, and strenuous efforts at red cell regeneration, greater numbers of normoblasts may appear in the peripheral blood; even younger red cell precursors back to erythroblasts may be seen, but this usually occurs only in extreme and unusual circumstances.†

MORPHOLOGIC ABNORMALITIES. Morphologic abnormalities of the circulating erythrocytes may give the lie to the presence of a hemolytic state. These abnormalities are usually associated with or caused by the specific hemolytic mechanism in operation and as such may provide strong evidence for a specific diagnosis. Under this heading come irreversibly sickled cells, target forms, budded cells (schistocytes), cells containing Heinz bodies, irregularly contracted cells, "moth-ball cells," stippled cells, pyknocytes, triangular cells, etc. Probably the most frequently seen, since it is the result of many different pathologic processes, is the spherocyte or microspherocyte—the small, densely staining, thick-appearing cell. This may be seen both in hereditary hemolytic anemia, where the abnormality is intrinsic to the cell, and in various forms of acquired hemolytic anemias, where the change is secondary to an extrinsic abnormality such as a chemical or antibody.

SUMMARY. In summary of the above, the definitive diagnosis of the presence of a hemolytic process ultimately depends on the demonstration of a decreased erythrocyte survival time. In actual practice satisfactorily strong evidence for the existence of a hemolytic process may be obtained from persistent reticulocytosis, jaundice of the acholuric type, and erythrocyte abnormalities. These are determinations that can be readily made in most situations. The other tests mentioned above (the van den Bergh test, the E/M ratio, and tests to detect hemoglobinuria, hemoglobinemia, methemalbuminemia, decreased plasma haptoglobin, increased urobilinogen excretion, hemosiderinuria, etc.) are in general more difficult to perform, are usually required only for problem or borderline cases, and actually

* Since the life span of a reticulocyte has been estimated between 1 and 3 days (i.e., at this time reticulum is no longer detectable by the usual techniques and the cell is morphologically classified as mature), this undoubtedly means that most but not all cells are delivered to the peripheral blood as reticulocytes; some must be delivered as cells that appear mature by the usual morphologic criteria. Some cells may lose their reticulum before nuclear extrusion takes place and therefore never qualify as reticulocytes.

† Red cell precursors (erythroblasts, normoblasts, reticulocytes) may also be seen in conditions associated with bone marrow "irritation" such as myelophthisis, metastases, and in myeloid metaplasia, where anemia and hemolysis may be very minor components if present at all.

form beginning investigative studies concerning the etiology of the hemolytic process or attempts to establish the diagnosis of a specific hemolytic disease entity. Although many clinical laboratories are now equipped to perform a red cell survival study by Cr^{51} techniques, obviously it is not always feasible to make such a determination. However, in many circumstances it should be remembered that a reasonably accurate estimate of bone marrow function and hemolytic rate may be obtained from the transfusion requirements of a patient. In the normal individual approximately 1 per cent of the red cell mass, or 5.6 to 6.7 Gm of hemoglobin, is removed and replaced daily. This amounts to approximately 250 ml of red blood cells (500 ml of whole blood) every 10 days. In the absence of external blood loss, if more than 1 pt of blood per week is required to maintain a stable circulating hemoglobin level, the presumption is justified that abnormal hemolysis is taking place.

Aplastic Crisis

There is ample evidence that an aplastic crisis (temporary bone marrow failure, cessation of hematopoiesis, hypoplastic crisis, aregenerative crisis) may occur in hematologically normal individuals in association with a toxic, inflammatory, or allergic process. In this situation it is seldom of significant clinical consequence. However, such a marrow response occurring in an individual with a hemolytic disorder always presents a potentially dangerous situation necessitating careful observation and frequently constitutes a dangerous situation necessitating immediate remedial therapy. In the so-called aplastic crisis, the marrow essentially shuts down and ceases delivery of cells to the peripheral blood (107). This is most often seen in relation to red cell production but may also involve leukocyte and/or platelet production. Because of the relatively long life span of

the erythrocyte in the normal individual, changes in the hemoglobin level of the circulating blood and in the red cell count are difficult to discern during the usually short periods of bone marrow inhibition that occur unless careful, repeated counts are done or ferrokinetic and erythrokinetic observations are made. With a loss of erythrocytes and hemoglobin of only approximately 1 per cent per day at the normal removal rate, appreciable time must elapse before significant changes in the peripheral counts can be detected by the usual tests (114). Not so, however, for the patient with a hemolytic process. For with a shortened erythrocyte survival time, precipitous falls may occur in the hemoglobin level of the circulating blood because of lack of replacement during a period of continuing rapid hemolysis. The marrow shuts down; no new cells are delivered to the peripheral blood; hemolysis continues at the usual increased rate. In some hemolytic anemias it has been documented that the peripheral hemoglobin may drop to one-half the usual value within 48 hours—a fall from perhaps a borderline 6 Gm to a critical 3 Gm per 100 ml. This abrupt fall can best be appreciated when it is remembered that the erythrocyte survival curve usually shows a rapid fall-off in the first portion of the curve, with subsequent flattening. If marrow function is totally inhibited, varying degrees of leukopenia and thrombocytopenia also occur. Such crises have been demonstrated in many of the chronic hemolytic disorders: hereditary spherocytosis, sickle cell anemia and its variants, thalassemia major, paroxysmal nocturnal hemoglobinuria, acquired hemolytic anemia (symptomatic or idiopathic and autoimmune), hereditary nonspherocytic hemolytic anemia, erythroblastosis fetalis, etc. There is reason to suppose that this phenomenon may occur in all hemolytic disorders (Figure 3.4).

The sequence of events and changes that is observed can be accurately predicted from a consideration of the basic pathophysiology (93, 241). The rate of red cell destruction is not increased above that usually seen for the particular individual. Indeed the absolute number of cells destroyed per day decreases since fewer cells are available every day for destruction according to the curve of erythrocyte life span. This means that less hemoglobin is catabolized than usual, and consequently *less* bilirubin and urobilinogen are produced. Clinically it has been noted that icterus recedes; the unconjugated bilirubin in the plasma progressively falls and the fecal urobilinogen may reach very low values. With cessation of erythropoiesis, reticulocytes disappear from the peripheral blood and values of zero are not unusual. (The inhibition may, of course, not be complete; the resultant changes are altered proportionately.) This reticulocytopenia may persist for varying lengths of time, usually 5 to 10 days, but periods up to a month have occurred. The plasma iron concentration, which is usually somewhat elevated in hemolytic anemia, remains elevated during an aplastic crisis. This is presumably so because erythrocyte destruction continues, but with no new cell and hemoglobin production, iron utilization by the marrow is at a minimum and little is removed from the plasma by this ordinarily major route.

The leukocyte and thrombocyte count may fall but changes in these elements are not regularly seen. Descriptions in the literature of the bone marrow alterations are not uniform, but this may be due to the specimens' having been obtained at different times during a changing picture. It seems likely that early in the course, at the maximal effect of initial inhibition, an aplastic, acellular marrow is present with very few erythrocyte precursors. Specimens obtained later are interpreted as showing "maturation arrest," with large primitive proerythroblasts but a striking lack of later red cell precursors. Just prior to, and then simultaneous with, the reticulocytosis that follows release of the marrow, enormous normoblastic hyperplasia occurs. This may be accompanied by severe bone pain originating in sites of active marrow and presumably resulting from an increase in the intramedullary pressure secondary to the rapid increase in the volume of regenerating red cell precursors (155). The reticulocyte peak may achieve levels of 60 to 80 per cent followed by re-establishment of the patient's usual hemoglobin, leukocyte, and platelet levels. It is evident that the severity of the anemia and the rapidity of the development is directly related to the erythrocyte life span. In severe hemolytic anemia due to an erythrocyte life span of 14 days and a complete cessation of red cell production, all cells would theoretically be removed from the peripheral blood by 2 weeks. Transfusions obviously are mandatory to maintain life until regeneration takes place.

The etiology of these episodes is unknown. They may occur for no discernible reason but are usually associated with various types of infections (usually viral) and may run sequentially through several members of a family in which hemolytic anemia is found. Episodes have been described secondary to anaphylactic and toxic reactions, and a somewhat similar sequence of events has been well documented during the administration of chloramphenicol to apparently hematologically normal individuals (279).

More recently it has been noted that hematologic responses may follow the administration of large, so-called "pharmacologic," doses of folic acid, and it has been hypothesized that in the presence of increased red cell turnover "relative deficiencies" of hematopoietic substances may occur, i.e., with increased demands, supernormal amounts of certain nutrients may be necessary (47, 249b). It is also possible that an unknown folic acid antagonist may develop (47a) to aggravate a "subclinical" folic defect.

CLASSIFICATION OF HEMOLYTIC DISORDERS

The classification of hemolytic disorders presented in Table 9.1 is based upon the location of the defect responsible for the shortening of the erythrocyte life span: intracorpuscular or extracorpuscular.

From the table it is also apparent that in most hemolytic disorders resulting from intracorpuscular defects the abnormalities are heritable (inborn errors of metab-

olism) and are associated with alterations in the red cell stroma, hemoglobin production, intracellular energy metabolism, or porphyrin synthesis. The striking exception is paroxysmal nocturnal hemoglobinuria, in which the defect is clearly intracorpuscular, yet apparently acquired. It is not surprising that acquired nutritional deficiencies (vitamin B_{12}, folic acid, iron) result in the faulty production of erythrocytes afflicted with a built-in defect responsible for shortened survival.

TABLE 9.1.   Classification of hemolytic disorders

I. Intracorpuscular abnormalities
   A. Hereditary defects of red blood cells
      1. Hereditary spherocytosis
      2. Ovalocytosis
      3. Stomatocytosis
      4. Thalassemia
      5. Hereditary nonspherocytic disease
         a. Defect in Embden-Meyerhof pathway (pyruvate kinase deficiency)
         b. Defect in pentose phosphate pathway (primaquine-sensitive anemia)
         c. Defect(s) unknown
      6. Hemoglobinopathy (see Table 3.1)
         a. Sickle cell anemia (homozygous hemoglobin S disease)
         b. Sickle cell-hemoglobin C disease
         c. Sickle cell-hemoglobin D disease
         d. Sickle cell-hemoglobin E disease, etc.
         e. Hemoglobin C disease (homozygous hemoglobin C disease), etc.
      7. Combination of hemoglobinopathy plus other defect
      8. Erythropoietic porphyria
   B. Acquired defects of red blood cells
      1. Paroxysmal nocturnal hemoglobinuria
      2. Nutritional deficiencies
         a. Vitamin B_{12} deficiency
         b. Iron lack
         c. Folic acid deficiency

II. Interaction of intra- and extracorpuscular abnormalities
   A. Acquired extracorpuscular defect; hereditary intracorpuscular defect
      1. Primaquine-sensitive hemolytic anemia (glucose–6–phosphate dehydrogenase deficiency)
      2. Favism (glucose–6–phosphate dehydrogenase deficiency)
   B. Acquired intra- and extracorpuscular defects
      1. Lead poisoning
      2. Burns
      3. Hemolytic disease of the newborn induced by vitamin K and related compounds (glucose deficient)
      4. Pernicious anemia (vitamin B_{12} deficiency, folic acid deficiency)
      5. Infantile pyknocytosis

TABLE 9.1 (*continued*)

III. Extracorpuscular abnormalities
    A. Acquired defects associated with demonstrable antibodies
        1. Hemolytic disorders caused by iso-antibodies
            a. Erythroblastosis fetalis and most hemolytic transfusion re-
               actions (caused by anti-A, anti-B, and Rh (D) reactions)
            b. Reaction to subgroup factor
        2. Autoimmune hemolytic disease ("autoaggression")
            a. Paroxysmal cold hemoglobinuria caused by cold agglutinin
               (idiopathic or secondary to viral infection)
            b. Paroxysmal cold hemoglobinuria caused by cold hemolysin
               (luetic or nonluetic)
            c. Secondary, or symptomatic, acquired hemolytic anemia
               ("warm" antibody type) (secondary to leukemia, lymphoma,
               disseminated lupus erythematosus, drug, etc.)
            d. Idiopathic acquired hemolytic anemia ("warm" antibody
               type)
            e. Thrombotic thrombocytopenic purpura (rare)
    B. Acquired defects not associated with demonstrable antibodies
        1. Hemolytic disorders caused by chemicals toxic to normal cells,
           such as heavy metals, arsine, naphthalene, phenylhydrazine,
           oxidant compounds, surface-active compounds, water (intra-
           venous)
        2. Hemolytic disorders caused by physical agents, such as thermal
           injury, ionizing radiation
        3. Hemolytic disorders caused by infectious agents, such as bac-
           terial toxins or hemolysins (*Cl. welchii*, bacterioides, hemo-
           lytic streptococcus, etc.) and red cell parasites (associated
           with malaria and Bartonella infection)
        4. Hemolytic disorders caused by unknown mechanisms
            a. Associated with malignant tumors
            b. Associated with acute and chronic infections
            c. Associated with acute and chronic renal disease
            d. Associated with chronic inflammatory disorders (rheumatic
               fever, etc.)
            e. Associated with congestive splenomegaly or splenic reticulo-
               endothelial hyperplasia (liver disease), acute fatty changes,
               cirrhosis, histiocytosis (lipoid dystrophy), splenic vein
               thrombosis, myeloid metaplasia, infection, etc.
            f. Hemolytic anemia uremic syndrome
            g. Thrombotic thrombocytopenic purpura
            h. Infantile pyknocytosis
            i. Acanthocytosis

On the other hand, in the majority of disorders resulting from extracorpuscular defects the abnormalities are not heritable but, at present, appear in one way or another to be *acquired*. Thus another classification of hemolytic anemias as "acquired" and "hereditary" has come into fairly common usage. As usually presented the two classifications obviously do not coincide and are not interchangeable.

HEMOLYTIC DISEASES CAUSED BY INTRACORPUSCULAR DEFECTS
Hereditary Spherocytosis[*]

CLINICAL MANIFESTATIONS AND LABORATORY FINDINGS. This is a heritable disease characterized by (a) acholuric jaundice; (b) erythrocytes that are spherocytic, abnormally fragile under osmotic

[*] Formerly and less properly termed congenital hemolytic jaundice.

stress, and intrinsically defective in metabolism or structure; (c) splenomegaly; and (d) a hemolytic process or anemia that varies considerably from patient to patient but which is (e) invariably abolished by splenectomy although the intrinsic red cell abnormality persists. The disease is generally concluded to be inherited as a single Mendelian dominant factor (260). However, almost every series reported contains deficiencies in the expected number of affected siblings and one or more families in which both parents of a proband and available relatives have no demonstrable abnormality on repeated testing (353). There is, however, no deficiency in the expected number of affected offspring of patients known to have the disease. Since the exceptions to the proposed single dominant mode of inheritance appear too numerous to be explained by mutations, the problem must be kept under continued study. There is no predilection by sex and although not racially restricted (49), the disease is most frequently seen in people of (northern) European origin.

The existence of the disease may be first suspected and recognized at any age —from newborn to 85 years—so its variability is evident (36, 42, 308). The diagnosis is usually made in any one individual because of studies pursuant to the findings of anemia, splenomegaly, jaundice, or gallstones. It may be established as an incidental finding on a routine examination or because of investigations undertaken relative to an affected member of the family. On the other hand, it may be arrived at because of severe anemia, jaundice, and/or splenomegaly in the newborn, or because of severe anemia associated with an infection and/or cholelithiasis at almost any age. Although occasionally severe, the anemia is usually mild; a well-compensated hemolytic process *without* anemia may be present (96). If severe anemia and jaundice become established at any time, they seem likely to persist until splenectomy is accomplished.*

There may be a history of gallstones (pigment stones), and intractable leg ulcers comparable to those seen in sickle cell anemia have been described (17). Accounts of transitory episodes of increased jaundice and signs and symptoms probably associated with lowered hemoglobin levels are usually difficult or impossible to interpret. Such episodes have, however, been documented as "hyperhemolytic" on rare occasions (57). Once the diagnosis is established, retrospective history elicited by direct questioning frequently reveals that from time to time relatives or friends have commented on yellow eyes and/or pallid skin, perhaps occurring following strenuous exercise or with excessive fatigue.

Cholelithiasis is reported to occur in up to 85 per cent of adults at some time during the course of the disease (13). Pigment stones have been found in children as young as 3 years of age, and the incidence progressively increases with age.

The physical findings vary according to the severity of the hemolytic process. Scleral icterus is usually present when carefully looked for, and the spleen is frequently readily palpable. It is probably invariably enlarged (500 to 2,000 Gm) but on unusual occasions not sufficiently enlarged to be palpable. Associated congenital abnormalities have been described but are unusual.

Examination of the peripheral blood by routine methods discloses a variable degree of anemia (if any) characterized by normocytic, "hyperchromic" indices (MCHC may be 37 to 40 per cent) and sustained reticulocytosis of 2 to 20 per

---

* The advisability of splenectomy in childhood and infancy has been questioned because of reported increases in incidence of severe infections after the operation. There are no adequate controls for the observations and the question remains unsettled (33, 103, 115, 182, 200, 236, 274, 303, 305).

cent, usually less than 10 per cent. Erythrocytes examined in a stained film of the peripheral blood show only slightly greater-than-normal variations in size and shape. The characteristic cell is, of course, the spherocyte. This cell is significantly smaller in diameter, appears thicker, and takes a more intense stain than the normal erythrocyte. Usually there is no evidence of central pallor or biconcavity. Although by convention it is called a microspherocyte since it covers a smaller-than-normal area in the blood film, because it is a thick cell its volume (CV) is normal. The extent of the cellular abnormality as determined by examination of the stained film of the peripheral blood varies considerably from individual to individual, from many obvious densely stained microspherocytes contrasting markedly with the macrocytic polychromatophilic cells to a very few discernible only after the diagnosis has otherwise been established. The leukocyte and platelet counts are within normal limits. Examination of the urine yields normal results. Even if the urine is more darkly pigmented than normal in association with rapid hemolysis, excessive urobilinogen and bile are not present unless there are hepatobiliary complications. The serum is icteric owing to an elevation of the unconjugated bilirubin fraction. All studies searching for extracorpuscular abnormalities (see pages 293 to 301) are negative. In individuals in whom a severe hemolytic process has become established early, skeletal changes may be detected by x-ray examination.

The history, physical signs, and laboratory findings outlined above are not unique to hereditary spherocytosis, but are also seen in other types of hemolytic disorders—various types of *acquired* hemolytic anemias or hereditary spherocytosis in association with another defect. Therefore, to make a definitive diagnosis and undertake treatment further studies must be done to certify the abnormality as hereditary spherocytosis and to exclude other factors.

Erythrocyte osmotic fragility test. The classic feature of this disease has been the presence in the peripheral blood of cells with abnormal geometric configurations —spherocytic erythrocytes, or more accurately, cells that in varying degrees are more nearly spheroidal and less distinctly disc-like than normal.* Various studies have demonstrated that a relation exists between the fragility of erythrocytes in hypotonic solutions and the geometric configurations of the cell (44, 145, 348). Under the conditions of the osmotic fragility test, there is essentially no exchange of electrolytes between the cell and its environment, and any changes are occasioned by the movement of water brought about by the osmotic characteristics of the cell relative to the suspending media. A normal red cell will, within limits, behave as a perfect osmometer and swell in a hypotonic medium, changing from its normal biconcave configuration until it has achieved a spherical form (121). At this stage the greatest volume is contained within the minimum surface area— a surface area actually equal to that of the formerly biconcave configuration. The membrane now behaves as though it were not elastic, and any further increase in volume induced by osmotic stress results in lysis, i.e., structural changes permitting leakage of hemoglobin and cell contents

---

* It should be pointed out that cells "more nearly spheroidal than normal" may be produced in a variety of ways. When exposed to hypotonic media, a normal cell will take in water and increase in size to become spherical; the MCV increases and the MCHC decreases; examined under the microscope the cell is a *macro*spherocyte. However, the cell of hereditary spherocytosis usually has a normal or low normal MCV and a higher-than-normal MCHC; examined under the microscope it is a *micro*spherocyte since it covers a smaller-than-normal area of the slide. This red cell of hereditary spherocytosis has become more nearly spheroidal in association with a decrease of surface area.

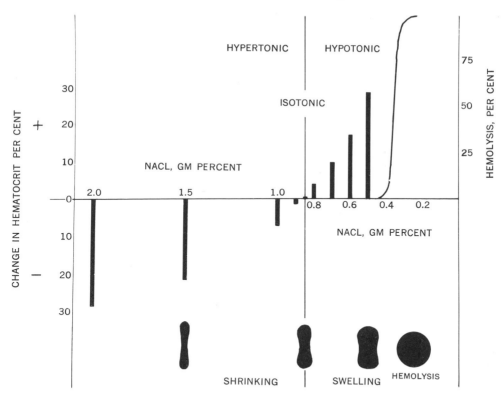

FIGURE 9.5. Behavior of normal cell in hyper- and hypotonic media. (From Castle, W. B., *in* Sodeman, W. A. (ed.), Pathologic Physiology: Mechanisms of Disease, ed. 3, p. 889, Saunders, Philadelphia, 1961)

(Figure 9.5). It is said that the membrane is "plastic but not elastic."* Susceptibility to hemolysis in hypotonic solutions is thus interpreted as a function of a cell's capacity to swell before reaching the critical spherical shape. This capacity would be less in a spheroidal than in a flat or biconcave cell. The decreased resistance to osmotic lysis seen in hereditary spherocytosis† is consistent with the observation that many of the cells are in a spherical or nearly spherical form in the circulating blood. Therefore, a classic confirmatory test for suspected hereditary spherocytosis has long been the demonstration of increased erythrocyte osmotic fragility. The red cells of the majority of patients with hereditary spherocytosis demonstrate an abnormally increased osmotic fragility (Figure 9.6); however, *in a small proportion of cases the osmotic fragility test yields results in the accepted normal range.*

The osmotic fragility test performed after sterile incubation of the blood sam-

* It should be remarked that this applies to the conditions of osmotic fragility as applied in the standard test. Here the osmotic stress is abrupt and extreme with minimum opportunity for electrolyte exchange between the cell and its altered environment. If osmotic hemolysis is induced by a gradual decrease in the ionic strength of the surrounding medium (76, 77), different results are obtained. The membrane is shown to be elastic to some extent, and the cell can continue to increase in size a small amount even after it has become spherical (169). Erythrocyte osmotic fragility is therefore dependent upon the gradient of osmotic pressure to which the cells are subjected and *also* on the rate of entry of water, lower rates of entry resulting in less hemolysis.

† Studies indicate that these cells also behave as perfect osmometers.

ple for 24 hours was introduced by Ham and Castle as a device to enhance a defect or uncover an otherwise latent abnormality. When normal red cells are sterilely incubated for 24 hours, they undergo metabolic changes that are not completely understood making them more fragile than previously.[*] This "shift" in osmotic fragility consequent to incubation has been quantitatively defined for the normal as shown in Figure 9.6 (92). In all instances of several large series, the osmotic behavior of the erythrocytes of hereditary spherocytosis became abnormal (more fragile than comparably treated normal erythrocytes, Figure 9.6) after the incubation procedure. As will be shown, erythrocytes in other hemolytic states may demonstrate a similar abnormality in this test so that by this means alone a positive diagnosis of hereditary spherocytosis cannot be made. However, if the described abnormality is *not* present, the diagnosis can be confidently excluded.

Another test that is subject to the same limitations and conditions relative to diagnostic interpretation is the determination of the erythrocyte mechanical fragility (255, 289). In this test a timed, standard amount of trauma (rolling glass beads) is inflicted upon a set volume of red cells contained in an Erlenmeyer flask. In the great majority of instances of hereditary spherocytosis so far reported the number of cells destroyed by this procedure has been greater than the established normal range, and 24 hours of sterile incubation enhances the abnormality.

The tests of erythrocyte osmotic and mechanical fragility can be employed to confirm or exclude a diagnosis but at this point must not be taken to indicate a specific red cell defect or to have specific pathophysiologic significance.

Autohemolysis test. Measurement of the amount of lysis occurring spontaneously when red cells are incubated sterilely for 48 hours at body temperature has been found useful in the investigation of certain hemolytic states (354). When normal cells are so treated, usually less than 6 per cent are lysed; this percentage is significantly decreased (to about 1 per cent) if glucose is added to the blood before incubation. Abnormally increased autohemolysis (about 20 per cent of cells) is most consistently demonstrated in hereditary spherocytosis but may also be found in other types of hemolytic disorders. The addition of glucose regularly causes marked reduction of autohemolysis in hereditary spherocytosis (hemolysis reduced to about 3 per cent; 206). Further studies and interpretation of the results in terms of possible defects in the erythrocyte of hereditary spherocytosis will be presented later. The results of this test correlate very closely with the

---

[*] Recent studies by Murphy (226) concerning the changes that occur during sterile incubation have shown that under controlled metabolic conditions the increase in erythrocyte osmotic fragility is directly correlated with loss of erythrocyte cholesterol. Erythrocyte cholesterol is ordinarily in equilibrium with free cholesterol in the serum. During incubation a heat-labile serum factor takes part in the esterification of the serum's free cholesterol, upsetting the cell-serum equilibrium so that cell cholesterol decreases. With this loss, the cell does not change in volume, but the surface area decreases, with consequent spheroidicity and increased osmotic fragility.

The changes in osmotic fragility, cell volume, and cation concentrations that ordinarily take place during the 24-hour incubation can be *prevented* if the serum is previously heated at 56°C for 30 minutes and the incubation performed at pH 7.5, reduced oxygen tension, sufficient glucose, and low hematocrit.

Erythrocytes incubated at pH 7.0 in heated serum or glucose-free heated serum show increased osmotic fragility, cation content, and cell volume, but *no* change in erythrocyte cholesterol. The increase in osmotic fragility associated with inhibition of glucose metabolism or following incubation with ouabain (to block active cation transport) occurs without change in erythrocyte cholesterol.

The complex changes that occur during incubation and result in increased osmotic fragility involve changes that occur in the serum as well as changes in the production and utilization of energy derived from glucose metabolism.

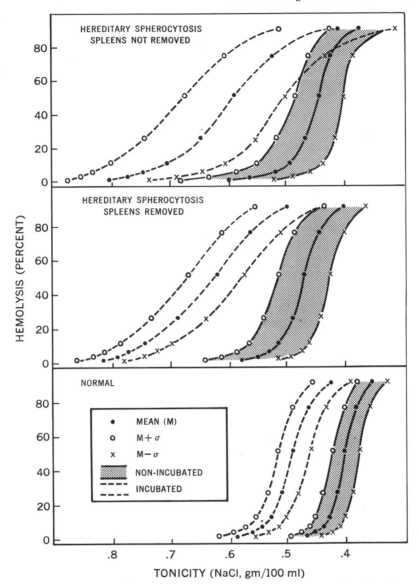

FIGURE 9.6.   Effect of incubation upon osmotic fragility of normal red cells and red cells of hereditary spherocytosis before and after splenectomy. (From Emerson, C. P., et al., A.M.A. Arch. Int. Med. 97:1, 1956)

results of the osmotic fragility test (especially the 24-hour incubation modification) in indicating the presence or absence of a cellular abnormality and are interpretable in much the same way.

CRITERIA FOR DIAGNOSIS. At present there is no one test upon which the diagnosis of hereditary spherocytosis can be certified; no unique structural, behavioral, or metabolic abnormality has been defined. Usually the diagnosis is obvious from the above-mentioned findings, but to prove it in a conclusive sense is elusive. The diagnosis becomes acceptable when the accumulation of positive evidence (familial, laboratory, clinical) and negative evidence (negative results on searching for antibodies and extracorpuscular lesions) becomes sufficient to be convincing.

MacKinney and coworkers (206) present a discussion concerning the problem of which tests are most valuable and how many of a group of selected tests are necessary to ascertain a diagnosis of hereditary spherocytosis in a situation where the disease is known to occur in the family under study. Their observations emphasize that there is no presently applicable test that cannot be perfectly mimicked by other forms of hemolytic anemia, but that once one acceptable diagnosis has been arrived at in a family by the usual constellation of positive and negative findings, various additional members can be determined as having or not having the disease usually on the basis of not more than four tests (spherocyte score, reticulocyte count, hemoglobin and bilirubin determinations). They find that these four tests account for 88 per cent of the variability between normal subjects and classic cases of hereditary spherocytosis.

LOCATION OF RED CELL DEFECT. Early clinical observations established that splenectomy consistently relieved the anemia and jaundice (288). A recent series of observations by Emerson (91) has clearly defined the *interdependence* of the intracorpuscular defect of hereditary spherocytosis and the spleen: the incompatibility of the cells and the spleen (Figure 9.7). Employing the Ashby technique and suitable cross transfusions, it was shown that normal cells survived normally in a patient with hereditary spherocytosis both before and after the spleen had been removed from the recipient. No abnormality existed that was either extracorpuscular or transferable from the patient's cells.* When erythrocytes were obtained from a patient with hereditary spherocytosis before splenectomy and again after the patient's spleen has been removed, the red cell survival time determined in one normal recipient was on both occasions abnormally short. An *intracorpuscular* abnormality was

thereby demonstrated that persisted despite the *absence* of the patient's spleen. When the erythrocytes from the patient with hereditary spherocytosis were transfused into a splenectomized recipient (normal except for post-traumatic splenectomy), the cell survival was prolonged and approached normal. Thus, for the intracorpuscular abnormality of hereditary spherocytosis to curtail the red cell life span, the presence of a (normal) spleen was necessary.

This series of observations concisely demonstrates in hereditary spherocytosis (a) the existence of a nontransferable intracorpuscular defect, (b) the absence of an extracorpuscular abnormality, and (c) the fact that spleen is required for abnormally rapid red cell destruction.

ROLE OF THE SPLEEN. The information lacking in the above study is due to the limitations of the Ashby technique, namely, the survival of the patient's cells in their natural habitat. When this information is added, it may be briefly stated that in hereditary spherocytosis the erythrocyte life span is decreased in a patient or a normal individual when the spleen is present; the life span is normal in a splenectomized patient or normal subject; and normal cells survive normally in a patient.

There is considerable additional evidence to indicate a specific interrelation and incompatibility between the erythrocyte of hereditary spherocytosis and the spleen (340). Pursuing the observation that remarkably little blood oozed from the cut surface of a spleen freshly removed from a patient with hereditary spherocytosis, Dacie attempted to clear out the red cells by saline perfusion. It

---

* Earlier workers had considered all or part of the abnormal hemolysis of hereditary spherocytosis to be due to "hypersplenism." These present studies clearly demonstrate the *absence* of any abnormal splenic function with respect to normal cells, and, moreover, show that the patient's spleen functions as does a normal spleen relative to the cells of hereditary spherocytosis.

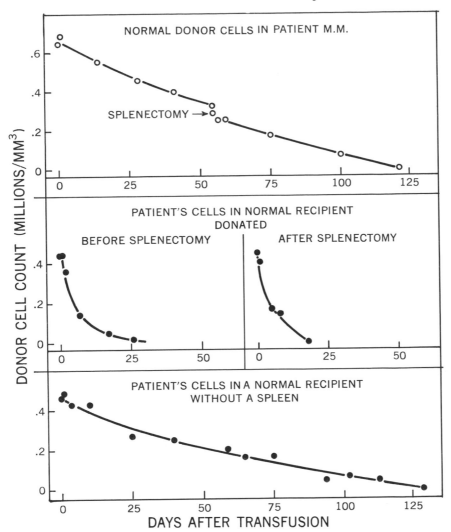

FIGURE 9.7.   Determination of red cell survival time in various circumstances, demonstrating incompatibility of the cells of hereditary spherocytosis and the spleen. (From Emerson, C. P., Boston Med. Quart. 5:65, 1954)

proved to be readily possible to remove normal cells from normal spleens by perfusion but impossible to achieve comparable results with specimens from patients with hereditary spherocytosis. Young (353) showed that if a normal spleen was perfused with a mixture of cells obtained from a normal donor and a patient with hereditary spherocytosis, the abnormal cells were selectively removed from the mixture and retained by the spleen. In vivo counterparts are avail-

able to give more physiologic significance to these in vitro observations. Following the radioactive labeling of erythrocytes from a patient with hereditary spherocytosis, directional tracking by collimated counters indicates that the abnormal cells are selectively removed from the circulating blood by the spleen and retained therein when the blood is either reinfused into the patient or transfused into a normal recipient.

But the spleen cannot simply continue

to trap and retain the abnormal erythrocytes without something giving way somewhere. Measurements of the bilirubin content of splenic vein blood show the values to be significantly higher than in the peripheral blood. Destruction of red cells and hemoglobin degradation must be occurring in the spleen at rates of considerable magnitude. The several lines of investigation concerning the precise mechanisms whereby this is brought about provide interesting evidence.

It is clear that the abnormal cells of hereditary spherocytosis are selectively removed from the circulation by the spleen and therein destroyed. Since splenectomy results in permanent cessation of the abnormal hemolysis, cell destruction must be dependent upon the peculiar structure and circulation of the spleen and its relation to the abnormal cell.

STRUCTURE AND CIRCULATION OF THE SPLEEN.* Blood enters through the splenic artery, which promptly branches into the trabecular arteries. These leave the trabeculae and enter the white pulp as central arteries. From the white pulp the blood flows through the red pulp, which, with a hand lens, may be recognized as made up almost entirely of (a) small cucumber-shaped spaces (blood vessels called splenic sinuses or sinusoids) and (b) thin plates or partitions that lie between the sinuses (blood-containing tissues called splenic cords or Billroth's cords). From the red pulp the blood is collected into veins, which then enter the trabeculae and join at the hilum to form the splenic vein. There has been considerable disagreement concerning the so-called intermediate circulation of the spleen; the connections to the splenic sinuses and cords; and whether the circulation is open, closed, or mixed (27, 174, 307, 344). However, the recent studies by Weiss and coworkers (56, 341, 342) employing electron microscopic techniques constitute most valuable contributions to this problem and necessitate a re-evaluation of the findings obtained by usual fixation and light microscopy for both normal splenic circulation and that of hereditary spherocytosis (347). For example, empty splenic sinuses, described as typical of hereditary spherocytosis, are not seen by electron microscopy and are probably artifacts of conventional fixation techniques.

There are no cells known to be unique to the spleen; classic morphologic techniques and electron microscopy indicate that all the cells contained in the spleen are present in various other areas of the body but in dissimilar architectural arrangement. Consequently the structure of the spleen and the relation of the peculiar structure to function is of paramount interest.

The central artery of the white pulp gives rise to branches which often take off at right angles to the main stem, and some of these appear to contain only plasma so that it is possible that in these vessels some partition of cells and plasma takes place. Moreover, the central artery and its branches have a cuboidal or even columnar endothelium, which may partly or completely impede the flow of corpuscles. These branches of the central arteries continue into (a) the white pulp, where they terminate as capillaries; (b) the red pulp; and (c) the marginal zone, where they empty into the transitional tissue between white and red pulp. Most of the arterial terminations in the spleen end in the marginal zone (a large vascular space transitional between white and red pulp) by funnel-shaped orifices or by direct opening into a sinus of the red pulp that comes directly into the marginal zone. The cords of the red pulp are directly continuous with this marginal zone.

The red pulp is virtually entirely made up of two vascular structures, the splenic

* The material contained in this section is largely taken, by permission, from a privately printed syllabus, Notes on the Spleen, by Leon Weiss, 1961.

sinuses and cords. The sinuses are composed of living cells and a basement membrane. They are long (several hundred micra), tortuous vascular channels of large but variable diameter (40 to 50 μ), which represent the first collecting venous vessels in the spleen. The lining cells are elongate reticular cells flattened to endothelial form. Since they are oriented to the long axes of the sinus, in cross section they appear cuboidal in shape. The luminal surface is made highly irregular by delicate and variable cytoplasmic projections and gaps between lining cells. Blood cells are often seen traversing the sinus walls. Occasionally a lining cell is absent, leaving an even larger gap in the wall. The basement membrane is reduced to reticular strands that present a well-developed latticed appearance. Defects in the continuity of the endothelium and small apertures through the entire sinus wall are common. By almost insensible transition the sinuses become tributaries to the veins of the red pulp, which empty into trabecular veins that are made up of typical squamous endothelium, unperforated basement membrane, etc. Some sinuses may contain a disproportionate volume of plasma; others may be packed with white cells.

The cords of Billroth lie between the sinuses. They are also lined by reticular cells and share a basement membrane with the contiguous sinus. Passing across splenic cords and sinuses, the following sequence will be found: sinus lumen, sinus endothelium, fenestrated basement membrane, cord endothelium, cord lumen, cord endothelium, fenestrated basement membrane, sinus endothelium, sinus lumen, etc. The cords often contain blood, and most arterial vessels not opening into the marginal zone open into the cords. They are regarded as vascular spaces, since they receive blood and are lined by a cell characteristic of certain blood vessels. Slender reticular fibers span the lumen of the cords, dividing it up rather regularly into openly communicating compartments. The reticular lining cells of the cords tend to be much flatter than those of the sinuses. These cord cells appear to become phagocytic more readily than the sinus endothelium, and the cords may appear as a pure tissue of macrophages filled with damaged red cells.

The cords communicate with the sinuses through the endothelial gaps and the fenestrated basement membrane. The communications may be 2 to 3 μ in diameter or even larger. The cords then are vascular spaces capable of receiving a great volume of the splenic arterial blood. They may sequester cells and permit the transformation of lymphocytes and monocytes into plasma cells and macrophages. The cords are in communication with the marginal zone and with the sinuses.

After distributing branches to the white pulp, red pulp, and marginal zone, the central artery continues into the red pulp as the artery of the red pulp. This vessel may branch into several slender vessels called *penicilli*, which may terminate as such or form the finer arterial capillaries. Because of a high endothelium, the lumen of these vessels is often absent or virtually absent. A basement membrane is present but usually incomplete. Almost all the terminal arterial capillaries are enveloped in an elliptical or cylindrical sheath of closely packed phagocytic cells and reticular fibers—the sheaths of Schweigger-Seidel. These possess a remarkable ability to take up particulate or colloidal material. In the red pulp proper almost all the terminal vessels end in the cords; very few have direct connections with the sinuses.

The normal paths of circulation through the spleen are not known with certainty, and indeed it seems likely that the pathways are in a dynamic state of change, with sinuses, cords, and marginal zone functioning differently in different areas of the organ. Thus, for example, some sinuses may contain little other than plasma, some many macrophages, and others the usual blood cells.

The red pulp in the human being is an enormous vascular bed of splenic sinuses and splenic cords that constitute the intermediate blood vessels of the spleen. They may be patent or collapsed in varying degrees, share common walls, or communicate with one another through anastomotic apertures. So constructed, the red pulp is able to concentrate the formed elements of the blood and the plasma itself: to retain selectively rigid particles in excess of a certain diameter or a particular type of cell. For example, studies by Weiss (341) following the intra-arterial injection of starch granules of known dimensions showed that 81 per cent of the granules with a diameter of 5 μ were retained in the sinuses, whereas only 5 per cent of the granules 1 μ in diameter were retained by the sinus walls (see also reference 27).

Studies concerning the intrasplenic biochemical environment of the erythrocytes are preliminary and fragmentary. They indicate the existence of blood-containing spaces in the spleen which are not in equilibrium with the arteriovenous system.* That the concentration of glucose in the splenic vein is higher than that in the blood derived from spleen itself speaks for fast-circulating by-passes in the spleen (258). Other observations indicate that the hematocrit is markedly increased, the pH decreased, lactic acid content increased four times that of the venous blood, and the carbon dioxide–combining power only 50 per cent that of venous blood (226). All these changes point to an environment predictably *unfavorable* for the erythrocyte. However, by techniques so far reported, red cells from the splenic artery and vein differ only slightly in chemical content (diphosphoglycerate, inorganic phosphate, ATP, total lipids, cholesterol) from cells obtained from the cut surface of the freshly

excised spleen; the latter do have a slightly increased total sodium and potassium cation content (258).

There is no question that the spleen so constructed can selectively remove from circulation and sequester the abnormal erythrocytes of hereditary spherocytosis. The mechanism by which this is done is not clear. It has been proposed that because of its shape (especially thickness), the spheroidal cell cannot pass through specific splenic structures and apertures, particularly since it cannot be as easily distorted as a normal discoidal cell. The millipore filter, for example, prevents the passage of spheroidal cells (160). There is similar in vivo and in vitro evidence that selection and sequestration of other abnormal erythrocytes occurs because of shape, size, agglutination, or rigidity. Studies by Paolino (243) showed that even the reticulocytes of patients with hereditary spherocytosis were somewhat increased in thickness as compared with normal reticulocytes. Thus, one theory proposed that spheroidicity per se was essential to the mechanism of sequestration.

Spheroidal cells are undoubtedly sequestered by the spleen, but although this is a major factor in the decreased survival time of the erythrocytes of hereditary spherocytosis, it is unlikely that spheroidicity itself is the entire story and it is not necessarily the initial critical determinant. Prankerd (258) studied a patient with hereditary spherocytosis whose cells demonstrated no increase in their unincubated osmotic fragility. Although subsequently destroyed in the spleen, these cells were not at first delayed in passage or sequestered by the spleen. Spherocytic, osmotically fragile cells from another patient were initially delayed in passage, were sequestered, and had a similarly

---

* Studies in dogs (300) using S^{35}-labeled sulfate and I^{131} iodinated albumin to evaluate extracellular space versus vascular space supply evidence for a functional closed circulation in the spleen.

shortened life span (131). Normal erythrocytes, heat-treated to produce comparable spheroidicity and osmotic fragility changes, were delayed in initial passage through the spleen but thereafter survived normally. In addition, there has been no good correlation in this disease between osmotic fragility and spheroidicity on the one hand and rate of red cell destruction. Accordingly investigations have been undertaken attempting to demonstrate abnormalities other than geometric that might place the cell at a disadvantage in terms of survival ability.

RESULTS OF SPLENECTOMY. The erythrocytes of patients with hereditary spherocytosis remain abnormal after splenectomy, as is clearly shown by their shortened survival time when transfused into a normal recipient. Splenectomy then does *not* abolish the intracorpuscular defect. Examination of the peripheral blood after operation shows normal hemoglobin and reticulocyte concentration and a normal hematocrit; the total bilirubin content is within normal limits as is the result of the van den Bergh partition. But the cells are still *abnormally spherocytic* and retain their *abnormal osmotic and mechanical fragility* characteristics. The persistence of these measurable defects provides some insight into the pathophysiology of cell destruction. Since cells with abnormally increased osmotic and mechanical fragility can survive normally in a splenectomized patient or subject, the mechanism of cell destruction cannot depend solely on these characteristics. The buffeting about which the mechanically fragile cell receives in the circulation exclusive of the spleen does not prematurely disrupt it. The osmotic stresses the fragile cell endures in the circulation exclusive of the spleen are not sufficient to lyse it. This is the reason it was formerly stated that the abnormal results of these tests must not be used at this point to indicate other than the existence of an abnormal cell; specifically they are not to

be interpreted in terms of a mechanism of cell destruction. It is only in combination with unique splenic functions that such pathophysiologic interpretations may be essayed. The mechanism of abnormal blood destruction in hereditary spherocytosis must be investigated by studying the function of the spleen relative to the abnormal red cell.

PROGRESSIVE CONDITIONING OF CELLS. Careful examination of precisely plotted erythrocyte osmotic fragility curves in hereditary spherocytosis prior to splenectomy reveals that in most patients the pattern is asymmetric and biphasic (Figure 9.8), with a portion of the cell population (10 to 20 per cent) exhibiting marked increase in susceptibility to lysis. Following splenectomy the osmotic fragility curve becomes symmetrical and monophasic owing to the rapid (2 to 3 days) elimination of the highly abnormal cells from the peripheral blood. Based on the cross-transfusion survival time studies outlined earlier in this chapter, it is reasonable to presume that the cell types produced by the marrow are the same postoperatively as preoperatively. Granting this, the highly abnormal cell fragility must have resulted from red cell–spleen interaction. When the mechanical and osmotic fragility characteristics of the intrasplenic erythrocytes are determined (by postoperative recovery from minced spleen), these cells are found to be more grossly abnormal than the erythrocytes in the peripheral blood. A large proportion of the population (70 per cent and greater) is extremely fragile. This is not observed except in trace amounts when normal cells are recovered postoperatively from minced spleen. These changes have been demonstrated to take place in the abnormal erythrocyte of hereditary spherocytosis and not in the normal erythrocyte by means of cross transfusions between patients with hereditary spherocytosis and subjects with normal spleens. Thus, the spleen pulp invariably contains

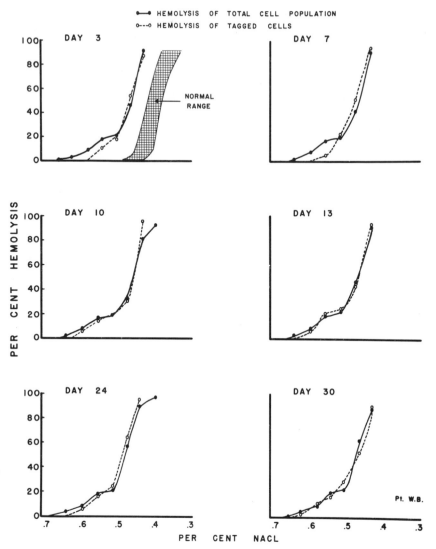

FIGURE 9.8.   Progressive increase in osmotic fragility related to in vivo erythrocyte aging in hereditary spherocytosis. (From Griggs, R. C., et al., J. Clin. Invest. 39:89, 1960)

not only a higher proportion of abnormal cells (selective trapping) but also cells with more abnormal osmotic and mechanical fragility than is observed in the peripheral blood cells.

These extreme changes are regarded as evidence that the cells have been sequestered and held in a deleterious environment, a process to which the term "conditioning" has been applied. That such changes in erythrocyte osmotic and

mechanical fragility do take place in vivo has been demonstrated recently in hereditary spherocytosis.

By means of radioactive iron an identifiable phalanx or cohort of newly formed red cells of very restricted age span was tagged so that cell characteristics could be followed as the group aged (119). By external counting it was possible to track the cells during their stay in the vascular system. The osmotic fragility of the *newly formed* cells was demonstrated to be similar to that of the majority of the unlabeled peripheral erythrocytes, but none of the labeled cells was as fragile as some of the "conditioned" (more markedly fragile) cells of the peripheral blood. As cells aged, a progressive increase in osmotic and mechanical fragility occurred in a portion of the population until in 10 days the labeled cells demonstrated the same asymmetrically abnormal osmotic fragility curve as the cells of the peripheral blood. During this time a build-up of radioactivity occurred over the spleen area indicating sequestration. It is not known how long the cells are retained in the spleen for conditioning (or destruction) or what proportion is released from the spleen to show up in the peripheral blood as the markedly fragile, conditioned cells. Observations on the survival of cells recovered from the spleen indicate that the conditioned cells have a very short life span even in a spleenless circulation. There is, therefore, in vivo evidence that in patients with hereditary spherocytosis a significant proportion of the red cells is sequestered and conditioned in the spleen over a period of days. Some are destroyed in the spleen giving rise to the increased splenic vein bilirubin, some are released back to the peripheral blood as the markedly fragile cells destined for rapid destruction or perhaps reprocessing by the spleen giving rise to a continuous daily production of cells with increased spheroidicity.

It is thus possible to define in a fairly quantitative fashion the *circumstances* of the erythrocyte-spleen interaction that are necessary for the abnormally rapid red cell destruction demonstrated in hereditary spherocytosis. But what exactly happens to a red cell during conditioning by the trapping and sequestering spleen is not known. In hereditary spherocytosis there is a notable lack of evidence indicating phagocytosis or antibody-complement lysis. If osmotic or mechanical

fragility played a role of significant magnitude in intravascular lysis, an increase in extracellular hemoglobin in the peripheral blood would be expected, but is not found. Measurements of haptoglobin levels yield significantly subnormal values. The significance of this finding is obscure, however, since the level is also depressed in other situations where extravascular hemolysis is presumed to exist. There is no information concerning the presence of these factors in splenic effluent, but to account for the rate of destruction sometimes seen, the spleen would have to possess an enormous efficiency for processing and degrading free hemoglobin, something it does not possess in other situations known to be accompanied by intravascular hemolysis. Because of this, observations have been made concerning enzyme activities and erythrocyte metabolism in hereditary spherocytosis.

AUTOHEMOLYSIS. As outlined above, the observations of Ham and Castle demonstrated that during 24 hours of sterile incubation normal cells become progressively more susceptible to osmotic lysis; in the same procedure the cells of hereditary spherocytosis become significantly more susceptible to osmotic lysis than the normal. During the first 24 hours of incubation, there is an influx of sodium and a lesser efflux of potassium so that a net gain of electrolytes and water occurs. Swelling of the cells of hereditary spherocytosis occurs at about the same rate as normal, but hemolysis occurs earlier in the incubation. Dacie (72) showed that during a second 24-hour period of incubation both types of cells *shrank* to approximately their original volumes but that during this period the cells of hereditary spherocytosis underwent lysis some five to ten times more rapidly than normal cells. He concluded that the lysis was due to a "defective cell membrane" which underwent "degenerative and irreversible shrinkage" more rapidly than normal.

It was then observed that the "autohemolysis"—lysis occurring during sterile incubation—could be markedly reduced by the addition of glucose. Subsequent observations showed that the glucose effect could be blocked by fluoride or iodoacetate and that adenosine and guanosine substantially reduced autohemolysis. Since abnormal behavior had been found in the cells of hereditary spherocytosis by this test, numerous studies were undertaken into the various pathways by which the erythrocyte provides energy for self-maintenance.

BIOCHEMISTRY OF THE SPHEROCYTE. Concerning possible biochemical abnormalities, it has been known for some time that the hemoglobin concentration is frequently higher than normal and that the potassium and water content is diminished (156, 256). More recently it has been demonstrated that although the sodium concentration is normal, the rate of sodium turnover is high (21). These alterations, plus the effect of glucose upon abnormal autohemolysis, have directed attention to glucose metabolism in the hereditary spherocyte. The over-all rates of glucose consumption and phosphate exchange were found to be normal, but the movement of phosphates into the various intermediates was distinctly different from the normal (315). In some of the studies the addition of adenosine reverted the alteration toward normal. However, the interpretation of these findings is unclear at present since there is no agreement concerning the size of the pool of intermediates (ATP, ADP, 2, 3-phosphoglycerate, and inorganic phosphate), a factor which could, of course, alter the P^{32} distribution in the compartments. Tanaka (318) has recently reported that all intermediates of the Embden-Meyerhof pathway, as well as G-6-PD and enolase, are normally active or increased in activity.

Surprisingly little work has been done concerning the structure and composition of the red cell stroma. In 1937 Erikson studied the cell lipids from four patients with hereditary spherocytosis and found a significant deficiency. This finding has more recently been interpreted as correlating with the reduced surface area of the spherocyte, and the suggestion has been made that during maturation there is a disproportionately great loss or deficient replacement of the materials that compose the cellular surface so that the characteristic microspherocyte results. It is now clear that many erythrocyte phospholipids are in a dynamic exchange with plasma components and that the mechanism of exchange is dependent upon the metabolism of the erythrocyte itself, specifically its glucose utilization (265). Since a specific enzymatic defect has not been established for the red cell of hereditary spherocytosis, it has been suggested that there is a defective tie-up between the normally produced energy and the lipid exchange that is important to the integrity of the red cell (265). The recent report of Allison (5), purporting to show a block in the production of phosphatidyl ethanolamine with consequent decrease in this compound and increase in a precursor compound, lysophosphatidyl ethanolamine, capable of inducing spherocytosis of normal cells, is provocative but has not been reproduced by the studies of Phillips and Roome (249a), who found no abnormality employing methods to avoid possible methodologic difficulties that might have given rise to Allison's results.

SUMMARY. In attempting to give an account of the mechanism of cell destruction in hereditary spherocytosis, it is well to start with the conclusion firmly based on the sound evidence obtained from determination of erythrocyte survival times: namely, that the abnormal degree of red cell destruction seen in hereditary spherocytosis is dependent upon a specific interrelation and incompatibility between the intrinsically defective erythrocyte and the spleen. The striking findings are that following splenectomy the abnormal hemolysis is relieved, the erythrocyte survival time returns to within the normal (or very nearly normal) range, and this occurs *despite* the persistence of the primary intrinsic cellular abnormalities—be they metabolic or structural. These metabolic and structural abnormalities cannot therefore be, by themselves, held accountable for the cell destruction. The crucial point of the pathophysiology of this disease is the relation of the abnormal erythrocyte of hereditary spherocytosis to the spleen.

Since Prankerd's work does not support the concept that the abnormal geometric configuration of the hereditary spherocyte is the factor initially responsible for progressive damage and eventual cell destruction, and since the hereditary spherocyte is known to be abnormally susceptible to glucose deprivation because of either metabolic or structural deviations, the following sequence has been proposed (160). A *randomly* selected minor population of erythrocytes is subjected to repetitive episodes of glucose deprivation in the "sluggishly flowing backwaters" of the spleen, where even minor metabolic or structural deviations would be expected to invoke significant physiologic disadvantages over the normal. By this means a minor population of erythrocytes is continuously generated that becomes progressively more and more spheroidal during several days of circulation. These cells have been "conditioned" by the spleen. It is clear that *these* are the cells now susceptible to selective (not random) removal from the peripheral circulation and sequestration by the spleen; it is likely but not completely necessary* that the selection of the spheroidal cell is determined by the biophysical characteristics of the cell per se (its spheroidal shape), but the possibility exists that selection and sequestration may in addition or alternatively be brought about by its biochemical charac-

teristics. This sequestration by the spleen leads to the final events responsible for cell destruction. These are still unknown.

Primaquine-sensitive Hemolytic Anemia†

GENETIC MECHANISMS AND DISTRIBUTION. Formerly, hemolytic anemias associated with drug or chemical administration were classified among the extracorpuscular abnormalities. In the past few years, however, evidence has accumulated that establishes the existence of a previously unknown type of intrinsic abnormality of the red cell—an enzyme abnormality that is usually harmless unless the cell is exposed to one of many otherwise nontoxic agents. Although demonstrably abnormal on specific testing, the erythrocytes of such an affected individual function and survive adequately unless challenged by the administration of a specific agent, at which point destruction of the sensitive cell (hemolysis) occurs.†† Since this type of cell destruction was first clearly described in association with the administration of the antimalarial agent, primaquine, the designation "primaquine-sensitive hemolytic anemia" has come into general use. It is now used as a generic term for the hemolytic process produced in susceptible individuals by a growing list of chemical agents. The phenotypic designation primaquine-sensitive should probably be retained in preference to glucose-6-phosphate dehydrogenase deficiency until the basic biochemical and genetic defect is established.

* Jacob and Jandl (148), for example, have reported that cells treated with a nonhemolyzing, nonsphering amount of sulfhydryl-blocking agents are removed from circulation by the spleen; splenectomy results in a thirtyfold increase in cell survival.
† Also called glucose-6-phosphate dehydrogenase (G-6-PD) deficiency.
†† This situation is not too dissimilar from that seen in hereditary spherocytosis; the erythrocyte, although demonstrably abnormal by fragility and chemical tests, functions and survives adequately in an asplenic circulation.

Although it had long been known that an acute hemolytic process might result in some individuals from exposure to ordinarily nontoxic drugs, it was usually concluded that such a reaction was due to individual "idiosyncrasy" or "hypersensitivity." Following the more detailed delineation of the abnormalities associated with primaquine-sensitive hemolytic anemia, they were found to have, first, a racial predilection and, more recently, a familial tendency with a specific pattern of inheritance (53). It is, therefore, proper to designate this as another example of an inborn error of metabolism. Various in vitro tests have been used to determine the presence (and to some degree the extent) of the intracorpuscular defect. The available evidence indicates the mode of inheritance to be a sex-linked gene with intermediate dominance. Thus the *homo*zygous female, (X) (X), and the *hemi*zygous male, (X)Y, show full expression, while the *hetero*zygous female, (X)X, shows only an intermediate expression of the abnormality.* However, it is apparent that the in vitro tests currently employed do not necessarily and invariably yield a basis for accurate prediction of in vivo hemolysis following the administration of a suitable drug, so that final determination of the mode of genetic transmittance must await more definitive genetic, biochemical, and phenotypic data.

The trait responsible for the development of primaquine-sensitive hemolytic anemia is ubiquitous. Since the number of drugs capable of substituting for primaquine is considerable and growing, and since they are frequently employed, a large volume of case reports has accumulated in a relatively short span of time. The incidence of the trait varies in racial and ethnic groups and among Caucasians is roughly related to the degree of skin pigmentation. In Caucasians of non-Mediterranean origin the incidence is less than 1 per cent; among Kurdish Jews the incidence is approximately 60 per cent. It is estimated that the defect probably affects more than 100 million people (!) throughout the world. Like sickle cell disease and thalassemia, it seems to confer the biologic advantage of mitigating the severity and decreasing the mortality of malaria due to *Plasmodium falciparum* in infants and young children (6, 54).

In the American Negro acute hemolysis that may destroy half the circulating red cells in a few days occurs in 10 to 15 per cent of males and 1 to 2 per cent of females given test doses of primaquine; intermediate degrees of hemolysis can be expected in an additional 16 to 18 per cent of females.

COURSE OF THE HEMOLYTIC REACTION. In an otherwise healthy individual the clinical course of the hemolytic reaction is fairly consistent when 30 mg of primaquine base is administered (Figure 9.9).

Acute hemolytic phase. No sign of hemolysis becomes evident until 1 to 3 days after the first dose of the drug. Unlike immunologic sensitivity, the latent period is the same whether the drug is being administered for the first or subsequent time. Early in the onset of hemolysis Heinz bodies (101) appear in many of the red cells; these are coccoid-appearing bodies not visible in the blood film prepared with Wright's stain but readily demonstrable with supravital techniques ("wet" preparations) using crystal blue, crystal violet, etc. Later in the process they are not found. After 2 or 3 days of drug administration, the urine begins to darken. Specific tests show evidence of increased red cell destruction with falling

---

* Beutler et al. (25) have applied the "mosaic" hypothesis to the heterozygous female to suggest the intriguing possibility of the presence of two genetically different red cell populations, one normal and one deficient in G-6-PD. However, analysis of survival curves of DFP[32]-labeled erythrocytes during primaquine-induced hemolysis (32) was interpreted as showing no cell behavior comparable to that of controls, so that all erythrocytes were thought to be involved in the genetic defect.

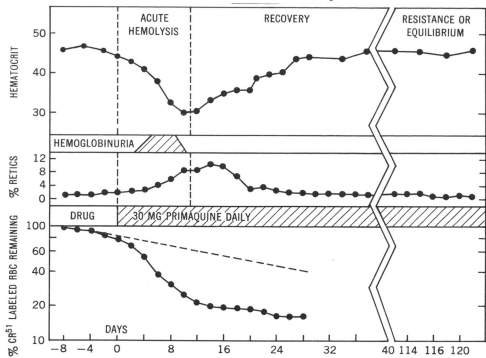

FIGURE 9.9.   Course of experimentally induced hemolytic anemia in primaquine-sensitive individual. (From Alving, A. S., et al., Bull. World Health Organ. 22:621, 1960)

hemoglobin concentration and hematocrit, increased plasma and urine hemoglobin, decreased plasma haptoglobin, and increased methemalbuminemia. The plasma bilirubin content increases more gradually (van den Bergh partition shows approximately equal distribution of conjugated and unconjugated bilirubin), and clinical icterus may become evident. The hemoglobin depression becomes most severe by the eighth to twelfth day. Systemic symptoms may be absent or the patient may feel weak and complain of abdominal or back pain; the sclerae may become icteric and the urine nearly black.

Recovery phase. After 7 to 10 days, *despite continued administration of the drug*, hematologic recovery begins with reticulocytosis and elevation of hemoglobin and hematocrit. The patient feels better, the urine color returns to normal, and the clinical icterus subsides. A normal peripheral blood picture is re-established.

Equilibrium phase. Even though drug administration is continued at the same dose level, there is no anemia or acute hemolysis. However, specific tests demonstrate a shortened survival of the patient's erythrocytes and increased erythropoiesis compensating for the increased destruction. A compensated hemolytic process is present. If, at this point, the dose of the drug is increased, a new episode of acute hemolysis is brought on, followed by recovery and a new level of equilibrium between increased destruction and production evidenced by a further decrease in erythrocyte life span and a further increase in erythropoiesis (171). If drug administration is stopped, hemolysis continues in lessening degrees for 36 to 56 hours and a new hemolytic process will not be initiated by readministering the same dose until a few weeks have elapsed beween stopping and restarting the agent.

AGENTS CAPABLE OF INDUCING HEMOLYSIS. Over forty drugs are now known to produce somewhat comparable processes in sensitive individuals (Figure 9.10). A partial list of the most commonly incriminated includes *antimalarials* like primaquine and quinine; *sulfonamides* such as sulfanilamide, sulfamethoxypyridazine (Kynex, Midicel), and sulfisoxazole (Gantrisin); *nitrofurans* like nitrofurantoin (Furadantin) and nitrofurazone (Furacin); *antipyretics and analgesics* like aspirin, acetophenetidin (Phenacitin); *sulfone* like sulfoxone (Diasone); and *other compounds* such as naphthalene, acetylphenylhydrazine, vitamin K, quinidine. In general, sulfonamide, sulfone, benzene, and quinoline derivatives are potentially toxic.

LABORATORY FINDINGS. When not challenged by drug administration, the sensitive individual has a normal peripheral blood count and red cell indices. Cellular morphology is normal in the stained film of the peripheral blood. The hemoglobin migration is normal on electrophoresis, and the erythrocytes show a normal mechanical fragility and a slightly increased resistance to osmotic stress (a *decreased* osmotic fragility). No cellular or circulating antibodies are demonstrable. Recent studies (30) reveal a shortened life span of the sensitive cell (95 to 110 days as opposed to 110 to 120 days for normal cells in the same environment), approximately a 25 per cent shorter span even in

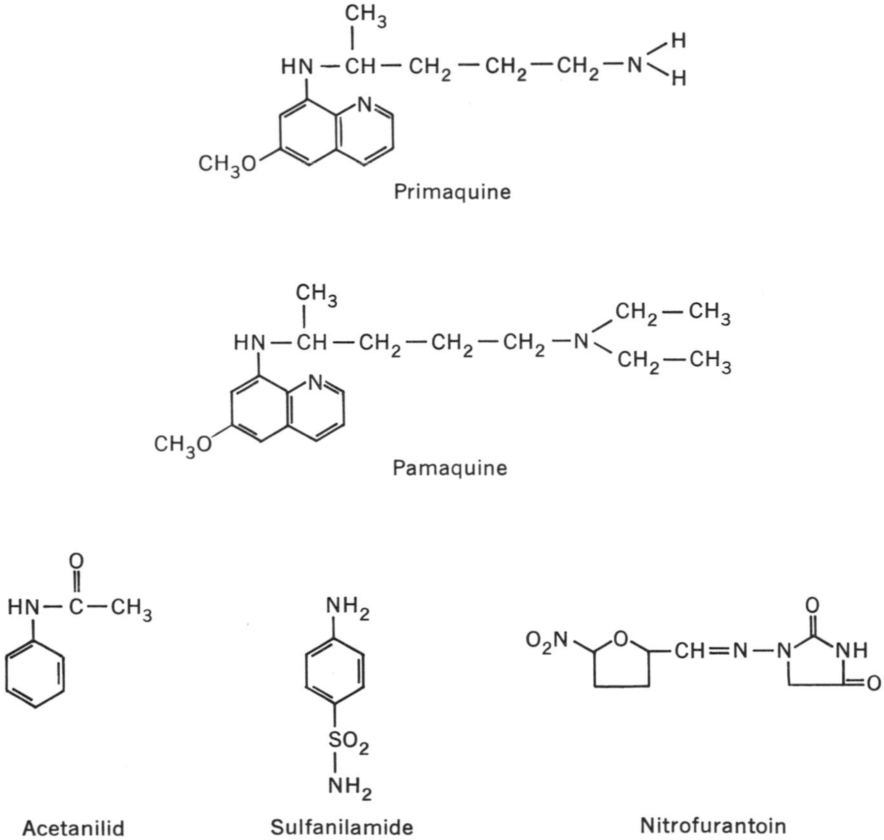

Primaquine

Pamaquine

Acetanilid   Sulfanilamide   Nitrofurantoin

FIGURE 9.10.   Types of compounds involved in production of hemolysis in primaquine-sensitive individuals. (From Beutler, E., *in* Stanbury, J. B., et al. (ed.), The Metabolic Basis of Inherited Disease, p. 1031, McGraw-Hill, New York, 1960)

the *absence* of drug administration. Thus a chronic compensated hemolytic process is present.

LOCATION OF RED CELL DEFECT. Basic cross-transfusion studies have localized the fundamental defect responsible for red cell lysis in the red cell itself: an intrinsic red cell abnormality. Red cells from sensitive individuals were labeled with Cr^{51} and transfused into normal recipients. The labeled cells survived adequately until primaquine was administered to the recipients. Rapid destruction of the donor cells was thereafter demonstrated. That the spleen plays no essential role in this hemolytic process is shown by the lack of accumulation of radioactivity over the splenic area during the rapid destruction of a large portion of erythrocytes and the rapid destruction of sensitive red cells in a splenectomized recipient receiving primaquine. When Cr^{51}-labeled cells from a normal donor were transfused into a sensitive individual, they survived normally despite the administration of primaquine and the development of a hemolytic process due to the destruction solely of the patient's own erythrocytes. The sensitivity to primaquine is nontransferable, is not due to abnormal metabolism of the drug or the development of immune mechanisms by sensitive individuals, but rather resides in the cell itself regardless of its environment.

But what of the self-limited nature of the disease as revealed by the "recovery phase" that occurs despite the continued administration of primaquine? It has been demonstrated by cross-transfusion studies using Cr^{51} that a sensitive individual in the recovery phase subsequent to a hemolytic episode retains an undiminished capacity to destroy transfused sensitive cells from another donor. Moreover, the red cells of such an individual in the recovery phase are not sensitive to the same dose of primaquine even when circulating in a recipient who had never previously been given the drug. There-

fore the change in reactivity of the red cell cannot be due to altered metabolism of primaquine leading to the recovery phase but rather, again, to changes in the cell population itself regardless of its environment.

By means of radioactive iron, a restricted population of cells of narrow age range was labeled and its reactivity to primaquine followed during the aging of this phalanx of tagged red cells. Young cells were found to be relatively resistant to the hemolytic action of primaquine; older cells were demonstrated to be highly sensitive.

Based on these observations the events occurring during the hemolytic and recovery phase can be reconstructed. When the drug is first administered, the older portion of the red cell population is most sensitive and is destroyed rapidly over the course of some 7 days. At the end of this time only the younger, relatively insensitive cells remain. These, of course, age and become susceptible of destruction but this occurs at a rate not exceeding normal. The new cells produced by the bone marrow in increased numbers in response to the anemia are also insensitive until they become some 60 days old. This acquisition of sensitivity is such a gradual process that it is *clinically* imperceptible and is compensated for by the increased bone marrow activity. Hence the terms recovery and equilibrium phase are used. If the dose of the drug is increased, a larger proportion of the cells are affected and the drug can reach further back, so to speak, into the otherwise less susceptible younger cells to effect destruction.

Here then is indisputable evidence that the administration of a drug to a susceptible patient induces a hemolytic process because of an intrinsic cellular abnormality that becomes manifest during the latter portion of the red cell life span so that only the older erythrocytes are susceptible to abnormal destruction.

BIOCHEMICAL AND ENZYMATIC ABNOR-MALITIES. *Heinz-body production.* Studies were undertaken relative to the presence of the Heinz bodies that had been noted early in the hemolytic episodes. It was found that when incubated in the presence of oxygen with various chemicals (phenylhydrazine, acetylphenylhydrazine, ascorbic acid, etc.), sensitive cells developed a different pattern of Heinz-body formation than did nonsensitive cells. Under controlled conditions (control of pH, glucose, and reducing agent) five or more Heinz bodies are consistently found in *more than* 40 per cent of the erythrocytes of sensitive patients; *less than* 30 per cent of the red cells from nonsensitive subjects contain five Heinz bodies. Since somewhat inconsistent results have been obtained by various workers, the test has recently been modified to control also the hematocrit and the oxygen tension.

Because it had previously been demonstrated that the addition of sulfhydryl binders (iodoacetate, arsenite) to normal cells caused them to react in Heinz-body formation like the more recently described sensitive cells, investigations were undertaken into the sulfhydryl-containing compounds present in primaquine-sensitive red cells.

Glutathione content and instability. The first biochemical abnormality described for the primaquine-sensitive cell was a decreased content of reduced glutathione (GSH).* Moreover, when the GSH levels were studied in vivo during a hemolytic episode or in vitro during exposure of sensitive cells to acetylphenylhydrazine, the levels of red cell glutathione were observed to drop markedly. The GSH content of the primaquine-sensitive cell was accordingly unstable or vulnerable during drug exposure. It is known that the ratio of oxidized to reduced glutathione is maintained in the red cells by an enzyme, glutathione reductase, for which TPNH functions as coenzyme

(Figure 8.4). When glutathione reductase was found to be increased in sensitive cells, the TPNH/TPN ratio was determined; TPNH was found decreased while TPN was reciprocally increased (198, 286).

Pentose phosphate pathway. This abnormality indicated defective glucose metabolism, specifically a defective pentose phosphate pathway, since TPNH is therein generated. It may be recalled that in the erythrocyte the Embden-Meyerhof pathway of glycolysis, wherein glucose is converted to lactate, results in the generation of ATP and DPNH, while the pentose phosphate shunt is the only known sequence whereby TPNH is formed (Figure 8.4). Glucose-6-phosphate dehydrogenase (G-6-PD) initiates the pentose phosphate pathway, and primaquine-sensitive cells were found to be markedly deficient in this enzyme activity. Its activity is reduced to some 10 per cent of normal. This is the most severe defect known and may well represent the primary defect. Accordingly the disease is also designated glucose-6-phosphate dehydrogenase deficiency. As pointed out under Aging of the Red Cell, in Chapter 8, G-6-PD is one of the enzymes whose activity is known to decrease progressively with age in the normal red cell. This same fall-off is found in accelerated degree in the primaquine-sensitive erythrocyte. This accounts for the greater susceptibility of older cells to primaquine lysis.

Responsiveness of pentose phosphate pathway. With such a marked deficiency, a compromise in the energy made available to the red cell by means of the pentose phosphate pathway would be expected and has been demonstrated. The normal red cell increases its oxygen con-

* Reduced glutathione is in a dynamic state in the erythrocyte. Employing N^{15}-labeled glycine it was shown (85) that the half life of the N^{15} in GSH was 4 days. It is not known, however, if the entire molecule is synthesized or if there is a glycine interchange.

sumption and glucose utilization when exposed to methylene blue;* the primaquine sensitive red cell shows a diminished responsiveness to this stimulation, and the pentose phosphate pathway thus demonstrates an inability to respond under stress (172). Despite the increase in the obligate coenzyme of G-6-PD, TPN, brought about by methylene blue, the activity of G-6-PD is so deficient that a normal response cannot occur and TPNH is not regenerated rapidly enough to attain normal or adequate levels.

The primaquine-sensitive red cell therefore has a diminished TPNH content and cannot, under redox stress, rapidly generate this compound that along with GSH is essential as an intracellular reducing agent.

Consequences of diminished responsiveness of pentose phosphate pathway. The mechanisms whereby this defect plays a role in destruction of primaquine-sensitive erythrocytes has been investigated by several workers proceeding along similar lines (15, 29, 128, 130, 157, 176). Reducing systems are necessary in the red cell because if a redox equilibrium is permitted, electrons will flow from the red cell constituents (globin, GSH) to oxygen, thereby effecting spontaneous oxidation. Continuous generation of reducing agents is necessary and is brought about by glucose metabolism. The drugs and chemicals active in producing primaquine-sensitive hemolysis have the property of reacting with molecular oxygen to form actual or potential redox intermediates between oxygen and hemoglobin and other intracellular components. They thereby transmit the high oxidation potential of oxygen to cellular components by bridging what is otherwise a relative obstruction in the electron flow. If the cell is unable to increase its reducing capacity sufficiently to prevent the electron flow, oxidative destruction of the cellular components takes place.

Allen and Jandl (3) studied the effects of phenylhydrazine and related compounds on solutions of crystalline human hemoglobin and demonstrated the in vitro production of Heinz bodies by the following mechanism. Methemoglobin was formed followed by the appearance of a hemoglobin component with altered electrophoretic and chromatographic mobility. Irreversibly denatured hemoglobin derivatives such as sulfhemoglobin could at this point be detected, which then precipitated into coccoid bodies 2 to 3 μ in diameter with properties identical to those of Heinz bodies.

Within the red cell the sequence appears to be that as GSH is oxidized to GSSG, a portion of the GSH becomes bound to the hemoglobin by forming mixed disulfides with globin sulfhydryl groups. Hemoglobin is converted to methemoglobin. The two reactive sulfhydryl groups of hemoglobin are oxidized, resulting in loss of the normal configuration of the molecule. The oxygen dissociation curve is altered, and electrophoretically and chromatographically abnormal components appear. Other reactive groups of the globin become susceptible to oxidation, and "sulfhemoglobin-like" compounds are produced. The denatured hemoglobin molecules polymerize and precipitate as coccoid granules, or Heinz bodies.

Since methemoglobin appears to be one obligate intermediary in the sequence outlined above, it might well be asked if methemoglobin is seen during a hemolytic episode brought on by primaquine. As is pointed out in Chapter 8, intracellular methemoglobin is reduced by enzymes which are dependent upon DPNH and TPNH as cofactors. However, met-

* An increased rate of oxidation of glucose to carbon dioxide but no increase in the rate of conversion of glucose to lactic acid can be induced in human erythrocytes by a variety of "physiologic" compounds (cysteine, ascorbic acid, pyruvate) and "nonphysiologic" compounds (phenylhydrazine, primaquine, fava bean extract, etc.; 314).

hemoglobin is not usually found during the hemolytic sequence, and the observation has frequently been made that on a clinical basis methemoglobinemia and hemolysis appear to be dissociated both in occurrence and in type of drug responsible for their induction. The explanation for this now seems to be that primaquine-sensitive erythrocytes are more susceptible to the induction of methemoglobin than normal cells but that (as with normal cells) methemoglobin is preferentially formed in the older cells. These are the cells that are the most promptly destroyed during a drug-induced hemolytic episode, and methemoglobin consequently does not accumulate in sufficient amounts to permit detection by the usual methods (31).

Decreased catalase content. One other biochemical abnormality of the primaquine-sensitive erythrocyte deserves comment at this point. Assay for catalase, an enzyme capable of destroying peroxides, shows a decrease in activity: a 20 to 40 per cent reduction (319). The explanation for this is not known, but the decrease could play a significant role in the enhanced erythrocyte destruction brought about by drug administration since the reactive intermediate peroxides formed by the presence of the drug or derivatives in the red cell would not be readily destroyed. Actually the decrease is not found in all heterozygous females and the presence of catalase in sufficient quantity apparently accompanies decreased susceptibility to hemolysis. It has been postulated that as a heme-protein complex (Fe^{++}) it, like hemoglobin, would be susceptible of oxidation to the inactive met- form (Fe^{+++}), perhaps irreversibly so. In precise sequence studies catalase activity has been shown to decrease before other enzymes.

✓ *Summary.* In summary, the erythrocytes of primaquine-sensitive individuals have deficient activity of glucose-6-phosphate dehydrogenase, catalase, and re-

duced glutathione. They are unable to regenerate TPNH sufficiently rapidly to combat the effects of actual or potential redox derivatives of administered drugs that serve as intermediates between oxygen and cell components. In the presence of these redox intermediates, GSH, hemoglobin (Fe^{++}), globin, and perhaps catalase (Fe^{++}) are oxidized. The GSH combines with the hemoglobin (Fe^{++}) to take part in its initial denaturation as it is changed to methemoglobin (Fe^{+++}), sulfhemoglobin-like compounds, and finally polymerizes into the coccoid Heinz bodies at irreversible denaturation.

This, of course, does not necessarily account for the destruction of the erythrocyte. A decrease in ATP (217) and amount or availability of DPNH (310) has been demonstrated during in vitro exposure of sensitive cells to acetylphenylhydrazine, and alterations in potassium content and ion exchange have been shown upon in vitro exposure of sensitive (and normal) cells to primaquine (337, 338; Table 9.2). It has been postulated (148) that structural components essential for membrane integrity may be affected by oxidative denaturation as is hemoglobin and thereby be responsible for the cell's destruction.

VARIANTS OF G-6-PD DEFICIENCY. The above account of primaquine-sensitive hemolytic anemia is drawn from studies made on the American Negro. It now appears that there are four tentatively accepted variants of G-6-PD deficiency (177).

A. The primaquine sensitivity as seen in the American Negro is associated with a reduction of G-6-PD activity not due to a qualitative abnormality of the enzyme molecule. It is a generalized body disorder, as evidenced by a decreased rate of glucose oxidation in males (43) even though the defect has been demonstrated only in non-nucleated cells, erythrocytes, lens tissue, and perhaps platelets.

B. In a few males with partially ex-

TABLE 9.2.   Biochemical and metabolic abnormalities of primaquine-sensitive erythrocytes

I. Abnormalities of the pentose phosphate pathway
   A. Deficient glucose–6–phosphate dehydrogenase activity
   B. Diminished TPNH, increased TPN
   C. Inadequate responses to stimulation
      1. Oxygen consumption
      2. Glucose utilization
      3. TPNH regeneration
      4. Methemoglobin reduction
      5. Pentose formation
   D. Consequences of defective and inadequately responsive pentose phosphate pathway
      1. Decreased GSH
      2. GSH instability
      3. Increased GSH reductase activity
      4. Increased methemoglobinemia
      5. Oxidation of hemoglobin; Heinz-body formation
      6. Decreased lipid content
      7. Decreased catalase activity and further fall with drug administration (?)

II. Abnormalities of the Embden-Meyerhof pathway
   A. Increased aldolase activity
   B. Decreased DPNH, increased DPN
   C. Fall of ATP content in vitro on exposure to drug

Adapted from Tarlov, A. R., et al., A.M.A. Arch. Int. Med. 109:209, 1962.

pressed defect the enzyme has differed in some physical properties from the normal.

C. In primaquine-sensitive Caucasians, a more severe hemolytic process is usually seen, and the G-6-PD activity may be completely absent. Its deficiency has been demonstrated in tissues other than the erythrocyte: ectodermal (lens, salivary gland, skin); endodermal (liver); and mesodermal (erythrocytes, leukocytes, platelets). A G-6-PD activator may be absent from red cell stroma (209, 210, 261, 272). Morphologically the erythrocytes, although temporally young, appear old (progeria) by electron microscopic techniques (78).

D. In some of the hereditary nonspherocytic hemolytic anemias (see below) there may be complete or almost total lack of activity of the red cell G-6-PD enzyme, which appears qualitatively abnormal (178). A continuing mild hemolytic anemia exists.

INFLUENCE OF EXTRACORPUSCULAR FACTORS. One final important point should be emphasized. The above outline of the primaquine-induced hemolytic process applies only to otherwise healthy individuals. Patients ill with infections or metabolic derangements may develop an accentuated, fulminating hemolytic process upon drug administration (173). Thus, extracorpuscular factors may in one way or another influence the course of the hemolysis. In renal disease (321),* liver dysfunction, or altered absorptive mechanisms the metabolism of the drug may be altered or its concentration in the blood increased; in diabetic acidosis TPNH levels are demonstrably low and the cells apparently hypersusceptible; in the newborn with physiologic hypoglycemia (358) the red cell behaves as though sensitive with an unstable GSH. Hyper-

* In renal insufficiency the GSH stability is decreased; the G-6-PD is increased because the cell population is younger than normal.

thyroidism is associated with a twofold *increase* in G-6-PD and may afford some protection (229, 246, 250). However, no drugs or procedures are known that will alleviate the hemolysis.

OTHER TYPES OF DRUG-INDUCED HEMO-LYTIC ANEMIAS. It should not be inferred from what has been described in the previous sections that all drug-induced hemolytic anemias work through this mechanism and are associated with defective red cell enzymes. Some chemical agents—phenylhydrazine and acetylphenylhydrazine, for example—will produce a hemolytic anemia in anyone if given in sufficient quantity. Most of the agents assumed on the basis of clinical observation or laboratory experimentation to be similar to those compounds are oxidants with resonating benzene rings. These chemicals are capable of producing lysis in vitro as well as in vivo. Moreover, unlike the hemolytic process associated with primaquine-sensitive cells, a marked increase in erythrocyte osmotic and mechanical fragility and many bizarre shapes and distorted red cells are seen when these agents are administered to man. Also, unlike the former disorder some abnormal degree of methemoglobin is likely to be formed intracellularly. There is also another type of drug-induced hemolytic anemia in which a serum factor or antibody is involved in such a fashion that the agglutinin, lysin, or sensitizing agent is not functional *unless* the drug (or derivative) is also present in vitro and in vivo (133, 203, 222). Apparently, hemolytic anemia can be induced by (a) chemicals that affect all cells, (b) chemicals that affect only cells with a defective enzyme system, and (c) chemicals that work in conjunction with abnormal serum factors (antibodies).

Hereditary Nonspherocytic Hemolytic Anemia

The term hereditary nonspherocytic hemolytic anemia (59, 69, 82, 273, 284) has long been used as a "wastebasket" category for a heterogenous group of familial and congenital hemolytic disorders that could not be made to fit into other more clearly defined syndromes such as hereditary spherocytosis, thalassemia, hemoglobinopathy, etc. Originally classified by Dacie (72) on the basis of response to the autohemolysis test and morphologic abnormalities of the erythrocytes into two types, a new classification is presently emerging based on the presence or absence of a demonstrable defect in glucose metabolism and, if present, on its location in the pentose phosphate pathway or the Embden-Meyerhof pathway. As might be expected, no uniform description can be given that adequately encompasses the various types of cases seen that fall into that category. All, however, do have in common the early establishment of a hemolytic process on the basis of an intracorpuscular abnormality. However, the severity of hemolysis varies from a degree leading to marked anemia requiring repeated transfusions to a degree readily compensated by moderately increased erythropoiesis. Abnormal hemoglobins have not been reported; abnormal antibodies have not been demonstrated; and there is lack of spherocytosis, lack of increased osmotic fragility, and lack of response to any known therapeutic agent. Despite splenomegaly, it is unusual for splenectomy to afford a permanent, beneficial effect.

There is typically present the full range of findings previously described for overt hemolysis: alterations in pigment metabolism associated with extravascular red cell destruction and alterations resulting from compensatory attempts by the bone marrow. Despite considerably accelerated red cell destruction, the plasma hemoglobin content is not markedly, if at all, increased, and there is usually no build-up of radioactivity over a particular organ that would indicate a site of sequestration or destruction when body-surface scanning is combined with radioactive labeling of red cells and autosurvival techniques. The erythrocytes of an affected individual have a shortened survival time when circulating in either the patient himself or in a normal individual. Normal erythrocytes typically survive normally in the patient. Because these patients have been only sporadically reported, the natural history of these diseases is not well known but is obviously variable. Some patients do not survive the neonatal period; most die in childhood; a few survive to adult age and are able to transmit the disease.

When a defect in glucose metabolism is present and located in the pentose phosphate pathway, there has been found either absence or near absence of G-6-PD activity and extreme glutathione instability, or increased G-6-PD activity, low GSH, and abnormal glutathione stability. In some, the G-6-PD appears qualitatively as well as quantitatively abnormal (178). Presumably the defect in the pathway is so severe that augmented erythrocyte destruction occurs even without the added injurious effect of a drug (294). The erythrocyte morphology varies from patient to patient: normocytic to macrocytic, ovalocyte, or target forms; hypochromic to normochromic; present or absent inclusion bodies or basophilic stippling. The available evidence indicates that the disorders are inherited as a Mendelian dominant. They form *part* of the group classified as type I by Dacie, having normal autohemolysis on incubation but a less-than-normal inhibition of the autohemolysis when incubated with added glucose.

When the defect is located in the Embden-Meyerhof pathway (317, 327) the enzyme pyruvate kinase is deficient; impaired regeneration of ATP and shortened erythrocyte survival result (Figure 8.4). All other enzymes tested in the pathways of glucose metabolism are present in normal or increased amounts. The erythro-

cytes of patients with this defect show a marked uniform macrocytosis with (postsplenectomy) numerous Pappenheimer bodies. Family data and biochemical data are consistent with an autosomal recessive mode of transmission; the heterozygotes are clinically and hematologically normal except for possessing only about one-half the normal level of pyruvate activity (317). They appear to be identical with the group classified as type II by Dacie, having an increased autohemolysis on incubation not corrected by the addition of glucose but corrected by the addition of ATP (82).

An additional group, probably heterogeneous, remains (apparently coinciding with part of those classified as type I by Dacie) in whom no defect in glucose metabolism has been demonstrated. In these patients the erythrocyte morphology is variable, the pathogenesis remains completely obscure, and several disorders are probably represented. In one family a chronic, fairly well compensated nonspherocytic hemolytic anemia was found to be associated with a very low (absent?) reduced glutathione content of the erythrocytes in four siblings. The mode of inheritance is obscure. In view of the important position assigned to reduced glutathione in maintaining the "integrity of the red cell," the mild nature of the hemolytic process is of interest; glutathione reductase and G-6-PD were present in normal amounts (237).

Hemoglobin H Disease

Up to this point hemolytic mechanisms have been illustrated by considering diseases in which there have been (a) a hemoglobin belonging to an abnormal molecular species that upon deoxygenated polymerization distorts the erythrocyte so that it cannot normally survive (sickle cell anemia), (b) a basic incompatibility between the spleen and a structurally or biochemically abnormal erythrocyte (hereditary spherocytosis), (c) a biochemically defective cell that is rapidly destroyed upon exposure to chemicals because it cannot adequately respond to oxidative stress (primaquine-sensitive hemolytic anemia), and (d) a cell so biochemically defective that it cannot survive even in a normal environment (hereditary nonspherocytic hemolytic anemia). A disease mechanism has now been unraveled that almost unbelievably seems to depend upon all four processes: a real tour de force of nature in which an abnormal hemoglobin molecule requires high levels of reducing and stabilizing substances to prevent its oxidation and irreversible denaturation and consequent erythrocyte destruction by the spleen.

Since the first description in 1955 of hemoglobin H disease, this rare disorder has been found in wide racial and geographic distribution. Basically it is a hemoglobinopathy; up to 40 per cent of the hemoglobin migrates at a rate faster than normal and undergoes spontaneous irreversible oxidative denaturation. Hemoglobin H is known to be composed of four β-polypeptide chains (β_4^H). The most probable genetic basis is the heterozygous occurrence of both the gene for hemoglobin H and the gene for thalassemia (181).

The clinical manifestations are chronic refractory anemia with reticulocytosis, bilirubinemia, decreased erythrocyte osmotic fragility, and splenomegaly. The blood smear exhibits marked anisocytosis, teardrop cells, target cells, polychromatophilia, and stippling. Upon incubation, the red cells develop inclusion bodies—rapidly if cresyl blue is present.

Transfusion studies have demonstrated an intrinsically defective erythrocyte. The electrophoretically abnormal hemoglobin in the red cell undergoes a spontaneous denaturation and precipitation that is greatly increased by oxidation to methemoglobin. This hemoglobin probably owes its instability to its composition of four β-polypeptide chains. Its oxygen dissociation curve is abnormal, having ten times the affinity for oxygen as the normal, and lacks evidence for heme-heme interaction, since the curve is hyperbolic and not sigmoidal (18). It also shows *reversible* precipitation upon deoxygenation.

Enzyme assays for G-6-PD, methemoglobin reductases, and catalase have yielded normal results, and no GSH instability was noted. The enzyme content is high in young cells and decreases with age, but unlike the normal, GSH content also decreases with age (271). It has been suggested that the abnormally unstable structure of hemoglobin H necessitates higher levels of reducing and stabilizing factors to maintain it and that at a cell age of 40 to 45 days, because of the usual age-dependent fall-off of enzyme activity, a critically low level is reached, at which point rapid irreversible denaturation of hemoglobin H takes place.

Labeling studies indicate that such cells forming intraerythrocytic inclusions at 40 to 45 days of age are rapidly destroyed by the spleen. Splenectomy is followed by an increase in the red cell life span, improvement in well-being, and increase in hemoglobin level, and cells with inclusion bodies are then found in the peripheral blood. Some random destruction of erythrocytes continues, presumably because of the reversible precipitation of hemoglobin H upon deoxygenation in capillaries, which leads to stagnation (270).

It would be expected that such patients would be susceptible to hemolytic episodes induced by exposure to primaquine-like drugs or by infections that would enhance the hemoglobin instability, and this has been found true.

Hemoglobin Zürich Syndrome

A somewhat similar situation is found in association with an abnormal hemoglobin tentatively designated Zürich (104). Inherited according to a dominant pattern it has been found in fifteen members of four generations of one Swiss family. The hemoglobin is of interest because in spite of no defects in the erythrocyte's enzyme complement, severe hemolytic crises have occurred after sulfonamide administration, at which time large inclusion bodies were found in all red cells. Here again, because of its globin abnormality, hemoglobin is unstable and can exist only in a cell that is not subjected to adverse redox stress.

Favism

Favism is the name given to the acute hemolytic anemia that results from the singular combination of an inborn error of red cell metabolism and a sensitivity to the fava bean, *Vicia fava* (164, 202). The metabolic error is apparently the same as that seen in primaquine-sensitive hemolytic anemia and has the same mode of inheritance (313); the allergy or hypersensitivity is apparently of the antibody type. Hemolysis is therefore dependent upon the coincidence of a genetically determined intracorpuscular abnormality and the development of an extracorpuscular abnormality that results from a peculiar individual reactivity to factors present in raw or lightly cooked fava beans or to the pollen of *Vicia fava*.

Only a small number of cases have been described from the United States, but the incidence is of considerable significance in the countries of the Mediterranean littoral. In Sardinia, reports indicate 5 cases annually per 1,000 population, with a mortality rate of 8 per cent among those affected (164).

When due to pollen inhalation, the hemolytic episode may begin within a matter of minutes; after bean ingestion there is usually a lag period of 5 to 24 hours. It is said that no reaction follows a first exposure. The illness begins suddenly with anorexia, weakness, pain in the abdomen, and malaise. Repeated yawning, nausea and vomiting, chills and fever, and diarrhea frequently develop. Pallor and headache may occur, followed by hemoglobinuria and jaundice. The acute illness usually lasts for 3 or 4 days during which time the spleen and/or liver may enlarge. The episodes vary greatly in intensity.

The decreases in hemoglobin concentration and red cell count are proportionate, and a fall to less than 1 million per cubic millimeter is not unusual. There is usually transitory leukopenia and thrombocytopenia followed by leukocytosis and eosinophilia. Although apparently only recently looked for, Heinz bodies develop in the red cells. No other morphologic abnormalities occur. The erythrocyte fragility is normal or slightly decreased. Hemoglobinemia and hemoglobinuria are almost constant findings, and the predictable changes in hemoglobin transport, excretion, and bilirubin metabolism follow. During the recovery phase polychromatophilic cells (reticulocytes) and normoblasts appear in the peripheral blood.

Reports concerning the detection of abnormal factors present in the circulating blood or adsorbed to the red cells have been quite variable. In this country, for example, the Coombs test has been consistently negative, and searches for serum factors have been unrewarding. A number of positive reactions to the direct and indirect Coombs tests have been reported in the European literature. In the light of recent findings this apparent discrepancy is probably due to the transitory nature of the abnormal factors in the circulating blood. Thus, Kantor and Argesman (166) have demonstrated that during the onset of the acute hemolytic episode, and only then, a factor is present in the serum that agglutinates red cells that have been coated with an extract of the fava bean. Although a hypersensitivity reaction is presumed responsible for the development of the factor in the peripheral blood, the nature of the reaction is unknown. Positive skin tests and passive transfer have been demonstrated in some patients. A provocative study by Roth and Frumin (277) showed that normal plasma prevented the sensitization of erythrocytes upon their exposure to fava-bean extract; no such effect could be demonstrated employing plasma from the one patient studied, whether his disease was in remission or relapse. Thus a serum *deficiency* was demonstrated to be perhaps of more importance in the causation of favism. The serum deficiency was not present in the patient's father, who was deficient in G-6-PD and consumed fava beans, but who had never suffered hemolysis. Some individuals may apparently eat fava beans and be exposed to pollen for years without adverse effect and then suddenly become reactive. The experimental feeding of one bean is said to be capable of producing a severe hemolytic episode; hemolysis has been described in a nursing infant whose mother ingested fava beans (90). Whatever the nature of the reaction, it now seems clearly established that an extracorpuscular abnormality develops (in the nature of a circulating blood factor) in response to ingestion of the fava bean or inhalation of its plant's pollen.

For many years it has been known that following an acute hemolytic episode a peculiar anergic state exists so that for a limited time further exposure to the noxious agent does not result in adverse reaction. It would now seem likely that this can be explained on the basis of the demonstrated intracorpuscular defect, namely (as in primaquine-sensitive hemolytic anemia), all the sensitive or susceptible cells have been destroyed, and a new population must be matured to replenish them.

Recent studies and sufficiently extensive surveys have now established that favism occurs only in individuals who have metabolically abnormal red cells and that the abnormality is apparently the same as that seen in primaquine-sensitive hemolytic anemia: low GSH level, GSH instability, and deficiency of G-6-PD. Moreover, the genetic mode of transmittance of the abnormality is the same: a sex-linked factor of intermediate dominance. Szeinberg and Marks (314) have recently described stimulation of glucose catabolism by the pentose phosphate pathway when erythrocytes are exposed to fava-bean extracts. Erythrocytes deficient in G-6-PD are not capable of normal responses to such exposure. As in the drug-induced hemolytic anemia, it must be acknowledged that the exact mechanism of red cell destruction is unknown, but whereas in primaquine-sensitive hemolytic anemia a good account can be given of the mechanism by which the drug or derivative stresses a relatively unresponsive pentose phosphate pathway, here the exact relations between the defective shunt, possible serum factors, and hypersensitivity to the fava bean are unknown.

Studies employing erythrocytes labeled with radioactive chromium have demonstrated (331) the normal survival of normal cells even in an acutely ill patient experiencing a hemolytic episode induced by fava-bean ingestion (no extracorpuscular factor capable of affecting *normal* erythrocytes). Labeled erythrocytes from susceptible patients survived adequately in normal recipients and in susceptible patients not concurrently exposed to the fava bean (no intracorpuscular abnormality capable of seriously compromising the cell in a normal environment). However, erythrocytes from a susceptible person did undergo increased destruction when injected into acutely hemolytic recipients. *Only in some instances* did cells from susceptible persons show a similarly increased rate of destruction when transfused into normal recipients who had ingested fava beans.* Thus, for hemolysis to take place there must occur the highly improbable coincidence of a misbegotten red cell circulating in an environment altered by a hypersensitivity phenomenon.

Although cortisone has been used in the treatment of the disorder, its effects in a process such as this, that is usually self-limited, are most difficult to evaluate. Transfusions are required in severe instances and, of course, should be of blood proved nonsensitive by appropriate tests.

Thalassemia

Thalassemia is a heritable disorder characterized by increased hemolysis based on an intracorpuscular defect; hypochromic, microcytic red cells; splenomegaly; and ineffective erythropoiesis with abnormalities in hemoglobin biosynthesis and red cell formation. Although this disorder is usually considered with the diseases associated with abnormal types of hemoglobins, no abnormal hemoglobin has as yet been described in the uncomplicated cases.† Unusually large amounts of hemoglobin F and hemoglobin A_2 have been found in some patients with apparently pure thalassemia, but these are *normal* hemoglobins appearing in *abnormal quantities and at unusual ages.*

GENETIC MECHANISMS AND DISTRIBUTION. With few exceptions, American workers consider that two main divisions exist in uncomplicated thalassemia: the major and the minor forms. This classification is, in the main, comparable to that of uncomplicated sickle cell disease with its subdivisions of sickle cell anemia and sickle cell trait. Extensive studies indicate that the population genetics are similar (Figure 3.3): a single incompletely dominant abnormal factor is present in thalassemia minor (heterozygous), and two incompletely dominant abnormal

alleles are present in thalassemia major (homozygous) (26).†† Numerous other names are also employed for this disease: Cooley's anemia and trait, Mediterranean anemia and trait, erythroblastic anemia, hereditary leptocytosis (target cell anemia), and familial microcytic anemia. Although it was first clearly delineated by Cooley in 1925 in America (60), the term thalassemia has been used most widely in recent years particularly with its discovered associations with many of the abnormal hemoglobins.

To avoid confusion, however, it must be pointed out that some workers in this country and many European workers believe that forms intermediate in hematologic and clinical manifestations between the anemia and the trait exist and are associated with several genetic factors rather than a single pair of alleles (thalassemia intermedia, minima, etc.). It would seem more sensible at the present time to await genetic and/or biochemical confirmation of this as the thalassemic syndromes are further clarified by various lines of study.

Until fairly recently the disorders were seldom described in patients whose ancestors did not originate from the northeastern shores of the Mediterranean. With more extensive surveys, particularly

* In a recent refinement of procedure, the same authors (242) have confirmed the above findings. Chromium-labeled erythrocytes from two patients with G-6-PD deficiency were transfused to six normals and eleven patients known to have favism. When fava juice was given orally, a higher rate of increased hemolysis was found in the patients known to have had favism in the past.

† Recently Fessas et al. (102) have described a hemoglobinopathy that resembles thalassemia in the heterozygous, homozygous, and double (with thalassemia) heterozygous state. The abnormal hemoglobin, tentatively called "Pylos," requires special electrophoretic procedures for its identification.

†† See below, under Genetics of Hemoglobin Components, for analysis of genetic mechanisms based upon the factors controlling α- and β-polypeptide chains of hemoglobin.

in association with searches for abnormal hemoglobins, the disease has been described as occurring in a wide band extending over northern Africa and southern Europe to Thailand and the Philippines (51), including the countries of Spain, Portugal, Italy, Greece, Syria, Turkey, Iran, Iraq, Egypt, Israel, Armenia, Indonesia, Ceylon, Burma, Malaya, Vietnam, China, Tunisia, Algeria, the Belgian Congo, and South Africa (Figure 9.11). Reports of isolated cases are available from most other countries of Europe and South America. Numerous instances have been reported of its occurrence in American Negroes, both with and without associated hemoglobinopathy (292). Among the various peoples involved, the trait exists with a frequency up to 50 per cent, usually under 5 to 8 per cent. It appears

likely that thalassemia minor carries with it a reduced morbidity and mortality from falciparum malaria in infants and young children.

CLINICAL MANIFESTATIONS. Thalassemia major (homozygous state) is a serious disorder that is usually recognized in early infancy and is frequently fatal in childhood. Some patients do survive into adult life (208), and a few females have gone through several successful pregnancies. Pallor is usually obvious early in the course. The descriptions of bouts of fever and of abdominal and joint pain found in the earlier literature need reevaluation in the light of the presently known association of thalassemia and sickle cell disease. Some degree of scleral icterus is usually present and overt jaundice may exist. The signs and symptoms

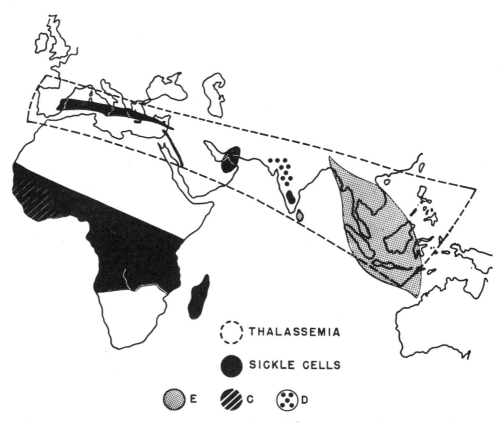

FIGURE 9.11.   Geographic distribution of major hemoglobin abnormalities. (From Lehmann, H., and Ager, J. A. M., *in* Stanbury, J. B., et al. (ed.), The Metabolic Basis of Inherited Disease, p. 1086, McGraw-Hill, New York, 1960)

are largely those associated with chronic severe anemia and the associated cardiorespiratory complications. Chronic or intermittent leg ulcers are sometimes seen, as in sickle cell anemia. The spleen is always enlarged, occasionally greatly so, and hepatomegaly may also occur. Cholelithiasis is found but much less frequently than in hereditary spherocytosis or sickle cell anemia. Skeletal lesions, evident on x-ray examination, are most prominent in the skull, spine, pelvis, and proximal long bones, and consist of widening of the medullary portions containing active marrow and thinning of the cortical bone (40). When the anemia is severe in childhood, transfusions are usually necessary to maintain the patient in relative health. Growth and development are usually fairly normal until adolescence, at which time there is little further growth and poor sexual development. The need for frequent transfusions raises the problem of induced iron overload; congestive heart failure associated with myocardial hemosiderosis is not an unusual cause of death (352) even in childhood (223, 266, 304).

LABORATORY FINDINGS. Examination of the blood reveals severe anemia with hypochromic and microcytic erythrocytes. The reticulocyte count is only moderately elevated, usually less than 10 per cent. Examination of the stained blood film reveals extreme variation in size and shape of cells, with many oval, target, stippled, and bizarre forms. Apparent fragments of cells may be present. The microcyte is the predominant form. The cells are very poorly and irregularly filled with hemoglobin so that only a thin rim of hemoglobin may be seen. Central or eccentric masses may in addition be found. Microspherocytes are rarely seen. Stippled cells are not unusual, and nucleated erythrocytes of various degrees of maturity are frequently seen. The predominant picture is hypochromicity in bizarrely shaped microcytes. The leuko-

cyte count is frequently slightly elevated; the platelet count is within normal limits. The icterus index is elevated mainly because of the disproportionate increase in the unconjugated bilirubin. The osmotic fragility of the erythrocytes is abnormal, but contrary to the findings in hereditary spherocytosis, the cells are *more* resistant (*less* fragile) to osmotic stress than normal. Following the 24-hour incubation procedure, a small proportion of the cells shows a slight increase in osmotic fragility (not into the abnormal range), while most of the cells become even more resistant than previously. In the few patients tested the mechanical fragility has been found slightly increased (167), with a less-than-normal increase following sterile incubation. In the absence of complicating factors (iron lack, infection, etc.), the serum iron content is higher than normal and the per cent saturation of the iron-binding globulin is also high. Examination of the bone marrow reveals normal leukocyte and platelet production with an increased proportion of red cell precursors. Basophilia persisting into late normoblasts with pyknotic nuclei indicates an abnormally delayed production of hemoglobin. Stains for iron show an amount of hemosiderin increased above normal. Despite morphologic similarities and comparable erythrocyte indices, there are numerous points on which thalassemia differs from iron-lack anemia: familial incidence, hyperbilirubinemia, reticulocytosis, chronicity, increased iron in plasma and bone marrow, and, of course, lack of response to adequate iron therapy.

Aplastic crises have been described in association with infection and toxicity, and a complication designated "relative folic acid deficiency" has been recognized in both thalassemia major and minor. Pregnancy may be an important component of this complication in adults, but a number of children have now been reported whose hemoglobin levels have been elevated following the administration of folic acid. The usual biochemical and morphologic concomitants of folic acid deficiency are usually *not* seen (155).

Thalassemia minor (39, 41) is, by and large, a clinically benign disorder. It is usually detected through a routine blood examination or through family studies carried out because of some other abnormality (301). However, a small but significant number of patients have a moderate degree of anemia and consequently have signs and symptoms appropriate to the hemoglobin lack. On occasion splenomegaly, minor bone changes, and/or a chronic acholuric type of jaundice of mild degree are found. It is evident that in some instances an exact differential diagnosis between thalassemia major and minor cannot be made without appropriate genetic studies. In thalassemia major (homozygous) both parents must have at least the trait and all offspring of the patient must bear the trait. In thalassemia minor (heterozygous) at least one parent must have the trait and normal offspring may result.

Examination of the peripheral blood shows the leukocytes and platelets to be quantitatively and qualitatively normal. The red cell indices usually indicate microcytosis and hypochromicity, although each is perhaps by itself of borderline significance. Examination of the blood film shows that the morphologic changes are disproportionate to the hemoglobin level. There is considerable variation in size and shape, and bizarre forms may be present; the over-all picture is that of moderate microcytosis and mild hypochromicity, as in a mild degree of iron-lack anemia. Reticulocytes are usually normal in numbers. The osmotic fragility characteristics of the red cells show changes similar to but not as extreme as those described for thalassemia major. The mechanical fragility is reported to be normal both before and after incuba-

tion (325). The serum iron content is usually normal but may be elevated, with nearly complete saturation of the iron-binding protein. The marrow contains normal or increased amounts of stainable iron.

LOCATION OF RED CELL DEFECT. The thalassemic syndromes are classified as hemolytic disorders with intracellular abnormalities since the erythrocytes from patients with thalassemia major have a shortened survival time when measured in the patient or in normal recipients (89, 167, 330). As in sickle cell trait, the erythrocyte survival time of patients with thalassemia minor is normal. In uncomplicated situations no extracorpuscular abnormality is demonstrable, but with marked splenomegaly there may be an increased destruction of normal donor cells. The patient therefore has a combined intra- and extracorpuscular hemolytic abnormality (50). Splenectomy may be of considerable benefit to this type of patient since in the severe forms repeated transfusions may be necessary to maintain life. Any maneuver to decrease transfusion requirement will lessen the iron overload and adverse transfusion reactions. Aside from these complications of hypersplenism, the anemia is not responsive to any known therapy. The survival time of the patient's cells in himself is not significantly altered by splenectomy.

PATHOGENESIS. *Mechanism of hemolysis.* No convincing evidence has been offered upon which can be based an account of the mechanism of erythrocyte destruction in this disease. Studies made at the time of splenectomy have provided evidence for a selective sequestration and conditioning of cells but in a degree far short of that seen in hereditary spherocytosis. Following splenectomy increased numbers of microspherocytes with increased osmotic fragility are found in the peripheral blood. This is probably at the most a minor component of the total hemolytic process. In support of this, unlike the findings in most hemolytic anemias with a demonstrable splenic mechanism, the spleen in thalassemia shows a conspicuous lack of iron-containing pigment despite excess iron elsewhere in the body. Moreover, radioactive labeling techniques and external body monitoring detect very little build-up of radioactivity over the spleen area, and the erythrocyte survival time is not influenced appreciably by the presence or absence of the spleen (except, of course, in connection with the extracorpuscular hypersplenic complications mentioned previously). Some workers describe two populations of red cells, one of which, with a mean life span of a few days, is taken up by the spleen (8). An unexplained finding is a minor degree of splenic sequestration of Cr^{51}-labeled erythrocytes in patients studied under conditions of low oxygen tension. Erythrocyte fragmentation has been proposed but not supported by evidence beyond that seen in peripheral blood morphology and the in vitro erythrocyte instability observed in various suspending media and dyes. The few reports available concerning the erythrocyte survival time in adults with severe iron-deficiency anemia and erythrocyte morphologic changes comparable to those seen in thalassemia major indicate a nearly normal survival time, so the bizzare shapes and extreme variations cannot per se be implicated in augmented destruction.

Several observers have reported an abnormal elevation of plasma hemoglobin level in thalassemia major (40 to 50 mg per 100 ml) as opposed to thalassemia minor (64, 79). However, these measurements were made in such a way that the total benzidine-reacting pigments are assayed and the actual amount of free and/or bound hemoglobin or methemalbumin making up the total benzidine-reacting pigments is not known. The plasma haptoglobin level is markedly subnormal. A stromal or developmental defect of the erythrocyte is, of course, presumed. In addition to the abnormal osmotic behavior found on incubation, abnormalities in the surface texture of the erythrocyte ghost have been demonstrated by electron microscopy to exist in thalassemia major but not minor and are interpreted as an "expression of an alteration in the molecular structure of their plasma membrane" (144).

Hemoglobin production. Observations have also been reported (7) concerning a defect in the maturation of the normoblast, based on the demonstration of a Periodic-Acid-Schiff-reacting mucopolysaccharide or glucomucoprotein not found in normal cells. But pathogenic interpretations of these findings are lacking, and the inclusions have been noted in other disorders.

Because of the morphologic similarity to iron-lack anemia, the excessive amount of tissue iron, and the increased erythrocyte protoporphyrin content, it has long been suspected that these cells are unable properly to utilize iron in hemoglobin biosynthesis. A direct approach to this problem has been made by Bannerman et al. (10, 120), who employed Fe^{59} and C^{14}-tagged glycine to measure the in vitro rate of heme biosynthesis in immature erythrocytes from patients with thalassemia. The results suggested a quantitative impairment of hemoglobin biosynthesis that is inherent in the cell and not influenced by normal or other plasma. There was no evidence of a specific alteration of globin biosynthesis, but the results did indicate a relatively slow rate of protoporphyrin production and a partial block in the combination of protoporphyrin and iron. Erlandson et al. (97), again by in vitro studies on erythrocytes, concluded that the relatively slow rate of heme production was due to a difficulty in the conversion of glycine to δ-aminolevulinic acid not correctable by pyridoxine or succinyl-CoA. These are important contributions to knowledge of the pathogenesis of thalassemia.

However, it is evident that some additional abnormality or some far-reaching undemonstrated effect secondary to the impaired hemoglobin biosynthesis must be present, for the paucity of hemoglobin per cell cannot account for the hemoglobin depression noted in the peripheral blood. Were the hypochromicity of each cell completely corrected by bringing its complement of hemoglobin up to 32 Gm per 100 ml, the hemoglobin level of the circulating blood in thalassemia major would be augmented by less than 30 per cent.

Attempts to study erythropoiesis by in vitro methods have not yielded clear-cut results but apparently implicate some maturation abnormality and impaired red cell production. By means of electron microscopy, an excess of iron-containing granules has been demonstrated in the developing and adult erythrocyte as ferritin and hemosiderin and also as "ferruginous micelles," interpreted as iron-laden mitochondria. More iron may be present in the stroma than in the hemoglobin. Consequently it may be concluded that transportation of iron to and into the erythrocyte is unimpeded but that a block exists in its subsequent utilization.

Erythropoietic response. Measurements of red cell destruction in thalassemia major indicate a rate of seven to ten times normal, estimated by Cr^{51} tagging. By the methods and calculations employed, this rate of destruction would not, of itself, be enough to result in the severe anemia regularly seen in this disease if the usual compensatory effort of a normal marrow occurred. Quantitation of the compensatory effort has been undertaken by ferrokinetic and erythrokinetic measurements (135, 207, 245, 248, 311). Blood production, as estimated by marrow morphology (E/M ratio), plasma iron turnover, and total urobilinogen excretion, was increased to the expected maximum (six to eight times normal). These parameters indicate the total erythropoiesis of the marrow irrespective of whether the hemoglobin-red-cell mass produced reaches the circulating blood or is partly destroyed and catabolized before reaching the peripheral blood. By determining the peripheral blood reticulocyte count, the red cell iron utilization, and the Cr^{51} survival time relative to the circulating red cell mass, an indication can be obtained of the quantity of cells and hemoglobin actually delivered from the marrow to the circulating blood: the "effective red cell production." Mildly anemic patients with thalassemia were found able to increase their effective red cell production only some four times normal; severely anemic patients were unable to exceed normal production. Thus, although the marrow is able to achieve the maximal degree of compensation seen in other hemolytic processes with respect to pigment production, it cannot deliver the pigment adequately packaged to the peripheral blood. An "intramarrow shunt" of ineffective erythropoiesis occurs, with diversion of heme pigment. This situation is comparable to that demonstrated in untreated pernicious anemia and folic acid deficiency and is termed dyshematopoiesis (135, 207). In view of the hematologic responses recently noted in some patients with thalassemia to the administration of folic acid, the question arises whether the dyshematopoiesis is a basic abnormality or partly a result of "relative folic acid deficiency." Although the latter possibility is considered unlikely, it cannot be ruled out at the present time.

The increased hemolysis seen in thalassemia contributes, of course, to the degree of anemia present, but the severity of the anemia is largely related to the production defect—the relative lack of increase in effective red cell production.

GENETICS OF HEMOGLOBIN COMPONENTS. At the beginning of this section it was stated that on the basis of extensive family and population surveys the conclusion was reached that thalassemia minor results from the inheritance of a single incompletely dominant abnormal autosomal factor (heterozygous state) and thalassemia major results from the inheritance of two incompletely dominant abnormal alleles (homozygous state). In terms of population genetics these statements are still accurate and are applicable in working out family trees in clinical situations. However, there has been growing evidence that there exists more than one genetically determined type of thalassemia: that the disease is genetically heterogeneous, with a given type following true to its pattern in any one family.

In addition to this, as in sickle cell disease, it must be acknowledged that on the basis of the structure of the hemoglobin molecule, cognizance must be taken of the fact that hemoglobin may no longer be considered under the control of a single genetic factor but rather under the control of the one-gene, one-polypeptide mechanism. Several workers have now analyzed the inheritance of thalassemia on the basis of its genetic heterogeneity and the genetics of the polypeptide chains of hemoglobin.

The normal individual possesses a major hemoglobin component, hemoglobin A, and several minor components hemoglobin F, A_2, A_3, etc. The genetics of the minor components is a relatively unexplored field at present, but hemoglobin A_2 has received more attention than the others. This hemoglobin is usually detected and quantitated by starch gel electrophoresis. One survey concerning the proportion of hemoglobin A_2 in twenty-three parents of children with thalassemia major (109) revealed that all parents had an increased amount.* The presence of an abnormally increased amount of

hemoglobin A_2 was then proposed as a specific biochemical criterion for the diagnosis of thalassemia. However, more extensive surveys revealed an occasional family in which *no* increase in A_2 percentage was found (46), and additional instances have been reported in association with various thalassemia-hemoglobinopathy combinations. It would therefore seem better to regard the presence or absence of an abnormal elevation of hemoglobin A_2 as evidence for more than one kind of thalassemia.

In genetic studies of thalassemia–sickle cell disease (mixed heterozygous condition) it has been clearly established that there are *two modes of inheritance* (230). In some families with thalassemia–sickle cell disease the abnormal traits behave as alleles (or closely linked) in that one trait or the other will go to an offspring but *not* both together (the traits segregate in the children); in other families a different genetic pattern is seen in that *both* traits or *neither* trait may go to one offspring (no segregation) and the factors cannot therefore be allelic, or closely linked.

Additional evidence for two types of thalassemia comes from families with mixed heterozygosity for thalassemia and hemoglobin S or C. In some families the abnormal hemoglobin (S or C) will consistently account for approximately 50 per cent of the total; in other families the abnormal hemoglobin will consistently make up 70 or 80 per cent of the total. In the latter situation the remaining hemoglobin is fetal in type, and *no* hemoglobin A is found. Here interaction is said to have taken place with the thalassemia factor, resulting in a lack of production of normal hemoglobin and consequently a

* Hemoglobin A_2 is not increased in thalassemia major, but the ratio of hemoglobin A_2 to hemoglobin F is increased. Increased amounts of A_2 have been found in a few acquired or transitory hematologic disorders: untreated pernicious anemia, malignant tumors, etc.

larger proportion of hemoglobin S or C. On re-examination of these families it was found that the amount of hemoglobin A_2 was abnormally elevated where interaction took place but not elevated where interaction did not take place. The division of thalassemia into two mutation types by these criteria would then be consistent (Table 9.3).

To account for the genetic heterogeneity of thalassemia, as described above, two suggestions have been advanced. In the first it was postulated that in thalassemia an abnormal hemoglobin is produced—a hemoglobin which, on complete chemical dissection of the amino acid sequence, structure, and folding of the polypeptide chains, will be demonstrated abnormal but which has an "electrophoretically silent substitution" because no charge difference is conferred on the polypeptide chain by the abnormally situated amino acid. The probability is high that such "hidden" amino acid substitutions will be found. For example, hemoglobin S and three hemoglobins D all migrate to the same zone on electrophoresis but contain differently substituted amino acids, some even on different polypeptide chains as in the D_a and D_β hemoglobins. By analogy with the production of other abnormal hemoglobins it was also proposed that the abnormal hemoglobin of thalassemia was synthesized at a decreased rate. If the mutation of thalassemia occurred at the genetic locus governing the production of the β^A chain, this polypeptide would then be in short supply as β^{Thal}. The production of α^A would be unaffected, as would the production of δ^{A_2}, γ^F, and β^S (when present). Accordingly the production of hemoglobin A^{Thal} ($\alpha_2^A\beta_2^{Thal}$) would be suppressed, but hemoglobins F ($\alpha_2^A\gamma_2^F$), A_2 ($\alpha_2^A\alpha_2^{A_2}$), and S ($\alpha_2^A\beta_2^S$) (if present) would be found in increased proportions. This would then be an interacting type, or β-thalassemia (Table 9.3).

Were the mutation to involve the genetic locus governing the production of the α^A chain (α^{Thal}), its production would be suppressed and no increase in the hemoglobins containing the α-chain would be found (A^{Thal}, A_2^{Thal}, F^{Thal}, S^{Thal}). This would be the noninteracting type, or α-thalassemia (Table 9.3).

In 1961 Rucknagel and Neel pointed out that "as matters stand at present it is

TABLE 9.3. Characteristics of two types of thalassemia classified on basis of hemoglobin components

Group I (β–thalassemia)	Group II (α–thalassemia)
1. Interaction with hemoglobin S or C (hemoglobin S or C 60–80% of total)	1. Noninteraction with hemoglobin S or C (hemoglobin S or C 40–50% of total)
2. Increased A_2 component	2. Normal A_2 component
3. Allelic, or closely linked, to hemoglobin S (traits segregate in children)	3. Nonallelic, or not closely linked, to hemoglobin S (both traits may go to same child)
4. Rarely found in hemoglobin H pedigrees	4. Commonly found in hemoglobin H pedigrees
5. Presumed β–chain abnormality (Hgb β^{Th}) or impaired production	5. Presumed α–chain abnormality (Hgb α^{Th}) or impaired production
6. Infrequently found in Negroes with thalassemia	6. Usually found in Negroes with thalassemia

possible to erect a conceptual framework wherein four genetic loci can control all known variations in human hemoglobin including the thalassemias" (280). However, since this proposal was made no abnormality in the hemoglobins of thalassemia has been described despite attempts at amino acid dissection. Although the lack of positive findings obviously does not rule out this first explanation of the types of thalassemia, it begins to lend support to the second hypothesis concerning the genetic heterogeneity of thalassemia. Moreover, difficulties with the first explanation have been encountered in the nature of patients with thalassemia characterized by an increase in hemoglobin A_2 but no increase in hemoglobin F, and the reverse (360). In addition, apparently otherwise normal individuals have been described who possess a genetically determined high fetal hemoglobin (28, 204, 236, 323).

According to the second hypothesis, there exist controller genes (as opposed to structural genes) that regulate the production of the various polypeptide chains.

With respect to thalassemia, a mutation might arise in the genetic locus that controls the production of the α^A-polypeptide chain or in the locus controlling the production of the β^A-polypeptide chain. By this mechanism no abnormality, "hidden" or otherwise, occurs in the various polypeptide chains, but because of altered production either the α^A- or β^A-polypeptide chain will be in short supply (or not produced) and consequently hemoglobins having these chains as components will be present in lesser proportion and the findings listed in Table 9.3 can be explained. In addition, alterations in the genetic loci controlling the production of the β^A-polypeptide chain could account for the variations in concentration of hemoglobin F seen in thalassemia and the high F syndrome (normal individuals except for persistence of high concentrations of fetal hemoglobin) by indirectly directing or permitting compensatory synthesis of γ-chains (287).

None of the proposed mechanisms have been established or accepted by all (230, 361), but they form a basis upon which to predict the findings in various genetic combinations and situations and so are susceptible to revision, discard, or validation.

Chronic Hemolytic Anemia with Paroxysmal Nocturnal Hemoglobinuria

CLINICAL MANIFESTATIONS AND LABORATORY FINDINGS. This uncommon acquired disorder is characterized by hemoglobinuria that is usually most pronounced at night, superimposed upon a chronic hemolytic anemia (61). Although it can become manifest in any decade of life, it is most commonly seen in adults at early middle age. Both sexes and many races are affected. There is no familial tendency. The severity may range from a mild defect, clinically benign and detectable only by special tests, to a life-endangering, chronically debilitating process. The course frequently appears to be fairly constant for long periods of time in any one individual. The onset is usually insidious and the established course prolonged, but there seems to be a tendency to remission with extended survival. Clinical remissions have been well documented in some instances with or without the persistence of abnormalities barely discernible by laboratory procedures. The usual complaints are weakness; sallow color; abdominal, back, or chest pains; and discolored urine. In the well-established disease, the nocturnal exacerbation of the hemoglobinuria may be lost or become so minor that it is not noted by the patient.

The complications most seriously to be feared are infections, aplastic crises, and thromboses. Infections of any type, even mild and ordinarily innocuous, may precipitate a severe exacerbation of the hemolytic process, with marked hemoglobinemia, hemoglobinuria, anemia, pain, and malaise. Aplastic or aregenerative crises may be associated with infections, as in other hemolytic disorders, and carry the same grave potential dangers. In some instances the aplasia, or aregenerative marrow complication, may persist for long periods of time for no evident cause (74). A number of patients have been followed for prolonged periods of time under the mistaken diagnosis of refractory anemia and pancytopenia (chronic bone marrow failure); they showed few or none of the changes usually associated with hemolytic disease, but the correct diagnosis was finally made on the basis of the pathognomonic test done on the patient's red cells.* In about 50 per cent of cases the cause of death is associated with a thrombotic episode, occurring in the portal, mesenteric, renal, cerebral, or extremity vessels. The disease definitely predisposes to thrombotic episodes, and such a complication is invariably serious.

The patients usually appear to have a background pallor with superimposed moderate jaundice or bronzed pigmentation. Except for this and splenomegaly, the physical examination is usually noncontributory. Indolent superficial ulcers may rarely be present on the lower legs, as in the other chronic hemolytic diseases.

Typically, pancytopenia is present, with a moderate but significant depression of the leukocyte and platelet counts. The leukocyte content of alkaline phosphatase is decreased below normal (316). The red cells are somewhat macrocytic, with some variation in size but little variation in shape; spherocytosis is not present. The proportion of polychromatophilic cells and reticulocytes present is usually elevated to 10 to 15 per cent. The erythrocyte mechanical and osmotic fragility is normal both before and after incubation. No hemoglobin abnormality has been detected. The plasma icterus index and the unconjugated bilirubin content

are elevated. The plasma may have the golden-brown color usually associated with the presence of small amounts of methemalbumin and extracorpuscular hemoglobin.

LOCATION OF RED CELL DEFECT AND BASIC PATHOPHYSIOLOGY. In vitro tests and in vivo survival studies clearly indicate an intracorpuscular abnormality. The in vitro studies by Ham (123–125) localized the basic abnormality in the erythrocyte by demonstrating that the cells, although they reacted normally to osmotic and mechanical stresses, lysed in vitro when incubated in the patient's or normal compatible serum at a slightly lowered pH. Clinical investigation then showed a diurnal variation in the level of plasma hemoglobin (reflected, of course, by urinary hemoglobin excretion) such that during sleep (irrespective of whether taken at night or day) significant elevations were demonstrated. On evidence that has never really been amplified, it was postulated that as a result of the decreased sensitivity of the respiratory center during sleep, the pH of the blood drops slightly, owing probably to carbon dioxide retention. In organs with slow blood flow or stasis, it is likely that the pH changes are more marked. Such increases in acidity would provide the medium suitable for increased destruction of the abnormal erythrocyte. These usual effects of sleep could be abolished by respirator-induced hyperventilation. The rate of cell destruction could also be increased by the administration of ammonium chloride or *temporarily* abolished by sodium bicarbonate.

The continued intravascular hemolysis of susceptible cells, with augmented destruction at night, results in significantly elevated levels of plasma hemoglobin and depletion of haptoglobin. Consequently

* Dacie (74) makes the suggestion that the causal mechanisms leading to marrow hypoplasia may in addition lead to the formation of erythrocytes with a defect indistinguishable from that of typical PNH.

methemalbuminemia, hyperbilirubine-mia, and hemoglobinuria are predictable. Owing to the renal tubular absorption of the hemoglobin passing the glomerulus and attempts at iron conservation, con-siderable amounts of ferritin and hemo-siderin are found in the tubular epithelial cells. Some of these compounds are ex-creted into the urine from the cells, some released into the urine when the cells slough, and some are apparently resorbed (147). A considerable amount of hemo-siderin is excreted, and indeed the full name of the disorder is "paroxysmal noc-turnal hemoglobinuria with perpetual he-mosiderinuria." This brings about an un-usually large loss of iron from the body, exceeding sometimes 20 mg per day, that may lead to superimposed iron-lack ane-mia (262).

Cross-transfusion studies (Figure 9.2) have confirmed the intracorpuscular locus of the abnormality by demonstrating nor-mal survival of normal cells in the patient but shortened survival of the patient's cells in himself or in a normal person. These latter observations also have dem-onstrated the existence of two popula-tions of cells: one very susceptible to de-struction, the other having an apparently normal survival (Figure 9.2). In vitro tests also have confirmed this by showing that a portion of the cells (so-called "sus-ceptible cells") are readily lysed in the acid hemolysis test, while the remaining cells are resistant to destruction by this technique. It is of considerable interest that the proportion of susceptible cells varies markedly from patient to patient but correlates well with the erythrocyte survival time and the clinical course of each patient (139).

Studies subsequent to these basic path-ophysiologic observations have attempted to define the mechanism of cell destruc-tion and the nature of the red cell defect. In this instance there is no good evidence that aging influences the susceptibility of the cell to acid lysis: apparently it does

not. There is, indeed, some in vitro and in vivo evidence that reticulocytes are most susceptible to destruction (214, 227).

NATURE OF RED CELL DEFECT. A physical defect in the membrane, a patchy, pitted surface with many clefts, has been dem-onstrated by electron microscopy. This finding has been by others both confirmed and denied as artifactitious. Various workers have found differences in the phospholipid content of cells of par-oxysmal nocturnal hemoglobinuria as op-posed to normal cells that could not be entirely accounted for by the younger age of the cells present in the PNH popula-tion. The cells show a decrease in phos-phoryl choline (phosphatidyl choline) and an excess of phosphoryl serine (phos-phatidyl serine), although the total phos-pholipid content is normal. An excess of arachidonic and pentanoic acids has been found and confirmed, as has a deficiency of oleic acid. Evaluation of the work must await further observations;* dietary in-take is known to affect red cell lipids, and it is not clear whether adequate dietary controls were in effect during the studies (12, 190, 224, 225). The recent observa-tions by Phillips (249a) revealed no devi-ation from the normal.

A decreased rate of entry of P^{32} into the cells and a decreased rate of efflux have been demonstrated. No defect in the phosphorylation of adenosine diphos-phate (ADP) has been found although apparently there is an increased turnover of the labile phosphate of adenosine tri-phosphate (ATP).

Acetylcholinesterase is an enzyme found exclusively in the stromal fabric.

* In the rare disorder called acanthocytosis (282) lipid defects are well established. These defects lead to morphologic changes in the eryth-rocytes ("spiny cells") and a hemolytic ane-mia. Lecithin and sphingomyelin are decreased (249) in the plasma, probably owing to a failure to synthesize the protein portion of the β-lipo-proteins. Because of the low plasma levels the equilibrium of lipids between erythrocytes and plasma is upset; the cells become deficient and short lived.

Its concentration is strikingly and consistently decreased* (usually less than 50 per cent of normal) in PNH cells, and such a decrease is seen consistently only in PNH cells (83, 127). This enzyme is known to be present in high concentrations in young normal cells and to decrease progressively with aging. It has been used as an indicator of bone marrow regeneration and red cell production. However, even in red cell preparations rich in PNH reticulocytes, the acetylcholinesterase activity is low. In this situation the existence of a factor inhibiting the activity of the enzyme is considered unlikely. The in vivo inhibition of acetylcholinesterase (215) in normal subjects did not influence the erythrocyte survival time, consequently normal amounts are not required for adequate survival. Moreover, acetylcholinesterase is absent from the erythrocytes of some animal species.

A curious behavior is exhibited by these cells toward iso-antibodies and other antibodies having both agglutinating and hemolytic activities (73, 194, 214). Normal cells are invariably more readily agglutinated than lysed by the techniques conventionally employed; PNH cells are lysed about as readily as they are agglutinated. Being much more susceptible to lysis than the normal, they are more sensitive indicators of lytic antibodies, as will be discussed later (page 306), and have been useful in detecting serum factors subliminal to other tests. Thus, the nature of the defect responsible for PNH remains as obscure as its intracorpuscular location is definite.

NATURE OF REQUISITE SERUM FACTORS. Investigations concerning the nature of the requisite serum factors and the serum-erythrocyte interaction have shown the following. There is a definite pH optimum for lysis that lies on the acid side of physiologic pH, drops off sharply on either side, but extends to some degree into the physiologic range. This reaction is temperature-dependent, being maximal at 37°C. Lysis depends on the presence of magnesium cations, does not depend upon calcium cations, and is inhibited by increased concentrations of calcium cations. It has long been known that lysis of PNH cells is dependent upon a heat-labile factor(s) present in normal serum. Recent studies by Hinz et al. (138) have demonstrated that properdin is necessary for serum lytic activity and that in every manner tested the PNH system is comparable in requirements and behavior to the properdin system with zymosan, bacteria, and viruses. Whether the components of the complement or other unknown serum factors make up the requisite serum constituents cannot be said with certainty at this time. So far, anything done to destroy the complement or remove one of its components abolishes the lytic activity of the serum. It should be noted that this reaction is dissimilar from usual antibody lysis in several ways: no abnormal antibody has been demonstrated on the red cell or in the plasma, calcium cations are inhibitory, and properdin is required.

Crosby has demonstrated that the addition of thrombin to acidified serum increases the hemolysis of PNH erythrocytes. It is not clear whether the thrombin acts upon clotting factors in the serum, upon requisite serum factors by activation or inactivation, upon the cell membrane, by the coincident addition of heterophilic antibodies, or by other mechanisms.

The two diagnostic procedures employed are the acid hemolysis or Ham test, which measures the lysis of red cells in acidified serum, and the thrombin activation test, which measures the *augmented* lysis of cells in acidified serum.

SUMMARY. In summary it may be said that lysis of PNH cells involves the interaction between an unknown intracellular

---

* An exceptional patient (with mild manifestations of the disease) has been found with normal levels of acetycholinesterase.

defect and several factors present in normal serum: magnesium cations, properdin, and "complement-like" components. The interaction leads to maximal lysis at a pH slightly lower than physiologic.

On the basis of the known thrombotic tendencies of these patients, several attempts have been made to implicate various clotting factors in the lytic action. As yet no clear-cut demonstration has been made that cannot be more consistently explained by the known greater susceptibility of PNH cells to lysis. It is curious that one of the drugs employed at times as a therapeutic agent effective against the hemolysis and clinical manifestations of PNH is Dicumarol. According to reports it has been used with variable success. Splenectomy is usually without very significant or prolonged beneficial effect, and ACTH or adrenal hormones have little to commend them on the basis of the few trials made. Dextran is reported to abolish hemolysis for short periods and may be considered in acute or critical situations.

Hemolytic Diseases Caused by Extracorpuscular Defects

Consideration has been given to examples of disorders resulting from (a) intracorpuscular abnormalities, either inherited (hemoglobinopathies, thalassemia, hereditary spherocytosis, hereditary nonspherocytic hemolytic anemia) or acquired (paroxysmal nocturnal hemoglobinuria); and (b) interaction of intracorpuscular abnormalities and an extracorpuscular factor (primaquine-sensitive hemolytic anemia, favism). A third group, wherein the life span of the red cell is shortened by an extracorpuscular factor, will now be discussed (Figure 9.1).

In some of the hemolytic diseases in this third group the existence of abnormal serum factors capable of interacting with erythrocytes can be clearly and readily demonstrated by in vitro tests. Examples are the agglutinins and/or lysins causing paroxysmal cold hemoglobinuria and the agglutinins and/or lysins causing so-called autoimmune hemolytic anemia of the idiopathic or symptomatic (secondary) type (333). In most disorders, however, the existence of abnormal extracorpuscular factors can be detected only by demonstrating that the life span of normal erythrocytes is shortened when the cells are transfused into a patient; it has not been possible to show, by presently available in vitro tests, abnormal tissue (see footnote, page 300) or serum factors. This latter type of hemolytic disease, due to an extracorpuscular abnormality but with no demonstrable serum factor, is by far the one most commonly encountered. The severity of the hemolysis may vary from a degree detectable only by precise studies of erythrocyte survival to an overt process that dominates the clinical picture.

Secondary Acquired Hemolytic Anemia without Demonstrable Serum Factor

Some degree of abnormal red cell destruction has been shown to occur in a large number of diseases that do not primarily affect erythropoiesis or the erythrocytes—secondary or symptomatic acquired hemolytic anemia. It is probably justified to say that in almost every disease that profoundly affects metabolism or is associated with generalized poisoning there occurs a shortening of the erythrocyte life span by mechanisms that are largely obscure.* A considerable number of diseases are quite regularly accompanied by a hemolytic process. The most frequently encountered are severe, acute, and chronic infections (159); malignant growths (particularly if widespread); acute leukemia; chronic leukemias of the aggressive types; uremia (165,

---

* Myxedema in humans (211) and hibernation in animals (34) are the only situations in which a prolongation of the red cell life span has been adequately documented.

196, 298); liver disease (150); and rheumatoid arthritis (212). Any disease that is accompanied by marked splenomegaly is very likely to have some associated hemolytic component (hypersplenism). In these situations it is rarely possible to demonstrate serum factors or tissue abnormalities that have any convincing etiologic relation to the red cell destruction. Although it is possible for an overt hemolytic process to be either the first manifestation of an underlying disease or the dominating feature of the clinical picture, in the vast majority of the patients, the process is hidden. Few of the usual findings indicative of hemolysis are present: there may be little or no increase in bilirubin content or reticulocyte count, and often the existence of hemolysis can be documented only by transfusion requirements or determination of erythrocyte survival time.

In most of these situations morphologic studies and ferrokinetic observations relative to red cell production indicate that there also exists depressed erythropoiesis. This is usually referred to as a "toxic depression of the marrow." These two factors (hemolysis and depression of marrow activity) combine in varying proportions to govern the level of hemoglobin in the circulating blood and the secondary manifestations of the resulting blood alterations. In some, the effects are determined by depressed bone marrow activity when this plays the major role; in others, both hemolysis and lack of bone marrow response play more nearly equal roles; in still others, the hemolytic component is dominant. In almost all situations, however, the bone marrow is unable to respond normally to the hemolytic process and a state of "relative bone marrow insufficiency" exists.

The anemia present in these disorders may then be said to result from a combination of hemolysis and bone marrow failure. In the majority of instances this cannot be demonstrated by the screening techniques usually available. It is obvious that these disorders account for a large number of frequently encountered clinical problems. The problems have been defined, but little can be said concerning the mechanism involved. Splenic sequestration is demonstrable to some extent in "hypersplenism," and there the hemolytic process is relieved in varying degree by splenectomy; otherwise no preferential site of erythrocyte sequestration or destruction is evident, and splenectomy is of no benefit. In Chapter 11 these disorders are individually considered in more detail as examples of bone marrow failure.

Secondary Acquired Hemolytic Anemia with Demonstrable Serum Factors

Many instances of overt hemolytic anemia and/or hemolytic anemia associated *with* demonstrable serum factors are secondary to lymphatic leukemia, a lymphoma, Hodgkin's disease, or disseminated lupus erythematosus (329). These associations have been known for some time. In addition to the above, a secondary or symptomatic hemolytic anemia may be seen in association with carcinoma, teratoma, pregnancy, tuberculosis, sarcoid, eosinophilic granuloma, polyarteritis, thrombotic thrombocytopenic purpura, infectious mononucleosis, drug ingestion, etc., or it may be idiopathic. Clinically, the hemolytic anemia may appear in several ways during the course of the underlying disease. Rarely, it may be the first sign.

Ordinarily, a slowly progressive anemia becomes apparent, jaundice is noted, and examination of the blood indicates the presence of a chronic hemolytic process. Exacerbations of the hemolytic process commonly parallel the manifestations of underlying disease. The hemolysis may subside when the underlying disease is brought under better control by appropriate therapy, but it is not unusual to have the first hemolytic episode follow shortly after therapy designed to decrease cell multiplication and curtail neoplastic growth. As a rule, no very distinctive changes are seen in the peripheral blood film. Abnormal variations in size and shape of the red cell are invariably present but may be no more than are seen in the uncomplicated disease itself. Reticulocytosis is usually moderate and a few spherocytes may be seen. Various types of serum factors and "antibodies" may be demonstrated in the patient's serum. Both "cold" type and "warm" antibodies have been found.* Most frequently the abnormal factor will have been taken up by (adsorbed to) the red cell, where it may be demonstrated by a positive reaction to the Coombs test. The results of other tests employed in attempts to elucidate the source, nature, and function of the abnormal serum factors and possible mechanisms of red cell destruction have been so variable and inconstant that as yet there is no discernible pattern. They will not be discussed here. In addition to supportive therapy (transfusions), treatment should be directed specifically against the primary disease (by means of ACTH or adrenal hormones, splenectomy, x-ray, or chemotherapy). When feasible, surgical removal of a tumor or tumor masses should be considered, because in a limited number of situations this may arrest the hemolytic process.

Mechanisms of Erythrocyte Destruction by Antibodies

Since the hemolytic processes resulting from ABO and D (Rh) blood group incompatibilities are best understood, they will be discussed as prototypes of the reactions occurring in so-called "auto-immune" hemolytic anemia (67, 146, 153, 154, 158, 179, 218).

CELL DESTRUCTION BY ABO ANTIBODIES. The hemolytic and/or agglutinating factors directed against the ABO-specific substances are termed iso-antibodies (iso-

agglutinin, iso-hemolysin). Although originally considered to be naturally occurring iso-antibodies because of their universal presence in appropriate situations, it is now generally accepted that they are immune antibodies that arise in response to repeated exposures to ABO substances present in various foods and exogenous substances. Chemically the ABO substances are mucopolysaccharides, and the antibodies directed against them are γ-globulins with variable characteristics such as molecular weight, sedimentation constants, electrophoretic migration, and chromatographic behavior (170). The interactions between the two closely resemble the characteristics of antigen-antibody interactions with respect to specificity, quantitative neutralization, nature of intermolecular bonds, fixation of complement components, thermal range, stability, etc.

An appalling number of mismatched transfusions have made possible many observations of the clinical consequences of this antigen-antibody reaction. When the antibodies are present in low concentrations, they appear to possess only agglutinating ability in vitro, hemolytic activity being subliminal with present techniques. When present in high concentrations and accompanied by the various components of the complement and a proper ionic constellation, the factors possess lytic activity. In heat-inactivated serum only the agglutinating property is present. The ultimate mechanism whereby the antibody effects lysis is unknown (see page 239 for discussion). Since in its activated form one of the components of complement, C'_1, possesses esterase activity, it has been presumed that lysis may result from "stromal dissolution" or disruption of restraining bonds.

* See below under Idiopathic Acquired Hemolytic Anemia (Autoimmune Antibody Type) for discussion of the nature, source, and possible etiologic significance of the various abnormal factors.

Observations have been made by Jandl et al. (153) and other workers on the fate of small volumes of Cr^{51}-labeled ABO-incompatible normal red cells infused into subjects in whom normal iso-agglutinin titers were present and in whom low iso-hemolysin activity was demonstrable in vitro. The incompatible red cells largely disappeared from the circulation within 2 minutes of the injection. This occurred concomitantly with an abrupt appearance of high levels of radioactivity over the liver, but not over the spleen, thorax, or lumbosacral areas. Immediately after injection of incompatible cells, Cr^{51} and extracellular hemoglobin appeared in the plasma,* reached maximum values in 5 to 6 minutes, and declined during the next several hours.

In subjects having normal iso-agglutinin titers but in whom no iso-hemolysin was demonstrable in vitro, the Cr^{51} and extracellular hemoglobin immediately rose to a low level but did not thereafter exceed this value. The removal of the cells from the peripheral blood was accompanied by marked and rapid accumulation of radioactivity in the liver.

In subjects having a high concentration of iso-hemolysin, hemoglobinemia was abrupt in onset, marked, and reached maximum values in less than 60 seconds. Over 80 per cent of the hemoglobin contained in the injected red cells could be accounted for in the circulating plasma. The hepatic accumulation of Cr^{51} was slower and less marked.

Thus, small volumes of ABO-incompatible red cells are destroyed abruptly in subjects with iso-agglutinin but no demonstrable iso-hemolysin. The destruction is accompanied by hepatic sequestration of the cells and moderate hemoglobinemia. In subjects in whom both agglutinin and hemolysin are demonstrable, red cell destruction is virtually instantaneous and presumably occurs within the general circulation, with prompt hemoglobinemia and a less pronounced hepatic accumulation of Cr^{51}. It seems probable that all normal persons possess some iso-hemolysin for ABO-incompatible cells even when not detected by standard in vitro procedures or that iso-hemolysin may be present in effective quantities in certain tissues. Cells not immediately lysed are sequestered, probably as agglutinates, in the liver.

Loutit made the observation that when red cells were agglutinated in vitro by anti-A serum and then infused into type A subjects, the survival of the cells was relatively normal. Presumably the agglutinates dispersed in the circulation. When Cr^{51} was employed in similar situations, about 25 per cent of the injected cells were almost immediately removed from the blood stream, and a small proportion of the Cr^{51} appeared extracellularly in the plasma. Hepatic radioactivity increased while splenic radioactivity remained low. During approximately a 2-hour period the Cr^{51} activity increased in the circulating red cells and returned to 93 per cent of the injected level. After this the erythrocyte survival was normal. Apparently here the agglutinates were filtered into the liver, a few cells were destroyed, and then the agglutinates dispersed, and the cells were redelivered to the peripheral blood none the worse for wear.

The above observations were made on small volumes of cells in an intended excess of antibody and serum factors but with possibly variable rates of dissociation of the antibody after infusion. Therefore, deviations from the results described above might be expected if large volumes of cells were involved that might exhaust one or another serum factor, result in less potent sensitization or complement fixation, or utilize or saturate all the avail-

---

* It is to be remembered that more than 90 per cent of the Cr^{51} is bound to the globin portion of the red cell's hemoglobin.

able sequestering capacity of the spleen or liver. For example, Castle et al. (45) observed that following a hemolytic transfusion reaction (resulting from the accidental administration of 500 ml of group A blood to a group O recipient whose serum contained only anti-A agglutinin activity*) small clumps of spheroidal red cells were demonstrable in the peripheral blood for 8 hours after the infusion.

When attempts were made to control antigen/antibody proportions and evaluate their influence on the kinetics of red cell destruction, it was demonstrated that with small antibody doses there was slow partial trapping by the spleen, with larger antibody doses a brisk trapping by the liver, while still larger doses caused intravascular hemolysis.

CELL DESTRUCTION BY RH ANTIBODIES. The composition of the antigenic substances responsible for the type specificity of red cells with respect to the Rh factors is not definitely known. Antibodies produced in response to immunization with CDE factors or erythrocytes in appropriate situations are globulins. The antibodies directed against the Rh system have never reliably been shown to possess lytic activity in vitro. Even with an extremely high titer of antibodies in the presence of fresh serum augmented with additional complement and various ions, no hemolytic activity is demonstrable. Only agglutinating capacities have been detected, and these may be of various types.

If the antibody produces red cell agglutination in saline dilutions, it is visualized as being bivalent, or capable of combining with two red cells, thereby producing agglutination. It is therefore termed a "complete" antibody or a "saline agglutinin." Other types of CDE antibodies combine with the specifically antigenic cell but produce no immediate, visible reaction. Their presence on the

cell may be demonstrated in a variety of ways. For example, the cells so affected can no longer be agglutinated by potent "saline agglutinating" anti-D sera; the saline agglutinin is somehow blocked from its usual activity, and the factor on the red cell responsible for this is thus termed a "blocking antibody." As another example, the cells so affected will agglutinate if suspended in a 20 per cent albumin solution or a similar medium. The antibody is visualized as being "univalent" and capable of combining with only one cell. When so combined, the cells do not agglutinate until the adsorbed "univalent" antibodies are bridged together by a serum factor or suitable environment that will complete their agglutinating potentialities. Such factors are termed "incomplete antibodies."

A sensitive and reliable way of detecting the presence of incomplete antibodies on red cells is by means of the Coombs, or antiglobulin, test. Since the incomplete antibodies are γ-globulins, antibodies directed against γ-globulins will combine with them on the surface of the red cell, presumably join together such antibodies on adjacent cells, and result in agglutination. The Coombs test depends on the use of an antiserum to human globulin (Coombs' serum) that is prepared by the injection of human globulin into rabbits. Antibodies are formed by the rabbits against the human globulin. At an appropriate time serum is obtained from the immunized animal. Coombs' serum is, therefore, a rabbit serum containing antibodies directed against human globulin. When sensitized cells (cells coated with incomplete antibodies) are suspended in the Coombs' serum, agglutination of the cells takes place. Normal cells so treated

---

* Ebert and others have shown that in the opposite situation, namely the injection of large amounts of group O plasma into A, B, or AB subjects, the hemolytic process thereby induced is also accompanied by an increased osmotic fragility of the recipient's red cells (281).

do not agglutinate. In dealing with the Rh antibody system, therefore, it must be kept in mind that (a) no lytic factors are known, (b) the antibody may be complete and saline agglutinating, or (c) incomplete and nonagglutinating.

When small volumes of Cr^{51}-labeled type-D-positive red cells are injected into recipients with a high titer of incomplete anti-D factor, rapid removal of the cells from the circulation occurs; half are gone in 14 minutes. There is an associated build-up of radioactivity in the *spleen* area and a lesser build-up over the liver. Little or no Cr^{51} or extracellular hemoglobin appears in the plasma. When larger volumes of cells are employed, the maximum levels of Cr^{51} and extracellular hemoglobin are attained about 1 hour after injection, but the levels represent only 5 per cent of the total amount infused.

When the recipient's serum contains agglutinating as well as incomplete antibodies, the events are quite similar except for a more rapid and pronounced *hepatic* sequestration of red cells.

By a procedure demonstrated not to affect erythrocyte survival time, D-positive cells were made to react with potent, incomplete antibodies. The coated, or sensitized, cells were then injected into normal recipients. Half of the injected cells were removed from the circulation in about 30 minutes. Very little Cr^{51} or extracellular hemoglobin appeared in the plasma. Shortly after the injection of the sensitized but unagglutinated cells, small numbers of red cell agglutinates and chains of cells were visible in the peripheral blood. A heavy build-up of Cr^{51} in the spleen area occurred with little evidence of hepatic accumulation. Further studies indicated that the rate and extent of destruction of the sensitized cells was proportional to the volume of antibody relative to the number of red cells employed, and presumably, then, to the degree of sensitization or antibody coating.

Thus, employing the Rh antigen-antibody system, it was again demonstrated that agglutinated red cells were sequestered rapidly, and primarily in the liver. Cells sensitized with an incomplete antibody were rapidly and almost totally sequestered in the spleen. In each instance the release of hemoglobin into the plasma was slow and of small degree.

As with the ABO antibodies, this pattern was modified by quantitative relation. When these were controlled in the experimental procedure it was demonstrated that with small and moderate amounts of incomplete anti-D iso-antibody a predominantly splenic pattern of destruction occurred; large amounts of the same antibody caused a moderate hepatic uptake in addition.

SUMMARY. In summarizing the kinetics of erythrocyte destruction as mediated by the ABO and Rh antibody systems (Figures 9.12 and 9.13) it is evident that the nature of the antibody plays an important role in the different routes of cell destruction but that the different routes are also modified by purely quantitative factors. In addition, it is most probable that the results obtained are modified and limited by the techniques employed for making the observations. The demonstration of splenic and hepatic sequestration by directional radioactive counting employing a collimated scintillation probe is successful because these organs represent concentrations of parts of the reticuloendothelial system in discrete anatomic structures. Were the structures not concentrated but spread out in thin layers over large areas pervading the body (even though retaining their peculiar circulatory and architectural organizations), it would be technically difficult if not impossible to demonstrate their sequestering functions. This is, of course, the situation for the reticuloendothelial system of the bone marrow, which bears

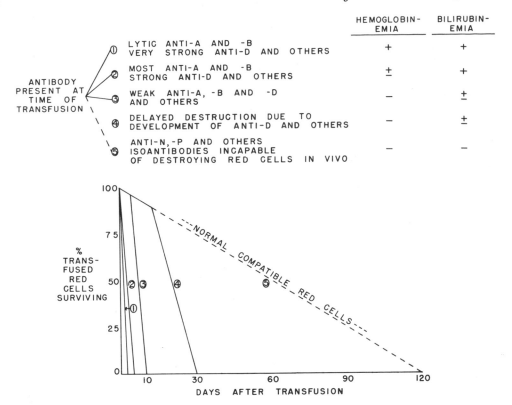

FIGURE 9.12. Red cell survival time and plasma pigment changes as determined by type and/or response of antibody involved. (From Mudge, G. H., Am. J. Med. 16:878, 1954)

a striking resemblance to that of the spleen. On the basis of a not very satisfactory analogy between rabbit and man, it has been estimated (89) that over one-third of physiologic red cell destruction would be expected to take place within the marrow of man. Were it technically possible to evaluate the role of the marrow in abnormal red cell destruction in terms of sequestration, it seems likely that additional modifications of the above conclusions would be necessary.

The mechanisms by which the spleen sequesters sensitized cells are not precisely known. The fact that agglutinates are seen in the peripheral blood indicates some procedure for completing the action of the sensitizing incomplete antibodies, and the observation that agglutinates are much more numerous in splenic blood

obtained at the time of operation makes it likely that this agglutination is effected in the spleen. The splenic hematocrit is appreciably higher than that of the peripheral blood, and the protein concentration of the intrasplenic plasma is also increased (299). From in vitro observations it is known that any increase in plasma globulins (including fibrinogen) induces or intensifies red cell agglutination, particularly of sensitized cells. Simple dehydration of plasma is very effective and forms the basis of some tests. It seems probable that by supplying the proper suspending media the spleen induces agglutination of sensitized cells, and because the proper anatomic structure for retention of agglutinated cells is provided, sequestration occurs. From many observations it is evident that sequestered

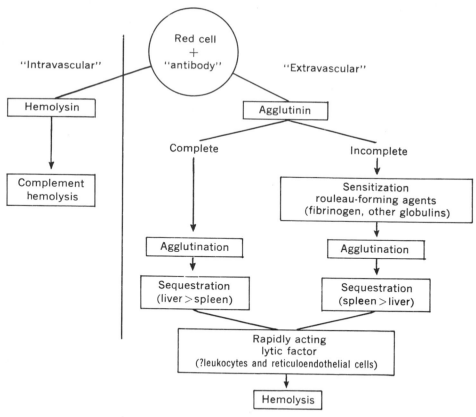

FIGURE 9.13.   Mechanisms of red cell destruction by iso-antibodies, through intra- and extravascular routes. (From Castle, W. B., *in* Sodeman, W. A. (ed.), Pathologic Physiology: Mechanisms of Disease, ed. 3, p. 889, Saunders, Philadelphia, 1961)

cells are not in a favorable environment.* Markedly increased osmotic fragility is noted, and many spherocytes appear. If these result from osmotic intake of water, at a high splenic hematocrit an appreciable plasma dehydration may be effected. This, in turn, favors agglutination and sequestration (Figure 9.13).

Once sequestration of sensitized red cells in the spleen has occurred by virtue of their agglutinability, it appears that their actual destruction follows in a matter of minutes. The average half-maximum plasma hemoglobin level follows the average red cell half-life survival time by less than 10 minutes. Moreover, the serum level of unconjugated bilirubin rises within 1 hour, and the rise quantitatively reflects the much greater breakdown of

larger amounts of hemoglobin than appear in the plasma. The spleen is able to sequester and destroy large amounts of red cells very rapidly and to catabolize the hemoglobin mainly *in situ* allowing

* Many substances having the capacity to destroy or "condition" (45) erythrocytes have been extracted from splenic tissue (as well as from brain, lung, liver, kidney, serum, red cell stroma, etc.). These usually coexist with substances that inhibit their lytic capacity. Over the years their potential role in in vivo erythrocyte destruction has interested many investigators whose views have been well summarized by Ponder (253). The most recent study relative to this problem is by Stefanini et al. (309), who found that in "nonimmunologic" hemolytic anemias the amount of extractable inhibitors was decreased and that the administration of steroids was accompanied by increases in inhibitor concentrations.

the escape of only a minor proportion of hemoglobin into the general circulation.

Clinical Entities Illustrating Secondary Acquired Hemolytic Anemia

From the heterogenous group of disorders included under the term "acquired hemolytic anemia associated with demonstrable serum factors" only a few can be separated out that form discrete clinical entities, readily identified by clinical course and specific laboratory tests. The remainder can be divided into subgroups only on the basis of fairly inconstant, probably artificial criteria, so that it is reasonable to consider them as one group. The two most obvious examples of secondary acquired hemolytic anemia are, of course, the hemolytic processes due to transfusion incompatibilities of various types and the maternal-fetal type-specific incompatibilities giving rise to erythroblastosis. These will not be discussed further.

PAROXYSMAL COLD HEMOGLOBINURIA ASSOCIATED WITH COLD HEMOLYSIN. One of the discrete entities that will be here considered is paroxysmal cold hemoglobinuria caused by a hemolysin. This is now a rare disease in which the striking manifestation is the passage of dark urine containing hemoglobin after local or general exposure of the body to cold. In some instances only brief exposure to moderate cold is necessary for the induction of an attack; in other instances prolonged and marked chilling is necessary. Systemic symptoms may appear during or up to 8 hours after the exposure to cold and consist of aching and pain in the abdomen, back, chest, and extremities; malaise; and even vomiting and diarrhea. A severe, shaking chill frequently occurs and is then followed by fever. Urine passed at this time is brown, red-brown, or black, but only a few subsequent specimens may be discolored before clearing takes place.* Prostration may be profound, and the patient usually notices subsequent weakness, shortness of breath, pallor, and perhaps some jaundice. Dermal manifestations in the form of wheals, urticaria, or acrocyanosis have been described.

The blood findings are those of an acute hemolytic anemia resulting from intravascular hemolysis; the severity of the changes reflect the severity of the attack. The hemoglobin in the circulating blood may be only slightly altered or decreased to one-third of the usual level. The plasma becomes red in an overt attack and hemoglobinuria follows depending upon the extent of plasma hemoglobin rise and the amount of red cell destruction. Methemalbumin becomes detectable and a rise in the unconjugated bilirubin level follows. Early in a paroxysm, erythrophagocytosis and marked leukopenia may be observed; the latter is soon replaced by leukocytosis (163). No morphologic changes are noted in the red cells. A positive reaction to the direct Coombs test is present during an acute attack but usually for only short periods thereafter. No change in the erythrocyte osmotic and mechanical fragility has been noted. The usual signs of blood regeneration (polychromatophilia, reticulocytosis) are found during the recovery phase. It is said that with repeated minor episodes a significant degree of anemia may develop associated with hemosiderinuria.

The demonstration of the Donath-Landsteiner hemolysin is the pathognomonic test of this disease (86). The unique hemolysin responsible for this reaction is effective against all normal erythrocytes (a panhemolysin) and requires the following conditions for its full activity: (a) complement must be present with the antibody; (b) the red cell–antibody system must be chilled to fix the antibody to the red cell; and (c) the sensitized cell–complement system

---

* Described by one patient as "the color of ox-blood shoe polish."

must then be warmed for hemolysis to take place. The Donath-Landsteiner reaction therefore involves a cold phase and a warm phase. In a recent detailed analysis of this hemolytic system by Hinz (140–142), employing a concentrated, partially purified antibody, the 11 S γ-globulin of Müller-Eberhard, and the various components of complement, it was shown that during the cold phase (optimal at 1°C) the antibody is fixed to the cell in the presence of the 11 S component, and C'_1 (or its activated esterase form) combines with the complex in the presence of calcium ions; during the warm phase (optimal at 37°C) C'_4, C'_2, magnesium cations, and C'_3, in sequence, are necessary for lysis (140, 141).

Griggs has recently demonstrated that employing either the patient's or normal erythrocytes, the cold hemolysin has a greater lytic capacity against the older erythrocytes than the younger. Weintraub et al. (339a) showed that on lipid analysis of the erythrocytes there was no evident gross abnormality but that patients' cells were always more susceptible to the hemolysin than normal cells. Beyond this little is known concerning the mechanism of hemolysis by this factor (269).

The Donath-Landsteiner hemolysin is usually but not always found in association with a positive reaction to the Wassermann test, resulting from congenital or acquired syphilis. It may be present only transiently but it usually persists for long periods of time. It may or may not disappear following antiluetic therapy, and it has been shown to be separate from the Wassermann factors responsible for the various biologic tests for syphilis. In a few instances, it has been demonstrated for short periods following infectious diseases (measles) (290). The reason for the development of the peculiar antibody in any of the situations in which it has appeared is not known. The clinical counterparts of the Donath-Landsteiner test responsible for producing a hemolytic episode appear obvious, and in many instances hemolytic episodes have been produced by the controlled chilling and warming of an extremity in a susceptible patient.

A peculiar property of the Donath-Landsteiner antibody is that while possessing considerable lytic activity, its agglutinating properties appear slight, if present at all. The cold agglutinin titer of serum containing the Donath-Landsteiner hemolysin is usually within the normal range. Practically all other antibodies exhibit a much greater capacity for agglutination than for lysis as assayed by the usual titration procedures.

PAROXYSMAL COLD HEMOGLOBINURIA ASSOCIATED WITH COLD AGGLUTININ. A second type of paroxysmal cold hemoglobinuria is distinguished by the presence of an abnormal amount of cold agglutinin. Curiously enough except under special conditions the agglutinin usually exhibits little or no lytic activity (68).

The clinical picture and the hematologic changes noted may mimic very closely those described above as occurring with the Donath-Landsteiner factor. The patients are more prone to develop dermal manifestations, Raynaud's phenomenon, frostbite, and even gangrene of the extremities (231). They are less likely to experience hemoglobinuria with each paroxysm and more likely to develop a chronically depressed hematocrit and hemoglobin concentration associated with reticulocytosis and hemosiderinuria. (The chronicity is obviously related to exposure and to the climate. In the Northern Hemisphere the changes may be noted only during the colder winter months.)

Extraordinarily high titers of the agglutinin, which is effective against all erythrocytes (panagglutinin)* have been

* Type I–negative erythrocytes are *not* agglutinated by the cold antibody, but since this blood type occurs in less than one in ten thousand individuals, for practical purposes the antibody can be considered a panagglutinin.

reported in association with the syndrome. Cold agglutinin may be detected in normal serum in titer of 1:8 or 1:16. In paroxysmal cold hemoglobinuria the reported titers range up to 1:1,000,000 but are usually around 1:30,000. When the agglutinin is present in high titer, it is frequently impossible to perform a red cell count unless warmed equipment and stages are used. Moreover, as the titer of the antibody is elevated, the thermal range of effective agglutination appears increased so that gross agglutination may be present in blood samples at room temperature. Normally the agglutinin is sought and quantitated by chilling to 5°C a small volume of normal type O cells in large volumes of serially diluted serum.

Cold agglutinin may be found in patients' sera in such large quantities that abnormal peaks are present in the electrophoretic pattern. These abnormal peaks can be specifically removed by adsorption of the cold antibody onto erythrocytes in the cold (116). In some patients they are described as being in the γ-globulin position, in others in the β-globulin range. There is evidence that the antibody is macromolecular, with a sedimentation constant of S_{20w} 16 to 19. The highest temperature at which cells are agglutinated in vitro is 28 to 32°C. The fact that the direct Coombs test is usually also positive in this disease is probably due to cooling of the blood below 37°C in peripheral cutaneous areas. Although the agglutinin is reversibly dissociated from the red cell by rewarming to 37°C, some sensitizing factor remains adsorbed to the red cell surface.* This appears to be made up largely of a component(s) of complement and apparently is responsible for the positive reaction to the direct Coombs test (192).

Although for many years this factor was thought to have agglutinating abilities only, recent studies have demonstrated the capacity for lytic action in the presence of complement, although the

serum may have to be suitably acidified (68).

The cause of the formation of the cold iso-antibody in such high titer is obscure. A moderate rise in titer is seen during various types of atypical or virus pneumonia; rarely, following such an infection the titer may increase remarkably and assume values known to be associated with clinical manifestations. If such patients are subjected to chilling episodes, hemolytic anemia associated with hemoglobinuria and hemoglobinemia may occur. In these instances the titer usually falls spontaneously, returning to normal in a matter of weeks or months. Some individuals may have a high titer from no known cause. The high titer may persist for many years. This is seen almost exclusively in elderly patients. In others the rise in titer is associated with the development of a neoplastic process, usually leukemia or lymphosarcoma. Moderate increases in cold agglutinin titer are frequently seen in patients with acquired hemolytic anemia with or without other demonstrable serum factors.

The strongly agglutinated cells are more susceptible to mechanical trauma in vitro. Such agglutinated cells have been seen in conjunctival and nail-bed capillaries on cooling, and concentration of Cr^{51} has been demonstrated in chilled body areas of patients whose cells have been so labeled. It would seem reasonable to suspect that the mechanical trauma inflicted *in situ* on these sequestered clumped cells would account for at least some of the hemolysis. The agglutinin also has lytic potentialities, but the in

* At one time it was suggested that an "incomplete cold agglutinin" remained fixed to the cell. In a study to determine if the serologic activity attributed to an "incomplete cold antibody" could be separated from the "complete" cold agglutinin antibody, Leddy et al. (187) could not achieve separation by zone electrophoresis, density gradient ultracentrifugation, and anion exchange chromatography. They concluded that only one antibody was involved, the cold agglutinin.

vivo significance of the finding is presently obscure. The role of the spleen in hemolytic antibody production or activation or as sequestering organ for the sensitized cells has not been adequately evaluated. In some patients splenectomy has had a beneficial long-term effect.

Idiopathic Acquired Hemolytic Anemia (Autoimmune Antibody Type)

Under this heading is included a considerable number of hemolytic anemias that are apparently of primary origin or at least of unknown etiology. For unknown causes, abnormal tissue or plasma factors develop that apparently play an active role in the destruction of the patient's own red cells.* These factors have agglutinating or lytic properties that may require one or more of a bewildering variety of techniques for demonstration and have accordingly been called antibodies. The disease is frequently referred to as idiopathic acquired hemolytic anemia of the autoimmune antibody type. As more careful and prolonged studies of patients with idiopathic acquired hemolytic anemia are made, more and more patients are found to have underlying diseases and their anemias are accordingly reclassified to the symptomatic group. However, some anemias run extended courses without discoverable underlying cause even on postmortem examination.

CLINICAL MANIFESTATIONS. For reasons not now definitely explicable these patients begin to destroy their own red cells at increased rates that may vary from those barely discernible by erythrocyte survival techniques to those that are rapidly fatal. The hemolysis may have an acute onset and run a brief course (Lederer's anemia in children); it may have an insidious onset and run a prolonged course; it may be characterized by exacerbations and remissions. The usual course is prolonged and the degree of hemolysis enough to produce signs and symptoms. Patients of all ages (235) and both sexes are affected,

but there is a slight predominance of females over males in various large series reported. Most of the patients described are of European extraction, but no familial tendency has been noted. The patients' symptoms are attributable to the anemia and the signs are those basic to hemolytic disorders: a variable but often severe degree of anemia, signs of increased bone marrow activity, acholuric jaundice, and splenomegaly.

LABORATORY FINDINGS. The peripheral blood findings are so numerous and variable and occur in so many combinations and permutations that they can only be summarized here. There usually is some degree of macrocytosis that becomes more prominent with increasing hemoglobin deficit. Spherocytes may be absent or they may constitute the predominant cell. They are usually somewhat macrocytic and consequently probably differ from the spherocyte of hereditary spherocytosis, which is of normal volume.† There is usually greater-than-normal variation in size and shape of the red cells, with some bizarre forms. Polychromatophilia and reticulocytosis are usually marked, but these cells may constitute anywhere between 1 and more than 85 per cent of the total cells. Nucleated red cells, usually of the late normoblastic stage, are frequently seen. Autoagglutination may be present (clumping of patient's red cells in his own plasma or serum), and the disease may be first suspected when it is found impossible to perform a red cell count by ordinary methods. The erythrocyte osmotic fragility may be increased, normal, or de-

---

* It must be pointed out that some patients develop an acquired hemolytic anemia of unknown etiology but *no* abnormal tissue or serum factors are demonstrable by available techniques. The course of this disease may be otherwise comparable in every way.

† It is not clear whether this represents a different mechanism of production (osmotic swelling *vs.* surface shrinkage) or whether it represents a spherocyte of younger age and consequently larger size.

creased; there is frequently a spread population of cells with both increased and decreased fragility after 24 hours of sterile incubation. The mechanical fragility is frequently increased, especially after incubation. The autohemolysis test is variable; in most instances hemolysis is somewhat increased with added glucose but hemolysis is usually decreased following the addition of adenosine (354).

The leukocyte and platelet counts are usually normal, although moderate leukocytosis is frequent in patients with the most rapid hemolysis. Leukopenia and thrombopenia are associated frequently enough, however, to make up a so-called "Evans syndrome" (99).

The serum bilirubin values most frequently range up to 4 mg per 100 ml. A slight elevation of plasma hemoglobin level is usually present, and marked hemoglobinemia, hemoglobinuria, and hemosiderinuria may be found, although usually only for short periods of time. The bone marrow is very active in all cell series but with a predominating normoblastic hyperplasia. Red cell maturation appears normal unless superadded deficiencies distort the picture. Aplastic crises are well documented in these disorders and are usually acute and transient (65, 216, 293, 349).

CHARACTERISTICS OF AUTOIMMUNE ANTIBODIES. The hallmark of this group of hemolytic anemias is, of course, the presence of abnormal tissue or serum factors usually called antibodies (55). The hemolytic anemias caused by cold antibodies have for convenience been dealt with separately. Pathogenically and etiologically this may be a completely artificial separation. In practice, any device, manipulation, or degree of ingenuity available is used to demonstrate abnormal behavior of cells or serum—cold, pH, specially treated cells, diseased cells, added chemicals, ions, drugs, complement, proteins, antibodies, cell extracts, polymers (153), etc.; all are designed to detect an abnormal cell factor or serum factor capable of producing or inducing erythrocyte agglutination, lysis, or other abnormal type of behavior.

The "cold" antibodies are usually present in the serum in easily detected quantities, presumably because the usual range of body temperature is such that the circulating factor is not bound to the red cells. The "warm" antibodies are less easy to detect and study because they are rarely found in high concentration in the serum. Presumably they are continuously adsorbed to the patient's own cells at body temperature. For many years the search for serum factors was only rarely rewarded with positive results when ordinary techniques were employed. After the Coombs antiglobulin test became available in 1945, it became possible for the first time to test for abnormal factors *on* the red cell. The most consistent immunologic finding in acquired hemolytic anemia is a positive response to the direct Coombs test. (This applies to the secondary as well as idiopathic variety.) Moreover, the test gives consistently negative results in the hereditary hemolytic anemias of all types and in those caused by acquired intracorpuscular defects (paroxysmal nocturnal hemoglobinuria and deficiency in vitamin B_{12}, iron, and folic acid). A positive result on the direct Coombs test is strong evidence for the presence of a so-called autoimmune acquired hemolytic process and in its simplest interpretation indicates the presence of an abnormal protein factor on the surface of the red cell. However, there is solid evidence that not all abnormal factors are detected by the Coombs test as usually performed. Since the original Coombs test was made using immune serum produced in rabbits by injection of *whole* human serum, the Coombs antiglobulin serum was much more than the antiserum to human globulin its name implied. Subsequently, Coombs serum has been produced by injecting "purified" human γ-globulin and much the same results are obtained. Moreover, the test can be neutralized by the addition of γ-globulin to the Coombs serum so that aside from the instances in which non-γ-globulin substances have been detected (β-globulins in some cold antibodies?) the presumption is good that a positive agglutination test indicates that a γ-globulin is present on the erythrocyte.

The antibodies are not irreversibly bound to the erythrocyte but under proper conditions (saline, serum, serum plus complement) may transfer to normal cells. The rate of transfer is apparently related to the concentration of the antibody present on the surface and can therefore be used to attempt to correlate disease activity with the antibody content. In serial observations in a small series of patients (99) the hemolytic severity did roughly parallel antibody content estimated by this method.

The factor has been eluted from the red cells in quantities sufficient for serologic tests, and the following characteristics have been noted. The factor appears to be a γ-globulin of small molecular weight (S_{20w} 7) (105). By and large, it is adsorbed to the red cells irrespective of the known blood groups. In a small but definite number of instances the factor behaves as if it were an Rh antibody directed against a cell carrying the same specific antigen. The incidence of the Rh-specific autoantibodies corresponds closely to the incidence of the Rh antigens in the population; anti-e is therefore most common. This may be of considerable practical importance in managing a particular patient, since blood lacking the specific antigen will be compatible. In dealing with panagglutinins or panlysins, antibodies directed against all cells (the usual situation), one frequently has to face the fact that all blood for required transfusions will be incompatible to some degree and that the cells will consequently have an abbreviated life span.

The serum factor almost always reacts as an incomplete antibody and it is for this reason that the Coombs serum is so valuable. For not only may abnormal substances be detected on the surface of the red cell, but by means of the indirect Coombs test, assay for serum factors may be made. In this latter procedure normal (various types) red cells are suspended in small quantities of the patient's serum, neat or diluted, and an incubation is carried out. (Appropriate manipulations are made with respect to pH, temperature, etc.) The cells are removed from the serum, washed free of nonspecifically or loosely adherent protein, and then tested by Coombs serum as before. Agglutination indicates the adsorption onto the red cell of an abnormal serum factor. It is also known that treatment of normal cells with various enzymes such as trypsin will alter them so that they agglutinate in the presence of an incomplete antibody without any additional manipulations.

It is rare to find a complete agglutinin or active lysin in the serum, although one or more of the various manipulations mentioned above may increase the sensitivity of the test to such an extent that its presence becomes evident.

For "supersensitive" detection of potentially lytic antibodies, trypsinized cells or erythrocytes from patients with paroxysmal nocturnal hemoglobinuria have been used. These cells are much more susceptible to lytic antibodies than normal cells and are therefore very good indicators. Normal cells, for example, are usually much more readily agglutinated than lysed. An A cell in fresh anti-A serum may be agglutinated to an antibody dilution of 1:64 but lysed only to 1:4; the erythrocyte from a patient with paroxysmal nocturnal hemoglobinuria may well show both agglutination *and* lysis in antibody dilutions of 1:64. Interpretation of results, except for the demonstrated presence of abnormal substance, becomes more and more difficult in terms of physiologic relevance with each additional manipulation.

Thus, the serology of the acquired hemolytic anemias has an awesome complexity (80, 98, 264). For almost every patient studied one or more factors may be demonstrated to differ in subtle ways from those described in other clinically comparable patients until it would seem that no common abnormality, no pattern, no consistent set of findings is discernible. Moreover, it is frequent that the positive reaction to the Coombs test persists after active hemolysis subsides and an otherwise complete remission of hematologic symptoms is present. It is likely that although any or all of the above serologic contortions definitely indicate abnormalities, the correct test to detect the basic common denominator, if any, has not yet been devised.

SITES OF RED CELL DESTRUCTION. By tagging the patient's red cells with Cr^{51} it is possible not only to measure the rate of red cell destruction but also to determine the main body sites of red cell sequestration and destruction. The rate of destruction reflects accurately the severity of the disease in general (Figure 9.14). By the mechanisms considered previously, the spleen has been found to be the main site of hemolysis in patients with incomplete warm antibodies. An increase in erythrocyte survival time usually occurs after splenectomy (Figure 9.3). Nevertheless, the liver is usually not completely passive, and after splenectomy the liver often becomes enlarged and appears to take on the role previously played by the spleen.

The etiology of this disease or group of diseases is under active investigation and debate. There are two main theories. The most prevalent and generally accepted is that it is a classic example of "autoimmunity" (339): that in exception to the normal processes of immune tolerance, an antibody is formed against some tissue of the self—in this instance the red cell. This could conceivably occur through alteration of the red cell surface so that in essence it becomes foreign; such changes might be brought about by faulty protein biosynthesis or by changes induced by infective agents, chemicals, enzymes, etc., which uncover normally hidden antigen sites. It might also occur by the emergence of previously suppressed "clones" of "immunologically competent" antibody-producing cells that have not acquired, or have lost through mutation, tolerance to the erythrocytes (37, 38). None of the proposed theories holds up completely on critical and detailed examination, but it is apparent that the main body of evidence in this and other fields of "autoimmunity" is moving in this direction. However, it seems equally possible at this time to conceive that the demonstrated serum factors and tissue factors are not antibodies in the classic sense of being specifically produced in response to a specific antigenic stimulus, but are simply abnormal proteins produced in response to as yet unknown stimuli (infections, chemical agents, neoplasms)—proteins that happen to have cross reactivity with the erythrocytes and thereby initiate the chain of events known as idiopathic or symptomatic acquired hemolytic anemia of the (so-called) autoimmune antibody type.

TREATMENT. There are several therapeutic possibilities available. Of prime importance is a critical and prolonged search for underlying disorders of etiologic significance and proper handling of them when potent measures are available.

Blood transfusions may be necessary but are of temporary benefit at best except in the rare instance of a type-specific antibody that can be circumvented. Usually, however, normal cells, compatible in terms of known major and minor

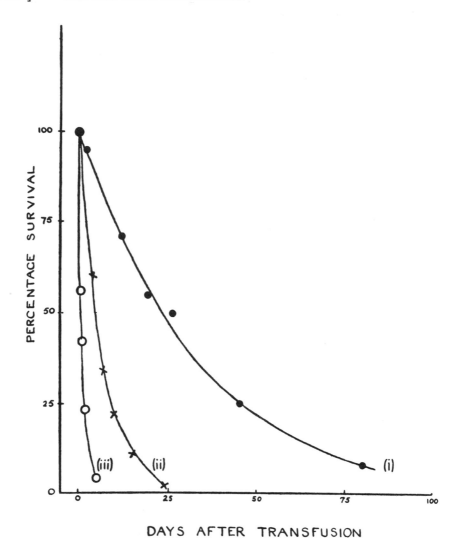

FIGURE 9.14.   Survival of transfused red cells (Ashby technique) in three cases of acquired hemolytic anemia: i, mild; ii, moderate; iii, severe. (From Mollison, P. L., Blood Transfusion in Clinical Medicine, Charles C. Thomas, Springfield, Ill., 1961)

blood types are rapidly destroyed by the extracorpuscular defect.

ACTH and steroid hormone preparations have been widely used since 1950. They are now the treatment of choice and many patients react favorably; some quickly experience a complete and lasting remission. Usually these preparations are capable of influencing the rates of red cell production and destruction so that a favorable balance is reached (10 or more Gm of hemoglobin per 100 ml blood) at

doses of the newer agents that are reasonably well tolerated by patients for prolonged periods. It is not at all clear how they work; in most patients the Coombs test remains positive and antibodies continue to be produced, although perhaps at lower levels. Other agents such as 6-mercaptopurine and heparin have been reported beneficial in some series of patients (213, 291).

Splenectomy is ordinarily reserved for patients failing to respond to steroid

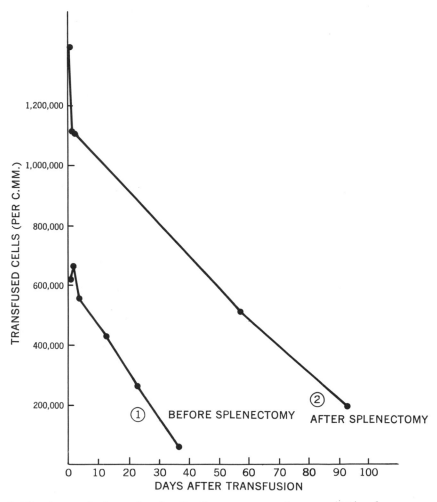

FIGURE 9.15.   Survival of transfused red cells in patient with acquired hemolytic anemia, with negative direct Coombs test (1) 5 months before splenectomy and (2) immediately following splenectomy. Initial fall in the concentration of transfused cells after transfusion (2) may have been related to changes in blood volume in period immediately following operation. (From Mollison, P. L., Blood Transfusion in Clinical Medicine, Charles C. Thomas, Springfield, Ill., 1961)

therapy or who require such large doses of the hormones for control that the metabolic side effects are objectionable (Figure 9.15). Splenectomy is effective in only about one-half the patients (good or fair results) and then not in those with the most active hemolysis. Temporary benefit may occur following splenectomy only to be superseded by relapse. There appears to be no consistently reliable way by which to predict the long-term response to therapy.

Bibliographic references for Chapter 9 begin on page 427.

CHAPTER TEN

POLYCYTHEMIA*

In its original, strict meaning, the term polycythemia denoted significant increase above normal in the number of red cells in the peripheral blood. Since blood volume observations were unavailable at the time the first clinical and laboratory descriptions of polycythemia were made (by Krehl in 1889 and Vaquez in 1892; 19, 73, 99), the term perforce referred to the number of red cells per unit volume of peripheral blood. It was not possible to make use of the concept now implied in "total red cell mass" as opposed to concentration per unit volume. However, by the time Osler (83) dealt with the topic (in 1903) he could sort out "two classes of polyglobulism—*relative,* in which the condition is due to a mininution in the quantity of the plasma of the blood and *true,* in which there is an actual increase in the number of blood corpuscles." Thus, *polycythemia* rather vaguely encompassed situations in which the number of cells per unit volume of blood was increased in association with a normal (perhaps even decreased) total red cell mass as well as situations in which the total red cell mass was increased in association with an increased (perhaps even normal) number of erythrocytes per unit volume of blood.

The difficulty is, of course, based in the presumption that these clinical states are the opposite of anemia and the fact that anemia has never been satisfactorily defined. There are those who would define anemia in terms of the *total mass* of functioning † hemoglobin present in the body and those who would define it in terms of *concentration* of functioning hemoglobin present in the peripheral blood. No one now, it would seem, defines anemia in terms of red cells, for although an abnormal increase of red cells invariably accompanies an increase of hemoglobin, the converse is not always true. With due reference to physiologic balances, adjustments, and controls, it is most reasonable at present to define anemia in terms of the concentration of functional hemoglobin in the circulating blood. In keeping with this the term polycythemia is now employed so that it refers to an increased concentration of circulating hemoglobin rather than of red cells.

Although numerous authors formally introduce the designations "erythrocytosis" or "erythrocythemia" for sustained polycythemia secondary to recognized causes, and "erythremia" for the disease of undetermined etiology (otherwise known as polycythemia (rubra) vera, or

* General references and review articles: 13, 16, 20, 24, 27, 31, 36, 41, 45, 49, 56, 60, 70, 71, 87, 90, 104, 111, 113, 120, 124, 125, 129, 130.

† Functioning in terms of oxygen uptake, transport, and delivery.

polycythemia vera), these introductions are usually the only places in which the words appear in the literature. Certainly they are seldom in common usage. Polycythemia may be classified as shown in Table 10.1.

RELATIVE POLYCYTHEMIA

In relative polycythemia the total blood volume is less than normal (60). This change is occasioned by a decrease in the plasma compartment, which is disproportionate to any change in the total hemoglobin-red-cell mass so that there results a *relative* increase in the concentration of hemoglobin (and red cells) per unit volume of peripheral blood. The cause of this type of polycythemia is almost invariably apparent from the patient's history and from clinical observation and is associated with excessive loss and/or shifts of body fluid: sweating, hyperemesis, fluid deprivation, diarrhea, burns, increased capillary permeability, etc.

Although the causes of relative polycythemia are usually readily apparent, patients are frequently seen who manifest relative polycythemia of undetermined origin, which is usually mild or moderate

in degree. These disorders have been variously reported as hypovolemic polycythemia, pseudopolycythemia, and stress erythrocytosis. By means of phosphorus-labeled red cells, Lawrence (60) showed that the total volume of red cells in the peripheral blood was within normal limits even though the venous hematocrit was in excess of 50 per cent. The calculated plasma volume was therefore below normal in every patient studied. Patients with relative polycythemia present a fairly uniform clinical picture (30). They are usually hyperactive, anxious males, with a ruddy cyanosis; about half are overweight and half are hypertensive. The symptoms are those seen in polycythemia vera (described below), but there is *no* splenomegaly, leukocytosis, or thrombocytosis.

In addition to blood volume characteristics that differentiate relative polycythemia from absolute polycythemia, there are significant physiologic differences: ferrokinetics are normal and there is no arterial hypoxemia. Treatment has been completely unsatisfactory, and the term stress polycythemia was derived from Lawrence's suggestion that the condition

TABLE 10.1.   Classification of polycythemias

I. Relative polycythemia (pachyhemia)
    A. Secondary to fluid loss or plasma shift
    B. Idiopathic (stress)
    C. Caused by unequal distribution of red cells in the vascular compartment

II. Absolute polycythemia
    A. Secondary (erythrocytosis, erythrocythemia)
        1. Caused by demonstrable hypoxemia resulting from
            a. Cardiac disorders
            b. Pulmonary disorders
            c. Respiratory center dysfunction
            d. Abnormal hemoglobin pigments: abnormal globin or abnormal cell enzymes
            e. High altitude
            f. Newborn
        2. Occurring in association with abnormalities of specific organs such as kidneys, central nervous system, ovaries, adrenals, etc.
        3. Caused by chemical agents such as cobalt
    B. Primary
        1. Polycythemia vera (polycythemia rubra vera, erythremia)
        2. Primary erythrocytosis of childhood

---

might be a reaction to the stress of daily living.

Recently (14) Lawrence's method of calculating plasma volume has been questioned, and some evidence has been put forward indicating a shift in the distribution of red cells as a cause of the polycythemia indicated by increased peripheral blood hematocrit in some patients. Since earlier work by Gibson had demonstrated the hematocrits of various organs to vary from 15 per cent in some vessels of the kidney to 82 per cent in the spleen, confirmation of the above findings will be of considerable interest. The cause of the shifts in red cell distribution in these patients is completely unknown.

ABSOLUTE SECONDARY POLYCYTHEMIA

In clear contradistinction to relative polycythemia, all the subtypes of absolute polycythemia are characterized by an *increase* in the total hemoglobin-red-cell mass. The plasma volume may be normal or, more usually, slightly diminished (119), but the hemoglobin-red-cell mass is always increased in absolute amount. These findings have been confirmed in many laboratories by various techniques.

Chief Cause (Demonstrable Hypoxemia)

The cause common to the great majority of patients with absolute secondary polycythemia is hypoxemia, and it is apparent that as a general rule the severity of the polycythemic changes can be correlated with the degree of hypoxemia. In this context it is of interest that in 1878 Paul Bert (9) predicted on the basis of his respiratory studies that the most ready and effective adjustment of an organism to existence at low oxygen tension would be made by a compensating increase in hemoglobin. The prediction was justified shortly thereafter by the demonstration of increased hemoglobin in animals existing at high altitudes and low oxygen tensions (10). The studies on man made and collected by Hurtado et al. (47) concerning high-altitude polycythemia illustrate this point very well. Figure 10.1 shows the inverse correlation between the concentration of hemoglobin in the peripheral blood and the percentage of oxygen saturation occasioned by residence at high altitude and indicates the existence of a precise mechanism for controlling hematopoiesis in terms of oxygen supply. In this type of polycythemia the total blood volume is increased, usually entirely because of the augmentation of the hemoglobin mass. Recent studies have also demonstrated an increase in concentration of myoglobin, and this too is proportional to the altitude of residence (114).

The clearest data on this phenomenon have come from studies of subjects with high-altitude polycythemia, but there is no reason to suspect that the basic pathogenesis is different in patients with hypoxemia due to other causes, however modified by the alterations peculiar to each situation. This type of polycythemia may be seen in any cardiovascular or pulmonary disorder that results in insufficient oxygenation of the arterial blood. It is classically seen in cyanotic congenital heart disease, where a portion of the blood passes into the aorta without traversing the normally functioning pulmonary capillary bed (109, 111). In acquired heart disease the hypoxemia usually results from secondary pulmonary dysfunction such as the thick alveolar membranes with diffusion abnormalities sometimes seen in association with chronic mitral stenosis. Less constantly, polycythemia occurs in various types of pulmonary diseases such as silicosis, emphysema,* Ayerza's disease, pulmonary

---

* Several studies have pointed out that polycythemia as judged by peripheral blood counts is rather infrequently seen in association with hypoxemic pulmonary emphysema (54, 63). More recent examinations of this problem indicated that the red cell volume is consistently and proportionately increased as predicted (127) but that because of plasma volume changes, the increase is not reflected by the peripheral blood counts (106).

ALTITUDE (THOUSANDS FEET)

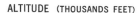

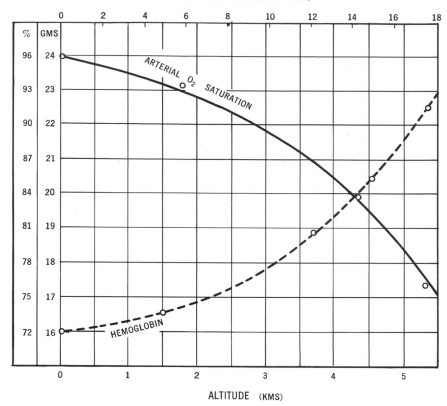

ALTITUDE (KMS)

Figure 10.1. Correlation between concentration of hemoglobin in peripheral blood and percentage of oxygen saturation of atmosphere at various altitudes. (From Hurtado, A., et al., Arch. Int. Med. 75:284, 1945)

hemangioma and arteriovenous fistulae, and disturbances in the alveolar membrane that impair the diffusion of oxygen through the alveolar walls into the capillary blood.

Polycythemia has been described in association with marked obesity (4) and attributed either to a mechanical impairment of respiration or to reflex abnormalities. This has been named the Pickwickian syndrome and may be corrected by weight reduction. Malfunction of the respiratory center or decreased sensitivity to normal stimuli (idiopathic or secondary to cerebrovascular disorders) may result in hypoventilation and hypoxemia (23, 84, 89). The polycythemia of the newborn is evidently due to the fact that *in utero* the infant's blood derives oxygen from the placental circulation and not from the aerated lung as it does after birth. During the neonatal period the polycythemia is readily corrected.

Former theories held that erythropoiesis was governed by a direct effect of oxygen (or its lack) on the bone marrow. More recent experiments have convincingly demonstrated that the increased proliferative activity of the erythropoietic tissue associated with hypoxemia is mediated through a humoral substance, probably produced mainly in the kidney but to limited extent elsewhere in the body. This distant effect and the existence of the humoral factor was neatly demonstrated by Reisman, who made one partner of parabiotic rabbits hypoxemic and found polycythemia and marrow erythrocytic hyperplasia in the demonstrably well-oxygenated animal. Studies on poly-cythemic patients with patent ductus ar-teriosus and reversed blood flow (101) have shown the well-oxygenated sternal marrow as well as the hypoxemic iliac crest marrow* to be erythropoietically hyperactive. Further discussion of the circulating factor now termed erythro-poietin appears in Chapter 6. Several ob-servers have demonstrated increased amounts of circulating erythropoietin in secondary polycythemia of this type.

Clinical Manifestations

Varying, of course, with the degree of elevation of the hemoglobin concentra-tion of the circulating blood and the de-gree of increase in the blood volume, the signs, symptoms, and complications of absolute secondary polycythemia are the same as those of polycythemia vera. However, symptoms such as myeloid metaplasia and terminal acute leukemia, which are *not strictly caused by* the cir-culatory changes, are not present. Gout (113) and thrombotic and hemorrhagic episodes are present to an abnormal de-gree. In addition, clubbing of the fingers and osteoarthropathy associated with the arterial hypoxemia, and symptoms sec-ondary to the primary disorder are evi-dent. Splenomegaly and hepatomegaly do not occur in the absence of other dis-ease.

Laboratory Findings

In the secondary forms of polycythemia, although the changes are seldom as se-vere as those in the primary, the red cells may reach values of 8 million per cubic millimeter. The increases in hematocrit may not be strictly proportional to the in-creases in hemoglobin concentration, so that slightly hypochromic and microcytic erythrocytes may be seen. Otherwise, the red cells are within normal limits. Reticu-locytosis and hyperbilirubinemia of mild degree are characteristic. Leukocytosis

and leukemoid changes do not occur and the platelet count is normal. Examina-tion of the bone marrow by aspiration or biopsy shows significantly increased ac-tivity in the production of the erythro-cyte series (normoblastic proliferation). Unless arterial hypoxemia is demon-strated, the diagnosis cannot be made with certainty. Arterial hypoxemia is best determined by blood-gas analysis and the finding of a hemoglobin saturation of 90 per cent or less (37). The diagnosis may be strongly suspected if the cyanosis is promptly abolished by the administration of oxygen, except, of course, in those pa-tients with alveolar diffusion abnormal-ities or large vascular shunts. Aside from the demonstration of minor decreases in affinity for oxygen in the hemoglobin of patients living at high altitudes, no other abnormalities have been described, and the pigment appears functionally normal (48).

Pathophysiology

Significant increases in absolute amount and peripheral concentration of red cells and hemoglobin could occur either by in-creased production *or* by a prolonged life span of the erythrocytes even though pro-duced at a normal rate. That the former is the true situation has been established by the repeated demonstration of normal red cell life span in polycythemia of this type by several different methods (92). Moreover, direct confirmatory evidence has been obtained through ferrokinetic studies revealing an increased metab-olism of iron compatible with the in-creased total hemoglobin mass (92). The iron level of the circulating plasma is in the normal range, but radioactive tracer studies have demonstrated the iron to be cleared through the plasma much more rapidly and incorporated into new red

* A hypoactive marrow may be found in situations where the hypoxemia is extreme, in confirmation of in vitro marrow-culture experi-ments, where it has been shown that cell growth is consistently retarded by low oxygen tension.

cells at a higher percentage of utilization than normal. A few observations have demonstrated normal ferrokinetic values during the administration of oxygen, when oxygen tension was high enough to abolish the arterial hypoxemia (59; Figure 10.4).

Other Causes

In a restricted number of special circumstances a proportion of the hemoglobin may become functionally inactive. This results in a diminished *effective* oxygen tension and saturation: anemic hypoxemia. The bone marrow responds by producing more hemoglobin to compensate for the changes brought about by the circulating but functionally inactive pigment. Polycythemia, in terms of the total amount and concentration of red cells and hemoglobin, results. This is seen in patients with hereditary methemoglobinemia, a disorder in which the red cell is unable to convert intracellularly formed methemoglobin back to the functional pigment (34). Usually, 30 per cent, more or less, of functionally inert methemoglobin and the induced change in the oxygen dissociation of the functional hemoglobin must be compensated for. This kind of polycythemia is less frequently seen and documented in *acquired* pigment abnormalities—principally methemoglobinemia, carboxyhemoglobinemia, and sulfhemoglobinemia resulting from chronic exposure to carbon monoxide or various aniline dyes and nitrates. After prolonged administration in high dosage, cobalt also can produce polycythemia in man and animals. The exact mechanism is unknown, although increased amounts of circulating erythropoietin have been shown to result from its administration. No abnormal hemoglobin pigments have been detected, so a cobalt-induced "histotoxic hypoxia" is presumed. Its effects can be abolished or prevented by the simultaneous administration of cysteine.

Androgenic substances also can consistently produce polycythemia in some patients, and if of adrenocortical origin, may help explain the mild polycythemia sometimes seen in Cushing's disease.

Recently there has been a revival of interest in a secondary form of polycythemia not associated with arterial hypoxemia or changes in the other formed elements of the blood (31). This polycythemia has been found in a group of patients who also had various renal abnormalities (61) such as renal tumors (15, 44), hydronephrosis (39, 70), and polycystic kidney disease, and in a much smaller group of patients with ovarian tumors, hepatoma (102), hamartoma of the liver (53), uterine fibroids (108), and subtentorial tumors or vascular anomalies (16, 100).* When occurring in connection with renal abnormalities, the condition is called "nephrogenic polycythemia." It is of considerable interest that prolonged remission of polycythemia may result from removal of the associated abnormality. The pathophysiology is unknown, although in a few instances erythropoiesis-stimulating factors have been extracted from the lesions.

Treatment

In all the above situations treatment of the secondary polycythemia is essentially that of the underlying disorder. In certain circumstances venesection and even marrow inhibition by chemotherapy or irradiation have been beneficially used. In the polycythemia of arterial hypoxemia, the increment in circulating hemoglobin increases the oxygen capacity. However, the increment of red cells also increases the viscosity of the blood, and at the higher hematocrit ranges (Figure 10.2) this increase in viscosity may impede cir-

* It should be pointed out that the percentage of patients with renal abnormalities, subtentorial tumors, vascular anomalies, etc., who have associated polycythemia, is very small—probably less than the estimated 1 or 2 per cent.

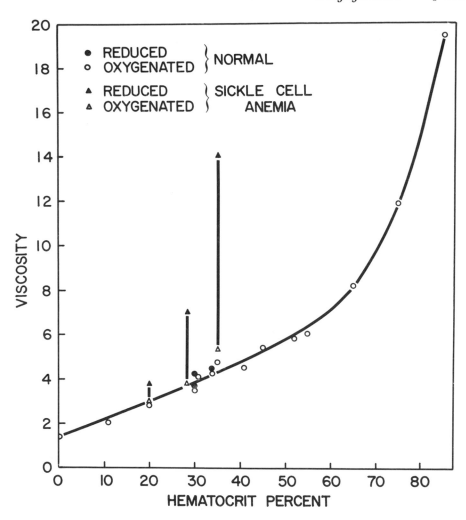

FIGURE 10.2.   Relation of blood viscosity to hematocrit. Viscosity indicated in figure is calculated relative to water at 37°C and determined in Ostwald viscometer

culation. Therefore, judicious reduction of the hematocrit results in subjective and objective benefit, even increased oxygen saturation (5).

ABSOLUTE PRIMARY POLYCYTHEMIA

Polycythemia vera is a chronic disease of unknown etiology, characterized by insidious onset and relentless progression through various stages. The early stages are distinguished by a sustained elevation of the hemoglobin level and red cell count accompanied often by leukocytosis and sometimes by thrombocytosis. Subse-

quently, more marked white cell alterations (leukemoid changes) usually occur, accompanied by myeloid metaplasia and splenomegaly that may become massive. Anemia invariably supervenes during the latter stages and may be associated with leukemic changes terminating in acute blastic crisis indistinguishable from that seen in acute leukemia. Many diverse clinical and hematologic pictures are encountered during the course of polycythemia vera, and evolutionary stages must be recognized for a proper comprehension of this disease. Unfortunately, no adequate observations of the natural history of the disease unaltered by therapeutic attempts of one kind or another have been recorded. In a critical review of the relation of polycythemia to leukemia, made in 1950, Schwartz and Ehrlich (104) were able to find only one acceptable, unequivocal case report of leukemia terminating the course of polycythemia in patients never treated with x-ray. This reflects the frequency with which ionizing radiation has been employed (it became available for clinical use before the disease was adequately delineated) rather than the infrequency of terminal leukemia. This lack of controls returns frequently to plague one during the study of polycythemia vera, particularly with respect to the fundamental nature of the disease and the beneficial, or possibly deleterious, effects of various therapeutic attempts.

Incidence

Polycythemia vera is by no means a rare disease, as is indicated by the number of cases reported from various large clinics by interested physicians: Reinhard and Hahneman, 279 patients (90); Lawrence, 269 (60); Wasserman and Bassen, 253 (124); Stroebel and Fowler, 230 (111); Damon and Holub, 197 (31); Tinney et al., 168 (117); Stecher et al., 130 (110); Videbaek, 125 (120); and Calabresi and Meyer, 107 patients (20, 21). Consequently, its various clinical and hematologic manifestations are well documented. Its course is of long duration—frequently 10, sometimes 20, years. Its onset is insidious, probably measured in several years. The average age at diagnosis is the latter forties; the range is from 20 to 80 years. Although reported in children (3, 42, 69), it is rare.* A definite familial or heritable tendency is most unusual (58, 80), but the disease is rare in some races (notably among Negroes) and the incidence is perhaps increased among

Jews (31). The male/female preponderance is 1.8:1.

Clinical Manifestations

Although typical symptoms are rarely seen in the presence of normal peripheral blood values (some patients may have increased blood volume in the presence of normal hemoglobin concentration), signs and symptoms are usually related to the magnitude of the blood changes and the stage to which the disease has progressed. Presenting complaints are usually weakness and fatigue, often associated with headache, dizziness, impaired mentation, paresthesias (especially pruritus on exposure to heat), and changes in the hue of complexion (13). Hemorrhagic or thrombotic episodes may first call attention to the disease. Cerebral, gastrointestinal, urinary, and nasal hemorrhages may occur at any time during the course. Minor wounds or surgical procedures (dental extraction) may provoke unusual loss of blood. Thrombosis of any vein or artery may occur, and embolic phenomena are not infrequent. The most common and serious of these occur in cerebral vessels, but thromboses are also seen in the branches of the portal or hepatic veins (85). The complexion changes consist of dusky-red or purplish colors most noticeable on the face, lips, hands and feet, and in the buccal cavity, a "ruddy cyanosis" and plethora that is aggravated by exposure to the cold. The

* As indicated in Table 10.1, a condition known as "primary erythrocytosis of childhood" has been described (57). Apparently most of the cases of polycythemia reported to occur in childhood belong in this category (especially if familial) or represent inadequately studied cases of hypoxemic secondary polycythemia. Knock concludes that a total of fifteen cases of erythrocytosis in childhood have been reported which appear to represent a primary disturbance of the total red cell mass. None of the patients showed elevations of white cells or platelets, and the disorder is compatible with prolonged survival. In earlier writing it is referred to as "benign familial polycythemia in childhood" (6, 80).

scleral vessels are suffused and plethoric, as are the retinal veins.

Splenomegaly occurs in the majority of patients. In some the spleen becomes so huge that it produces the "small stomach syndrome" and interferes with food intake. Even with no or only moderate splenomegaly, complaints referable to the gastrointestinal system (ranging from chronic indigestion to epigastric pain) are frequent. Although the extent of splenomegaly is originally due to engorgement with blood, it later is determined by reticular fibrous tissue proliferation and myeloid metaplasia. The liver is usually only minimally enlarged until late in the course. Clubbing of the fingers does not occur. The blood pressure, especially the systolic element, is elevated in nearly half of the patients.

Laboratory Findings

During the early phase of the disease the red cell count may number around 8 to 10 million per cubic millimeter; the hemoglobin level is also increased. The hematocrit is usually somewhat disproportionately more elevated, so that the red cells are somewhat microcytic and hypochromic* and show greater-than-normal variation in size and shape. Polychromatophilia (reticulocytosis) is mild, and occasional nucleated red cells can be found. Thrombocytosis and granulocytic leukocytosis are found in the majority of instances, roughly correlating with the increase in number of red cells (correlation index, 0.75); the granulocytes may demonstrate a shift toward immaturity, with metamyelocytes, myelocytes of various stages, and even myeloblasts being seen. Examination of the bone marrow (14) by aspiration or trephine biopsy or at autopsy shows a tissue active not only in the red cell series but in the granulocytic and megakaryocytic series as well. The tissue is increased in total volume,

replacing in varying degrees the yellow, fatty marrow. Aspiration biopsy usually yields a hypocellular preparation owing to admixture with an unusually large amount of peripheral blood because of rupture of the distended marrow capillaries (demonstrable by isotope techniques). There may be a slight but usually not significant increase in the proportion of red cell precursors (122). Marrow aspiration is seldom of *positive* diagnostic help or useful as a therapeutic guide; it may, however, be useful in ruling out other causes of a polycythemia seen occasionally as an early manifestation of leukemia or bone marrow malignancy. However, trephine biopsy furnishes a preparation of intact architecture, whose quantitative and qualitative changes are reported to be of diagnostic value. Routine urine tests frequently show mild albuminuria and a few red cells and leukocytes. These abnormalities may reverse with adequate treatment and control of polycythemia.

The above is largely a description of the polycythemic phase which may last for many years. However, a wide variety of hematologic and clinical pictures may be seen. By and large, these are due to the exhaustion, or "burning out," of one of the formed elements, or the aggravated proliferation of another, plus myeloid metaplasia. There may be thrombocytosis (even up to 2 million platelets per cubic millimeter), with bizarre large platelets and fragments of megakaryocytes in the peripheral blood, or thrombocytopenia. There may be qualitative and quantitative changes in the leukocyte series, even to simulating myelocytic leukemia. Any combination of changes plus the alterations induced by therapy may be encountered. If the patient survives long enough (5 to 25 years), almost with-

---

* Probably owing to relative iron deficiency brought about by previous unrecognized blood loss.

out exception an anemic phase occurs, usually spoken of as "burned out" or "spent" polycythemia. This may follow a period of so-called remission characterized by normal red cell and hemoglobin values. However, this remission phase is frequently unapparent.

During the anemic phase, the signs and symptoms are predominantly due to hemoglobin lack. To these may be added, if and when they develop, the signs and symptoms due to abnormalities in platelet and leukocyte production, hypermetabolism and organomegaly resulting from myeloid metaplasia. Transfusions may then become mandatory in an individual previously treated by vigorous, repeated venesections. The white cell and platelet abnormalities become more and more marked. Splenic enlargement may be rapid, probably secondary to myeloid metaplasia, so that erythrocyte abnormalities such as polychromatophilia, "teardrop" cells, elliptical cells, spherocytes, and other bizarre forms arise. At varying times during these progressive changes fibroblastic and even osteoblastic proliferation takes place in the marrow at the expense of the normal inhabitants, so that myelofibrosis and osteosclerosis occur. However, islands of active red marrow remain in varying degrees. Pancytopenia may accompany these changes to terminate in blastic crisis similar to that seen in acute leukemia. Alternatively the terminal crisis may follow a phase indistinguishable from myeloid leukemia.

These changes should not, strictly speaking, be considered *complications*, since they are really phases of polycythemia vera. It is obvious that polycythemia vera is an ever-changing and progressing disease which unfolds with a bewildering array of signs, symptoms, and findings. Moreover, it is seldom that the disease runs its course without considerable modification by various types of therapy or by the numerous complications to which these patients are predisposed.

Complications

THROMBOTIC. The complications that occur are mostly due to the hypervolemia and the hyperactivity of the hematopoietic tissues responsible for the abnormally augmented hemoglobin-red-cell mass. Debilitating or fatal hemorrhagic or thrombotic episodes occur frequently: in Wasserman's series (124), thrombosis occurred in 24 per cent and hemorrhage in 10 per cent (of these 56 per cent died). After adequate therapy, the incidence of complications was markedly reduced to 5.5 per cent and 2.2 per cent, respectively. Even higher incidences of these complications are recorded in some series, but with earlier therapy and better control of hemoglobin levels and hematopoiesis, there has been a definite decrease. On the basis of clinical and laboratory evidence, there is reason to connect the thrombotic episodes with the increase in blood viscosity that is dependent upon the elevation in red cell count. The relation of viscosity to hematocrit and red cell count is illustrated in Figure 10.2. Marked increase in viscosity occurs when the hematocrit exceeds 60 to 70 per cent.

Inadequately controlled polycythemia frequently results in a thick, viscous blood that is difficult to aspirate with a syringe and impossible to spread properly on a slide or cover slip. It has been proposed by some that the marked increase in platelets also contributes to the thrombotic tendency. Except in instances of extreme hematocrit elevations, the slow peripheral blood flow brought about by the viscosity increase does not impair delivery of oxygen to most tissues, since the increase in hemoglobin also enhances the oxygen-carrying capacity of the blood. The result is that the arterial and venous oxygen tensions are normal (3, 50). Kety (55, 81) states that the lowest recorded value for cerebral blood flow occurred in a patient with polycythemia vera, but that the amount of oxygen delivered was normal. The basal metabolic rate is usually increased so there is no evidence of over-all tissue anoxia (12, 70). Of course, these findings in no way deny small local areas of hypoxemia that might damage vascular endothelium and start thrombus formation. If such were the case, however, one would expect complications comparable in number and type in secondary polycythemia with its consistently more severe hypoxemia; such is not the case. Perhaps in keeping with modern views of panmyelopathy, the vascular endothelial (reticuloendothelial) system is also abnormal.

HEMORRHAGIC. Curiously enough, the factors responsible for thrombotic episodes probably also contribute to the hemorrhagic tendency, since the poor vascular elasticity resulting from the long-standing distention and engorgement of vessels produced by the excessive blood volume apparently renders hemostasis more difficult. Numerous studies have not revealed any consistent defects in the plasma clotting factors (1, 2, 11, 51, 96, 128). The most consistent findings have been relative fibrinogen deficiency and defective clot retraction during which the red cells fall out of the clot. The former exists because of relatively less plasma mass per unit of whole blood than normal and the latter because of a relatively increased red cell mass and a disorganized fibrin network (51). The above explanations are obviously first approximations, but whatever the reasons ultimately found, the defects have serious consequences. Impressive are the figures of Wasserman and Bassen (124) and Rigby and Leavell (96) for the complications encountered when surgery is performed during the uncontrolled polycythemic phase. Of twenty-six cases in Wasserman's study, 50 per cent had "se-

vere thrombotic and hemorrhagic complications," and 20 per cent died as a direct result; of thirteen cases adequately controlled preoperatively, complications occurred in only two.

GASTROINTESTINAL. During the long course of the disease repeated thrombotic episodes in the portal and hepatic radicles or the splenic vein may produce pressure changes sufficient to cause varices of the lower esophagus or upper stomach, with consequent liability to gastrointestinal hemorrhage. Peptic ulceration is seen in some 8 to 10 per cent of patients with polycythemia vera. Of these ulcers, nine out of ten are duodenal in location. This is about four times the expected frequency in the general population. The cause is obscure, but it is of interest to note that polycythemia experimentally induced in rats is likewise associated with a high incidence of peptic ulcer (28), and experienced workers indicate the incidence of peptic ulceration is increased in patients with high-altitude polycythemia (28). Although there is no direct evidence, most writers have accepted Boyd's suggestion that thrombosis of the small mesenteric vessels, impaired circulation in the dilated capillary vessels, and hyperacidity are the pathogenic findings.

Because of the hemorrhagic and thrombotic tendencies, surgery and the frequently suggested anticoagulant therapy must be undertaken with full appreciation of the possible consequences since they frequently raise as many, if not more, problems than they solve. The same complications, although in much diminished percentage, are associated with the polycythemia of hypovolemia and are reported to occur in high-altitude polycythemia.

BIOCHEMICAL. The hematopoietic hyperactivity has resulted in hyperuricemia in about 30 per cent of studied cases, with three times as many males affected as females. The incidence of clinical gout has been less, somewhere between 4 and 10 per cent in various series (113, 117, 120). Only about 1 per cent of patients developed renal calculi from uric acid. Although there is little doubt that the hyperuricemia is associated with the enormous anabolic and catabolic activity of nucleoproteins, no good correlation with the erythrocyte and leukocyte levels has been shown. However, following therapeutic bone marrow depression, a definite reduction in blood and urinary uric acid occurs. Metabolic studies employing N^{15}-labeled glycine (130) have demonstrated differences in the incorporation of the label into uric acid and its excretion in gout associated with secondary polycythemia and polycythemia vera as opposed to primary gout. In both situations the hyperuricemia and hyperuricosuria are attributable to overproduction of uric acid. In the primary gout the label promptly appears in the excreted uric acid by means of the "shunt" pathway. In the gout associated with polycythemia the label appears only after a delay during which it has been shown to be incorporated into nucleoproteins with subsequent degradation to purines and uric acid. Thus, the pathways of uric acid metabolism are demonstrably different.

Circulatory Dynamics

From what has been described above, it is obvious that polycythemia has a very marked effect on circulatory dynamics. For one thing, the amount of blood present in each unit weight of tissue is sometimes more than doubled, and the blood flow is consequently slower than normal. The circulation time is significantly prolonged, but the prolongation is due to the slow flow through the dilated capillary bed. Direct observation of nail-bed capillaries has shown a greatly diminished rate of flow through elongated, tortuous, distended venous segments (3). A number of studies have demonstrated marked increases in blood viscosity at the higher hematocrit values (Figure 10.2), and in view of the confirmatory in vivo studies demonstrating that flow and oxygen delivery are maximal at normal hematocrit values but fall off significantly in the higher or lower ranges (Figure 6.2), it appears justified to give physiologic relevance to these findings in terms of the known circulatory adjustments, signs, symptoms, and complications (especially thrombotic). Nevertheless, caution must be exercised in translating the crude experiments where viscosity is measured relative to water in rigid glass capillary tubes of fixed diameter under constant flow pressure into a situation where the flow is pulsatile, where the capillaries are variable in diameter and distensible, where axial streaming of cells may be of significance, and where the blood does not necessarily behave like water (i.e., is non-Newtonian) because of its macromolecules and formed elements (126).

Scattered studies done by various methods indicated a normal or increased cardiac output in polycythemia vera (3, 17, 40). More recent studies by Cobb et al. (26) described ten patients with polycythemia vera at a time when the blood volume and red cell mass were abnormally increased and reported a normal or elevated cardiac output and a consistently increased stroke volume. After the blood volume and red cell mass had been reduced by phlebotomy, in seven patients both the cardiac output and the stroke volume fell, suggesting a causal relationship. Previous short-term studies on dogs and man, in which the hematocrit was altered independently of the blood volume, suggested that the cardiac output and stroke volume were influenced by total blood volume and/or the plasma flow requirement of the body tissue. In this connection it was pointed out that as a consequence of the increased cardiac output, a normal plasma flow is maintained in polycythemia.

Altschule has recently pointed out that the frequently recurring statement that an increased blood volume "puts a strain on the heart" is grossly inaccurate because, when stabilized, blood volume does not per se determine the work of the heart. However, when associated with an increased cardiac output in the presence of an abnormally viscous fluid, an additional strain would be expected to be present. Nevertheless, cardiac decompensation, if it does occur in polycythemia, is usually brought on by accompanying hypertension and/or arteriosclerosis.

Cobb's studies also showed a good correlation between blood volume and oxygen consumption in the patients with polycythemia and a slight increase in oxygen consumption after phlebotomy. These findings suggest that the increased red cell mass, blood volume, and metabolic activity are manifestations of the bone marrow dysfunction.

Erythropoiesis

There are in general two opposing theories of the control of erythropoiesis in polycythemia vera: neoplastic and physiologic. Although neither is in complete command of the field, the position occupied by the neoplastic proponents would seem to be the more favorable at present. All agree that the increase in red cell mass is due to increased production of cells and hemoglobin rather than prolongation of the erythrocyte life span. Indeed, while some observers find a normal red cell life span by various methods (35, 52, 74, 95, 105), others, using the Ashby agglutination test and radioactive tracer techniques, report a significantly *shortened* life span (8) of at least a portion of the erythrocyte population. Data are not available to settle this, but it may well be that the erythrocyte life span is normal or shortened depending on the activity and phase of the disease. It follows, therefore, that erythropoiesis must be greater than normal to account for the augmented cell mass.

The findings of polychromatophilia, reticulocytosis, and the presence of nucleated red cells suggest increased erythropoiesis. Interpretation, however, is difficult because these changes could possibly result from bone marrow irritation secondary to the fibrosis that is known to be present in many cases. More direct measurements of erythropoiesis in untreated polycythemia vera have been made employing isotope procedures. When tracer amounts of radioactive iron are bound to transferrin and administered intravenously, the iron is removed or cleared from the plasma more rapidly than normal (10 to 60 minutes as opposed to 70 to 120 minutes for the normal 50 per cent clearance value). Although exceptions to the rule occur, in general an increased iron clearance indicates erythropoietic hyperactivity. Confirmatory is the finding that following adequate myelosuppressive therapy the iron clearance rate returns to or toward the normal. Interestingly, in hypoxemic polycythemia the rapid iron clearance rate is brought back to normal by the administration of oxygen (Figures 10.3 and 10.4); in polycythemia vera the abnormal iron clearance is *not* brought back to normal by the administration of oxygen (59). Certainly, then, this abnormality, presumably reflecting the increased erythropoiesis, is clearly not due to hypoxemia and is not under the usual physiologic controls, unless, of course, the increased erythropoiesis is due to local hypoxemia in the marrow (see below for evidence against this). By placing scintillation counters over bone marrow, liver, and spleen for in vivo tracking of radioactive iron, the sites of red cell formation can be demonstrated. In most patients with polycythemia vera the production of red cells

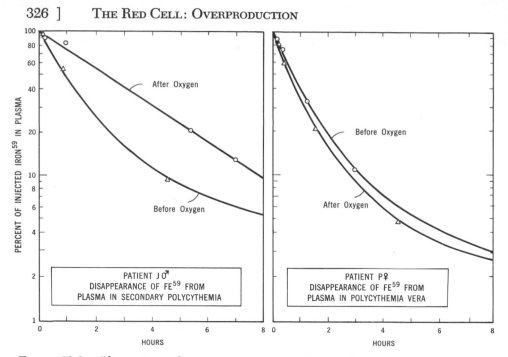

FIGURE 10.3.   Plasma iron clearance rates in secondary polycythemia and in polycythemia vera before and after oxygen inhalation. (From Lawrence, J. H., et al., Cardiologia 21:337, S. Karger, Basel/New York, 1952)

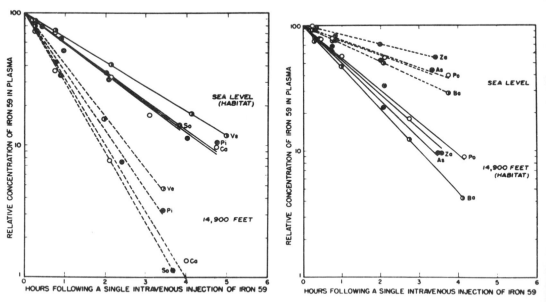

FIGURE 10.4.   Change in plasma iron clearance rates. (A) Change in four medical students caused by ascent to high altitude; (B) change in four Peruvian Indians caused by descent to sea level. (From Lawrence, J. H., Polycythemia, p. 97, Grune & Stratton, New York, 1955)

is confined to the bone marrow (2). However, when marrow fibrosis and splenic and liver myeloid metaplasia are present, radioiron fails to accumulate in the bone marrow but does so in spleen and liver.

An additional method useful in assessing erythropoiesis is the per cent utilization of injected radioactive iron, i.e., how much of the administered dose is effectively built into hemoglobin and delivered to the peripheral blood. In polycythemia vera the iron utilization is usually maximal: 90 per cent or more appears in the peripheral red cells. All the lines of evidence consistently point to increased erythropoiesis as the proximate cause of the increased red cell mass and exclude prolonged erythrocyte life span.

Pathophysiology

Since hypoxemia has been shown so consistently to result in polycythemia in other uncomplicated states, it is of interest to examine the possible mechanisms by which it might conceivably cause polycythemia vera. It is emphasized that in polycythemia vera the arterial oxygen saturation is consistently above 91 per cent* unless some complicating factor is present such as pulmonary dysfunction or insensitivity of the respiratory center. This has been a most reliable means of differentiating between polycythemia vera and hypoxemic secondary polycythemia. If the arterial oxygen saturation is above 91 per cent, hypoxemic polycythemia can be confidently excluded. The presence of adequate arterial saturation does not, however, differentiate between polycythemia vera and the polycythemia associated with renal tumors, etc.

Although this percentage indicates slight arterial unsaturation, it is not of the magnitude to indicate hypoxemia sufficient to account for the polycythemic responses usually present. The minor impairment of pulmonary function is un-doubtedly an effect rather than the cause of the increased red cell mass (116). Moreover, since the venous oxygen saturation studies indicate normal or near normal oxygen delivery (3, 50), there can be no body-wide increased tissue respiration leading to relative hypoxia in a specific erythropoiesis-controlling tissue, as had been proposed. Recent studies have shown a normal oxygen dissociation curve for polycythemic blood (22), so an abnormally functioning hemoglobin comparable to carboxyhemoglobin or methemoglobin can be excluded.

The physiology of oxygen transport is demonstrably normal down to the level of the bone marrow. If hypoxemia is a cause, it must be due to abnormalities located in the bone marrow or other controlling tissue. Some workers have proposed and others have tested the hypothesis of specific bone marrow hypoxemia. Reznikoff et al. (93) reported bone marrow capillary wall thickening and fibrosis resulting in inadequate oxygen diffusion. Further studies indicated the findings were peculiar to the particular group Reznikoff had available for study. The question of bone marrow hypoxia has been directly attacked by Berk et al. (7), Hecht and Samuels (43), and Schwartz and Stats (103), who found either normal or increased oxygen saturation values in bone marrow aspirates from patients with polycythemia vera. There is, therefore, no evidence for hypoxia of the bone marrow; neither is there direct evidence that some elements of the marrow (leukocytes) preferentially utilize oxygen at the expense of the erythrocytes.† It is still possible, in view of the normal or elevated oxygen saturation values, that some of the

---

* In ninety-nine patients with polycythemia vera, whose hematocrits ranged to 81 per cent, the arterial oxygen saturation varied from 91 to 98.3 per cent, with a mean of 93.3 per cent (124).

† In the studies by Berk et al. there was a suggestion of slightly lowered saturation value with high leukocyte counts (7).

bone marrow cells are abnormal or poisoned and therefore unable to utilize the oxygen conveyed to them. But the intracellular respiration of the marrow has not been shown abnormal in polycythemia vera (68). Nevertheless, Turnbull and others have noted that zones of increased hematopoietic activity may, by unknown mechanisms, surround discrete secondary metastases of neoplastic tissue in fatty marrow. Polycythemia has (rarely) been described as an early manifestation of multiple myeloma, lymphatic leukemia, histiocytic leukemia, and Hodgkin's disease, and is well known to occur transiently in some patients early in myelogenic leukemia.

Because of the lack of evidence for abnormal factors *in* the bone marrow, interest has recently turned again to possible peripheral blood factors derived from either sites or tissues. Shortly after intrinsic factor was described by Castle, an excess of intrinsic factor was hypothesized as causative of polycythemia, and a gastric hormonal factor, addisin, was also postulated. Gastrectomy, repeated gastric lavage, and gastric irradiation were employed ineffectively; the administration of gastric tissue, liver extract, and vitamin B_{12} in excessive amounts did not produce polycythemia. Although neither the findings nor the interpretations are accepted by all workers in this field, assays for erythropoietin in plasma have demonstrated abnormally high levels in some patients. When normal or only slightly elevated levels are found, they have been explained as resulting from increased utilization of the factor by the abnormally large and hyperactive marrow mass. A recent article by Noyes et al. (82a) summarizes the various findings to date and reports no increase in erythropoietin employing a very sensitive assay system.

The evidence is good that normal red cell production and the increased production of red cells seen in polycythemia secondary to hypoxemia are controlled by a circulating erythropoietic factor(s). However, difficulty is encountered in applying these findings to polycythemia vera. With the exceptions to be mentioned below, none of the erythropoietic factors described effect a change in the leukocytes and platelets. But involvement of leukocytes and platelets is an evident and essential part of polycythemia vera. In terms of marrow alteration, Parkes-Webber drew attention to the observation that granulocytic hyperplasia may exceed the erythrocytic hyperplasia, and Minot emphasized the megakaryocytic increases. Clearly there is involvement of three main cellular elements of the marrow: a *panmyelosis*. Something in addition to increased erythropoietin levels must be involved.

Work concerning the control of thrombocyte and leukocyte production in the human being is fragmentary and preliminary, but a humoral regulatory mechanism is suggested. Employing animals, Linman (66) has reported that the administration of batyl alcohol results in increased production of erythrocytes, leukocytes, and platelets. This is a compound that is present in bone marrow and blood, but to achieve significant increases in cellular production unphysiologic amounts must be administered. Recently, Linman (67) has reported that normal rats given multiple daily doses of plasma from rabbits with phenylhydrazine-induced anemia developed leukocytosis and thrombocytosis. The agent in the plasma was thermostable and active by oral and parenteral routes. On this basis it was suggested that a single factor may effect the proliferation of all blood cell precursors. The relation of this factor to batyl alcohol is presently unknown. If confirmed and extended to human studies, these observations are perhaps an important key to the understanding of polycythemia vera.

Because of the diverse findings in polycythemia vera (erythrocytosis, leukocytosis, thrombocytosis, myeloid metabolism, myelofibrosis, anemia, leukemia, and blastic crises) and the various stages through which the disease progresses, "myeloproliferative syndrome" has been employed as an over-all descriptive term.

Here it is postulated that a primary stimulus affects the primitive reticulum, stem, or multipotential cell. Variations in the stimulus to, or responsiveness of, the different maturation lines determine the resultant hematologic and pathologic changes. In polycythemia vera clinical and pathologic evidence indicates that cell proliferation begins simultaneously in the marrow, spleen, and probably liver. With the stimulus provoking all cell lines, polycythemia and myeloid metaplasia result. When one line takes over (usually at the expense of another), other stages and pictures are produced: fibroblastic and osteoblastic activity produce myelofibrosis (62) or osteosclerosis; megakaryoblastic activity leads to thrombocytosis; overproduction of white cell precursors results in leukemoid or leukemic changes. Any and all combinations of cellular activity may occur in no set sequence so that a variety of hematologic and pathologic patterns may result. Although this has been regarded as a "dynamic" viewpoint, it is little, if anything, more than a description of the interrelations of changing clinical and pathologic pictures and contributes little to an understanding of the mechanisms of the disease process.

As mentioned before, there are very few well-documented records of the natural course of polycythemia vera unaltered by therapy. Nevertheless, there are instances of leukemia developing in patients with no prior radiation therapy. It is clear that leukemia in one form or another is a naturally occurring late or terminal event in the course of polycythemia (71, 75, 97, 104, 109, 123, 124). Principally because of this, polycythemia is generally regarded as a neoplastic process

akin to leukemia. However, as Castle has stated, at least early in the course, erythropoiesis is still subject to some of the usual physiologic controls. Observations on the changes in hemoglobin and red cells that occur following the administration of iron to patients with polycythemia vera and superimposed iron lack show that the red cell count *falls* after maximal hemoglobin response. In addition, there are a few well-documented instances of anemia developing after thyroidectomy in polycythemia vera, with subsequent elevation of the hemoglobin in response to thyroid administration (64, 86). Nevertheless, even early in the course some of the usual physiologic controls are not effective; this is illustrated by the lack of change in the increased iron turnover when oxygen is administered (59) in contrast to other disorders characterized by increased erythropoiesis (72).

Chemical studies on the alkaline phosphatase score and/or content of the leukocytes consistently show high values comparable to those seen in pyogenic leukemoid response (76). It is only in the myeloid metaplasia and frankly leukemic phase that the alkaline phosphatase score falls into the range seen in the usual myeloid leukemia (76).

The nature of the disease, the factors involved in the changing picture, and the stimulus to increased red cell and hemoglobin formation are unknown. Accepted theory presently regards the disease as neoplastic.

Treatment

Treatment of the disease is obviously governed by the stage and the pathophysiology present at the time. Early in the course venesection must immediately be employed to correct hypervolemia and blood viscosity changes. In a small number of patients prolonged remission of a year or more may follow adequate venesection. It frequently is the best way to manage younger individuals or patients with mild polycythemia. Repeated venesections will result in a relative iron lack and the patient will then not be able to increase his hemoglobin production. Unfortunately, at this time he may show other manifestations of tissue iron depletion (such as glossitis and cheilosis) in addition to the picture of hypochromic, microcytic blood, and so may require iron administration to effect a rapid, apparently specific reversal of tissue changes but, of course, a subsequent rise in hemoglobin level. Instead of repeated removal of large volumes of blood (300 to 500 ml), hookworm infestation has been employed to induce chronic blood loss and iron lack (18, 79).

In the vast majority of patients some myelosuppressive therapy is required repeatedly during the chronic course. Although many agents have been used and found effective, the P^{32} therapy introduced by Lawrence in 1940 is probably the best standardized and most completely evaluated (20, 21, 24, 36, 60, 90, 112, 120, 124, 129). It usually must be combined with venesection, at least initially, since even with a significant reduction in the rate of red cell manufacture, a decrease to reasonable levels in the peripheral blood does not occur till after many weeks. With adequate therapy, prolonged remission of several years' duration frequently occurs. There is little question now but that the patient's life span can be significantly increased by these methods—13 or more years compared with 6 years with the forms of management employed before P^{32} became available.

As more and more data accumulate it is evident that an increasing percentage of patients are developing acute myeloblastic leukemia terminally—11 per cent of 64 persons followed to death (124). Because of the lack of suitable controls it is impossible to say whether (a) leukemia is the usual termination of polycythemia vera, and hemorrhagic and thrombotic complications are being prevented so that more patients are now living long enough to reach this stage; (b) the leukemia is induced or accelerated by long-term radiation therapy, or (c) radiation brings out a latent tendency. However, there is no question but that the combination of radiation therapy (preferably P^{32}) and venesection has beneficial effects, prolonged as they usually are, that vastly outweigh the possible deleterious effects. In recent years other myelosuppressive agents such as Myleran (56) and pyrimethamine (38) have become available, have been shown to be effective as immediate therapy, and are now being evaluated with respect to long-term management of the patient.

Bibliographic references for Chapter 10 begin on page 445.

PART VII] THE RED CELL: UNDERPRODUCTION

CHAPTER ELEVEN

THE ANEMIAS OF BONE MARROW FAILURE*

GENERAL CONSIDERATIONS

The erythropoietic abnormalities seen in bone marrow failure are best dealt with in terms of the basic considerations of normal red cell production developed in Chapter 6. These will be briefly recapitulated here.

Marrow responds according to the stimulation it receives from a circulating factor(s) (erythropoietin) and according to its own inherent capacity. As indicated in the erythrokinetic classification of anemias (Table 6.6), bone marrow failure may result from defective formation of the stimulating factor(s) or from defective marrow response to an apparently adequately produced stimulating factor. Bone marrow failure can be said to exist when, in absolute terms, a normal number of erythrocytes is not delivered to the peripheral blood. In addition bone marrow failure exists when the marrow does not *increase* its production as much as would a normal marrow in response to the same stimulus. Relative bone marrow failure (150) is present even though a marrow has increased its production (in absolute terms) two to three times normal because under comparably increased stimulation normal marrow would increase its production six to ten times the usual rate.

If an erythropoietic response does occur, it may be of two types: (a) an effective erythropoietic response in which functionally competent cells are delivered to the peripheral blood, and (b) an ineffective erythropoietic response in which the marrow is unable to deliver cells to the peripheral blood even though chemically and morphologically it may appear to be going through the motions of so doing. The total erythropoietic response is the sum of effective plus ineffective erythropoiesis.

Fundamental to bone marrow failure may be a lack of production of erythropoietic factor(s) or lack of responsiveness on the part of the marrow to adequately produced erythropoietic factor(s); if a response does take place, it may be inadequate in terms of the absolute or relative number of cells produced by effective or ineffective erythropoiesis.

Comparable evaluation of marrow adequacy or failure cannot yet be made with reference to leukocytes and platelets.

CLASSIFICATION OF THE ANEMIAS OF BONE MARROW FAILURE

In this chapter are considered the hematologic aspects of those diseases in which

* General references and review articles: 5, 24, 43, 51, 78, 79, 80a, 85, 88, 89, 99, 131, 148, 150, 151, 155, 169, 186, 191, 197, 211, 219.

a significant component of the total picture is contributed by failure of the bone marrow to fulfill its primary objective of producing and delivering to the peripheral blood adequate numbers of one or more of the formed elements. This component contributed by the bone marrow failure may vary from one that apparently dominates the picture, as in total hematopoietic failure of all marrow elements and severe peripheral blood pancytopenia with otherwise normally functioning organ systems, to one that is of secondary import, as in mild anemia associated with active rheumatoid arthritis. It was previously pointed out that almost any disease capable of producing profound body-wide metabolic alterations is also frequently associated with some shortening of the erythrocyte life span, alteration in iron metabolism, and impaired red cell production. Consequently, bone marrow failure is encountered in varying degrees of severity and may be produced by different pathogenic mechanisms in a large number of diverse situations. Largely for convenience, a limited number will be somewhat arbitrarily grouped together, as indicated in Table 11.1, and here dealt with briefly. Practically all these diverse clinical states have erythrokinetic alterations characterized by a slight shortening of the red cell life span and a relative or absolute depression of red cell production; these hematologic alterations are not corrected by the *usual* hematopoietic agents (iron, vitamins B_6 or B_{12}, folic acid).

APLASTIC ANEMIA

The concept of "aplastic anemia" was introduced by Ehrlich (56) in 1888 with the description of a rapidly fatal disease characterized by severe anemia, leukopenia and thrombocytopenia (pancytopenia), and an anatomically acellular (aplastic) bone marrow; the early descriptions indicate acceptance of the concept that the primary defect was decreased cell production *because* of the

TABLE 11.1. Classification of the anemias of bone marrow failure

   I. Aplastic anemia, acquired (idiopathic or secondary) or constitutional[a]

  II. Hypoplastic anemia, acquired (idiopathic or secondary) or constitutional

 III. Sideroachrestic anemia

  IV. Anemia associated with
       A. Malignancy
       B. Rheumatoid arthritis
       C. Renal disease
       D. Liver disease
       E. Chronic infection
       F. Endocrine abnormalities
       G. Ionizing radiation
       H. Myelophthisis, myelofibrosis, or osteopetrosis

[a] This term is used in the literature dealing with this topic to indicate a familial occurrence, frequently congenital but not proved to be on basis of inborn error that is heritable or genetically governed. Constitutional, as used, is largely interchangeable with congenital. Because other defects have not infrequently been present, the term Fanconi's syndrome has also been employed (15, 44). Fanconi's hypoplastic anemia is characterized by pancytopenia; hypoplastic bone marrow; pigmentation of skin; small stature; microcephaly; hypogenitalism; renal anomalies; hypoplasia or absence of thumbs and/or radii; syndactyly and other skeletal anomalies; mental retardation; and anomalies of eyes and ears.

physical lack of precursors. Aplastic anemia was initially a *morphologic* diagnosis. Since then two occurrences have broadened and altered the concept of aplastic anemia without, however, changing its name: (a) many patients have been encountered with similar peripheral blood pancytopenia without lymphadenopathy or splenomegaly, in whom the disease was chronic; (b) the major investigative efforts in hematology have progressed from descriptive morphology to dynamic physiology. Consequently, the initial designation was retained when patients with the characteristic pancytopenia and clinical course were found to have bone marrow that appeared normally cellular or even hypercellular. This marrow was evidently physiologically aplastic in terms of delivery of cells to the peripheral blood. By almost unapparent stages, and attended by not a little confusion in the literature, the disease acquired a *physiologic* designation instead of a *morphologic* one; the original name was retained but under a new definition. As it is now commonly employed in this context, "aplastic" refers to the physiologic, functional ability of the bone marrow to deliver cells to the peripheral blood and not to its morphologic or anatomic appearance. This general idea is expressed by other terms sometimes used, such as aregenerative anemia, refractory anemia, toxic paralytic anemia, and, probably best of all, chronic bone marrow failure; but aplastic anemia is the name most frequently employed in clinical discussion.

Clinical Course

Because of the variability in course, manifestations, remissions, and responsiveness to treatment, it is most probable that many diseases of different etiologies and biochemical abnormalities have been unwittingly lumped together (2, 24, 25, 45, 48, 85, 98, 99, 118, 126, 148, 158–160, 169, 171, 176, 179, 184, 186, 200, 205, 211, 217,

220). For convenience the picture presented by acquired aplastic anemia will be set forth and exceptions noted when appropriate. Present-day views of this topic are presented in reviews by Hasselback and Thomas (85), Havard (88), Israels and Wilkinson (99), Mohler and Leavell (148), Rankin (169), Scott et al. (186), Vilter et al. (211), and Wolff (220).

A slight preponderance of males over females has been noted in most series studied, and there is a definitely decreased incidence of the disease in Negroes compared with whites. Onset of the disease occurs in all decades. The course pursued varies tremendously, from one characterized by abrupt onset and rapid progression through fulminating, toxic symptoms to death in weeks or a few months, to one with insidious onset, mild and manageable disability, remissions and relapses of many months or years duration ending perhaps in complete and lasting remission or in death due to infection or hemorrhage 4 to 5 years after onset. The signs and symptoms are most frequently referable to the depression of the hemoglobin and the rapidity of the change, infectious complications associated with the leukopenia, or hemorrhagic phenomenon due to thrombocytopenia. In the chronic form, weight and general muscular strength are well maintained. Lacking complications, which usually appear later in the course and are due to infection, central nervous system hemorrhage, or iron overload partly from repeated transfusions, organ dysfunction is minimal; with an adequate transfusion program, many patients are readily able to pursue their usual occupations and activities.

Physical Findings

Splenomegaly is unusual enough to warrant re-evaluation of the diagnostic criterion when it is seen early in the course; hepatomegaly and splenomegaly are found in about one-third of patients who have been followed and treated for some time and are probably the consequences of iron overload and repeated transfusions. At the time of initial examination approximately 50 per cent of patients show hemorrhagic phenomena in retinae, skin, and/or mucous membranes. Although in children retarded growth is noted, the striking clinical impression among adults is that of a well-nourished, well-developed individual with no evidence of organ dysfunction except for the anemic pallor due to bone marrow failure.

Laboratory Findings

The classic laboratory findings are, of course, the triad of severe anemia, leukopenia, and thrombocytopenia: a pancytopenia reflecting failure of the marrow to produce and deliver the formed elements to the blood. The anemia is usually severe and is either normocytic or moderately macrocytic (MCV about 100 cu μ); the red cells show only slightly greater-than-normal variation in size and shape. (It must be remembered that to obtain the true picture counts must be obtained before transfusions are given.) Signs of new cell formation are characteristically lacking; the percentage of cells that are reticulocytes is frequently below normal and not unusually is zero. When calculated in absolute numbers, the reticulocyte count is significantly low. The presence of nucleated red cells in the peripheral blood is distinctly unusual. An absolute neutropenia of about 1,000 to 2,000 cells per cubic millimeter is the usual finding; lymphopenia, when present, is of minor degree. Blastic forms are "never" present. The thrombocytopenia is frequently marked, but the platelets are usually of normal appearance. It should be pointed out that although the classic finding is pancytopenia, patients are encountered who show selective depression of only one or two marrow elements (i.e., anemia alone, anemia plus thrombocytopenia, or anemia plus leukopenia) while fulfilling all the other disease criteria. The literature is difficult to deal with on this point because authors may select for reporting only those patients with full pancytopenia. It must be acknowledged that evaluation of marrow production is presently possible only with respect to the red cell through ferrokinetic and erythrokinetic measurements; the evaluation of leukocyte and thrombocyte production and destruction is quantitatively not feasible. Rather than set up precise morphologic criteria, it would seem better (while retaining subclasses) to include and report all patients with "bone marrow failure" of one degree or another and thereby hope to get a better picture of the full spectrum.

Bone Marrow Findings

Bone marrow aspiration usually yields a poorly cellular specimen. When the aspirate is adequate for differential counting, a relative lymphocytosis is frequently found. For true evaluation of the marrow cellularity, it is necessary to obtain a biopsy specimen with intact marrow architecture by formal surgical technique or modified Vim-Silverman needle. The marrow may be hypo-, normo-, or hypercellular. The differential count may not deviate greatly from the normal. Even in marrow that is severely hypocellular, with marked fat cell replacement, active cellular areas or islands are seen, and in some instances an increase of lymphocytes may be present; thus general cellularity must not be the only factor considered in evaluating the presence and activity of the marrow elements. In terms of red cell production and delivery to the peripheral blood, it is clear that a morphologically cellular, active-appearing marrow may be incapable of effective erythropoiesis. Although the same statement cannot be made with a similar degree of assurance relative to leukocytes and platelets, by analogy with the red cell findings, it is not unexpected to find cellular, active-appearing marrow accompanying a peripheral pancytopenia. Recently there has been re-emphasis on, and new findings concerning, maturation abnormalities in the red cell series relative to nucleic acid production, iron metabolism, hemoglobin formation, and cytoplasmic maturation. In some patients megaloblastic or "megaloblastoid" maturation is seen; in some, abnormal chromatin clumping in proerythroblasts and normoblasts is present; and in others, excessive numbers of large siderotic granules are scattered through the cell or arranged in a "perinuclear collar."

Two points should be here emphasized: these marrow abnormalities do not change in response to the usual hematopoietic agents, and increased numbers of leukocyte blastic forms are not seen.

The results of other laboratory procedures are usually unrewarding except insofar as they reflect the changes due to anemia and thrombocytopenia. The earlier accounts of increased incidence of liver dysfunction probably indicate changes secondary to repeated transfusion and iron overload rather than changes due to the disease process itself, since liver dysfunction is usually found late in the course. The changes in iron metabolism and pigment metabolism will be discussed later.

Differential Diagnosis

There are no specific morphologic or biochemical tests that will certify the diagnosis of bone marrow failure, and there are many disorders with which it can be associated. Consequently when presented with a patient with marrow failure of one form or another, one must be alert to and concerned with numerous diagnostic possibilities; the differential diagnosis ranges wide as illustrated in Table 11.2.

In most situations an orderly approach to the problem presented by the patient readily indicates the correct diagnosis and suggests appropriate therapy. Since there are no pathognomonic changes, the diagnosis of idiopathic bone marrow failure and of failure presumed secondary to drugs or chemicals, even though strongly suggested by characteristic clinical and laboratory findings, is one that in many instances is made largely by exclusion. The possibility that the bone marrow failure may be due to exposure to drugs or to some toxic compound in the environment is exceedingly important to determine and will be discussed later. Two conditions are notoriously difficult to exclude and must be constantly kept in mind: miliary tuberculosis and atypical leukemia.

Miliary (disseminated) tuberculosis involving the bone marrow has been shown to result in severe pancytopenia and bone marrow changes which, when evaluated by aspiration technique, are consistent with those sometimes seen in aplastic anemia (38, 50, 61, 65, 142). The basic disease may elude detection for long periods of time, pursuing a mildly febrile course for months without the usual involvement of the lungs or other organs. Bone marrow biopsy with examination of the intact architectural structure for granulomatous lesions almost invariably reveals the correct diagnosis; more recently the modified Vim-Silverman needle biopsy technique has been of value.

It is now well established that a picture indistinguishable from that usually presented in aplastic anemia may be an early atypical manifestation of leukemia (21, 24, 134, 141). Even when the patient is subjected on repeated occasions to the most searching studies now available the picture of well-developed leukemia may emerge only months or years after the initial manifestations of bone marrow failure. It cannot be stated whether the leukemia has been present all the time manifesting itself as bone marrow failure, whether the patient had both aplastic anemia and leukemia (from the same or

TABLE 11.2.   Disorders from which bone marrow failure must be differentiated

---

I. Atypical manifestation of leukemia ("aleukemic leukemia")

II. Myelophthisic anemia
   A. Metastatic carcinoma
      1. Bone marrow replacement
      2. Relative nutritional deficiency
   B. Multiple myeloma
   C. Hodgkin's disease, lymphosarcoma
   D. Myelofibrosis, myelosclerosis, agnogenic myeloid metaplasia
   E. Osteopetrosis

III. Infections
   A. Miliary (disseminated) tuberculosis
   B. Equine infectious anemia
   C. Disseminated fungus

IV. Disorders involving the spleen
   A. Congestive splenomegaly
   B. Reticulum cell sarcoma, lymphosarcoma, Hodgkin's disease
   C. Gaucher's disease, Niemann-Pick's disease, Letterer-Siwe's disease
   D. Kala-azar, sarcoid, miliary tuberculosis
   E. "Primary splenic panhematopenia"

V. Deficiency diseases
   A. Vitamin B_{12} deficiency
   B. Folic acid deficiency
   C. Vitamin B_6 abnormality
   D. Iron lack

VI. Paroxysmal nocturnal hemoglobinuria (rare manifestation)

VII. "Toxic depression" of bone marrow activity (associated with rheumatoid arthritis, renal disease, liver disease, chronic infection, malignancy (thymoma), endocrine deficiency)

VIII. Secondary to
   A. Drug (chloramphenicol, Mesantoin, etc., see Table 11.3)
   B. Chemical agent (benzol, organic arsenicals, radiomimetic agents, antimetabolites)
   C. Physical agent (ionizing radiation)

IX. Idiopathic
   A. Hypoplastic ("pure red cell defect")
      1. Constitutional (familial)
         a. Adult
         b. Childhood (Diamond-Blackfan syndrome; responsive to adrenal steroids)
      2. Acquired
         a. Adult (thymoma)
         b. Childhood (responsive to adrenal steroids)
   B. Aplastic
      1. Constitutional (familial) Fanconi
         a. Adult
         b. Childhood (responsive to combination of adrenal and androgenic steroids)
      2. Acquired
         a. Adult
         b. Childhood (responsive to combination of adrenal and androgenic steroids)

related cause), or whether some metabolic derangement associated with the aplastic anemia induced or provoked the leukemia. When it does become manifest, the leukemia is usually acute and blastic in type—most frequently myeloblastic. This possibility must always be kept in mind when following these patients.

Pathophysiology

As pointed out at the beginning of this section, all the conditions grouped under the general heading "bone marrow failure" have in common a variable degree of inadequate responsiveness of the erythropoietic system. It must be acknowledged that the basic underlying abnormality responsible for this defect is not known; indeed, it seems evident that more than one abnormality must exist to account for the diverse manifestations encountered. In addition to this defect in responsiveness of the marrow, a hemolytic component is not infrequently present. The balance between these two factors determines the severity of the anemia and to some extent the course and complications experienced by the patient. Extensive erythrokinetic observations have been frequently made, with essential agreement in several different laboratories, on patients with chronic bone marrow failure (aplastic anemia, idiopathic acquired or secondary to chemical exposure). These will be described here and will later serve as a basis for discussion of the significant alterations from the pattern seen in other types of marrow failure.

Erythropoietin Production

It was clearly indicated by Ehrlich's observations that the primary defect was decreased red cell production. Failure of production could eventuate either from an inadequate stimulus or from a lack of response to the stimulus (end-organ defect). The recent demonstration that erythropoietin is present in the blood and urine of a number of patients with aplas-

tic anemia tends to rule out failure of production of this factor thought to provide the stimulus essential to red cell production (121). Studies have not conclusively demonstrated that the erythropoietin is normal and unaltered, i.e., effective for human cells, but the presumption is justified that it is. Although it appears probable that there are multiple erythropoietic factors, there is no evidence concerning possible deficiencies of one or another component. Present evidence, then, places the defect(s) in the reactivity of the cells of the bone marrow.

Basic Abnormalities (Theories)

The nature of the defect(s) is obscure although several suggestions have arisen in relation to studies on specific cases. In general, the failure to produce and deliver cells to the peripheral blood has been attributed to (a) primary defect of blood formation or defective formation due to direct cytotoxicity of endogenous or exogenous agents or lack of normal detoxification (24); (b) autoimmune factors (antibodies) capable of attacking the precursor cells, thereby destroying or inhibiting them (76); (c) abnormalities of DNA metabolism, idiopathic or induced by a, b, or d (211); and (d) deficiency of an unidentified factor. With respect to this last possibility, it must be acknowledged that at one time the anemias associated with iron lack, vitamin B_{12} deficiency, and folic acid or vitamin B_6 abnormalities were considered to be refractory anemias of bone marrow failure.

Erythrokinetics

The studies relative to erythrokinetics and ferrokinetics have shown the following (78, 79, 155). The plasma iron content is usually elevated, with a normal or slightly decreased plasma iron-binding capacity. Some degree of tissue hemosiderosis is present due in part to the iron deviated from the peripheral blood, where it would normally be present in circulating hemoglobin, and in part from the iron derived from transfusions and/or enhanced absorption. Radioactive iron clearance studies have revealed two types of patterns: in one the iron is removed from the plasma at a very slow rate when calculated either in terms of the absolute amount of iron removed per unit of time or in terms of rate of disappearance of the radioactivity; in the second type the iron is rapidly removed from the plasma when calculated by either of the above methods. When the tagged iron is followed by external tracking, it is frequently found that an abnormally large proportion (sometimes the major portion) is apparently cleared from the plasma directly to the liver, with subnormal amounts going to the bone marrow. Determination of the rate and percentage reappearance of the tagged iron in the circulating red cells shows in all instances that the percentage of the administered dose utilized for new red cell formation is markedly subnormal and that the rate of reappearance is slowed. This affords direct evidence of a decreased ability of the marrow to produce new erythrocytes and deliver them as functional units to the peripheral blood: effective erythropoiesis is markedly diminished. In the patients demonstrating rapid clearance of iron, ferrokinetic studies plus urobilinogen measurements indicate that *total* erythropoiesis is not depressed and may indeed exceed the normal unstimulated rate. Iron and pigment studies indicate apparent hemoglobin biosynthesis but inadequate delivery of cells to the peripheral blood: ineffective erythropoiesis. The type of dyshematopoiesis seen in untreated pernicious anemia and thalassemia is present. Usually, in addition to being ineffective, the total marrow response does not equal the response that a normal marrow would achieve under the same stimulus. Thus, both relative bone marrow failure and ineffective erythropoiesis are involved. These changes are not influenced by administration of the usual hematopoietic agents. Although generally in aplastic anemia rapid clearance of iron from the peripheral blood is associated with ineffective erythropoiesis and normally cellular or hypercellular marrow, there has been no strict correlation between marrow morphology and erythrokinetic studies, which again illustrates the present difficulty in correlating function and morphology in this situation.

Erythrocyte Survival

Erythrokinetic studies employing the Ashby cross-transfusion method or the Fe^{59} or Cr^{51} autosurvival techniques usually show a nearly normal red cell life span or the presence of minor hemolytic processes resulting from an abnormality extrinsic to the red cell (155). The presence of an overt hemolytic component or marked shortening of the red cell life span is distinctly unusual in idiopathic or secondary aplastic anemia; as will be pointed out, the contribution made by accelerated rate of red cell destruction to the anemia is quite variable in the other instances of bone marrow failure to be considered and can be anything from overt hemolysis dominating the picture, as is sometimes the case in infections or liver disease, to minor degrees of increased destruction detectable only by survival techniques, as in mild anemia associated with malignancy or renal disease.

Erythrokinetic studies indicate that the marrow with respect to total erythropoiesis is in relative or absolute failure, that the erythropoiesis present may be significantly ineffective in character, and that some degree of shortening of the red cell survival time frequently exists.

Biochemical Abnormalities

There have been many searches into possible biochemical abnormalities relative to bone marrow failure. No abnormal hemoglobins have been detected, but on numerous occasions elevations in an al-kali-resistant hemoglobin, apparently the same as hemoglobin F of cord blood, have been demonstrated (192). Curiously, this hemoglobin is not equally distributed among all the cells, but rather is present in increased amounts in a relatively minor proportion suggesting two populations of cells. Recent observations on children made while their hematologic symptoms were apparently in remission showed the persistence of the high hemoglobin F levels. Several groups of workers have studied, in certain instances of bone marrow failure, the results of tryptophan-loading tests with respect to the urinary excretion of tryptophan metabolites (8, 135, 198). While there is no agreement among the various groups concerning specific derangements, there is concurrence in the opinion that abnormalities of tryptophan metabolism exist that are impossible to interpret at the present time. There is little doubt that these biochemical abnormalities should be explored and exploited as far as possible, both because they have intrinsic value and promise and because apparently no other comparable leads exist. In a study on detoxification mechanisms in children with aplastic anemia, Wagner and Smith (211a) could demonstrate no abnormalities in the mechanisms evaluated.

Etiologic Agents

Studies on bone marrow failure—particularly of the types seen in aplastic or hypoplastic anemia, acquired or constitutional —have been markedly hampered by a lack of naturally occurring suitable animal counterparts and the fact that animal marrow apparently reacts differently from human marrow to many chemical agents. Certain observations made in humans have been confirmed in animals under more satisfactory experimental conditions, but little new knowledge of value has been added. Benzene, ionizing radiation, radiomimetic drugs, and antimetabolites used in the chemotherapy of malignancies have long been known to produce bone marrow failure in humans and consistently produce bone marrow failure in animals when administered in sufficiently high doses. It is of interest that in the animal experiments employing estrogens and antifolic acid preparations, the marrow appears to become *hyper*plastic first, then progressively less cellular until frank morphologic aplasia has been produced (151). Although it is possible that the different marrow pictures seen in patients represent different stages in essentially the same pathologic process, clinical experience does not now substantiate this.

Most agents implicated in the production of aplastic anemia in humans fail to do so in animals. These agents are now being listed in ever-increasing number, and although the evidence is for the most part convincing that they do produce bone marrow failure in humans, the evidence is circumstantial. Experiments on human beings to verify the conclusions are obviously impracticable: the recovery rate in an individual with suspected drug poisoning is too slow and the possible consequence of re-exhibition of the drug too dangerous. Epidemiologic studies under present circumstances are not possible because there is no accurate way of determining the total number of individuals exposed to a given agent. Moreover, the reaction rate is probably too low to make such studies feasible: it has been estimated, for example, that aplastic anemia develops in only 1 of every 800,000 individuals given chloramphenicol, a drug for which there is good evidence concerning its relation to altered erythropoiesis. Rubin et al. (181) have shown that under certain circumstances the administration of chloramphenicol in usual dosage is accompanied by an elevated serum iron level, a decreased rate of clearance of iron from the plasma, and a decreased rate of radioiron incorporation into peripheral blood erythrocytes. These changes were noted to occur 7 to 10 days prior to a drop in the circulating hemoglobin level. In addition, the administration of chloramphenicol may be accompanied by morphologic changes in the red cell maturation series, intranuclear and cytoplasmic vacuolization being prominent (81, 182). The administration of very high doses of the drug in experiments on ducks, dogs, and human beings has resulted in some depression of bone marrow activity: leukopenia, thrombocytopenia, and vacuolization of marrow cells have been noted in humans (115). The evidence here is convincing that chloramphenicol is potentially toxic to bone marrow; actually the low incidence of serious complications is surprising.

Epidemiologic studies concerning the induction of aplastic anemia by Atabrine were possible because of controlled wartime circumstances (45). The incidence of aplastic anemia was significantly increased among service men in the theaters where Atabrine was employed for 4 to 14 months as a malarial suppressant compared with theaters not requiring its use; moreover, within a given area the number of cases found was demonstrated to be proportional to the dose administered and the duration of administration.

Except for occasional instances (prolonged nitrous oxide anesthesia, for example, 122, 218), the evidence incriminating drugs in the production of bone marrow failure is largely circumstantial. There is, however, little reason to doubt that many agents can produce aplastic anemia—perhaps on an idiosyncratic basis. The list of such agents is long (Table 11.3).

In a significant proportion (approximately 50 per cent) of all patients with *acquired* aplastic anemia no convincing history of exposure to a toxic agent can be demonstrated; these patients are presumed to have idiopathic bone marrow failure. In spite of this, in the management of a patient with aplastic anemia one must continually search for possibly injurious agents so that they may be immediately removed from the patient's environment. This is obviously the first step in the proper treatment. Thorough "in the home" and/or "on the job" surveys, although often inconclusive, are important, since change in environment is indicated even on the basis of suspicious findings. *All* medications the patient may have been receiving before the development of marrow failure should be discontinued unless deemed absolutely essential for specific reasons.

Treatment

Bone marrow failure cannot be reversed by any known agent. But since there is an apparent tendency to remission with prolonged survival, supportive therapy becomes extremely important. Evidence is now accumulating on the course taken by the disease, the complications to be anticipated, and the prognosis for the patient whose disease is modified by therapy. However, because of a skewed distribution curve it is difficult to estimate the average survival time and possible changes induced by therapy (186). In general, about 50 per cent of patients live for 2½ years and 40 per cent live for 4 years or longer. Again, it must be pointed out that the course may be extremely rapid, fulminant, and toxic, with death occurring in a few weeks, or may be indolent and prolonged, with sufficient recovery so that treatment is no longer needed.

At present, there is no way of knowing in any given individual whether the marrow damage is irreversible or not (43, 151). Exposure to possible offending agents must be stopped and prevented from recurring. Even the long-held general impression that a cellular marrow is more likely to be associated with remission and recovery is not well documented by adequate evidence. Repeated transfusions are usually necessary to maintain a hemoglobin level compatible with nor-

TABLE 11.3.　Agents associated with the occurrence of pancytopenia

Agents which regularly produce marrow hypoplasia and aplasia if a sufficient dose is given:
  Ionizing radiation (roentgen rays, radioactive phosphorus, gold, etc.)
  Mustards (sulfur and nitrogen mustards, triethylenemelamine (TEM), etc.)
  Urethan, Myleran
  Benzene

  Antimetabolites (antifolic acid compounds, 6–mercaptopurine, etc.)

Agents occasionally associated with hypoplasia or aplasia (idiosyncratic reaction?):

Class of compound	20 to 100 or more reported cases	Single or very few reports
Antimicrobial agents	Arsenobenzol Chloramphenicol	Inorganic arsenicals Streptomycin Sulfonamides Oxytetracycline Chlortetracycline
Anticonvulsants	Mesantoin (methyl-phenylethyl hydantoin)	Tridione (trimethadione) Nuvarone (methylphenyl hydantoin)
Antithyroid drugs		Carbimazole (carbethoxy-thiomethylglyoxaline) Tapazole (methylmercapto-imidazole)
Antihistaminics		Pyribenzamine
Insecticides		Chlorophenothane (DDT)
Miscellaneous agents	Gold preparations Trinitrotoluene	Quinacrine (Atabrine) Dinitrophenol Phenylbutazone Chlorpromazine and promazine Hair dyes Meprobamate Bismuth Mercury Colloidal silver Carbon tetrachloride

Adapted from Wintrobe, M. W., Clinical Hematology, ed. 5, p. 553, Lea & Febiger, Philadelphia, 1961.

mal or somewhat restricted activity. These confer a known hazard as well as benefit through the very real dangers of hepatitis, iron overload, and the development of subgroup incompatibilities. Iron overload is inevitable in a prolonged illness requiring frequent transfusions, and recent studies indicate that the incidence of hepatic, pancreatic, and cardiac complications (intractable congestive failure, recurrent pericarditis) rises in rough proportion to the number of transfusions (59, 149). The administration of fresh platelets is sometimes necessary; it is certainly feasible on a short-term basis and has occasionally been successful on a long-term basis (13). Despite the fact that leukopenia apparently confers a susceptibility to infection, "prophylactic" antibiotic therapy seems to lead only to further complications, emergence of resistant organisms, and increased incidence of fungal infections. Although there are case reports (usually single) recounting beneficial effects from one agent or another, or from combinations of agents such as cobalt (188, 204), riboflavin (66), cortisone, vitamin B_{12}, marrow transplantation (175, 188), etc., only steroid therapy and splenectomy appear to have sufficient merit to warrant discussion here.

SPLENECTOMY. The possible benefits from splenectomy have been recently reviewed (89, 91, 186), and therapeutic trial obviously warrants serious consideration. In the studies by Loeb et al. (131) cited above increased iron utilization and decreased hemolysis were in some instances documented. Most notable was a complete and lasting remission after splenectomy in a young male who had required over 600 transfusions. Heaton's (89) review of the results of splenectomy points out that the operation is frequently beneficial but that the benefit is usually of minor degree (slight elevation of hemoglobin level and/or decreased transfusion requirement). Though of minor degree, this is of major importance to the patient. Curiously, however, the beneficial effect seems frequently to be delayed 4 to 8 months before it is notable. Scott's (186) analysis of the results of splenectomy is in general agreement with that of Heaton, but the point is made that it is not yet possible to evaluate the effect of splenectomy on the life expectancy or survival time of these patients. From the data available it is *possible* that the patient's survival time is materially enhanced by splenectomy but critical statistical evaluation does not *support* this conclusion.

STEROID THERAPY. In adults the use of androgens has not been adequately evaluated but at present does not appear to have been beneficial in the limited number of trials attempted (see below for results in children).

The most physiologic evaluation of steroid therapy has been made by Loeb et al. (131), who measured ferrokinetics and red cell survival times before and after ACTH or corticosteroid therapy and also before and after splenectomy. A beneficial effect with reference to red cell production and destruction was noted with steroid therapy. Experience indicates that on occasion the beneficial effect is significant, resulting in elevation of hemoglobin level and decrease of transfusion requirements. It must be acknowledged that the likelihood of benefit from a trial of corticosteroid therapy is small in adults and that if a beneficial result does occur the change induced is usually minimal although definite. Against this must, of course, be balanced the real dangers of prolonged steroid therapy.

These considerations concerning the management of chronic aplastic anemia apparently apply equally to the idiopathic acquired type and the type secondary to drugs or chemical agents; they also apply to the constitutional forms of the disease, although experience with these forms is much more limited and the prognosis is significantly poorer (176). Fortunately it is now possible to state with good assurance that the situation is different with respect to the aplastic anemia of childhood, both the acquired and congenital types.

The mortality in this age group used to be extremely high, the number of spontaneous remissions low, and the number of sustained remissions extremely small. Corticosteroids have been tried, but no true remissions attributable to them have been noted, although hemorrhagic phenomena may have been slightly alleviated. When androgenic hormones are added (190, 191) to the corticosteroids, a slow, sustained reticulocytosis occurs in the majority of children, followed by increase in hematocrit and hemoglobin levels; normal values are reached only after several months of treatment. Leukocyte and platelet counts also increase. The speed of the response apparently varies with the state of the bone marrow, but the mechanism of action is completely obscure. Once remission is obtained in those with the *acquired* form of the disease, it is sustained even after hormone therapy is withdrawn.

Children with the congenital form (Fanconi's anemia; 86, 191) also frequently show a rapid reticulocyte response when testosterone is given along with corticosteroids. A slow rise in hemoglobin level follows, but testosterone therapy must be continued (although in diminished amounts), since relapse promptly follows withdrawal of the agent. Preliminary observations (189) indicate that it may be possible to use anabolic agents to obtain favorable hematologic responses; these preparations produce less of the undesirable androgenic effects than the ordinary testosterone preparations.

TREATMENT OF HYPOPLASTIC ANEMIA. Special mention must be made of the treatment of so-called hypoplastic anemia: pure red cell defect. In adults this is an unusual condition (60, 205) and in a number of instances has been associated with a thymoma (12, 37, 87, 100, 112, 124). Although removal of the thymoma does not usually change the hematologic status, there have been reported a few instances of remission following thymectomy—some sustained, some temporary. In adults the anemia is unresponsive to adrenal steroid therapy (60), but is perhaps benefited by androgenic hormones (124). When hypoplastic anemia occurs in childhood (not in association with thymoma), it is usually of the congenital type and has been designated the Diamond-Blackfan syndrome, or pure red cell defect (29, 54, 162). Splenectomy may be of some benefit and cortisone therapy is definitely of value. Allen and Diamond point out that most of the patients are responsive if treatment is instituted early in the course (5). Reticulocytosis is usually prompt (4 to 11 days), and the hemoglobin values become normal in 4 to 6 weeks.

SUMMARY. None of the anemias of bone marrow failure of the aplastic or hypoplastic types respond to the usual hematopoietic agents. In adults with aplastic anemia of the acquired idiopathic or secondary type, or of the congenital type, a transfusion program and general supportive therapy are the mainstay; splenectomy may be followed by moderate though significant beneficial effects or, rarely, by remission. Children with aplastic anemia of the acquired type have a good chance of experiencing sustained hematologic remission following treatment with corticosteroids and androgen preparations, even though the agents are later withdrawn. If the aplastic anemia is of the congenital type, hematologic benefit is unlikely to follow splenectomy but is likely to occur with corticosteroids and androgenic preparations. However, relapse follows withdrawal of the agents. Hypoplastic anemia in adults may subside following removal of an accompanying thymoma; hypoplastic anemia in childhood may benefit from splenectomy (67, 160) but usually responds to corticosteroids if the treatment is instituted early in the course. For those failing to respond to therapy the possibility of bone marrow transplantation (using fetal (187) or homologous (41, 62, 140, 175) marrow) may be kept in mind as an experimental procedure, recalling that while the prognosis is poor, the disease tends to remit with prolonged survival.

These disorders are the examples of anemias of bone marrow failure wherein the hematologic manifestations dominate the picture and are of major concern in the management of the patient. Several other examples of diseases of bone marrow failure in which the blood changes dominate the picture have been considered in detail in other chapters: iron-lack anemia, anemia secondary to vitamin B_{12} deficiency or folic acid abnormality, and thalassemia. The many additional anemias of bone marrow failure listed in Table 11.1 will be briefly characterized but not considered in detail.

THE ANEMIA ASSOCIATED WITH LIVER DISEASE

Clinical Manifestations and Laboratory Findings

Despite a considerable diversity in the pathogenic and etiologic processes (infectious, toxic, degenerative, deficiency) that can give rise to chronic liver disease, present evidence indicates that the associated anemias have, by and large, similar morphologic and pathophysiologic characteristics. This immediately suggests that the hematologic alterations are secondary not to the initiating causes but rather to the end result of the factors that initiate damage in an organ believed to be markedly restricted in the forms by which it can react to insult. At the outset it must be stated that the mechanisms are unknown whereby anemia is associated with liver disease; the anemia is unresponsive to the usual hematopoietic agents but is usually alleviated if and when liver function improves. It must, of course, be recognized that since chronic liver disease is not uncommon in the population, various types of anemia will be found that coexist with hepatic disease but are present on a statistical rather than a causal basis. One must, therefore, be ready to recognize the hematologic changes characteristic of iron lack, hemoglobinopathy, hereditary or acquired hemolytic disease, pernicious anemia, folic acid abnormality, bone marrow failure, etc., either expressed as such or somewhat modified by the superimposed changes of the anemia of liver disease.

The anemia associated with liver disease (most frequently chronic liver disease) is usually of significant degree (hemoglobin concentration about 10 Gm per 100 ml) but rarely severe (less than 5 Gm per 100 ml) unless complicated by other factors such as blood loss or folic acid abnormalities (93, 102, 103, 116, 143, 152, 193, 214). In the uncomplicated anemia the red cells are normocytic or even more typically somewhat macrocytic (MCV, 100 to 115 cu μ). When macrocytic, the appearance of the cells is not like that classically seen in pernicious anemia: the variations in size and shape are not as extreme, the macrocytes not as well filled with hemoglobin, and the leukocyte changes not found. Although the macrocyte seen in liver disease covers a large area of the cover slip, it does not appear thick as judged by focal plane adjustment; it is a "thin macrocyte" with no great increase in cell volume (17, 18, 82). A moderate degree of polychromatophilia (reticulocytes composing 2 to 5 per cent of red cells) is usually noted along with stippled cells and target forms. These morphologic changes may be present in the absence of significant depression of the circulating hemoglobin level but can be *roughly* correlated with the degree of liver damage. The platelet count is frequently low or low normal even in the absence of clinically detectable splenomegaly. The bone marrow has been described as occupying a larger-than-normal volume, containing decreased amounts of fat, and showing hypercellularity with a "macronormoblastic proliferation" (14, 105, 143, 157). The red cell precursors are large; some demonstrate abnormalities of nuclear chromatin, nuclear-cytoplasmic asynchrony, and abnormal mitoses such as are seen in megaloblastic maturation, but (contrary to the anemias of vitamin B_{12} or folic acid abnormalities) all stages of maturation are seen, with a preponderance, if any, of the more mature stages. Abnormalities of leukocyte maturation are not seen.

Osmotic fragility tests demonstrate an abnormality seen in several other types of anemia, usually hemolytic. The initial part of the curve lies within the normal range but the top portion is shifted into the range of increased resistance; after incubation an exaggerated picture of the changes seen in the unincubated sample is produced. The erythrocyte mechanical fragility is usually low normal before incubation and higher than normal after. These changes probably mean an abnormal loss of osmotically active material from the cell and/or marked membrane alteration. However, the biochemical or metabolic changes have not been further characterized.

Pathogenesis

In the early considerations of the possible pathogenesis of the anemia of liver disease, the superficial resemblance to pernicious anemia suggested a possible defect in hepatic storage of the antipernicious anemia factor. But as pointed out above, the morphologic changes are *not* similar upon critical examination; the anemia does not respond to the administration of liver extract or vitamin B_{12}; and the antipernicious anemia factor has been demonstrated present in the liver by clinical assay. More recently, vitamin B_{12} has been found present in chronically diseased liver. It must be acknowledged that the values are significantly subnormal and the form in which the vitamin exists is only incompletely explored. Nevertheless, the serum vitamin B_{12} level frequently is much elevated above normal in liver disease, with or without anemia (167, 199), so a true deficiency is unlikely. Absorption as assayed by the Schilling test is characteristically normal. The administration of folic acid or citrovorum factor induces no hematologic improvement in patients with uncomplicated anemia of liver disease, and the absorption, concentration in the blood, excretion, and metabolic derivatives of these preparations are characteristically normal. The serum iron levels are variable—normal or slightly elevated (frequently elevated in acute liver damage).

Erythrokinetics

Several workers have pointed out that although the circulating hemoglobin level may be decreased, this occurs because even though the red cell mass may be normal or even slightly increased the plasma volume is much increased above normal ("ascites of the blood"; 36, 57, 83). Apparently this is most likely to be true if esophageal varices or cyanosis is present (57).* Hemodilution probably plays a significant role in determining the peripheral blood values in a number of patients, but the characteristic cellular marrow of increased volume and peripheral blood reticulocytosis indicate a significant erythropoietic effort by the marrow. It has been known for some time that some patients with the anemia of liver disease excrete an increased amount of urobilinogen, both fecal and urinary (213), and numerous studies have more recently demonstrated decreased red cell survival. Because of the danger of transmitting hepatitis, no studies have been made to establish directly the presence of an intrinsic defect by observing the survival of a patient's cells after transfusion into a normal individual. However, Ashby and Cr^{51} techniques, by which the survival of normal cells or the patient's own cells is determined in the patient, demonstrate in most cases a significantly shortened survival time and an extracorpuscular abnormality (6, 34, 35, 83, 102, 110). The degree of anemia present correlates roughly with the shortening of the erythrocyte survival time (102). Characteristically, demonstrable circu-

* It has been shown that some degree of decreased arterial oxygen saturation exists in liver disease (1), probably on the basis of slight shift in the dissociation curve (114) but mainly because of venous admixture. The oxygen unsaturation does not correlate with the presence of clubbed fingers sometimes seen in liver disease (cirrhosis).

lating agglutinins and hemolysins are absent, and the survival time is unchanged by the administration of steroid preparations. Following transfusion of Cr^{51}-labeled autogenous cells, a considerable build-up of splenic radioactivity indicates the spleen as a major organ of erythrocyte destruction. Nevertheless, splenectomy is followed by little or no change in hemoglobin levels, and similar curves for red cell destruction are obtained.

The few direct measurements of the rate of marrow production in the anemia of liver disease confirm the indirect calculations made from erythrocyte survival curves and indicate in practically all instances an increase in total and effective erythropoiesis (79, 83). However, the increase is not equivalent to the capabilities of a normal marrow under similar stimulation so that some degree of bone marrow hypofunction, or relative bone marrow failure, exists.

Although most of the above conclusions have been drawn from studies made on patients with anemia associated with cirrhosis because of the relative stability of this situation, sufficient evidence is available to warrant applying the conclusions to the anemia of liver disease in general.

It must be pointed out that instances of classic, overt, acquired hemolytic anemia, with positive results in the direct and/or indirect Coombs tests have been seen, occasionally recurrent with exacerbations of the liver dysfunction. In addition, Zieve (113a, 221) described a syndrome consisting of jaundice, hyperlipemia, hypercholesterolemia, and hemolytic anemia that follows excessive alcohol intake and improves rapidly once the drinking stops. Liver biopsy shows fatty infiltration and minimal to moderate partial cirrhosis. Consequently it must be acknowledged that, exceptionally, hemolysis may become the dominant element (95).

Not so exceptionally, decreased bone marrow production may dominate the picture when folic acid abnormality results in megaloblastic changes. These patients are usually more severely anemic, frequently show evidence of other vitamin deficiencies, and usually give a history of inadequate dietary intake but markedly increased alcohol intake; their red cells appear markedly macrocytic (103, 116, 152, 214). Hematopoietic response apparently may follow (a) cessation of the alcohol intake, (b) change of diet, (c) bed rest, (d) administration of physiologic amounts of folic acid or citrovorum factor, or (e) no discernible change in the patient's routine. It is conceivable that alcohol increases the requirement for folic acid or one of its derivatives or acts as a toxic inhibitor of erythropoiesis. McCurdy et al. (139) have reported bone marrow alterations in acute alcoholism consisting essentially of nuclear and cytoplasmic vacuolizations such as are seen in chloramphenicol poisoning.

In general, however, it may be said that the anemia associated with liver disease is of unknown etiology, refractory to therapy, exaggerated by hypervolemia, and characterized by increased red cell destruction and relatively inadequate bone marrow response.

THE ANEMIA ASSOCIATED WITH INFECTION

Clinical Manifestations and Laboratory Findings

In association with infection (most frequently chronic) a morphologically nonspecific type of anemia often occurs that is not due to blood loss, overt hemolysis, deficiency of vitamin B_{12} or iron, or abnormality of folic acid metabolism, and that is refractory to the usual hematopoietic agents. The degree of anemia varies with the type, severity, and duration of the infection. Bacterial endocarditis is usually accompanied by significant anemia (hemoglobin concentration 10 Gm per 100 ml) and not infrequently by severe anemia (161); tuberculosis is seldom accompanied by a more than mild degree of anemia (27, 74, 145) except when miliary spread occurs (38, 61, 65, 142). Pyogenic suppurative infections (as in lung abscess and osteomyelitis) are likely to be accompanied by severe depression of hemoglobin level especially when caused by a mixture of organisms. Contracted plasma and blood volumes are usually present (33) except early in rheumatic fever, when the significant depression of the circulating hemoglobin level is apparently due to an increase in plasma volume (136); later on in the course of rheumatic fever the decreased circulating hemoglobin level can be attributed to a diminution in the red cell mass (94, 170).

Characteristically the anemia is of mild to moderate severity and most frequently normocytic and normochromic (33, 183, 208); rarely in chronic infection the cells may become slightly microcytic and hypochromic even when no response to administration of iron can be obtained and the iron stores appear adequate. The variation in size and shape of the red cells appears to be within normal limits and the proportion of reticulocytes is decreased. In general the anemia develops slowly during the course of an infection so that by a month or two after onset the hemoglobin concentration may have dropped to 10 to 11 Gm per 100 ml. With the more chronic infections an equilibrium is apparently reached at about this time so that no further change of significance takes place. However, with overwhelming sepsis and blood-stream invasion (by *Clostridium welchii, Escherichia coli,* streptococci, and staphylococci) anemia may develop very rapidly (in days) with no apparent equilibrium point to limit the severity.

The bone marrow usually shows a decrease in the proportion of red cell precursors, some increase in the proportion of immature cells, and poor hemoglobin production in the normoblasts as evidenced by a basophilic or darkly polychromatophilic cytoplasm.

Erythrokinetics

Although the mechanism whereby anemia occurs in association with infection is unknown, old and new evidence indicates that impaired erythrocyte production is the major component. It has long been known that an intercurrent infection will promptly suppress a reticulocyte response that is under way or that would otherwise be induced by the appropriate treatment of pernicious anemia or iron-lack anemia. By more direct and recent techniques, impaired utilization and delayed reappearance of radioiron (derived from damaged red cells) have been noted in the ferrokinetic studies evaluating erythropoiesis. While demonstrable in otherwise hematologically normal individuals, this "toxic depression" of bone marrow activity is seen in perhaps its most drastic form in the aplastic, or aregenerative, crisis of the various hemolytic anemias (144).

Accompanying the erythropoietic changes marked alterations in iron metabolism are regularly seen in infection or inflammation. The plasma iron level is consistently and significantly lowered; the iron-binding protein level is also depressed so that the per cent saturation may not be greatly altered (33). Even though, as indicated above, a diminished and delayed reutilization of iron from nonviable red cells occurs, the plasma clearance rates and utilization of transferrin-bound iron for new red cell formation are not impaired (30, 68).* Since destruction and breakdown of the red

* Earlier studies indicating impaired utilization of transferrin-bound iron were done employing large nontracer amounts and must be now considered invalid (33).

cells occur in the reticuloendothelial system, there appears to be a defect in the release of iron from the tissues to the iron-binding protein of the plasma. This combination of continuing utilization of transferrin-bound iron for red cell formation plus the decreased release of iron from tissues to transferrin is thought to account for the lowered plasma iron level seen in infection and inflammation. When severe bone marrow depression occurs, as in chloramphenicol poisoning during treatment of an infection, a marked elevation occurs in serum iron level; labeled iron is slowly cleared from the plasma and poorly utilized in red cell formation.

The normal rates of iron clearance from plasma and utilization in red cell production might at first be taken as evidence of unimpaired erythropoiesis, but when these are translated into absolute terms (amount of iron cleared per time unit and amount of iron utilized per day for hemoglobin production), a significantly impaired production is indicated in terms of the potential of the normal unimpeded marrow. The nature of the disturbance is not clear, but the alteration in iron metabolism and the fact that the erythrocyte protoporphyrin concentration is elevated in infection have been interpreted as pointing to a quantitative defect in the rate of conversion of protoporphyrin to hemoglobin (33, 207, 208). Since hypochromic erythrocytes are so infrequently found, a defect in cell production must also be assumed.

When the erythrocyte survival time is studied in the anemia of chronic infection, a modest hemolytic component is frequently demonstrable that is of the type due to an extracorpuscular defect (28). However, except in the unusual circumstances to be mentioned below, the shortening of the red cell survival time is of such minor degree that a normal uninhibited marrow would be expected to compensate very readily. Consequently, it is concluded that bone marrow failure is the principal cause of the anemia.

On occasion, overt hemolytic anemia may develop in association with infection and may even dominate the clinical picture and obscure the underlying disease. Jandl et al. (104) point out that at least four distinctive hemolytic syndromes may be delineated: (a) an acute, often lethal, intravascular hemolysis during bloodstream invasion by organisms (such as *Clostridium welchii*) that produce hemolysins; (b) direct infection of red cells by the red cell–adherent organism, *Bartonella bacilliformis*, causing splenic trapping and acute hemolytic anemia; (c) acute or chronic hemolytic anemia associated with the development of cold agglutinins or cold hemolysins; and (d) hemolytic anemia in which a minor population of spherocytes and increased splenic sequestration are the common features and are considered to result from a form of hypersplenism that occurs during prolonged pyrogenic stimulation of the reticuloendothelial system and is associated with an increased number of circulating mononuclear leukocytes.

THE ANEMIA ASSOCIATED WITH RHEUMATOID ARTHRITIS

The anemia seen in association with active rheumatoid arthritis appears to belong in the same general category as the anemia secondary to chronic infection or inflammation (10, 107, 109, 156, 168, 216). The severity of the anemia correlates closely with the degree of activity of the rheumatoid process as indicated by active joint involvement, but there is little correlation with the duration of the disease. The typical picture is a normochromic, normocytic anemia of mild degree. The serum iron level is usually moderately decreased (180) even in patients with adequate amounts of marrow hemosiderin (55, 69, 180); the iron-binding protein is variable (55, 216). The clearance of transferrin-bound radioactive iron from plasma is within normal limits (55, 69), and the utilization of iron in red cell production is either normal (55, 69) or occasionally slightly impaired (216). The gastrointestinal absorption of iron is normal (108, 180, 216).

The usual tests for demonstrating abnormal substances on the red cells are negative. However, employing a dextran-cell, latex-fixation test, Finkelstein et al. (63a) have demonstrated a substance coating the red cells that is similar to the rheumatoid factor of serum. Red cell survival studies of normal erythrocytes transfused into a patient (Ashby selective agglutination technique) show a moderately shortened life span (4, 69, 128, 138); however, survival times determined by autotransfusion (patient's cells labeled with radioactive chromium circulating in the patient) are within normal limits (16, 55, 128, 174, 216). Only a rare patient shows a significantly increased rate of destruction by the chromium technique. These results suggest the unusual occurrence of a process in the patient with active rheumatoid arthritis that by an extrinsic abnormality shortens the life span of normal donor cells but not the patient's own cells. The main, if not the only, cause of the anemia associated with rheumatoid arthritis is apparently marrow failure. The anemia is almost always responsive to steroid therapy, but the hemoglobin level soon falls to its former value after steroids are discontinued. Anemia of arthritis is seldom treated per se, since it is usually moderate and treatment of the joint disease is far more important.

In *some* surveys of patients with chronic rheumatoid arthritis a significant number of patients have been found with a hypochromic, microcytic anemia. In about half of those with hypochromic changes, the anemia was responsive to the administration of iron (but reportedly only to iron given parenterally), while in the rest the anemia was refractory even to parenteral iron therapy (196). Marrow studies may show no stainable iron (173). In these patients chronic blood loss has usually not been eliminated as a cause of the blood changes apart from the effect of the active rheumatoid arthritis, so ferrokinetic studies are presently impossible to evaluate. In general, if a severe degree of anemia is found, it is usually hypochromic and microcytic, and etiologic factors must be searched for in addition to the rheumatoid arthritis.

The Anemia Associated with Renal Disease

Clinical Manifestations and Laboratory Findings

Both acute and chronic renal insufficiency are usually accompanied by profound alterations in erythrokinetics (113, 117, 209). Red cell aplasia (morphologic erythroblastopenia) has been shown to occur in acute renal failure (172), and anemia regularly develops shortly after the metabolic alterations secondary to renal shutdown (202). In some instances the bone marrow failure appears to be the most important factor; in others a hemolytic component may be evident, with vigorous attempts at red cell regeneration, as in the so-called hemolytic uremia syndrome, usually seen in children (7, 75, 106, 119), in which the findings indicative of overt hemolytic anemia (pigment alterations, reticulocytosis, nucleated red cells, and "small irregularly contracted red cells") are accompanied by thrombocytopenia.

Almost invariably some degree of anemia develops in chronic renal failure regardless of its etiology and may be the main factor producing symptoms that first cause the patient to seek medical help (9). In general the anemia of chronic renal disease is normocytic and normochromic, but in the more chronically and severely anemic individuals, mild macrocytosis may be seen. Usually only moderate variation in the size and shape of the red cells is seen, but when the impairment of renal function results in an elevation of the blood urea nitrogen to the level of 150 mg or over, bizarre, irregularly contracted red cells (3, 130) are almost invariably seen in the blood film (spiny cells, burr cells, triangle cells, tricorn-hat cells, etc.). These cells are not pathognomonic of renal disease and may also be found in malignancy, gastrointestinal hemorrhage, thrombotic thrombocytopenic purpura, etc. (185). The severity of the anemia is in general correlated with the degree of elevation of nitrogen retention: the higher the blood urea nitrogen or nonprotein nitrogen levels, the. lower the hemoglobin level (177). However, this is a statistical correlation; many individual exceptions are seen, and no causal relation is implied. It is now clear that anemia may develop on the basis of renal disease before significant retention of nitrogenous substances is detectable.

Erythrokinetics

Studies evaluating the erythrocyte life span uniformly show an increased rate of red cell destruction of the type due to extracorpuscular abnormality (35, 52, 58, 111, 113, 132, 168). The degree of shortening of the red cell survival time is usually mild but may on occasion be marked (58). The red cells show a decreased glutathione content and glutathione stability but the G-6-PD activity is elevated because the cell population is younger than normal (203). Reticulocytes may on occasion be slightly increased in numbers in the peripheral blood, but a lower-than-normal value is the usual finding. The bone marrow picture is variable (32); there may be marked normoblastic hyperplasia, but more frequently there is depressed red cell activity with poor hemoglobin formation in the normoblasts. Marked erythroblastopenia may occur in severe azotemia

and early in acute renal failure (172). The serum iron level follows no consistent pattern, but the iron-binding protein is usually lower than normal (132). Fluid retention, with plasma volume changes, have made exact erythrokinetic studies difficult, but there is general agreement that erythropoiesis is impaired so that adequate compensation for decreased red cell survival is not possible. Iron incorporation into erythrocytes is uniformly decreased (111, 113, 132, 168), and increased storage of the iron takes place in the liver and spleen. Accumulating evidence indicates that the kidneys are a major source of erythropoietin, so chronic renal damage could be expected to interfere with production of this factor (154). Assays to determine the level of erythropoietin in the plasma in acute and chronic renal disease (or following bilateral nephrectomy in animals) indicate markedly decreased content, but the assay procedure is difficult because of the inhibitory nature of the serum demonstrated by in vivo and in vitro techniques. It seems likely that decreased production of erythropoietin plays a significant role in the lack of bone marrow response. However, to be certain that this is the only factor, the anemia must be shown to respond to the administration of erythropoietin when a potent human preparation becomes available.

THE ANEMIA ASSOCIATED WITH MALIGNANCY

Clinical Manifestations and Laboratory Findings

The anemia associated with malignancy has been characterized by both morphologic and erythrokinetic studies; when uncomplicated it most nearly resembles the anemia due to infection. Both are usually slight or moderate in degree; both are normochromic and normocytic (rarely, slightly hypochromic and microcytic); both show evidence of decreased red cell production and moderately increased hemoglobin breakdown (53, 96, 97, 146, 178); and both are refractory to the usual hematopoietic agents. It is clear that the inability of the marrow to produce erythrocytes and deliver them to the peripheral blood is the major defect. However, superimposed complications that modify the basic picture are encountered more frequently and are more varied in malignancy; these are blood loss with or without iron depletion, overt hemolysis, vitamin B_{12} or folic acid abnormality, and, most frequently, changes induced by neoplastic invasion of the bone marrow—myelophthisic or myelopathic changes (129, 165).

When the first three complications occur, the peripheral blood takes on the expected characteristics; when the fourth complication (myelophthisis) occurs, the peripheral blood is distinguished by the presence of increased numbers of polychromatophilic cells (reticulocytes), nucleated red cells, a shift toward immaturity of leukocytes, and more-than-normal variation in size and shape of adult erythrocytes, which become slightly macrocytic. The anemia has been explained on the basis of a mechanical "crowding out" of the cells concerned with red cell production. Indeed, histologic examination of the marrow in leukemia and extensive carcinomatosis may well raise the question how any red cells are produced. But the mechanical explanation cannot obtain in the vast majority of circumstances since the severity of the anemia does not correlate with demonstrable bone marrow involvement. Moreover, one study of patients with bone marrow metastases found that approximately 50 per cent were anemic and 50 per cent were not anemic (194).

Erythrokinetics

When erythrocyte survival studies are done, evidence is usually found indicating a definite, though mild, hemolytic process of the type resulting from extracorpuscular defect. Although the marrow can increase its production rate somewhat, it cannot achieve the rate of production expected of a normal marrow under similar stimulation, so relative bone marrow failure exists. The mechanism effecting the increased red cell destruction is obscure, although not infrequently in lymphatic leukemia, Hodgkin's disease, lymphosarcoma, etc., an autoimmune process is presumed in association with abnormal factors demonstrable by a positive reaction to the Coombs test or other manipulations. This hemolytic component may be of rather mild degree or may dominate the clinical picture.

In unusual instances widespread bone marrow neoplasia may in unknown fashion (possibly parasitic) preferentially take up folic acid or vitamin B_{12} and leave the red cell series relatively deficient. Some benefit in the form of reticulocytosis and modest increases in hemoglobin may follow the administration of folic acid or vitamin B_{12}.

Cobalt and Androgen Therapy

In considering the anemias associated with renal disease, chronic infection and inflammation, and malignancy, it should be pointed out that the administration of cobalt in large doses may be followed by reticulocytosis and an increase in hemoglobin levels (71). The more nearly normal hemoglobin levels frequently do not seem to be of significant clinical benefit to the patient or to alter the course of the underlying disease, but on occasion the significant benefit of a reduced transfusion requirement may be achieved. Androgenic steroids in pharmacologic doses (72) have been tried on a limited basis in some of these situations and may also improve the hemoglobin values. Clinically beneficial results have fairly regularly been observed in multiple myeloma.

The mechanisms of action of both cobalt and androgens are unknown.

THE ANEMIA ASSOCIATED WITH ENDOCRINE ABNORMALITIES

In connection with endocrine disorders, a severe degree of anemia is most likely to be seen in association with hypothyroidism; moderate or slight anemia may sometimes be associated with pituitary deficiency or Addison's disease (47, 80, 195, 201).

Thyroid Abnormality

The anemia associated with myxedema is characteristically normocytic and normochromic, and a normoblastic type of maturation is found in the hypocellular marrow (11). The blood volume and red cell mass are decreased (153). An unusually high proportion of patients with myxedema have severe anemia that is either macrocytic or hypochromic and microcytic and results from superimposed deficiency of vitamin B_{12} (206a) or iron. About 50 per cent of patients with myxedema have been demonstrated to have gastric anacidity, and, more recently, impaired absorption of vitamin B_{12} usually corrected by intrinsic factor (206). The finding of a megaloblastic type of maturation in the bone marrow indicates vitamin B_{12} deficiency, and a hematopoietic response can be expected to follow vitamin B_{12} therapy. The incidence of true pernicious anemia is disproportionately high in myxedema. The finding of a hypochromic, microcytic anemia is due to iron lack secondary to the menorrhagia or metrorrhagia that may accompany hypothyroidism. In view of the decreased absorption of food iron and vitamin B_{12} (125) demonstrated in myxedema, the occurrence of complicating deficiencies may not be as coincidental as formerly presumed.

When uncomplicated, the anemia of hypothyroidism is undoubtedly due to lack of production. There is no evidence for an increased rate of erythrocyte destruction; indeed, in this situation the red cell survival time has been shown to be longer than normal (137). It has long been considered that this anemia represents an adjustment to the decreased metabolic demands of the body. With decreased oxygen consumption, but constant blood flow, relative hyperoxia occurs, and red cell production is appropriately lowered (23). Disappearance of hematologic symptoms follows the administration of thyroid extract, but it is well established that the response is slow: a low, late reticulocytosis occurs followed by a slow rise in hemoglobin level and hematocrit. After the abnormal oxygen utilization has been corrected, frequently many months pass before normal hemoglobin levels are re-established. This should not be interpreted to mean that in hypothyroidism red cell and hemoglobin production is slow but rather that the final hemoglobin level attained is consistent with oxygen supply and demand. Evidence for this is found in the observation that when iron (or vitamin B_{12}) depletion is superimposed on the anemia of hypothyroidism, administration of iron (or vitamin B_{12}) is followed by an adequate hematologic response and an increase in the hemoglobin up to the limit set by the hypothyroidism. In addition, an individual with the anemia of hypothyroidism subjected to acute hemorrhage (123) shows an adequate bone marrow response by reticulocytosis and hemoglobin production.

When a patient with hypothyroidism was made hypermetabolic by the administration of dinitrophenol, the oxygen requirement of the patient was increased without change in the I^{131} uptake by the thyroid gland or elevation of the peripheral blood thyroxin level (215). Along with the increase in oxygen requirement, the red cell mass also rose significantly (153). The degree of thyroid hormone deficiency does not, therefore, impair red cell and hemoglobin production, but rather adjusts and sets the limit within which erythropoiesis takes place through re-establishment of a new level of oxygen requirement.

Pituitary Abnormality

Following destruction of the anterior lobe of the pituitary, or with its hypofunction, a normocytic, normochromic anemia frequently develops that is usually moderate, rarely severe. The signs of blood regeneration are minimal and the bone marrow is hypocellular. No hemolytic component has been demonstrated, and since the anemia responds to the administration of thyroid, testosterone, and corticosteroids, it appears to represent an adjustment to the decreased metabolic demands resulting from deficiency of the secretion of target glands regulated by the pituitary rather than a specific pituitary defect.

Adrenal Abnormality

In Addison's disease the normocytic, normochromic anemia appears mild as judged by the circulating hemoglobin level because of the significant decrease in plasma volume and hemoconcentration that are characteristic of the disease. As would be predicted from other known functions of adrenal steroids, there is also leukopenia, increase in eosinophils, and relative lymphocytosis. All are slowly corrected with adequate replacement therapy.

THE SIDEROACHRESTIC ANEMIAS

Clinical Manifestations and Laboratory Findings

This anemia is refractory to all therapeutic efforts so far tested and is chiefly characterized by abnormally large amounts of nonhemoglobin iron in the erythrocyte precursors. Since diverse clinical manifestations and morphologic changes have been described, it is likely that several disorders of different etiologies are represented (20, 31, 44, 46, 70, 77, 90, 133). Although a few cases have been reported in which the anemia is present early in life, it is usually of sporadic occurrence, showing up in the third or fourth decade. It is apparently transmitted through the female and may affect multiple male members of a family. The number of affected males reported greatly exceeds the number of females. The anemia is usually severe; the erythrocytes are definitely hypochromic and mildly microcytic; and evidence of blood regeneration is minimal. No abnormal hemoglobins have been described for these patients; the levels of hemoglobins A_2 and F are not abnormal. The disorder does not appear to be part of the thalassemia spectrum. The serum iron level is high, with almost complete saturation of the iron-binding protein. Marked hemosiderosis is present in many tissues; in some instances the amount of iron present apparently far outweighs that derived from transfusions. Consequently iron absorption must be greatly increased for prolonged periods of time despite tissue overload and markedly depressed erythropoietic activity. The bone marrow is most frequently cellular, with normoblastic maturation (some maturation abnormalities are occasionally detected). The amount of marrow hemosiderin is tremendously increased, and the developing erythrocytes contain large numbers of iron granules (sideroblasts) in the cytoplasm forming a ring surrounding the nucleus (26). The younger (non-nucleated) erythrocytes in the peripheral blood may also contain iron granules (siderocytes), but adult cells do not unless the spleen has been removed. The ferrokinetic studies are difficult to interpret because of the excess iron stores and uptake by erythrocyte precursors of iron not incorporated into hemoglobin. By and large the studies have shown a normal or rapid rate of clearance of radioiron from the peripheral blood, build-up in the bone marrow, then a rapid shift to the liver. Since a large but unknown quantity is nonhemoglobin iron, the rate of reappearance of the iron is largely uninterpretable at present, even though the siderotic granules do not persist in the cells but are apparently removed by the so-called "pitting" function of the spleen (42). The few studies reported show minimal, if any, shortening of the erythrocyte life span, and studies of pigment excretion are not remarkable. No response is elicited by the administration of the usual hematopoietic agents. The basic abnormality of the disease is unknown, but some speculation is possible on the following considerations. About eighty patients have now been shown to have a similar type of anemia and similar abnormalities of iron metabolism that respond partly or adequately to the administration of pyridoxine. Although usually of sporadic occurrence in adult males (84, 92), familial occurrences are known affecting both male (19) and female (39) and during childhood. Vitamin B6 is known to be essential for heme biosynthesis and also affects iron metabolism and absorption. In the sideroachrestic anemias absorption of iron into the body through the mucosal cells is excessive, and absorption of iron into the developing red cell is also excessive. Moreover, once in the cell the iron is not properly incorporated into hemoglobin but rather aggregates within the cytoplasm. The biochemical defects in the sideroachrestic anemias therefore apparently lie in the biosynthesis of heme and in the largely unknown areas whereby the cell processes absorbed iron for incorporation into hemoglobin.

HEMATOLOGIC EFFECTS OF IONIZING RADIATION AND PRODUCTION OF TEMPORARY OR PROLONGED BONE MARROW FAILURE

When calculated in terms of the absorbed dose (rad), the biologic effect of ionizing radiation is the same regardless of whether it is derived from an alpha-, beta-, or gamma-ray emitting source. Within the sublethal range of total-body irradiation, direct damage of the adult circulating blood cells is not important. Studies now indicate that the critical injury resulting from ionizing radiation is that inflicted upon the factors that control both DNA biosynthesis and the onset of mitosis. It is believed that these effects are most likely due to the induced formation of peroxides within the cell that inhibit biosynthesis of DNA by the nucleus and consequently prevent replication and mitosis. The effects of ionizing radiation depend upon many factors: radiosensitivity of the cells, regenerative capacity of the tissue, and the life span of the cell in question. Rapidly multiplying cells are a most sensitive indicator of radiation damage. Based on experiments on animals and observations on humans, the tissues most readily reflecting change induced by radiation are, in order: (a) germinal epithelium (spermatogenesis), (b) hematopoietic tissue, (c) epithelium of the intestinal crypts of the small intestine, (d) epithelium of the stomach and colon, and (e) basal layers of the skin. It now appears well established that within the hematopoietic tissue the order of sensitivity of the various cells is as follows: (a) lymphocyte series (very readily affected), (b) erythrocyte series (equally or almost equally sensitive), (c) granulocyte series, (d) monocyte series, and (e) megakaryocyte series.

The reticulum cells and plasma cell series appear to be very radioresistant. Because of limitations of knowledge about the life span and pool size of the leukocytes and because of the changes in capillary permeability, with consequent relocation of cells and fluid, that occur at some dose levels, the sequence of events cannot be predicted with great accuracy, but the following general trends can be charted for total-body irradiation by 200 to 400 r (22, 101, 147, 212). The lymphocyte series is exquisitely sensitive, and the lymphocyte count begins to decrease immediately after exposure. Various morphologic changes (fissured nuclei, cytoplasmic refractile granules) may be observed soon after exposure. Significant lymphopenia is detectable by 24 hours and may persist for many weeks. The lymphocyte response is so uniform that it may be used as a rough index of absorbed dose. However, the depression is maximal at about 200 to 250 r, and greater doses do not further depress the count.

An early (1 to 3 days after exposure) rise in the granulocyte count is thought to be due to stress phenomena and radiation sickness and is followed by a depression of the granulocyte count on the fourth or fifth day. This depression is followed by a transient rise at about the tenth to fifteenth day followed by a more severe depression, with the lowest counts reached about 4 to 6 weeks after exposure. Beginning at about the sixth week the granulocyte count rises toward the normal range.

After a probable (but poorly documented) rise, the platelets fall progressively, reaching their lowest values around the tenth to fourteenth day. Hemorrhagic phenomena are probably due to thrombocytopenia and endothelial damage in capillaries; lacking hepatic injury, there is no good evidence for the development of deficiencies of other factors involved in coagulation. Recovery from the platelet depression begins around the twenty-fifth to the thirty-fifth day.

Because of the prolonged life span of the adult erythrocyte, changes in the circulating hemoglobin level are slow to take place, and recovery may occur before the normal rate of red cell destruction (less than 1 per cent per day) produces a reliably detectable drop in the peripheral blood level. Nevertheless, the extreme sensitivity of the erythrocyte series can be detected by significant decreases in the rate of clearance of radioiron from the plasma when this agent is employed to indicate changes in erythropoiesis following irradiation (127). Changes in rate of reappearance of radioiron in the red cells have been shown to occur but apparently are not as reproducible. The reticulocyte level is somewhat depressed in the first few days. Anemia, if it develops, reaches its maximum severity at about the twentieth to thirtieth day, when the platelets and granulocytes are increasing toward normal values. At about 6 or 7 weeks a spontaneous, brisk reticulocytosis may indicate the recovery phase.

Again it must be stressed that the sequence of events is not as orderly as that presented above and that "the greater the dose, the more profound is the blood damage, the more rapidly it develops, and the more slowly it is repaired" (147). The lymphocyte count returns toward a normal value first, followed by the granulocyte, platelet, and red cell counts.

In the bone marrow, changes in the erythrocyte precursors have been documented shortly after exposure: there are pyknosis and decrease in the mitotic index (64). The precursor cells in the marrow mature and are then delivered to the peripheral blood so that the number of developing erythrocytes diminishes rapidly. The granulocyte precursors diminish next in order; the last cells to decrease are the megakaryocyte precursors, which reach maximal depression at the sixth to seventh day. The rate at which the cells decrease in the marrow does not appear to depend upon the dose administered, but the duration of depression is prolonged with increasing doses.

The induced damage may be irreversible (presumably due to stem cell depletion) or prolonged periods of time may be required before recovery takes place, and the picture of aplastic anemia may be found. The anemia described for those patients with radium poisoning (largely resulting from the painting of luminous instrument dials) was severe and associated with leukopenia but no great degree of thrombocytopenia. It appeared only many years after the absorption of the radium, which (handled by the body similarly to calcium) located in the skele-

ton, where it could produce a cumulative effect upon the bone marrow. Although aplastic anemia has been described in the survivors of Nagasaki (120) and in patients treated by x-ray to the spine for ankylosing spondylitis (40), the incidence is very low (less than the incidence of induced leukemia) and, strictly speaking, not demonstrated to be causally related to the radiation.

Bibliographic references for Chapter 11 begin on page 451.

REFERENCES

GENERAL REFERENCES

1. Allen, F. H., Jr., and Diamond, L. K.: Erythroblastosis Fetalis: Including Exchange Transfusion Technic, Little, Brown, Boston, 1958.
2. Cartwright, G. E.: Diagnostic Laboratory Hematology, Grune & Stratton, New York, 1958.
3. Castle, W. B.: Disorders of the blood, *in* Sodeman, W. A. (ed.), Pathologic Physiology: Mechanisms of Disease, ed. 3, ch. 28, Saunders, Philadelphia, 1961.
4. Dacie, J. F.: The Haemolytic Anaemias, Congenital and Acquired, Grune & Stratton, New York, 1954.
5. Dacie, J. F.: The Haemolytic Anaemias, Congenital and Acquired: Part I. The Congenital Anaemias, ed. 2, Grune & Stratton, New York, 1960.
6. Dacie, J. F.: The Haemolytic Anaemias, Congenital and Acquired: Part II. The Auto-immune Haemolytic Anaemias, ed. 2, Grune & Stratton, New York, 1962.
7. Daland, G. A.: Color Atlas of Morphology, with a Guide to Clinical Interpretation, Harvard University Press, Cambridge, Mass., 1959.
8. DeGruchy, G. C.: Clinical Haematology in Medical Practice, Blackwell, Oxford, 1958.
8a. Goldberg, A., and Rimington, C.: Diseases of Porphyrin Metabolism, Charles C. Thomas, Springfield, Ill., 1962.
9. Hayhoe, F. G. J. (ed.): Lectures on Haematology, Cambridge University Press, London, 1960.
10. Herbert, V.: The Megaloblastic Anemias: Modern Medical Monographs, Grune & Stratton, New York, 1959.
11. Ingram, V. M.: Haemoglobin and Its Abnormalities, Charles C. Thomas, Springfield, Ill., 1960.
12. Jonxis, J. H. P., and Delafresnaye, J. F. (ed.): Abnormal Haemoglobins: A Symposium, Blackwell, Oxford, 1959.
13. Lajtha, L. G.: Use of Isotopes in Haematology, Blackwell, Oxford, 1961.
14. Leavell, B. S., and Thorup, O. A.: Fundamentals of Clinical Hematology, Saunders, Philadelphia, 1960.
15. MacFarlane, R. G., and Robb-Smith, A. H. T. (ed.): Functions of the Blood, Academic Press, New York, 1961.
16. Miale, J. B.: Laboratory Medicine: Hematology, ed. 2, Mosby, St. Louis, 1962.
17. Mollison, P. L.: Blood Transfusion in Clinical Medicine, Charles C. Thomas, Springfield, Ill., 1961.
18. Page, L. B., and Culver, P. J. (ed.): Syllabus of Laboratory Examinations in Clinical Diagnosis, Harvard University Press, Cambridge, Mass., 1960.
19. Prankerd, T. A. J.: The Red Cell: An Account of Its Chemical Physiology and Pathology, Blackwell, Oxford, 1961.
20. Schwartz, S. O., Hartz, W. H., and Robbins, J. H.: Hematology in Practice, McGraw-Hill, New York, 1961.
21. Smith, C. H.: Blood Diseases of Infancy and Childhood, Mosby, St. Louis, 1960.

22. Thompson, R. B.: Haematology, Lippincott, Philadelphia, 1961.
23. Wallerstein, R. O., and Mettier, S. R. (ed.): Iron in Clinical Medicine, University of California Press, Berkeley, 1958.
24. Whitby, L. E. H., and Britton, C. J. C.: Disorders of the Blood: Diagnosis, Pathology, Treatment, Technique, Grune & Stratton, New York, 1953.
25. Wintrobe, M. M.: Clinical Hematology, ed. 5, Lea & Febiger, Philadelphia, 1961.

CHAPTER ONE

HEME BIOSYNTHESIS, THE PORPHYRIAS AND PORPHYRINURIA

1. Ackner, B. G., Cooper, J. E., Gray, C. H., Kelly, M., and Nicholson, D. C.: Excretion of porphobilinogen and delta-aminolevulinic acid in acute porphyria, Lancet 1:1256, 1961.
2. Akson, A., von Ehrenstein, G., and Theorell, H.: Life span of myoglobin, Arch. Biochem. 91:310, 1960.
3. Aldrich, R. A., Hawkinson, V., Grinstein, M., and Watson, C. J.: Photosensitive or congenital porphyria with hemolytic anemia: I. Clinical and fundamental studies before and after splenectomy, Blood 6:685, 1951.
4. Aldrich, R. A., Labbe, R. F., and Talman, E. L.: Review of porphyrin metabolism with special reference to childhood, Am. J. M. Sc. 230:675, 1955.
5. Anderson, J. A.: Lead poisoning, in Nelson, W. E. (ed.), Textbook of Pediatrics, ed. 6, p. 630, Saunders, Philadelphia, 1954.
6. Ashe, W. F.: Industrial lead poisoning as clinical syndrome, J. Indust. Hyg. & Toxicol. 25:55, 1943.
7. Aub, J. C., Fairhill, L. T., Minot, A. S., and Reznikoff I.: Lead poisoning, Medicine 4:1, 1925.
8. Baetjer, A. M.: Effects of season and temperature on childhood plumbism, Indust. Med. 28:137, 1959.
9. Bariety, M., Gajdos, A., Gajdos-Török, M., Thibault, P., and Leymarios, J.: Essai thérapeutique de la porphyrie idiopathique par l'acide adenosine monophosphorique, Presse méd. 68:825, 1960.
10. Barnes, H. D.: Excretion of porphyrins and porphyrin precursors by Bantu cases of porphyria, South African M. J. 33:274, 1959.
11. Bashour, F. A.: Lead intoxication, increased porphobilinogen, urinary uroporphyrin, porphobilinogen and coproporphyrin excretion in lead-exposed workers, J. Lab. & Clin. Med. 44:764, 1954.
12. Bashour, F. A.: Lead poisoning with special reference to porphyrin metabolism, Bull. Minn. Hosp. & Med. Found. 26:423, 1955.
13. Beck, E., Lanini, G., and Berand, T.: Iron metabolism in lead poisoning, Helvet. med. acta 22:442, 1955.
14. Berger, H., and Goldberg, A.: Hereditary coproporphyria, Brit. M. J. 2:85, 1955.
15. Bessis, M., and Breton-Gorius, J.: Etude au microscope électronique du sang et des organes hématopoïétiques dans le saturnisme expérimental (cycle du fer figure), Semaine hôp. Paris, path. et biol. 33:411, 1957.
16. Blackman, S. S., Jr.: Intranuclear inclusion bodies in the kidney and liver caused by lead poisoning, Bull. Johns Hopkins Hosp. 58:384, 1936.
17. Blanchard, T. P.: Isolation from mammalian brain of coproporphyrin III and a uro-type porphyrin, Proc. Soc. Exper. Biol. & Med. 82:512, 1953.
18. Bogorad, L.: Enzymatic synthesis of porphyrins from porphobilinogen: I. Uroporphyrin I, J. Biol. Chem. 233:501, 1958.
19. Bogorad, L.: Enzymatic synthesis of porphyrins from porphobilinogen: II. Uroporphyrin III, J. Biol. Chem. 233:510, 1958.

20. Bogorad, L.: Enzymatic synthesis of porphyrins from porphobilinogen: III. Uroporphyrinogens as intermediates, J. Biol. Chem. 233:516, 1958.

21. Boyd, P. R., Walker, G., and Henderson, I. N.: Treatment of tetraethyl lead poisoning, Lancet 1:181, 1957.

22. Boyett, J. D., Pittman, J. A., Jr., and Butterworth, C. E., Jr.: Effects of chronic lead intoxication upon iron metabolism, Clin. Res. 8:52, 1960.

22a. Boyett, J. D., and Butterworth, C. E., Jr.: Lead poisoning and hemoglobin synthesis, Am. J. Med. 32:884, 1962.

23. Brown, E. G.: Evidence for involvement of ferrous iron in biosynthesis of δ-aminolevulinic acid by chicken erythrocyte preparations, Nature 182:313, 1958.

24. Brown, E. G.: Relationship of the tricarboxylic acid cycle to the synthesis of δ-aminolevulinic acid in avian erythrocyte preparations, Biochem. J. 70:313, 1958.

25. Brugsch, H. G.: Fatal nephropathy during edathamil therapy in lead poisoning, Arch. Indust. Hyg. 20:285, 1959.

26. Byers, R. K., and Lord, E. E.: Late effects of lead poisoning on mental development, Am. J. Dis. Child. 66:471, 1943.

27. Byers, R. K.: Lead poisoning, Pediatrics 23:585, 1959.

28. Canivet, J., and Pelhard-Considère, M.: Etude de l'hémolyse dans deux cas de porphyrie congénitale, Rev. franç. étude clin. biol. 3:27, 1958.

29. Cantorow, A., and Trumper, M.: Lead Poisoning, Williams & Wilkins, Baltimore, 1944.

30. Chisolm, J. J., and Harrison, H. E.: Treatment of acute lead encephalopathy in children, Pediatrics 19:1, 1957.

31. Clark, P., and Walsh, R. J.: Haem synthesis in vitro: Studies with mammalian and avian erythrocytes, Australian J. Exper. Biol. & M. Sc. 38:135, 1960.

32. Cookson, G. H., and Rimington, C.: Porphobilinogen, Nature 171:875, 1953.

33. Cremer, J. E.: Biochemical studies on the toxicity of tetraethyl lead and other organo-lead compounds, Brit. J. Indust. Med. 16:191, 1959.

34. Cummings, J. M.: Heavy Metals and the Brain, Charles C. Thomas, Springfield, Ill., 1959.

35. Dean, G., and Barnes, H. D.: Inheritance of porphyria, Brit. M. J. 2:89, 1955.

36. Dean, G.: Pursuit of a disease, Scient. American 196:133, 1957.

37. Dean, G., and Barnes, H. D.: Porphyria in Sweden and South Africa, South African M. J. 33:246, 1959.

38. Denny-Brown, D. D., and Sciarra, D.: Changes in the nervous system in acute porphyria, Brain 68:1, 1945.

39. Drabkin, D. L.: Metabolism of hemin chromoproteins, Physiol. Rev. 31:374, 1951.

40. Dresel, E. I. B., and Falk, J. E.: Studies on the biosynthesis of blood pigments: I. Biochem. J. 56:156, 1954; II. Biochem. J. 63:72, 1956; III. Biochem. J. 63:80, 1956; IV. Biochem. J. 63:87, 1956; V. Biochem. J. 63:388, 1956.

41. Eales, L.: The porphyrins and the porphyrias, Ann. Rev. Med. 12:251, 1961.

42. Eriksen, L.: Lead intoxication: I. The effect of lead on the in vitro biosynthesis of heme and free erythrocyte porphyrins, Scandinav. J. Clin. & Lab. Invest. 7:80, 1955.

43. Falk, J. E., Porra, R. J., Brown, A., Moss, F., and Larmine, H. E.: Effect of oxygen tensions on haem and porphyrin biosynthesis, Nature 184:1217, 1959.

44. Fischer, H., and Orth, H.: Die Chemie des Pyrrols, Pyrrolfarbstoffe: II. Erste Hälfte, Akademische Verlagsgesellschaft, Leipzig, 1937.

45. Fratianne, R. B., Griggs, R. C., and Harris, J. W.: Autosurvival of erythrocytes treated in vitro with lead chlorides, Clin. Res. 7:384, 1958.

46. Fullerton, J. M.: Value of haematology in diagnosis of chronic plumbism, Brit. M. J. 2:117, 1952.
47. Gajdos, A., and Gajdos-Torok, M.: Les systèmes enzymatiques de la biosynthèse de l'hème, Sang 30:445, 1959.
48. Gajdos, A., and Gajdos-Torok, M.: Porphyrie expérimentale observée chez le rat blanc à la suite de l'intoxication par l'hexachlorobenzene, Rev. franç. étude clin. biol. 6:549, 1961.
49. Gajdos, A., and Gajdos-Torok, M.: Therapeutic effect of adenosine-5-monophosphoric acid in porphyria, Lancet 2:175, 1961.
50. Gajdos, A., and Gajdos-Torok, M.: Action thérapeutique de l'acide adenosine-5-monophosphorique sur la porphyrie expérimentale de rat blanc due à l'intoxication par l'hexachlorobenzene, Rev. franç. étude clin. biol. 6:553, 1961.
51. Gajdos-Torok, M., Gajdos, A., and Benard, H.: Etude par le fer radioactife de l'enzyme catalysant la biosynthèse de l'hème, Sang 30:459, 1959.
52. Gajdos-Torok, M.: Localization of the inhibition of the synthesis of heme by lead, Compt. rend. Soc. biol. 154:508, 1960.
53. Gibb, J. W. G., and MacMahon, J. F.: Arrested mental development induced by lead-poisoning, Brit. M. J. 1:320, 1955.
54. Gibson, J. B., and Goldberg, A.: Neuropathology of acute porphyria, J. Path. & Bact. 71:495, 1956.
55. Gibson, K. D., Neuberger, A., and Scott, J. J.: Purification and properties of δ-aminolaevulinic acid dehydrase, Biochem. J. 61:618, 1955.
56. Gibson, K. D., Laver, W. G., and Neuberger, A.: Initial stages in the biosynthesis of porphyrins: II. The formation of δ-aminolaevulinic acid from glycine and succinyl–coenzyme A by particles from chicken erythrocytes, Biochem. J. 70:71, 1958.
57. Gibson, K. D., Laver, W. G., and Neuberger, A.: Properties of an enzyme system forming δ-ALA (δ-aminolevulinic acid), Fed. Proc. 17:228, 1958.
58. Gibson, K. D., Matthew, M., Neuberger, A., and Tait, G. H.: Biosynthesis of porphyrins and chlorophylls, Nature 192:204, 1961.
59. Goldberg, A., Paton, W. D. M., and Thompson, J. W.: Pharmacology of the porphyrin and porphobilinogen, Brit. J. Pharmacol. 9:91, 1954.
60. Goldberg, A.: Acute intermittent porphyria: A clinical and experimental study, Scottish M. J. 4:331, 1955.
61. Goldberg, A., Ashenbrucker, H., Cartwright, G. E., and Wintrobe, M. M.: Studies on the biosynthesis of heme in vitro by avian erythrocytes, Blood 11:821, 1956.
62. Goldberg, A.: Acute intermittent porphyria, Quart. J. Med. 18:183, 1959.
63. Granati, A., and Scavo, D.: Behavior of amino acids in urine in occupational lead poisoning, Folia med. 40:832, 1957.
64. Granick, S.: Enzymatic conversion of δ-aminolevulinic acid to porphobilinogen, Science 121:878, 1955.
65. Granick, S., and Vanden Schrieck, H. G.: Porphobilinogen and δ-aminolevulinic acid in acute porphyria, Proc. Soc. Exper. Biol. & Med. 88:270, 1955.
66. Granick, S.: Porphyrin biosynthesis in erythrocytes: I. Formation of δ-aminolevulinic acid in erythrocytes, J. Biol. Chem. 232:1101, 1958.
67. Granick, S., and Mauzerall, D.: Porphyrin biosynthesis in erythrocytes: II. Enzymes converting δ-aminolevulinic acid to coproporphyrinogen, J. Biol. Chem. 232:1119, 1958.
68. Granick, S., and Mauzerall, D.: Enzymes of porphyrin synthesis in red blood cells, Ann. New York Acad. Sc. 75:115, 1958.

69. Gray, C. H., and Neuberger, A.: Effect of splenectomy in a case of congenital porphyria, Lancet 1:851, 1956.

70. Gray, C. H.: Porphyrias, *in* Thompson, R. H. S., and King, F. S. (ed.), Biochemical Disorders of Human Disease, p. 658, Academic Press, New York, 1957.

71. Greengard, J., Rowley, W., Elam, H., and Perlstein, M.: Lead encephalopathy in children: Intravenous use of urea in its management, New England J. Med. 264:1027, 1961.

71a. Greengard, J., Voris, D. C., and Hayden, R.: Surgical therapy of lead encephalopathy, J.A.M.A. 180:92, 1962.

72. Griggs, R. C., and Harris, J. W.: Erythrocyte survival and heme synthesis in lead poisoning, Clin. Res. 6:188, 1958.

73. Grinstein, M., Aldrich, R. A., Hawkinson, V., Lowry, P., and Watson, C. J.: Photosensitive or congenital porphyria with hemolytic anemia: II. Isotopic studies of porphyrin and hemoglobin metabolism, Blood 6:699, 1951.

74. Grinstein, M., Bannerman, R. M., and Moore, C. V.: Utilization of protoporphyrin 9 in heme synthesis, Blood 14:476, 1959.

75. Haeger, B.: Increased content of δ-aminolevulinic acid-like substance in urine from workers in lead industry, Scandinav. J. Clin. & Lab. Invest. 9:211, 1957.

76. Haeger, B.: Studies on a δ-aminolevulinic acid-like substance in urine from lead workers, Scandinav. J. Clin. & Lab. Invest. 10:229, 1958.

77. Haeger, B.: Urinary δ-aminolaevulinic acid and porphobilinogen in different types of porphyria, Lancet 2:606, 1958.

78. Haeger-Aronsen, B.: Studies on urinary excretion of δ-aminolaevulinic acid and other haem precursors in lead workers and lead-intoxicated rabbits, Scandinav. J. Clin. & Lab. Invest. 12, Suppl. 47, 1960.

79. Harris, J. W., and Greenberg, M. S.: Erythrocyte fragilities in lead poisoning, Clin. Res. Proc. 2:55, 1954.

79a. Hellman, E. S., Tschudy, D. P., and Bartter, F. C.: Abnormal electrolyte and water metabolism in acute intermittent porphyria, Am. J. Med. 32:734, 1962.

80. Henderson, D. A.: Follow-up of cases of plumbism in children, Australasian Ann. Med. 3:219, 1954.

81. Hess, J. W.: Lead encephalopathy simulating subdural hematoma: A case report, New England J. Med. 274:382, 1961.

82. Holecek, V.: Excretion of urinary coproporphyrin in lead poisoning, Brit. J. Indust. Med. 14:198, 1957.

83. Holti, G., Rimington, C., Tate, B. C., and Thomas, G.: Investigation of "porphyria cutanea tarda," Quart. J. Med. 27:1, 1958.

84. Indust. Med. 28:94, 1959 (lead conference issue).

85. Iodice, A. A., Richert, D. A., and Schulman, M. P.: Copper content of δ-aminolevulinic acid dehydrase, Fed. Proc. 17:248, 1958.

86. Joyce, C. R. B., Moore, H. L., and Weatherall, M.: Effects of lead, mercury, and gold on the potassium turnover of rabbit blood cells, Brit. J. Pharmacol. 9:463, 1954.

87. Kark, R. M.: Clinical aspects of the major porphyrinopathies, Med. Clin. North America 39:11, 1955.

88. Kassenaar, A., Morell, H., and London, I. M.: Incorporation of glycine into globin and the synthesis of heme in vitro in duck erythrocytes, J. Biol. Chem. 229:423, 1957.

89. Kench, J. E., Gillam, A. E., and Lane, R. E.: Haemopoiesis in lead poisoning, Biochem. J. 36:384, 1942.

90. Kench, J. E., Langley, F. A., and Williamson, J. F.: Biochemical and pathological studies of congenital porphyria, Quart. J. Med. 22:285, 1953.
91. Kikuchi, G., Kumar, A., Talmage, P., and Shemin, D.: Enzymatic synthesis
of δ-aminolevulinic acid, J. Biol. Chem. 233:1214, 1958.
92. Kline, T. S.: Myocardial changes in lead poisoning, A.M.A. Am. J. Dis. Child.
99:48, 1960.
93. Krueger, R. C., Melnick, I., and Klein, J. R.: Formation of heme by broken-
cell preparations of duck erythrocytes, Arch. Biochem. 64:302, 1956.
94. Labbe, R. F., Talman, E. L., and Aldrich, R. A.: Porphyrin metabolism: II.
Uric acid excretion in experimental porphyria, Biochim. et biophys. acta
15:590, 1954.
95. Lamont, N. McE., Hathorn, M., and Joubert, S. M.: Porphyria in the African:
Study of 100 cases, Quart. J. Med. 30:373, 1961.
96. Landing, B., and Nakai, H.: Histochemical properties of renal lead-inclusions
and RNA demonstration in urinary sediment, Am. J. Clin. Path. 31:499, 1959.
97. Lascelles, J.: Synthesis of porphyrins by cell suspensions of tetrahymena
vorax: Effect of members of the vitamin B group, Biochem. J. 66:65, 1957.
98. Laver, W. G., Neuberger, A., and Udenfriend, S.: Initial stages in the biosynthesis of porphyrins, Biochem. J. 70:4, 1958.
99. Leckie, W. J. H., and Tompsett, S. L.: Diagnostic and therapeutic use of
edathamil calcium disodium (EDTA, versenate) in excessive inorganic lead
absorption, Quart. J. Med. 27:65, 1958.
100. Lochhead, A. C., and Goldberg, A.: Enzymatic formation of haem by human
and rat tissues, Biochem. J. 78:146, 1961.
101. Lockwood, W. H., and Rimington, C.: Purification of an enzyme converting
porphobilinogen to uroporphyrin, Biochem. J. 67:8P, 1957.
102. London, I. M., West, R., Shemin, D., and Rittenberg, D.: Porphyrin formation and hemoglobin metabolism in congenital porphyria, J. Biol. Chem.
184:365, 1950.
103. Lottsfeldt, F. I., Labbe, R. F., and Aldrich, R. A.: Effects of inosine on heme
synthesis in experimental porphyria, J.A.M.A. 178:928, 1961.
104. Lowry, P. I., Hawkinson, V., and Watson, C. J.: Isotopic study of type III
porphyrins and hemoglobin metabolism in an unusual case of "mixed" porphyria, Metabolism 1:149, 1952.
105. Ludwig, G. D.: Saturnine gout, A.M.A. Arch. Int. Med. 100:802, 1957.
106. Ludwig, G. D.: Hyponatremia in acute intermittent porphyria due to probable inappropriate secretion of antidiuretic hormone, Clin. Res. 9:340, 1961.
107. Ludwig, G. D., and Epstein, I. S.: A genetic study of two families having the
acute intermittent type of porphyria, Ann. Int. Med. 55:81, 1961.
108. MacGregor, A. G., Nichols, R. E. H., and Rimington, C.: Porphyria cutanea
tarda, A.M.A. Arch. Int. Med. 90:483, 1952.
109. Magnus, I. A., Porter, A. D., and Rimington, C.: Action spectrum for skin
lesions in porphyria cutanea tarda, Lancet 1:912, 1959.
110. Magnus, I. A., Jarrett, A., Prankerd, T. A. J., and Rimington, C.: Erythropoietic protoporphyria: A new porphyria syndrome with solar urticaria due to
protoporphyrinaemia, Lancet 2:448, 1961.
111. Malooly, D. A., and Hightower, N. C., Jr.: Quantitative determination of
porphobilinogen and delta-aminolevulinic acid in the urine, J. Lab. & Clin.
Med. 59:568, 1962.
112. Mann, T. S.: Lead intoxication in the surgical wards, Scottish M. J. 7:36,
1962.
113. Markowitz, M.: Acute intermittent porphyria: A report of five cases and a
review of the literature, Ann. Int. Med. 41:1170, 1954.

114. Marsden, H. B., and Wilson, V. K.: Lead-poisoning in children: Correlation of clinical and pathological findings, Brit. M. J. 1:324, 1955.
115. Marsh, J. B., and Drabkin, D. L.: Biosynthesis of cytochrome C in vivo and in vitro, J. Biol. Chem. 224:909, 1957.
116. Martin, W. J., and Heck, F. J.: The porphyrins and porphyria, Am. J. Med. 20:239, 1956.
117. Mauzerall, D., and Granick, S.: Occurrence and determination of δ-amino-levulinic acid and porphobilinogen in urine, J. Biol. Chem. 219:435, 1956.
118. McFadzean, A. J. S., and Davis, L. J.: On the nature and significance of stippling in lead poisoning, with reference to the effect of splenectomy, Quart. J. Med. 18:57, 1949.
119. Melby, J. C., Street, J. P., and Watson, C. J.: Chlorpromazine in the treatment of porphyria, J.A.M.A. 162:174, 1956.
120. Mellinkoff, S. M., Halpern, R. M., Frankland, M., and Greipel, M.: Abnormal urinary amino acid patterns in acute intermittent porphyria, J. Lab. & Clin. Med. 53:358, 1959.
121. Minakami, S., Yoneyame, Y., and Yoshikawa, H.: On the biosynthesis of heme and hemoproteins in liver cell, Biochim. et biophys. acta 18:447, 1958.
122. Muir, H. M., and Neuberger, A.: Biogenesis of porphyrins: I. The distribution of [15]M in the ring system, Biochem. J. 45:163, 1949.
123. Muir, H. M., and Neuberger, A.: Biogenesis of porphyrins: II. The origin of the methene carbon atoms, Biochem. J. 47:97, 1950.
124. Nemeth, A. M., Russell, C. S., and Shemin, D.: The succinate-glycine cycle: II. Metabolism of δ-aminolevulinic acid, J. Biol. Chem. 229:415, 1957.
125. Neuberger, A., Muir, H. M., and Gray, C. H.: Biosynthesis of porphyrins and congenital porphyria, Nature 165:948, 1950.
126. Neuberger, A.: Aspects of the metabolism of glycine and of porphyrins, Biochem. J. 78:1, 1961.
127. Neve, R. A., Labbe, R. F., and Aldrich, R. A.: Reduced uroporphyrin III in the biosynthesis of heme, J. Am. Chem. Soc. 78:691, 1956.
128. Nishida, G., and Labbe, R. F.: Heme biosynthesis in experimental hepatic porphyria, Clin. Res. 6:74, 1958.
129. Ockner, R. K., and Schmid, R.: Acquired porphyria in man and rat due to hexachlorobenzene intoxication, Nature 189:499, 1961.
130. Passow, H., and Tillman, K.: Untersuchungen über den Kaliumverlust bleivergifteter Menschenerythrocyten, Arch. ges. Physiol. 262:23, 1956.
131. Perkoff, G. T., Schwartz, H. C., and Tyler, F. H.: Incorporation of radioiron into myoglobin in an in vitro system, J. Clin. Invest. 38:1599, 1959.
132. Peters, H. A., Woods, S., Eichman, P. L., and Reese, H. H.: Treatment of acute porphyria with chelating agents: A report of twenty-one cases, Ann. Int. Med. 47:889, 1957.
133. Peters, H. A., Eichman, P. L., and Reese, H. H.: Therapy of acute, chronic and mixed hepatic porphyria patients with chelating agents, Neurology 8:621, 1958.
134. Pinto, S. S., Einert, C., Roberts, W. J., Winn, G. S., and Nelson, K. W.: Coproporphyrinuria, A.M.A. Arch. Indust. Hyg. 6:496, 1952.
135. Porphyria in Ireland (editorial), Lancet 2:636, 1960.
136. Porphyria in South Africa (editorial), Lancet 2:93, 1959.
137. Quastel, J. H., and Schalefield, P. G.: Biochemical aspects of cerebral dysfunction, Am. J. Med. 25:420, 1958.
138. Radin, N. S., Rittenberg, D., and Shemin, D.: Role of glycine in the biosynthesis of heme, J. Biol. Chem. 184:745, 1950.
139. Redeker, A. G., Sterling, R. E., and Archer, B.: Porphyria cutanea tarda, A.M.A. Arch. Int. Med. 104:779, 1959.

140. Richards, F. F., and Scott, J. J.: Glycine metabolism in acute porphyria, Clin. Sc. 20:387, 1961.

141. Richert, D. A., and Schulman, M. P.: Vitamin interrelationships in heme synthesis, Am. J. Clin. Nutrition 7:416, 1959.

142. Rimington, C.: Haems and porphyrins in health and disease, Acta med. scandinav. 143:161, 177, 1952.

143. Rimington, C., and Booij, J. L.: Porphyrin biosynthesis in human red cells, Biochem. J. 65:3P, 1957.

144. Rimington, C.: Some aspects of haemoglobin biosynthesis and their importance to medicine, Brit. M. J. 2:1017, 1958.

145. Rimington, C.: Biosynthesis of haemoglobin, Brit. M. Bull. 15:19, 1959.

146. Robinson, M. J., Karpinski, F. E., Jr., and Brieger, H.: Concentration of lead in plasma, whole blood and erythrocytes of infants and children, Pediatrics 21:793, 1958.

147. Roxburgh, R. C., and Haas, L.: Glycosuria as an early sign of lead poisoning, Arch. Dis. Childhood 34:70, 1959.

148. Rubino, G. F., Pagliardi, E., Prato, V., and Giangrandi, E.: Erythrocyte copper and porphyrins in lead poisoning, Brit. J. Haemat. 4:103, 1958.

149. Rubino, G. F., Prato, V., and Fiorina, L.: Anemia of lead poisoning: Its nature and pathogenesis, Folia med. 42:1, 1959.

149a. Runge, W., and Watson, C. J.: Experimental production of skin lesions in human cutaneous porphyria, Proc. Soc. Exper. Biol. & Med. 109:809, 1962.

150. Saint, E. G., Curnow, D., Paton, R., and Stokes, J. B.: Diagnosis of acute porphyria, Brit. M. J. 1:1182, 1954.

151. Saint, E. G., and Curnow, D.: Porphyria in western Australia, Lancet 1:133, 1962.

152. Salomon, K., and Cowgill, G. R.: Porphyrinuria in lead-poisoned dogs, J. Indust. Hyg. & Toxicol. 30:114, 1948.

153. Schiffmann, E., and Shemin, D.: Further studies on the utilization of δ-aminolevulinic acid for porphyrin synthesis, J. Biol. Chem. 225:623, 1957.

154. Schlenker, F. S., Davis, C. L., and Kitchell, C. L.: Plasma porphyrin, Am. J. Clin. Path. 36:31, 1961.

155. Schmid, R., Schwartz, S., and Watson, C. J.: Porphyrins in the bone marrow: Circulating erythrocytes in experimental anemias, Proc. Soc. Exper. Biol. & Med. 75:705, 1950.

156. Schmid, R., Hanson, B., and Schwartz, S.: Experimental porphyria: I. Isolation of uroporphyrin I from bone marrows of lead poisoned rabbits, Proc. Soc. Exper. Biol. & Med. 79:459, 1952.

157. Schmid, R., and Schwartz, S.: Experimental porphyria: III. Hepatic type produced by sedormid, Proc. Soc. Exper. Biol. & Med. 81:685, 1952.

158. Schmid, R., and Shemin, D.: Enzymatic formation of porphobilinogen from δ-aminolevulinic acid and the conversion to protoporphyrin, J. Am. Chem. Soc. 77:506, 1955.

159. Schmid, R., and Schwartz, S.: Studies of some liver heme proteins and porphyrins in experimental sedormid porphyria, *in* Wolstenholme, G. E. W., and Millar, E. C. P. (ed.), Porphyrin Biosynthesis and Metabolism: Ciba Foundation Symposium, Churchill, London, 1955.

160. Schmid, R., Schwartz, S., and Sundberg, H. D.: Erythropoietic (congenital) porphyria: A rare abnormality of normoblasts, Blood 10:416, 1955.

161. Schmid, R.: Cutaneous porphyria in Turkey, New England J. Med. 263:397, 1960.

162. Schmid, R.: The porphyrias, *in* Stanbury, J. B., Wyngaarden, J. B., and Fredrickson, D. S. (ed.), The Metabolic Basis of Inherited Disease, p. 939, McGraw-Hill, New York, 1960.

163. Schulman, M. P., and Richert, D. A.: Heme synthesis in vitamin B_6 and pantothenic acid deficiencies, J. Biol. Chem. 226:181, 1957.

164. Schwartz, G. A., and Moulton, J. A. L.: Porphyria: A clinical and neuropathological report, A.M.A. Arch. Int. Med. 94:221, 1954.

165. Schwartz, S., Keprios, M., and Schmid, R.: Experimental porphyria: II. Type produced by lead, phenylhydrazine and light, Proc. Soc. Exper. Biol. & Med. 79:463, 1952.

166. Schwartz, S.: Clinical aspects of porphyrin metabolism, Veterans Admin. Tech. Bull. TB 10–94, 6:1, 1953.

167. Scott, J. J.: Metabolism of δ-aminolaevulinic acid, *in* Wolstenholme, G. E. W., and Millar, E. C. P. (ed.), Porphyrin Biosynthesis and Metabolism: Ciba Foundation Symposium, Churchill, London, 1955.

168. Seven, M. J., and Johnson, L. A.: Metal-binding in Medicine, Lippincott, Philadelphia, 1960.

169. Shemin, D., and Rittenberg, D.: Utilization of glycine for synthesis of A-porphyrin, J. Biol. Chem. 159:567, 1945.

170. Shemin, D., and Rittenberg, D.: Biological utilization of glycine for the synthesis of protoporphyrin of hemoglobin, J. Biol. Chem. 166:621, 1946.

171. Shemin, D., and Kumin, S.: Mechanism of porphyrin formation: The formation of a succinyl intermediate from succinate, J. Biol. Chem. 198:827, 1952.

172. Shemin, D., and Russell, C. S.: δ-aminolevulinic acid: Its role in the biosynthesis of porphyrins and purines, J. Am. Chem. Soc. 75:4873, 1953.

173. Shemin, D., Abramsky, T., and Russell, C. S.: Synthesis of protoporphyrin from delta-aminolevulinic acid in a cell-free extract, J. Am. Chem. Soc. 76:1204, 1954.

174. Shemin, D.: The succinate-glycine cycle: The role of aminolevulinic acid in porphyrin synthesis, *in* Wolstenholme, G. E. W., and Millar, E. C. P. (ed.), Porphyrin Biosynthesis and Metabolism: Ciba Foundation Symposium, p. 4, Churchill, London, 1955.

175. Shemin, D., Russell, C. S., and Abramsky, T.: The succinate-glycine cycle: I. The mechanism of pyrrole synthesis, J. Biol. Chem. 215:613, 1955.

176. Shemin, D., and Kikuchi, C.: Enzymatic synthesis of δ-aminolevulinic acid, Ann. New York Acad. Sc. 75:122, 1958.

177. Shiels, D. V.: Elimination of lead in sweat, Australasian Ann. Med. 3:225, 1954.

178. Solomon, A. K.: Permeability of the human erythrocyte to sodium and potassium, J. Gen. Physiol. 36:57, 1952.

179. Stich, W.: Die kongenitale Porphyrie, eine erythropathische hämolytische Anämie (porphyrocytose), Schweiz. med. Wchnschr. 88:1012, 1958.

180. Sunderman, F. W., Jr., and Sunderman, F. W.: Practical considerations of diseases of porphyrin metabolism, Am. J. Clin. Path. 25:1231, 1955.

181. Sutherland, D. A., and Eisentraut, A. M.: Direct Coombs test in lead poisoning, Blood 11:1024, 1956.

182. Talman, E. L., Labbe, R. F., Aldrich, R. A., and Sears, D.: Porphyrin metabolism: V. The metabolism of purines in experimental porphyria, Arch. Biochem. 80:446, 1959.

183. Ten Eyck, F. W., and Martin, W. J.: Acute porphyria: Necropsy studies in nine cases, Proc. Staff Meet. Mayo Clin. 36:409, 1961.

184. Tio (Tiong Hoo), Leijnse, B., Jarrett, A., and Rimington, C.: Acquired porphyria from a liver tumour, Clin. Sc. 16:517, 1957.

185. Tishkoff, G. H., Granville, N. G., Rosen, B., and Dameshek, W.: Excretion of δ-aminolevulinic acid in lead intoxication, Acta haemat. 19:321, 1958.

186. Travers, E., Rendle-Short, J., and Harvey, C. C.: The Rotherham lead-poisoning outbreak, Lancet 2:113, 1956.
187. Varadi, S.: Haematological aspects in a case of erythropoietic porphyria, Brit. J. Haemat. 4:270, 1958.
188. Viglioglia, P. A., Viglioglia, J., Linares, R. O., and Vidiella, J.: Multilating porphyria, Prensa méd. argent. 45:3671, 1958.
189. Vincent, P. C., and Blackburn, C. R. B.: Effects of heavy metal ions on the human erythrocyte: I. Comparison of the action of several heavy metals, Australian J. Exper. Biol. & M. Sc. 36:471, 1958.
190. Vincent, P. C., and Blackburn, C. R. B.: Effects of heavy metal ions on the human erythrocyte: II. Effects of lead and mercury, Australian J. Exper. Biol. & M. Sc. 36:589, 1958.
191. Vincent, P. C.: Effects of heavy metal ions on the human erythrocyte: III. Inhibition of the effects of lead and mercury, Australian J. Exper. Biol. & M. Sc. 37:83, 1959.
192. Vogel, W., Richert, D. A., Pixley, B. Q., and Schulman, M. P.: Heme synthesis in iron-deficient duck blood, J. Biol. Chem. 235:1769, 1960.
193. Vogt, E. C.: Roentgenologic diagnosis of lead poisoning in infants and children, J.A.M.A. 98:125, 1932.
194. Waldenström, J.: The porphyrias as inborn errors of metabolism, Am. J. Med. 22:758, 1957.
195. Waldenström, J.: Recent observations in porphyria, Nord. med. 40:1443, 1959.
196. Waldman, R. K., and Bonnan, E. K.: Note on serum transaminase activity after lead absorption, A.M.A. Arch. Indust. H. 19:431, 1959.
197. Watson, C. J.: The erythrocyte coproporphyrin, Arch. Int. Med. 86:797, 1950.
198. Watson, C. J., Lowry, P. T., Schmid, R., Hawkinson, V. E., and Schwartz, S.: Manifestations of the different forms of porphyria in relation to chemical findings, Tr. A. Am. Physicians 64:345, 1951.
199. Watson, C. J.: Some studies on nature and clinical significance of porphobilinogen, A.M.A. Arch. Int. Med. 93:643, 1954.
200. Watson, C. J.: Porphyrin metabolism in the anemias, A.M.A. Arch. Int. Med. 99:323, 1957.
201. Watson, C. J.: Porphyrin metabolism, *in* Duncan, G. (ed.), Diseases of Metabolism, ed. 3, Saunders, Philadelphia, 1959.
202. Watson, C. J.: The problem of porphyrin: Some facts and questions, New England J. Med. 263:1205, 1960.
203. Watson, C. J., Berg, M. H., Hawkinson, V. E., and Bossermaier, I.: Studies on uroporphyrins: VI. Isomer composition of the "Waldenström porphyrins," effect of heat and the significance of porphyrinogen, Clin. Chem. 6:71, 1960.
204. Watson, C. J., Bossermaier, I., and Cardinal, R.: Acute intermittent porphyria, J.A.M.A. 175:1087, 1961.
205. Watson, R. J., Decker, E., and Lichtman, H. C.: Hematologic studies on children with lead poisoning, Pediatrics 21:40, 1958.
206. Weatherall, M.: Fate of intravenously administered coproporphyrin III in normal and lead-treated rabbits, Biochem. J. 52:683, 1952.
207. Whitaker, J. A., and Vietti, T. J.: Fluorescence of the erythrocytes in lead poisoning in children: An aid to rapid diagnosis, Pediatrics 24:734, 1959.
208. Widman, D. E., Newton, B. W., Sunshine, I., Griggs, R. C., and Harris, J. W.: Effect of lead ingestion on the daily urinary excretion of δ-aminolevulinic acid, porphobilinogen, coproporphyrin III and lead, Clin. Res. 6:393, 1958.
209. Wilson, V. K., Thomson, M. L., and Dent, C. E.: Amino-aciduria in lead poisoning, Lancet 2:66, 1953.

210. Wittenberg, J. B.: Formation of the porphyrin ring, Nature 184:876, 1959.
211. Wranne, L.: Free erythrocyte copro- and protoporphyrin, Acta paediat. 49:1, 1960.
212. Wriston, J. C., Lack, L., and Shemin, D.: Mechanism of porphyrin formation: Further evidence on the relationship of the citric acid cycle and porphyrin formation, J. Biol. Chem. 215:603, 1955.
213. Wyllie, J.: Urinary porphyrins in lead absorption, A.M.A. Arch. Indust. H. 12:396, 1955.

CHAPTER TWO
IRON METABOLISM AND IRON-LACK ANEMIA

1. Achlorhydria and anaemia (editorial), Lancet 2:27, 1960.
2. Allen, D. W., and Jandl, J.: Kinetics of intracellular iron in rabbit reticulocytes, Blood 15:71, 1960.
3. Alpen, E. L., and Cranmore, D.: Cellular kinetics and iron utilization in bone marrow as absorbed by Fe^{59} radioautography, Ann. New York Acad. Sc. 77:753, 1959.
4. Awai, M., and Brown, E. B.: Studies on the metabolism of human transferrin, J. Lab. & Clin. Med. 58:797, 1961.
5. Badenoch, J., and Callender, S. T.: Use of radioactive iron in the investigation of anaemia, Brit. J. Radiol. 27:381, 1954.
6. Badenoch, J., Evans, J. R., and Richards, W. C. D.: The stomach in hypochromic anaemia, Brit. J. Haemat. 3:175, 1957.
7. Bessis, M., and Breton-Gorius, J.: Iron particles in normal erythroblasts and normal and pathological erythrocytes, J. Biophys. & Biochem. Cytol. 3:503, 1957.
8. Bessis, M., and Breton-Gorius, J.: Studies of the iron-containing granules in normal and abnormal erythrocytes by means of the electron microscope, Rev. hémat. 12:43, 1957.
9. Bessis, M., Breton-Gorius, J., Dreyfus, J. C., and Schapira, G.: Appearance by electron microscopy of apoferritin more or less saturation with iron: Comparison between chemically prepared and cellular forms, Rev. franç. étude clin. biol. 3:981, 1958.
10. Bessis, M.: Erythropoiesis as seen with the electron microscope, in Stohlman, F., Jr. (ed.), Kinetics of Cellular Proliferation, p. 22, Grune & Stratton, New York, 1959.
11. Bessis, M. C., and Breton-Gorius, J.: Ferritin and ferruginous micelles in normal erythroblasts and hypochromic hypersideremic anemias, Blood 14:423, 1959.
12. Bessis, M.: Blood cells and their formation, in Brachet, J., and Mirsky, A. E. (ed.), The Cell, vol. V, part 2, p. 163, Academic Press, New York, 1961.
12a. Bessis, M. C., and Breton-Gorius, J.: Iron metabolism in the bone marrow as seen by electron microscopy: A review, Blood 19:635, 1962.
13. Beutler, E., Drennan, W., and Black, M.: Bone marrow and liver in iron deficiency anemia, J. Lab. & Clin. Med. 43:427, 1954.
14. Beutler, E.: Clinical evaluation of iron stores, New England J. Med. 256:692, 1957.
15. Beutler, E.: Iron content of haemoglobin in iron deficiency, Nature 181:837, 1958.
16. Beutler, E.: Red cell indices in the diagnosis of iron-deficiency anemia, Ann. Int. Med. 50:313, 1959.
17. Beutler, E., Larsh, S., and Tanzi, F.: Iron enzymes in iron deficiency: VII. Oxygen consumption measurements in iron-deficient subjects, Am. J. M. Sc. 239:759, 1960.

18. Beutler, E.: Iron metabolism, Ann. Rev. Med. 12:195, 1961.
19. Bohannon, R. A., Hutchison, J. L., and Townsend, S. R.: Use of radioiron in the study of anemia, Ann. Int. Med. 55:975, 1961.
20. Bonnet, J. D., Hagedorn, A. B., and Owen, C. A., Jr.: Quantitative method for measuring gastrointestinal absorption of iron, Blood 15:36, 1960.
21. Bonnet, J. D., Orun, A. L., Hagedorn, A. B., and Owen, C. A.: Rate of loss of radioiron from mouse and man, Am. J. Physiol. 198:784, 1960.
22. Bothwell, T. H., and Mallett, B.: Diurnal variation in the turnover of iron through the plasma, Clin. Sc. 14:235, 1955.
23. Bothwell, T. H., Mallett, B., Oliver, R., and Smith, M. D.: Inability to assess absorption of iron from plasma radio-iron curves, Brit. J. Haemat. 1:352, 1955.
24. Bothwell, T. H., Callender, S., Mallett, B., and Witts, L. T.: Study of erythropoiesis using tracer quantities of radioactive iron, Brit. J. Haemat. 2:1, 1956.
25. Bothwell, T. H., and Finch, C. A.: The intestine in iron metabolism, Am. J. Digest. Dis. 2:145, 1957.
26. Bothwell, T. H., Hurtado, A. V., Donohue, D. M., and Finch, C. A.: Erythrokinetics: IV. Plasma iron turnover as measure of erythropoiesis, Blood 12:409, 1957.
27. Bothwell, T. H., Pirzio-Biroli, G., and Finch, C. A.: Iron absorption: I. Factors influencing absorption, J. Lab. & Clin. Med. 51:24, 1958.
28. Bothwell, T. H., Pirzio-Biroli, G., and Finch, C. A.: Iron absorption: II. The absorption of radioiron administered with a standard meal in man, J. Lab. & Clin. Med. 51:37, 1958.
29. Brown, E. B., Dubach, R., and Moore, C. V.: Studies in iron transportation and metabolism: XI. Critical analysis of mucosal block by large doses of inorganic iron in human subjects, J. Lab. & Clin. Med. 52:335, 1958.
30. Brown, E. B., Jr., and Justor, B. W.: In vitro absorption of radioiron by everted pouches of rat intestine, Am. J. Physiol. 194:319, 1958.
31. Brummer, P.: Significance of achlorhydria for the etiology of iron-deficiency anemia, Acta. med. scandinav. 137:43, 1950.
32. Burko, H., Mellins, H. Z., and Watson, J.: Skull changes in iron deficiency anemia simulating congenital hemolytic anemia, Am. J. Roentgenol. 86:447, 1961.
33. Callender, S. T.: Iron absorption, Brit. M. Bull. 15:5, 1959.
34. Cappell, D. F.: Some aspects of iron metabolism, in University of London, British Postgraduate Medical Federation, Lectures on the Scientific Basis of Medicine, vol. 8, Athlone Press, London, 1960.
35. Cartwright, G. E., Huguley, C. M., Ashenbrucker, H., Fay, J., and Wintrobe, M. M.: Studies on free erythrocyte protoporphyrin, plasma iron, and plasma copper in normal and anemic subjects, Blood 3:501, 1948.
36. Castle, W. B.: Erythropoiesis: Normal and abnormal, Bull. New York Acad. Med. 30:827, 1954.
37. Chodos, R. B., Ross, J. F., Apt, L., Pollycove, M., and Halkett, T. A. E.: Absorption of radio iron labeled foods and iron salts in normal and iron-deficient subjects and in idiopathic hemochromatosis, J. Clin. Invest. 36:314, 1957.
38. Clark, P., and Walsh, R. J.: Synthesis of haem by circulating blood cells, Nature 184:1730, 1960.
39. Cohen, E., and Elvehjem, C. A.: Relation of iron and copper to the cytochrome oxidase content of animal tissues, J. Biol. Chem. 107:97, 1934.
40. Coleman, D. H., Stevens, A. R., Jr., and Finch, C. A.: Treatment of iron deficiency anemia, Blood 10:567, 1955.

41. Conrad, M. F., and Benjamin, N. R.: Hematologic changes induced by progressive iron depletion, *in* Proceedings, Seventh Congress of the International Society of Hematology, p. 191, Grune & Stratton, New York, 1958.
42. Crosby, W. H.: Evidence on the recycling of siderocyte iron, J. Clin. Invest. 38:997, 1959.
43. Davidson, W. M. B., and Markson, J. L.: Gastric mucosa in iron deficiency anaemia, Lancet 2:639, 1955.
44. Davis, A. E.: Relationship of disturbed pancreatic function to haemosiderosis, Lancet 2:749, 1961.
45. Demulder, R.: Iron metabolism, biochemistry, and clinical pathological physiology: Review of recent literature, A.M.A. Arch. Int. Med. 102:254, 1958.
46. Dowdle, E. B., Schachter, D., and Scherker, H.: Active transport of Fe^{59} by everted segments of rat duodenum, Am. J. Physiol. 198:609, 1960.
47. Drabkin, D. L.: Metabolism of the hemin chromoproteins, Physiol. Rev. 31:374, 1951.
48. Dubach, R., Moore, C. V., and Minnich, V.: Utilization of intravenously injected radioactive iron for hemoglobin synthesis, J. Lab. & Clin. Med. 31:1201, 1946.
49. Dubach, R., Callender, S. T. E., and Moore, C. V.: Studies in iron transportation and metabolism: VI. Absorption of radioactive iron in patients with fever and with anemias of varied etiology, Blood 3:526, 1948.
50. Dubach, R., Moore, C. V., and Callender, S. T. E.: Studies in iron transportation and metabolism: IX. The excretion of iron as measured by the isotope method, J. Lab. & Clin. Med. 55:599, 1955.
51. Endicott, K. M., Gillman, T., Brecker, G., Ness, A. T., Clark, F. A., and Adamik, E. R.: Study of histochemical iron using tracer methods, J. Lab. & Clin. Med. 34:414, 1949.
52. Faber, M., and Falbe-Hansen, I.: Nonhaem iron in erythrocytes as a precursor for haemoglobin, Nature 184:1043, 1959.
53. Farrant, J. L.: Electron microscopic study of ferritin, Biochim. et biophys. acta 13:569, 1954.
54. Fay, J., Cartwright, G. E., and Wintrobe, M. M.: Studies on free erythrocyte protoporphyrin, plasma iron, serum iron, serum iron binding capacity and plasma copper during normal pregnancy, J. Clin. Invest. 28:487, 1949.
55. Finch, C. A., Gibson, J. G., Peacock, W. C., and Fluharty, R. G.: Iron metabolism: Utilization of intravenous radioactive iron, Blood 4:905, 1949.
56. Finch, S. C., Haskins, D., and Finch, C. A.: Iron metabolism: Hematopoiesis following phlebotomy: Iron as a limiting factor, J. Clin. Invest. 29: 1078, 1950.
57. Finch, C. A.: Body iron exchange in man, J. Clin. Invest. 38:392, 1959.
58. Finch, C. A., and Noyes, W. D.: Erythrokinetics in diagnosis of anemia, J.A.M.A. 175:1163, 1961.
59. Finch, S. C., and Finch, C. A.: Idiopathic hemochromatosis, an iron storage disease: A. Iron metabolism in hemochromatosis, Medicine 34:381, 1955.
60. Freireich, E. J., Miller, A., Emerson, C. P., and Ross, J. F.: Effect of inflammation on utilization of erythrocyte and transferrin-bound radioiron for red cell production, Blood 12:972, 1957.
61. Garby, L., and Sjolin, S.: Absorption of labelled iron in infants less than three months old, Acta paediat. 48:24, 1959.
62. Giblett, E. R., Coleman, D. H., Pirzio-Biroli, G., Donohue, D. M., Motulsky, A., and Finch, C. A.: Erythrokinetics: Quantitative measurements of red cell production and destruction in normal subjects and patients with anemia, Blood 11:291, 1956.

63. Gibson, J. G., II, Weiss, S., Evans, R. D., Peacock, W. C., Irvine, J. W., Good, W. M., and Kip, A. F.: Measurement of the circulating red cell volume by means of two radioactive isotopes of iron, J. Clin. Invest. 25:616, 1946.

64. Gillman, T., and Hathorn, M.: Intracellular iron-containing enzymes, Brit. M. J. 2:635, 1958.

65. Gitlin, D., Janeways, C. A., and Farr, L. E.: Studies on the metabolism of plasma proteins in the nephrotic syndrome: I. Albumin, γ-globulin and iron-binding globulin, J. Clin. Invest. 35:44, 1956.

66. Goldberg, A.: Enzymic formation of haem by the incorporation of iron into protoporphyrin: Importance of ascorbic acid, ergothioneine and glutathione, Brit. J. Haemat. 5:150, 1959.

67. Granick, S.: Structure and physiologic functions of ferritin, Physiol. Rev. 31:489, 1951.

68. Granick, S.: Iron metabolism, Bull. New York Acad. Med. 30:81, 1954.

69. Granick, S.: Iron transport mechanisms in the intestinal tract, in Metabolism and Function of Iron (report of Nineteenth Ross Pediatric Research Conference), p. 15, Ross Laboratories, Columbus, Ohio, 1956.

69a. Greenough, W. B., III, Peters, T., Jr., and Thomas, E. D.: An intracellular protein intermediate for hemoglobin formation, J. Clin. Invest. 41:1116, 1962.

70. Hagberg, B.: Studies on the plasma transport of iron, Acta paediat., Suppl. 93, 1953.

71. Hahn, P. F., Bale, W. F., Ross, J. F., Hettig, R. A., and Whipple, G. H.: Radioiron in plasma does not exchange with hemoglobin iron in red cells, Science 92:131, 1940.

72. Hallberg, L.: Regulation of iron absorption, Acta haemat. 24:29, 1960.

73. Hallberg, L., and Sölvell, L.: Iron absorption studies, Acta med. scandinav., Suppl. 358, 1960.

74. Hallgren, B.: Haemoglobin formation and storage iron in protein deficiency, Acta Soc. med. 59:79, 1954.

75. Hamilton, L. D., Gubler, C. J., Cartwright, G. E., and Wintrobe, M. M.: Diurnal variation in the plasma iron level of man, Proc. Soc. Exper. Biol. & Med. 75:65, 1950.

76. Hansen, H. A., and Weinfeld, A.: Hemosiderin estimations and sideroblast counts in the differential diagnosis of iron deficiency and other anemias, Acta med. scandinav. 165:331, 1959.

77. Harrison, P.: Structures of ferritin and apoferritin: Some preliminary x-ray data, J. Med. Biol. 1:69, 1959.

78. Haskins, D., Stevens, A., Jr., Finch, S., and Finch, C. A.: Iron metabolism: Iron stores in man as measured by phlebotomy, J. Clin. Invest. 31:543, 1952.

79. Heath, C. W., and Patek, A. J., Jr.: The anemia of iron deficiency, Medicine 16:267, 1937.

80. Heilmeyer, L., Keller, W., Vivell, O., Keiderling, W., Betke, K., Wöhler, F., and Schultze, H. E.: Congenital transferrin deficiency in a seven-year-old girl, German Med. Monthly 6:385, 1961.

81. Heilmeyer, L., Keller, W., Vivell, O., Betke, K., Wöhler, F., and Keiderling, W.: Die kongenitale Atransferrinämie, Schweiz. med. Wchnschr. 91:1203, 1961.

82. Hitzig, W. H., Schmid, M., Betke, K., and Rothschild, M.: Erythroleukemia with hemoglobin disorders and disorders of iron metabolism, Helvet. paediat. acta 15:203, 1960.

83. Hobbs, J. R.: Iron deficiency after partial gastrectomy, Gut 2:141, 1961.

84. van Hoek, R., and Conrad, M. E.: Iron absorption: Measurements of ingested iron[59] by a human whole-body liquid scintillation counter, J. Clin. Invest. 40:1153, 1961.

85. Huff, R. L., Hennessey, T. G., Austin, R. E., Garcia, J. F., Roberts, B. M., and Lawrence, J. H.: Plasma and red cell iron turnover in normal subjects and in patients having various hematopoietic disorders, J. Clin. Invest. 29:1041, 1950.

86. Huff, R. L., Elmlinger, P. J., Garcia, J. F., Oda, J. M., Cockrell, M. C., and Lawrence, J. H.: Ferrokinetics in normal persons and in patients having various erythropoietic disorders, J. Clin. Invest. 30:1512, 1951.

87. Huff, R. L., and Judd, O. J.: Kinetics of iron metabolism, *in* Lawrence, J. H., and Tobias, C. A. (ed.), Biological and Medical Physics, vol. IV, p. 223, Academic Press, New York, 1956.

88. Hynes, M.: The iron reserve of a normal man, J. Clin. Path. 2:99, 1949.

89. Ingalls, R. L., and Johnson, F. A.: Iron from gastrointestinal sources excreted in the feces of human subjects, J. Nutrition 53:351, 1954.

90. Iron content of sweat in anemia, Nutrition. Rev. 17:295, 1959.

91. Jandl, J. H., Inman, J. K., Simmons, R. L., and Allen, D. W.: Transfer of iron from serum iron-binding protein to human reticulocytes, J. Clin. Invest. 38:161, 1959.

92. Jandl, J. H., and Katz, J. H.: Plasma-to-cell cycle of transferrin in iron utilization, Tr. A. Am. Physicians 74:72, 1961.

93. Jarnum, S., and Lassen, N. A.: Albumin and transferrin metabolism in infectious and toxic diseases, Scandinav. J. Clin. & Lab. Invest. 13:357, 1961.

94. Jones, N. L.: Irreversible shock in haemochromatosis, Lancet 1:569, 1962.

95. Josephs, H. W.: Absorption of iron as a problem in human physiology, Blood 13:1, 1958.

96. Kaldor, I.: Studies on intermediary iron metabolism: XII. Measurement of the iron derived from water soluble and water insoluble non-haem compounds (ferritin and hemosiderin iron) in liver and spleen, Australian J. Exper. Biol. & M. Sc. 36:173, 1958.

97. Katz, J. H.: Iron and protein kinetics studied by means of doubly labeled human crystalline transferrin, J. Clin. Invest. 40:2143, 1961.

98. Kerr, D. N. S., and Davidson, Sir Stanley: Gastrointestinal intolerance to oral iron preparations, Lancet 2:489, 1958.

99. Kerr, D. N. S., and Muir, A. R.: Demonstration of the structure and disposition of ferritin with human liver cell, J. Ultrastructure Res. 3:313, 1960.

100. Kistler, P., Nitschmann, H., Wyttenbach, A., Studer, M., Niederost, C., and Mauerhoffer, M.: Humanes Siderophilin: Isolierung mittels Rivanol aus Blutplasma und Plasmafraktionen, analytische Bestimmung und Kristallisation, Vox sang. 5:403, 1960.

101. Labbe, R. F.: An enzyme which catalyzes the insertion of iron into protoporphyrin, Biochim. et biophys. acta 31:589, 1959.

102. Labbe, R., and Hubbard, N.: Preparation and properties of the iron protoporphyrin chelating enzyme, Biochim. et biophys. acta 41:185, 1960.

103. Laurell, C. B.: Studies on transportation of metabolism of iron in body, with special reference to iron-binding component in human plasma, Acta physiol. scandinav. 14, Suppl. 46, 1947.

104. Laurell, C. B.: What is the function of transferrin in plasma? Blood 6:183, 1951.

105. Laurell, C. B.: Plasma iron and the transport of iron in the organism, Pharmacol. Rev. 4:371, 1952.

106. Laurell, C. B.: Diurnal variation of serum iron concentration, Scandinav. J. Clin. & Lab. Invest. 5:118, 1953.

107. Ley, A. B.: Relation of erythropoiesis to iron absorption, J. Clin. Invest. 39:1006, 1960.

108. Lochhead, A. C., and Goldberg, A.: Transfer of iron to protoporphyrin for haem biosynthesis, Lancet 2:271, 1959.

109. Loftfield, R. B., and Eigner, E. A.: Time required for synthesis of a ferritin molecule in rat liver, J. Biol. Chem. 231:925, 1958.

110. Mandel, E. E.: Serum iron and iron-binding capacity in clinical diagnosis, Clin. Chem. 5:1, 1959.

111. Manis, J. G., and Schachter, D.: Active transport of iron in vitro by duodenal segments and the "mucosal block," J. Clin. Invest. 40:1060, 1961.

112. Martin, C. M., and Jandl, J. H.: Inhibition of virus multiplication by transferrin, J. Clin. Invest. 38:1024, 1960.

113. Mazur, A., Baez, S., and Shorr, E.: Mechanism of iron release from ferritin as related to its biological properties, J. Biol. Chem. 213:147, 1955.

114. Mazur, A., Green, S., Sake, A., and Carleton, A.: Mechanism of release of ferritin iron in vivo by xanthine oxidase, J. Clin. Invest. 37:1809, 1958.

115. Mazur, A., Green, S., and Carleton, A.: Mechanism of plasma iron incorporation into hepatic ferritin, J. Biol. Chem. 235:595, 1960.

116. Mazur, A., Carleton, A., and Carlsen, A.: Relation of oxidative metabolism to the incorporation of plasma iron into ferritin in vivo, J. Biol. Chem. 236:1109, 1961.

117. Mazur, A., Carleton, A., and Carlsen, A.: Relation of ferritin to heme synthesis, Fed. Proc. 21:70, 1962.

118. Mendel, G. A.: Studies on iron absorption: I. Relationships between the rate of erythropoiesis, hypoxia and iron absorption, Blood 18:727, 1961.

119. Minot, G. R., and Heath, C. W.: Response of the reticulocytes to iron, Am. J. M. Sc. 183:110, 1932.

120. Minot, G. R., and Castle, W. B.: Interpretation of reticulocyte reactions, Lancet 2:319, 1935.

121. Mitchell, J., Halden, E. R., Jones, F., Bryan, S., Stirman, J. A., and Muirhead, E. E.: Lowering of transferrin during iron absorption in iron deficiency, J. Lab. & Clin. Med. 56:555, 1960.

122. Moore, C. V., Doan, C. A., and Arrowsmith, W. R.: Studies in iron transportation and absorption: II. The mechanism of iron transportation: Its significance in iron utilization in anemic states of varied etiology, J. Clin. Invest. 16:627, 1937.

123. Moore, C. V., Arrowsmith, W. R., Welch, J., and Minnich, V.: Studies in iron transportation and metabolism: IV. Observations on the absorption of iron from the gastrointestinal tract, J. Clin. Invest. 18:553, 1939.

124. Moore, C. V., and Dubach, R.: Observations on the absorption of iron from foods tagged with radioiron, Tr. A. Am. Physicians 64:245, 1951.

125. Moore, C. V., and Dubach, R.: Absorption of radioiron from foods, Science 116:520, 1952.

126. Moore, C. V., and Dubach, R.: Studies on iron metabolism using radioiron, in Wilkinson, J. F. (ed.), Modern Trends in Blood Diseases, Hoeber, New York, 1955.

127. Moore, C. V., and Dubach, R.: Metabolism and requirements of iron in the human, J.A.M.A. 162:197, 1956.

128. Moore, C. V.: Importance of nutritional factors in the pathogenesis of iron deficiency anemia, Scandinav. J. Clin. & Lab. Invest. 9:292, 1957.

129. Moore, C. V.: Iron and the essential trace elements, in Wohl, M. G., and

Goodhart, R. S. (ed.), Modern Nutrition in Health and Disease, ed. 2, Lea & Febiger, Philadelphia, 1960.

130. Moore, C. V.: Iron metabolism and nutrition, Harvey Lectures, series 55, 1959–1960.

131. Morgan, E. H., and Carter, G.: Plasma iron and iron-binding capacity levels in health and disease, with an improved method for the estimation of plasma iron concentration and total iron-binding capacity, Australasian Ann. Med. 9:209, 1960.

132. Morgan, E. H.: Factors regulating plasma total iron-binding capacity in rat and rabbit, Quart. J. Exper. Physiol. 47:57, 1962.

133. Nevé, R. A.: Enzymatic incorporation of iron into protoporphyrin, *in* Falk, J. E., Leuberg, R., and Morton, R. K. (ed.), Haematin Enzymes, p. 207, Pergamon Press, London, 1961.

134. Nishide, G., and Labbe, R. F.: Heme biosynthesis: On the incorporation of iron into protoporphyrin, Biochim. et biophys. acta 31:519, 1959.

135. Paoletti, C.: Rôle des β-globulines plasmatiques dans le transport du fer utilisé par les cellules érythroformatrices, Compt. rend. Acad. sc. 245:377, 1957.

136. Paterson, J. C. S., Marrack, D., and Wiggins, H. S.: Hypoferremia in the human subject: The importance of diurnal variation, Clin. Sc. 11:417, 1952.

137. Paterson, J. C. S., Marrack, D., and Wiggins, H. S.: Diurnal variation of the serum iron level in erythropoietic disorders, J. Clin. Path. 6:105, 1953.

138. Paterson, J. C. S.: Disappearance of radioactive iron from plasma by day and by night, Proc. Soc. Exper. Biol. & Med. 96:97, 1957.

139. Pirzio-Biroli, G., and Finch, C. A.: Treatment of iron deficiency anemia in the adult, J. Chronic Dis. 6:302, 1957.

140. Pirzio-Biroli, G., Bothwell, T. H., and Finch, C. A.: Iron absorption: II. The absorption of radioiron administered with a standard meal in man, J. Lab. & Clin. Med. 51:37, 1958.

141. Pirzio-Biroli, G., and Finch, C. A.: Iron absorption: III. The influence of iron stores on iron absorption in the normal subject, J. Lab. & Clin. Med. 55:216, 1960.

142. Pollycove, M.: Ferrokinetics: Techniques. Eisenstoffweschel, Beitrage zur forschung und klinik, p. 20, Thieme, Stuttgart, 1959.

143. Pollycove, M.: Presence of an erythropoietic labile iron pool, J. Clin. Invest. 40:1071, 1961.

144. Pollycove, M., and Mortimer, R.: Quantitative determination of iron kinetics and hemoglobin synthesis in human subjects, J. Clin. Invest. 40:753, 1961.

145. Powell, J. F.: Serum-iron in health and disease, Quart. J. Med. 13:19, 1944.

146. Price, D. C., Reizenstein, P. G., Cohen, S. H., Cronkite, E. P., and Wasserman, L. R.: Method for studying iron absorption and loss by whole body counting, Clin. Res. 9:165, 1961.

147. Rabinovitz, M., and Olson, M. E.: Participation of reticulocyte microsomes in the incorporation of iron into hemoglobin, Nature 181:1665, 1958.

148. Ramsay, W. N. M.: Plasma iron, Advances Clin. Chem. 1:1, 1958.

149. Rath, C. E., and Finch, C. A.: Serum iron transport measurements of iron-binding capacity of serum in man, J. Clin. Invest. 28:79, 1949.

150. Richter, G. W.: Study of hemosiderosis with the aid of electron microscopy, with observations on the relationship between hemosiderin and ferritins, J. Exper. Med. 106:203, 1957.

151. Richter, G. W.: Electron microscopy of hemosiderin: Presence of ferritin and occurrence of crystalline lattices in hemosiderin depots, J. Biophys. & Biochem. Cytol. 4:55, 1958.

152. Riegel, C., and Thomas, D.: Absence of beta-globulin fractions in the serum-protein of a patient with unexplained anemia, New England J. Med. 255:434, 1956.

153. Rossi-Fanelli, A., and Antonini, F.: Dissociation of hematin from hemoproteins at neutral pH, J. Biol. Chem. 235:4, 1960.

154. Sargent, T., Pollycove, M., Carpe, L., and Lawrence, J.: Dynamics of total body iron: Gastrointestinal, blood storage, and "fixed" components, Clin. Res. 10:78, 1962.

155. Schwaber, J. R., and Blumberg, A. G.: Papilledema associated with blood loss anemia, Ann. Int. Med. 55:1004, 1961.

156. Schwartz, H. C., Cartwright, G. E., Smith, E. L., and Wintrobe, M. M.: Studies on the biosynthesis of heme from iron and protoporphyrin, Blood 14:486, 1959.

157. Schwartz, H. C., Goudsmit, R., Hill, R. L., Cartwright, G. E., and Wintrobe, M. M.: Biosynthesis of hemoglobin from iron, protoporphyrin and globin, J. Clin. Invest. 40:188, 1961.

158. Schulz, J., and Smith, N. J.: Quantitative study of the absorption of food iron in infants and children, A.M.A. Am. J. Dis. Child. 95:109, 1958.

159. Shoden, A., Gabrio, B. W., and Finch, C. A.: Relation between ferritin and hemosiderin in rabbits and man, J. Biol. Chem. 204:823, 1953.

160. Shoden, A., and Richter, G. W.: On the extraction and staining of ferritin, Folia haemat. (N F) 4:180, 1960.

161. Shoden, A., and Sturgeon, P.: Hemosiderin: I. A physico-chemical study, Acta haemat. 23:376, 1960.

162. Shoden, A., and Sturgeon, P.: Formation of haemosiderin and the relation to ferritin, Nature 189:846, 1961.

163. Smith, M.D.: Iron metabolism: A review in relation to clinical problems, Scottish M. J. 4:467, 1959.

164. Sondhaus, C. A., and Thorell, B.: Microspectrophotometric determination of non-heme iron in maturing erythroblasts and its relationship to the endocellular hemoglobin formation, Blood 16:1285, 1960.

165. Steinkamp, R., Dubach, R., and Moore, C. V.: Studies in iron transportation and metabolism: VIII. Absorption of radioiron from iron-enriched bread, A.M.A. Arch. Int. Med. 95:181, 1955.

166. Suit, H. D., Lajtha, L. G., Oliver, R., and Ellis, F.: Studies on Fe^{59} uptake by normoblasts and the failure of x-irradiation to affect uptake, Brit. J. Haemat. 3:165, 1957.

167. Szur, L., and Smith, M. D.: Red-cell production and destruction in myelosclerosis, Brit. J. Haemat. 7:147, 1961.

168. Turnbull, A., and Giblett, E. R.: Binding and transport of iron by transferrin variants, J. Lab. & Clin. Med. 57:450, 1961.

169. Van Bruggen, E. F. J., Wiebenya, E. H., and Gruber, M.: Electron micrographs of ferritin and apoferritin molecules, J. Molecular Biol. 2:81, 1960.

170. Vannotti, A., and Delachaux, A.: Iron Metabolism and Its Clinical Significance, Grune & Stratton, New York, 1951.

171. Verloop, M. C., Meeuwissen, T. J. E., and Blokhuis, E. W. M.: Comparison of the "iron absorption test" with the determination of the iron-binding capacity of serum in the diagnosis of iron deficiency, Brit. J. Haemat. 4:70, 1958.

172. Vogel, W., Richert, D., Pixley, B. Q., and Schulman, M. P.: Heme synthesis in iron deficient duck blood, J. Biol. Chem. 235:1769, 1960.

173. Wallerstein, R. O., and Mettier, S. R. (ed.): Iron in Clinical Medicine, University of California Press, Berkeley, 1958.

174. Walsh, R. J., Thomas, E. D., Chow, S. K., Fluharty, R. C., and Finch, C. A.: Iron metabolism: Heme synthesis *in vitro* by immature erythrocytes, Science 110:396, 1949.
175. Walsh, R. J., Kaldor, I., Brading, I., and George, E. P.: Availability of iron in meat: Some experiments with radioactive iron, Australasian Ann. Med. 4:272, 1955.
176. Wasserman, L. R., Rashkoff, I. A., Leavitt, D., Mayer, J., and Port, S.: Rate of removal of radioactive iron from the plasma: An index of erythropoiesis, J. Clin. Invest. 31:32, 1952.
177. Wells, C. L., and Wolher, J. J.: Analysis of porphyrin in hemosiderin by microspectrophotometry, Fed. Proc. 20:70, 1961.
178. Wheby, M. S., Conrad, M. E., Hedberg, S. E., and Crosby, W. H.: Role of bile in the control of iron absorption, Gastroenterology 42:319, 1962.
179. Wöhler, F., Heilmeyer, L., Emrich, D., and Kang, S. H.: Zür Funktion des Ferritins bei der Eisenresorption, Arch. exper. Path. u. Pharmakol. 230:107, 1957.
180. Wöhler, F.: Über die Natur des Hämosiderins, Acta haemat. 23:242, 1960.
181. World Health Organization: Iron Deficiency Anemia, Report No. 182, 1959.
182. Wynder, E. L., and Fryer, J. H.: Etiologic considerations of Plummer-Vinson (Patterson-Kelly) syndrome, Ann. Int. Med. 49:1106, 1958.
183. Zizza, F., and Black, M.: Interrelationships of the serum iron, iron binding capacity and tissue iron, Acta haemat. 25:1, 1961.

CHAPTER THREE
GLOBIN BIOSYNTHESIS AND SICKLE CELL DISEASE

1. Allen, D. W., and Wyman, J., Jr.: Equilbre de l'hémoglobine de drépanocytose avec l'oxygène, Rev. hémat. 9:155, 1954.
2. Allen, D. W., Schroeder, W. A., and Balog, J.: Observations on the chromatographic heterogeneity of normal adult and fetal human hemoglobin: A study of the effects of crystallization and chromatography on the heterogeneity and isoleucine content, J. Am. Chem. Soc. 80:1628, 1958.
3. Allen, D. W.: Amino acid accumulation by human reticulocytes, Blood 16:1564, 1960.
4. Allen, E. H., and Schweet, R. S.: Role of transfer ribonucleic acid in hemoglobin synthesis, Biochim. et biophys. acta 39:185, 1960.
5. Allison, A. C.: Properties of sickle-cell haemoglobin, Biochem. J. 65:212, 1957.
6. Allison, A. C.: Recent developments in the study of inherited anemias, Eugenics Quart. 6:155, 1959.
7. Anderson, M., Went, L. N., MacIver, J. E., and Dixon, H. G.: Sickle-cell disease in pregnancy, Lancet 2:516, 1960.
8. Aschkenasy, A.: On the pathogenesis of anemias and leukopenias induced by dietary protein deficiency, Am. J. Clin. Nutrition 5:14, 1957.
9. Atwater, J., Schwartz, I. R., Erslev, A. J., Montgomery, T. L., and Tocantins, L. M.: Sickling of erythrocytes in a patient with thalassemia–hemoglobin I disease, New England J. Med. 263:1215, 1960.
10. Atwater, J., Schwartz, I. R., and Tocantins, L. M.: A variety of human hemoglobin with four distinct electrophoretic components, Blood 15:901, 1960.
11. Baglioni, C.: A chemical study of hemoglobin Norfolk, J. Biol. Chem. 237:69, 1962.
12. Bale, W. F., Yuile, C. L., DeLaVergne, L., Miller, L. L., and Whipple, G. H.: Hemoglobin labeled by radioactive lysine erythrocyte life cycle, J. Exper. Med. 90:315, 1949.
13. Bauer, J., and Fisher, L. J.: Sickle-cell disease with special regard to its non-anemic variety, Arch. Surg. 47:553, 1943.
14. Beaven, G. H., and Gratzer, W. B.: Critical review of human haemoglobin variants, J. Clin. Path. 12:1, 101, 1959.
15. Beaven, G. H., Ellis, M. J., and White, J. C.: Studies on human foetal haemoglobin: I. Detection and estimation, Brit. J. Haemat. 6:1, 1960.
16. Beaven, G. H., Ellis, M. J., and White, J. C.: Studies on human haemoglobin: II. Foetal haemoglobin levels in healthy children and adults and in certain haematological disorders, Brit. J. Haemat. 6:201, 1960.
17. Becklake, M. R., Griffiths, S. B., McGregor, M., Goldman, H. I., and Schreve, J. P.: Oxygen dissociation curves in sickle cell anemia and in subjects with the sickle cell trait, J. Clin. Invest. 34:751, 1955.
18. Beet, E. A.: Genetics of the sickle-cell trait in a Bantu tribe, Ann. Eugenics 14:279, 1949.

19. Bernstein, J., and Whitten, C. F.: Histologic appraisal of the kidney in sickle cell anemia, A.M.A. Arch. Path. 70:407, 1960.

20. Bessis, M., Nowarski, G., Thiery, J. P., and Breton-Gorius, J.: Etudes sur la falciformation des globules rouges au microscope polarisant et au microscope électronique: II. L'intérieur du globule: Comparaison avec les cristaux intra-globulaires, Rev. hémat. 13:249, 1958.

21. Beutler, E., and Mikus, B. J.: Effect of methemoglobin formation in sickle cell disease, J. Clin. Invest. 40:1856, 1961.

22. Bishop, J., Leahy, J., and Schweet, R.: Formation of the peptide chain of hemoglobin, Proc. Nat. Acad. Sc. 46:1030, 1960.

23. Bishop, J., Favelukes, G., Schweet, R., and Russell, E.: Control of specificity in haemoglobin synthesis, Nature 191:1365, 1961.

24. Bogoch, A., Casselman, W. G. B., Margolies, M. P., and Bockus, H. L.: Liver disease in sickle cell anemia: A correlation of clinical, biochemical, histologic and histochemical observations, Am. J. Med. 19:583, 1955.

25. Borsook, H., Deasy, C. L., Haagen-Smith, A. J., Keighley, G., and Lowy, P. H.: Incorporation in vitro of labeled amino acids into proteins of rabbit reticulocytes, J. Biol. Chem. 196:669, 1952.

26. Borsook, H., Fischer, E. H., and Keighley, G.: Factors affecting protein synthesis in vitro in rabbit reticulocytes, J. Biol. Chem. 229:1059, 1957.

27. Brachet, J.: Ribonucleic acids and the synthesis of cellular proteins, Nature 186:194, 1960.

28. Bragg, W. L., and Perutz, M. F.: External form of the haemoglobin molecule; Acta crystallog. 5:323, 1952.

29. Braunitzer, G., Liebold, B., Müller, R., and Rudloff, V.: Der Homologe chemische aufbau der Peptidketter im human Hämoglobin A, Ztschr. Physiol. Chem. 320:170, 1960.

30. Braunitzer, G., Hilschmann, M., Rudloff, V., Hilse, K., Liebold, B., and Muller, R.: The haemoglobin particles: Chemical and genetic aspects of their structure, Nature 190:480, 1961.

31. Braunsteiner, H., Fellinger, K., and Pakesch, F.: Über die Struktur der Reticulozyten, Acta haemat. 16:322, 1956.

32. Brown, H., and Brown, J.: Hemoglobin peptides used in hemoglobin synthesis, Metabolism 6:587, 1960.

33. Brunner, A., Jr., and Vallejo-Friere, A.: Electron microscopic observations on granules and filaments (reticulosomes) of reticulocytes, Exper. Cell Res. 10:55, 1956.

34. Callender, S. T. E., Nickel, J. F., and Moore, C. V.: Sickle-cell disease studied by measuring the survival time of transfused red blood cells, J. Lab. & Clin. Med. 34:90, 1949.

35. Carrington, H. T., Ferguson, A. D., and Scott, R. B.: Studies in sickle cell anemia: XI. Bone involvement simulating aseptic necrosis, A.M.A. Am. J. Dis. Child. 95:157, 1958.

36. Chalfu, D.: Difference between young and mature rabbit erythrocytes, J. Cell. & Comp. Physiol. 47:215, 1956.

37. Chatterjee, S. N., Sadhukaw, P., and Chatterjee, J. B.: Electron microscope studies on the haemoglobin molecules, J. Biophys. & Biochem. Cytol. 10:113, 1961.

38. Constituents of human haemoglobin: 1. Separation of the peptide chains of human haemoglobin (V. M. Ingram); 2. Comparison of normal adult human haemoglobin with hemoglobin I by finger printing (M. Murayama); 3. Formation of normal and doubly abnormal haemoglobin by recombination

of hemoglobin I with S and C (H. A. Itano and E. Robinson), Nature 183:1795, 1959.

39. Crick, F. H. C., Barnett, L., Brenner, S., and Watts-Tobin, R. J.: General nature of the genetic code for proteins, Nature 192:1227, 1961.

40. Crone, R. I., Jefferson, S. C., Pileggi, V. J., and Lowry, E. C.: Gross hematuria in sickle cell trait: A report of eight cases, A.M.A. Arch. Int. Med. 100:597, 1957.

41. Crosby, W. H., and Dameshek, W.: Significance of hemoglobinemia and associated hemosiderinuria with particular reference to various types of hemolytic anemia, J. Lab. & Clin. Med. 38:829, 1951.

42. Crosby, W. H.: Metabolism of hemoglobin and bile pigment in hemolytic disease, Am. J. Med. 18:112, 1955.

43. Cruz, W. O., Hawkins, W. B., and Whipple, G. H.: Acetylphenylhydrazine anemia: 2. Bile pigment elimination and new hemoglobin reconstruction in bile fistula dog, Am. J. M. Sc. 203:848, 1942.

44. Curtis, E. M.: Pregnancy in sickle cell anemia, sickle cell–hemoglobin C disease, and variants thereof, Am. J. Obst. & Gynec. 77:1312, 1959.

45. Daland, G. A., and Castle, W. B.: A simple and rapid method for demonstrating sickling of the red blood cells: The use of reducing agents, J. Lab. & Clin. Med. 33:1082, 1948.

46. de Torregrosa, M. V., Dapena, R. B., Hernandez, H., and Ortiz, A. O.: Association of salmonella-caused osteomyelitis and sickle-cell disease, J.A.M.A. 174:354, 1960.

47. Diggs, L. W.: Crisis in sickle cell anemia: Hematologic studies, Am. J. Clin. Path. 26:1109, 1956.

48. Dintzis, H. M., Borsook, H., and Vinograd, J.: Microsomal structure and hemoglobin synthesis in the rabbit reticulocyte, in Roberts, R. B. (ed. for the Biophysical Society), Microsomal Particles and Protein Synthesis, p. 95, Pergamon Press, New York, 1958.

49. Drabkin, D. L., and Wise, C. D.: Independent biosynthesis of hemin and globin in hemoglobin, Science 132:1491, 1960.

50. Edington, G. M.: Pathology of sickle-cell haemoglobin C disease and sickle cell anaemia, J. Clin. Path. 10:182, 1957.

51. Eriksen, L.: Evidence for the cytoplasmic formation of hemoglobin, Exper. Cell Res. 13:624, 1957.

52. Erlandson, M. E., Schulman, I., and Smith, C. H.: Studies on congenital hemolytic syndromes: III. Rates of destruction and production of erythrocytes in sickle cell anemia, Pediatrics 25:629, 1960.

53. Ferguson, A. D., and Scott, R. B.: Studies in sickle-cell anemia: XII. Further studies on hepatic function in sickle-cell anemia, A.M.A. Am. J. Dis. Child. 97:418, 1959.

54. Field, E. O., and O'Brien, J. R. P.: Dissociation of human haemoglobin at low pH, Biochem. J. 60:656, 1955.

55. Fink, A. I., Funahashi, T., Robinson, M., and Watson, R. J.: Conjunctiva in sickle cell disease, A.M.A. Arch. Ophth. 66:824, 1961.

56. Fowler, N. O., Smith, O., and Greenfield, J. C.: Arterial blood oxygenation in sickle cell anemia, Am. J. M. Sc. 234:449, 1957.

57. Fraimow, W., Rodman, T., Close, H. P., and Cathcart, R.: Oxyhemoglobin dissociation curve in sickle cell anemia, Am. J. M. Sc. 236:225, 1958.

58. Geeraets, W. J., and Guerry, D.: Angioid streaks and sickle cell disease, Am. J. Ophth. 49:450, 1960.

59. Geeraets, W. J., and Guerry, D.: Elastic tissue degeneration in sickle cell disease, Am. J. Ophth. 50:213, 1960.

60. Gerald, P. S., and Ingram, V. M.: Recommendations for the nomenclature of hemoglobins, J. Biol. Chem. 236:2155, 1961; Blood 19:124, 1962.

61. Golding, J. S. R., MacIver, J. E., and Went, L. M.: Bone changes in sickle-cell anaemia and its genetic variants, J. Bone & Joint Surg. 41B:711, 1959.

62. Goodman, G., von Sallmann, L., and Holland, M. G.: Ocular manifestations of sickle-cell disease, A.M.A. Arch. Ophth. 58:655, 1957.

63. Granick, S.: Chemistry and functioning of the mammalian erythrocyte, Blood 4:404, 1949.

64. Greenberg, M. S., and Kass, E. H.: Studies on the destruction of red blood cells: XIII. Observations on the role of pH in the pathogenesis and treatment of painful crisis in sickle-cell disease, A.M.A. Arch. Int. Med. 101:355, 1958.

65. Greer, M., and Schotland, D.: Abnormal hemoglobin as a cause of neurological disease, Neurology 12:114, 1962.

66. Griggs, R. C., and Harris, J. W.: Biophysics of the variants of sickle-cell disease, A.M.A. Arch. Int. Med. 97:315, 1956.

67. Haggard, M. E., and Schneider, R. G.: Sickle cell amenia in the first two years of life, J. Pediat. 58:785, 1961.

68. Hahn, E.V. and Gillespie, E. B.: Sickle-cell anemia: Report of a case greatly improved by splenectomy, Arch. Int. Med. 39:233, 1927.

69. Ham, T. H., and Battle, J. D.: Viscosity of sickle cells: A thirty-four-year study of an Italian family with sickle-cell and thalassemia traits: Splenectomy in two members, Tr. Am. Clin. & Climatol. Assoc. 68:146, 1957.

70. Hammarsten, E., Thorell, B., Aquist, S., Eliasson, N., and Ackerman, L.: Studies on the hemoglobin formation during regenerative erythropoiesis, Exper. Cell Res. 5:404, 1953.

71. Harris, J. W.: Studies on the destruction of red blood cells: VIII. Molecular orientation in sickle-cell hemoglobin solutions, Proc. Soc. Exper. Biol. & Med. 75:197, 1950.

72. Harris, J. W., Brewster, H. A., Ham, T. H., and Castle, W. B.: Studies on the destruction of red blood cells: X. The biophysics and biology of sickle-cell disease, A.M.A. Arch. Int. Med. 97:145, 1956.

73. Harris, J. W.: Role of physical and chemical factors in the sickling phenomenon, Progr. Hemat. 2:47, 1959.

74. Hasserodt, U., and Vinograd, J.: Dissociation of human carbonmonoxyhemoglobin at high pH, Proc. Nat. Acad. Sc. 45:12, 1959.

75. Hawkins, W. B., Sribhishaj, K., Robscheit-Robbins, F. S., and Whipple, G. H.: II. Bile pigment and hemoglobin interrelation in anemic dogs, Am. J. Physiol. 96:463, 1931.

76. Hawkins, W. B., and Johnson, A. C.: Bile pigment and hemoglobin interrelation in anemic dogs, Am. J. Physiol. 126:326, 1939.

77. Heller, P., Yakulis, V. J., and Josephson, A. M.: Immunologic studies of human hemoglobins, J. Lab. & Clin. Med. 59:401, 1962.

78. Henderson, A. B., Prince, A. E., and Greene, J. B.: Sickle-cell-disease variants and pregnancy, New England J. Med. 264:1277, 1961.

79. Herman, E. C., Jr.: Serum haptoglobins in hemolytic disorders, J. Lab. & Clin. Med. 57:834, 1961.

80. Herrick, J. B.: Peculiar elongated and sickle-shaped red corpuscles in a case of severe anemia, Arch. Int. Med. 6:517, 1910.

81. Hilkovitz, G.: Sickle-cell disease: The "aplastic crisis" and erythroid maturation defect occurring simultaneously in three members of a family, A.M.A. Arch. Int. Med. 105:76, 1960.

81a. Hill, R. J., Konigsberg, W., Guidotti, G., and Craig, L. C.: Structure of human hemoglobin: I. The separation of the α- and β-chains and their amino acid composition, J. Biol. Chem. 237:1549, 1962.

82. Hill, R. L., and Schwartz, H. C.: A chemical abnormality in haemoglobin G, Nature 184:641, 1959.

83. Hoagland, M. B.: Nucleic acids and proteins, Scient. American 20:55, 1959.

84. Holloway, B. W., and Ripley, S. H.: Nucleic acid content of reticulocytes and the relation to uptake of radioactive leucine in vitro, J. Biol. Chem. 196:695, 1952.

85. Hook, E. W., Campbell, C. G., Weens, H. S., and Cooper, G. R., Salmonella osteomyelitis in patients with sickle-cell anemia, New England J. Med. 257:403, 1957.

86. Hook, E. W., and Cooper, G. R.: Clinical manifestations of sickle cell hemoglobin C disease and sickle cell anemia, South. M. J. 51:610, 1958.

87. Huisman, T. H. J., Horton, B., and Sebens, T. B.: Identity of the α-chains of the minor human haemoglobin components A_2 and $A_2{}^1$ with the α-chains of human haemoglobin A and F, Nature 190:357, 1961.

88. Hunt, J. A.: Identity of the α-chains of adult and fetal human hemoglobins, Nature 183:1373, 1958.

89. Hurwitz, J., and Furth, J. J.: Messenger RNA, Scient. American 206:41, 1962.

90. Ingram, V. M.: Gene evolution and the haemoglobins, Nature 189:705, 1961.

91. Ingram, V. M.: Hemoglobin and Its Abnormalities, Charles C. Thomas, Springfield, Ill., 1961.

92. Ingram, V. M., and Stretton, A. O. W.: Human haemoglobin A_2: Chemistry, genetics, and evolution, Nature 190:1079, 1961.

93. Itano, H. A.: The human hemoglobins: Their properties and genetic control, Advances Protein Chem. 12:215, 1957.

94. Itano, H. A., and Robinson, E.: Specific recombination of the subunits of hemoglobin, Ann. New York Acad. Sc. 88:642, 1960.

95. Itano, H. A., and Robinson, E. A.: Genetic control of the α- and β-chains of hemoglobin, Proc. Nat. Acad. Sc. 46:1492, 1960.

96. Jandl, J. H., Greenberg, M. S., Yonemato, R. H., and Castle, W. B.: Clinical determination of the sites of red cell sequestration in hemolytic anemias, J. Clin. Invest. 35:842, 1956.

97. Jandl, J. H., Simmons, R. L., and Castle, W. B.: Red cell filtration and the pathogenesis of certain hemolytic anemias, Blood 18:133, 1961.

98. Jenkins, M. E., Scott, R. B., and Baird, R. L.: Studies in sickle cell anemia: XVI. Sudden death during sickle cell anemia crises in young children, J. Pediat. 56:30, 1960.

99. Jensen, W. N., Rucknagel, D. L., and Taylor, W. J.: In vivo study of the sickle cell phenomenon, J. Lab. & Clin. Med. 56:854, 1960.

100. Jensen, W. N.: The hemoglobinopathies, Disease-a-Month, p. 1, Feb. 1961.

101. Jonsson, U., Roath, O. S., and Kirkpatrick, C. I. F.: Nutritional megaloblastic anemia associated with sickle cell states, Blood 14:535, 1959.

102. Jonxis, J. H. P., and Huisman, T. H. J.: A Laboratory Manual on Abnormal Hemoglobins, Blackwell, Oxford, 1958.

103. Jonxis, J. H. P., and Delafresnaye, J. F. (ed.), Abnormal Haemoglobins: A Symposium, Blackwell, Oxford, 1959.

104. Jordan, R. A.: Cholelithiasis in sickle cell disease, Gastroenterology 33:952, 1957.

105. Kass, E. H., Geiman, Q. M., Ingbar, S. H., Ley, A. B., Harris, J. W., and Finland, M.: Some diseases which may be activated by ACTH: Observations on sickle cell anemia and malaria, in Proceedings, Second Clinical

ACTH Conference on Therapeutics, vol. 2, p. 376, Blakiston, Philadelphia, 1951.

106. Kassenaar, A., Morell, H., and London, I. M.: Incorporation of glycine with globin and the synthesis of heme in duck erythrocytes, J. Biol. Chem. 229:423, 1959.

107. Keitel, H., and Blakely, J.: Plasma hemoglobin concentration in sickle cell disease, A.M.A. Am. J. Dis. Child. 92:511, 1956.

108. Keitel, H. A., Thompson, D., and Itano, H. A.: Hyposthenuria in sickle cell anemia: A reversible renal defect, J. Clin. Invest. 35:998, 1956.

109. Kennedy, J. J., and Cope, C. B.: Intraocular lesions associated with sickle cell disease, A. M.A. Arch. Ophth. 58:163, 1957.

110. Klinefelter, H. F.: The heart in sickle cell anemia, Am. J. M. Sc. 203:34, 1942.

111. Lagerlof, B., Thorell, B., and Akerman, L.: Heme and dry mass formation during red cell development, Exper. Cell Res. 10:752, 1956.

112. Lange, R. D., Minnich, V., and Moore, C. V.: Effect of oxygen tension and of pH on the sickling and mechanical fragility of erythrocytes from patients with sickle cell anemia and the sickle cell trait, J. Lab. & Clin. Med. 37:789, 1951.

113. Lathem, W., and Jensen, W. N.: Plasma hemoglobin-binding capacity in sickle cell disease, Blood 14:1047, 1959.

114. Lathem, W., and Jensen, W. N.: Renal excretion of hemoglobin in sickle cell anemia, with observations on spontaneously occurring hemoglobinemia and methemalbuminemia, J. Lab. & Clin. Med. 59:137, 1962.

115. Leight, L., Snider, T. H., Clifford, G. O., and Hellems, H. K.: Hemodynamic studies in sickle cell anemia, Circulation 10:653, 1954.

116. Levin, W. C., Baird, W. D., Perry, J. E., and Zung, W. W. K.: Experimental production of splenic sequestration of erythrocytes in patients with sickle cell trait, J. Lab. & Clin. Med. 50:926, 1957.

117. Levin, W. C.: "Asymptomatic" sickle cell trait, Blood 13:904, 1958.

117a. Levin, W. C., Thurm, R. H., Ozer, F. L., and DeGroot, W.: Chronic hypoxia and heterozygous S hemoglobinopathies, J. Lab. & Clin. Med. 59:792, 1962.

118. Lichtman, H., Shapiro, H., Ginsberg, V., and Watson, J.: Splenic hyper-function in sickle cell anemia, Am. J. Med. 14:516, 1952.

119. Lieb, W. A., Geeraets, W. J., and Guerry, D., III: Sickle cell retinopathy, Acta ophth., Suppl. 58, 1959.

120. Liekin, S. L., and McCoo, J. W., Jr.: Sickle-cell anemia in infancy, A.M.A. Am. J. Dis. Child. 96:51, 1958.

121. London, I. M., Shemin, D., and Rittenberg, D.: In vitro synthesis of heme in the human red blood cell of sickle-cell anemia, J. Biol. Chem. 173:797, 1948.

122. London, I. M., Morell, H., and Kassenaar, A.: Incorporation of glycine into globin and the synthesis of heme in duck erythrocytes and rabbit reticulo-cytes, *in* National Research Council, Division of Medical Sciences, Conference on Hemoglobin (NAS-NRC Publication 557), Washington, D.C., 1958.

123. Lowenstein, L. M.: The mammalian reticulocyte, Internat. Rev. Cytol. 8:135, 1959.

124. MacIver, J. E., and Went, L. N.: Sickle-cell anaemia complicated by megalo-blastic anaemia of infancy, Brit. M. J. 1:775, 1960.

125. MacIver, J. E., and Parker-Williams, E. J.: Aplastic crisis in sickle-cell anaemia, Lancet 1:1086, 1961.

126. Malassenet, R.: Les hémoglobines humaines, Rev. hémat. 12:64, 1957.

127. Margolies, M. P.: Sickle cell anemia: A composite study and survey, Medicine 30:357, 1951.

128. Martin, W. W., Jr., Kough, R. H., and Branche, G. C., Jr.: Hereditary sphero-cytosis-sicklemia in the Negro, Blood 14:688, 1959.

129. Matsuda, G., Schroeder, W. A., Jones, R. T., and Weliky, N.: Is there an "embryonic" or "primitive" human hemoglobin? Blood 16:984, 1960.

130. McCormick, W. F.: Abnormal hemoglobins: II. The pathology of sickle cell trait, Am. J. M. Sc. 241:329, 1961.

131. McCurdy, P. R., Pearson, H., and Gerald, P. S.: A new hemoglobinopathy of unusual genetic significance, J. Lab. & Clin. Med. 58:86, 1961.

132. McKellar, M., and Dacie, J. V.: Thromboplastic activity of the plasma in paroxysmal nocturnal haemoglobinuria, Brit. J. Haemat. 4:404, 1958.

133. Mehta, S. R., and Jensen, W. N.: Haptoglobins in haemoglobinopathy: A genetic and clinical study, Brit. J. Haemat. 6:250, 1960.

134. Middlemiss, J. H.: Sickle cell anemia, J. Fac. Radiologists 9:16, 1958.

135. Moon, J. H.: Tactoid formation in deer hemoglobin, Am. J. Physiol. 199:190, 1960.

136. Moseley, J. E.: Patterns of bone changes in sickle cell states, J. Mt. Sinai Hosp. 26:424, 1959.

137. Moser, K. M., Luchsinger, P. C., and Katz, S.: Pulmonary and cardiac function in sickle cell lung disease: Preliminary report, Dis. Chest 37:637, 1960.

138. Muir, H. M., Neuberger, A., and Peronne, J. C.: Further isotopic studies on haemoglobin formation in the rat and rabbit, Biochem. J. 52:87, 1952.

139. Muller, C. J., and Jonxis, J. H. P.: Identity of haemoglobin A_2, Nature 188:949, 1960.

140. Nathan, D. G., Piomello, S., and Gardner, F. H.: Synthesis of heme and globin in the maturing human erythroid cell, J. Clin. Invest. 40:940, 1961.

141. National Research Council, Division of Medical Sciences: Conference on Hemoglobin (NAS-NRC Publication 557), Washington, D.C., 1958.

142. Neel, J. V.: Inheritance of the sickling phenomenon with particular reference to sickle-cell disease, Blood 6:389, 1951.

143. Neel, J. V.: Genetics of human hemoglobin differences, problems and perspectives, Ann. Human Genet. 21:1, 1956.

144. Neel, J. V.: The hemoglobin genes: A remarkable example of the clustering of related genetic functions on a single mammalian chromosome, Blood 18:769, 1961.

145. Nizet, A.: Recherches sur les relations entre les biosynthèses de l'hème et de la globine, Bull. Soc. chim. biol. 39:265, 1957.

146. Ober, W. B., Bruno, M. S., Simon, R. M., and Weiner, L.: Hemoglobin S–C disease with fat embolism: Report of a patient dying in crisis: Autopsy findings, Am. J. Med. 27:647, 1959.

147. Ober, W. B., Bruno, M. S., Weinberg, S. B., Jones, F. M., and Weiner, L.: Fatal intravascular sickling in a patient with sickle cell trait, New England J. Med. 263:947, 1960.

148. Oliner, H. L., and Heller, P.: Megaloblastic erythropoiesis and acquired hemolysis in sickle-cell anemia, New England J. Med. 261:19, 1959.

149. Paton, D.: Angioid streaks and sickle cell anemia, A.M.A. Arch. Ophth. 62:852, 1959.

150. Pauling, L., Itano, H. A., Singer, S. J., and Wells, I. C.: Sickle-cell anemia: A molecular disease, Science 110:543, 1949.

151. Pauling, L.: Abnormality of hemoglobin molecules in hereditary hemolytic anemias, Harvey Lectures, p. 216, 1953–1954.

152. Pease, D. C.: Electron microscopic study of red bone marrow, Blood 11:501, 1956.

153. Pierce, L. E., McCoy, K. H., and Rath, C. E.: A new hemoglobin causing sickling, Clin. Res. 10:57, 1962.

153a. Pierce, L. E., and Rath, C. E.: Evidence for folic acid deficiency in the genesis of anemic sickle cell crisis, Blood 20:19, 1962.

154. Prins, H. K.: Separation of different types of human haemoglobin, J. Chromatog. 2:445, 1959.

155. Rabinovitz, M., and Olson, M. E.: Evidence for a ribonucleoprotein intermediate in the synthesis of globin by reticulocytes, Exper. Cell Res. 10:747, 1956.

156. Rabinovitz, M., and Olson, M. E.: Participation of reticulocyte microsomes in the incorporation of iron into haemoglobin, Nature 181:1665, 1958.

157. Rabinovitz, M., and Olson, M. E.: Protein synthesis by rabbit reticulocytes: I. Kinetics of amino acid incorporation in vitro into protein fractions of intact cells, J. Biol. Chem. 234:2085, 1959.

158. Rabinovitz, M., and McGrath, H.: Protein synthesis by rabbit reticulocytes: II: Interruption of the pathway of hemoglobin synthesis by a valine analogue, J. Biol. Chem. 234:2091, 1959.

159. Raper, A. B., Gammack, D. B., Huehns, E. R., and Shrotes, E. M.: Four haemoglobins in one individual: A study of the genetic interaction of haemoglobin G and haemoglobin C, Brit. M. J. 2:1257, 1960.

160. Rappaport, D. A., and Sewell, B. W.: Metabolic changes induced in mammalian erythrocytes by whole x-irradiation, Nature 184:846, 1959.

161. Rebuck, J. W., Sturrock, R. M., and Monto, R. W.: Sequential electron micrography of sickling, Lab. Invest. 4:175, 1955.

162. Rhinesmith, H. S., Schroeder, W. A., and Martin, N.: N-terminal sequence of the beta chains of normal adult human hemoglobin, J. Am. Chem. Soc. 80:3358, 1958.

163. Ricks, P., Jr.: Sickle cell anemia and pregnancy, Obst. & Gynec. 17:513, 1961.

164. River, G. L., Robbins, A. B., and Schwartz, S. O.: S–C hemoglobin: A clinical study, Blood 18:385, 1961.

165. Robinson, E. A., and Itano, H. A.: Identification of the recombinant products of canine and human haemoglobins, Nature 188:798, 1960.

166. Rodman, T., Close, H. P., Cathcart, R., and Purcell, M. K.: Oxyhemoglobin dissociation curve in the common hemoglobinopathies, Am. J. Med. 27:558, 1959.

167. Rowe, C. W., and Haggard, M. E.: Bone infarcts in sickle cell anemia, Radiology 68:661, 1957.

168. Rucknagel, D. L., and Neel, J. V.: The hemoglobinopathies, in Steinberg, A. G. (ed.), Progress in Medical Genetics, vol. I, p. 158, Grune & Stratton, New York, 1961.

169. Schlitt, L. E., and Keital, H. G.: Renal manifestations of sickle cell disease: A review, Am. J. M. Sc. 239:773, 1960.

170. Schroeder, W. A.: Chemical structure of the normal human hemoglobins, Progr. Chem. Organic Natural Products 17:323, 1959.

171. Schweet, R., Lamfron, H., and Allen, E.: Synthesis of hemoglobin in a cell-free system, Proc. Nat. Acad. Sc. 44:1029, 1958.

172. Schweiger, H. G., Rappaport, S., and Schölzel, E.: Role of non-protein nitrogen in the synthesis of haemoglobin in the reticulocytes in vitro, Nature 178:141, 1956.

173. Scott, R. B., Freeman, L. C., and Ferguson, A. D.: Studies in sickle cell anemia: Effect of age (maturation) on incidence of the sickling phenomenon, Pediatrics 14:209, 1954.

174. Scott, R. B., and Ferguson, A. D.: Studies in sickle-cell anemia: XIV. Management of the child with sickle-cell anemia, A.M.A. Am. J. Dis. Child. 100:85, 1960.

175. Scott, R. B., and Kessler, A. D.: Sickle Cell Anemia and Your Child: Questions and Answers on Sickle Cell Anemia for Parents (13-page booklet), Howard University College of Medicine, Washington, D.C., 1960.

176. Scrimshaw, N. S., and Béhar, M.: Protein malnutrition in young children, Science 133:2039, 1961.

177. Shapiro, N. D., and Poe, M. F.: Sickle cell disease: An anesthesiological problem, Anesthesiology 16:771, 1955.

178. Sharpe, A. R., Jr., Fox, P. G., Jr., and Dodson, A. I.: Unilateral renal hematuria associated with sickle cell C disease and sickle cell trait: Study of five patients and review of literature, J. Urol. 81:780, 1959.

179. Shelley, W. M., and Curtis, E. M.: Bone marrow and fat embolism in sickle cell anemia and sickle cell–hemoglobin C disease, Bull. Johns Hopkins Hosp. 103:8, 1958.

180. Shemin, D., London, I. M., and Rittenberg, D.: Synthesis of protoporphyrin in vitro by red blood cells of the duck, J. Biol. Chem. 183:757, 1950.

181. Shen, S. C., Fleming, E. M., and Castle, W. B.: Studies on the destruction of red blood cells: V. Irreversibly sickled erythrocytes: The experimental production in vitro, Blood 4:498, 1949.

182. Sherman, I. J.: The sickling phenomenon, with special reference to differentiation of sickle cell anemia from the sickle cell trait, Bull. Johns Hopkins Hosp. 67:309, 1940.

183. Sherman, M.: Pathogenesis of disintegration of the hip in sickle cell anemia, South. M. J. 52:632, 1959.

184. Shubin, H., Kaufman, R., Shapiro, M., and Levinson, D. C.: Cardiovascular findings in children with sickle cell anemia, Am. J. Cardiol. 6:875, 1960.

185. Silver, H. K., Simon, J. L., and Clement, D. H.: Salmonella osteomyelitis and abnormal hemoglobin disease, Pediatrics 20:439, 1957.

186. Singer, K., Robin, S., King, J. C., and Jefferson, R. N.: Life span of the sickle-cell and the pathogenesis of sickle-cell anemia, J. Lab. & Clin. Med. 33:975, 1948.

187. Singer, K., Motulsky, A. G., and Wile, S. A.: Aplastic crisis in sickle cell anemia: A study of its mechanism and its relationship to other types of hemolytic crises, J. Lab. & Clin. Med. 35:721, 1950.

188. Singer, K.: Hereditary hemolytic disorders associated with abnormal hemoglobins, Am. J. Med. 18:633, 1955.

189. Singer, S. J., and Itano, H. A.: On the asymmetrical dissociation of human hemoglobin, Proc. Nat. Acad. Sc. 45:174, 1959.

190. Smith, E. W., and Conley, C. L.: Clinical features of the genetic variants of sickle cell disease, Bull. Johns Hopkins Hosp. 94:289, 1954.

191. Smith, E. W., and Conley, C. L.: Sicklemia and infarction of spleen during aerial flight: Electrophoresis of the hemoglobin in 15 cases, Bull. Johns Hopkins Hosp. 96:35, 1955.

192. Smith, E. W., and Conley, C. L.: Sickle cell–hemoglobin D disease, Ann. Int. Med. 50:94, 1959.

193. Smith, E. W., and Krevans, J. R.: Clinical manifestations of hemoglobin C disorders, Bull. Johns Hopkins Hosp. 104:17, 1959.

194. Sproule, B. J., Halden, E. R., and Miller, W. F.: Study of cardiopulmonary alterations in patients with sickle cell disease and its variants, J. Clin. Invest. 37:486, 1958.

195. Sribhishaj, K., Hawkins, W. B., and Whipple, G. H.: I. Bile pigment and hemoglobin interrelations in normal dogs, Am. J. Physiol. 96: 449, 1931.

196. Tanaka, K. R., Clifford, G. O., and Axelrod, A. R.: Sickle cell anemia (homozygous S) with aseptic necrosis of femoral head, Blood 11:998, 1956.

197. Thorell, B.: Studies on the formation of cellular substance during blood cell production, Acta med. scandinav., Suppl. 200, 1947.

198. Tuttle, A. H., and Koch, B.: Clinical and hematological manifestations of hemoglobin C–S disease in children, J. Pediat. 56:331, 1960.

199. Undritz, F., Betke, K., and Lehman, H.: Sickling phenomenon in deer, Nature 187:332, 1960.

200. Vinograd, J. R., Hutchinson, W. D., and Schroeder, W. A.: C^{14} hybrids of human haemoglobins: II. The identification of the aberrant chain in hemoglobin S, J. Am. Chem. Soc. 81:3168, 1959.

201. Vinograd, J., and Hutchinson, W. D.: Carbon-14 labelled hybrids of haemoglobin, Nature 187:216, 1960.

202. Von Ehrenstein, G., and Lipmann, F.: Experiments on hemoglobin biosynthesis, Proc. Nat. Acad. Sc. 47:941, 1961.

203. Walsh, R. J., Thomas, E. D., Chow, S. K., Fluharty, R. G., and Finch, C. A.: Iron metabolism: Heme synthesis in vitro by immature erythrocytes, Science 110:396, 1949.

204. Walters, J. H.: Vascular occlusion in sickle cell disease, Proc. Roy. Soc. Med. 51:646, 1958.

205. Watson, J., Stalman, A. W., and Bitello, F. W.: Significance of the paucity of sickle cells in newborn Negro infants, Am. J. M. Sc. 215:419, 1948.

206. Watson, R. J., Burko, H., Megas, H., and Robinson, M.: The hand-foot syndrome in sickle cell disease in children, A.M.A. Am. J. Dis. Child. 102:603, 1961.

207. Weatherall, D. J., and Boyer, S. H., IV: Evidence for the genetic identity of alpha chain determinants in hemoglobins A, A_2 and $F^{1, 2}$, Bull. Johns Hopkins Hosp. 110:8, 1962.

208. Weisman, R., Jr., Hurley, T. H., Harris, J. W., and Ham, T. H.: Studies of the function of the spleen in the hemolysis of red cells in hereditary spherocytosis and sickle-cell disorders, J. Lab. & Clin. Med. 42:965, 1954.

209. Whipple, G. H., and Robscheit-Robbins, F. S.: Amino acids and hemoglobin production in anemia, J. Exper. Med. 71:569, 1940.

210. Whipple, G. H.: Hemoglobin and plasma proteins: Their production, utilization and interrelation, Am. J. M. Sc. 203:477, 1942.

211. Whitten, C. F., Younes, A. A., and Frazaier, G.: Comparative study of renal concentrating ability in children with sickle cell anemia and in normal children, J. Lab. & Clin. Med. 55:400, 1960.

212. Whitten, C. F.: Growth status of children with sickle cell anemia, A.M.A. Am. J. Dis. Child. 102:101, 1961.

213. Whitten, C. F.: Studies on serum haptoglobin: A functional enquiry, New England J. Med. 266:529, 1962.

214. Wilden, A. L., and Cardon, L.: *Salmonella typhimurium* osteomyelitis with sickle cell–hemoglobin C disease: A review and case report, Ann. Int. Med. 54:510, 1961.

215. Wilson, S., and Smith, D. B.: Separation of the valyl-leucyl and valyl-glutamyl polypeptide chains of hemoglobins by fractional precipitation and column chromatography, Canad. J. Biochem. & Physiol. 37:405, 1959.

216. Wintrobe, M. M.: Cardiovascular system in anemia, with a note on the particular abnormalities of sickle cell anemia, Blood 1:121, 1946.

217. Wolpers, C.: Elektronenmikroskopische Untersuchungen der Innenstrukturen kernloser Erythrocyten: I. Reticulocyten und Pseudoreticulocyten, Klin. Wchnschr. 34:61, 1956.
218. Wright, C. S., and Gardner, E.: Study of the role of acute. infections in precipitating crises in chronic hemolytic states, Ann. Int. Med. 52:530, 1960.
219. Wyman, J., Jr., and Allen, D. W.: Problem of the heme interactions in hemoglobin and the basis of the Bohr effect, J. Polymer Sc. 7:499, 1951.
220. Zamecnik, P. C.: The microsome, Scient. American 198:118, 1958.
221. Zuelzer, W. W., and Robinson, A. R.: Haemoglobin F: Its significance in the genetics and evolution of haemoglobin, Nature 19:237, 1961.
222. Zuelzer, W. W., Robinson, A. R., and Booker, C. R.: Reciprocal relationship of hemoglobins A_2 and F in beta chain thalassemias: A key to the genetic control of hemoglobin F, Blood 17:393, 1961.

CHAPTER FOUR
EFFECTS OF ANEMIA

1. Abramson, D. I., Fierst, S. M., and Flachs, K.: Resting peripheral blood flow in the anemic state, Am. Heart J. 25:609, 1943.
2. Abramson, D. I., Landt, H., and Benjamin, J. E.: Peripheral vascular response to acute anoxia, A.M.A. Arch. Int. Med. 71:583, 1953.
3. Bing, R. J., Hammond, M. M., Handelsman, J. C., Powers, S. R., Spencer, F. C., Eckenhoff, J. E., Goodale, W. T., Hafkenschiel, J. H., and Ketz, S. S.: Measurement of coronary blood flow, oxygen consumption, and efficiency of the left ventricle in man, Am. Heart J. 38:1, 1949.
4. Bing, R. J., and Daley, R.: Behavior of the myocardium in health and disease as studied by coronary sinus catheterization, Am. J. Med. 10:711, 1951.
5. Bishop, J. M., Donald, K. W., and Wade, O. L.: Circulatory dynamics at rest and on exercise in the hyperkinetic states, Clin. Sc. 14:329, 1955.
6. Blumgart, H. L., Gargill, S. L., and Gillman, D. R.: Studies in the velocity of blood flow: XV. Velocity of blood flow and other aspects of the circulation in patients with "primary" and secondary anemia and in two patients with polycythemia vera, J. Clin. Invest. 9:679, 1931.
7. Blumgart, H. L., and Altschule, M. D.: Clinical significance of cardiac and respiratory adjustments in chronic anemia, Blood 3:329, 1948.
8. Bradley, S. E., and Bradley, G. P.: Renal function during chronic anemia in man, Blood 2:192, 1947.
9. Bradley, S. E., Bradley, G. P., Tyson, C. J., Curry, J. J., and Blake, W. D.: Renal function in renal diseases, Am. J. Med. 9:766, 1950.
10. Brannon, E. S., Merrill, A. J., Warren, J. V., and Stead, E. A., Jr.: Cardiac output in patients with chronic anemia as measured by the technique of right atrial catheterization, J. Clin. Invest. 24:332, 1945.
11. Crowell, J. W., Ford, R. C., and Lewis, V. M.: Oxygen transport in hemorrhagic shock in function of hematocrit ratio, Am. J. Physiol. 196: 1033, 1959.
12. Duke, M., and Abelmann, W. H.: Central blood volume in the high output state of anemia, Clin. Res. 9:327, 1961.
13. Ebert, R. V., Stead, E. A., and Gibson, J. G.: Response of normal subjects to blood loss, Arch. Int. Med. 68:578, 1941.
14. Ellis, L. B., and Faulkner, J. M.: The heart in anemia, New England J. Med. 220:943, 1939.
15. Fowler, N. O., Franch, R. H., and Bloom, W. L.: Hemodynamic effects of anemia with and without plasma volume expansion, Circulation Res. 4:319, 1956.
16. Gibson, J. G., II, Harris, A. W., and Swigert, V. W.: Clinical studies of the blood volume: VIII. J. Clin. Invest. 18:621, 1939.
17. Goodale, W. T., Martin, L., Eckenhoff, J. E., Hafkenshiel, H., and Bonfield, W. G., Jr.: Coronary sinus catheterization for studying coronary blood flow and myocardial metabolism, Am. J. Physiol. 152:340, 1948.
18. Gregersen, M. I., and Rawson, R. A.: Blood volume, Physiol. Rev. 39:307, 1959.

19. Gupta, N. N.: Observations on renal function in anemias, J. Indian M.A. 14:297, 1945.

20. Guyton, A. C., Lindsey, A. W., Kaufman, B. N., and Abernathy, J. B.: Effect of blood transfusion and hemorrhage on cardiac output and on the venous return curve, Am. J. Physiol. 194:263, 1958.

21. Hunter, A.: The heart in anemia, Quart. J. Med. 15:107, 1946.

22. Jasinsk, B.: Pathologic electrocardiogram in deficiency anemias (iron deficiency, sprue, pernicious anemia) and its pathogenesis, Cardiologia 27:215, 1955.

23. Kennedy, A. C., and Valtis, D. J.: Oxygen dissociation curve in anemia of various types, J. Clin. Invest. 33:1372, 1954.

24. Kety, S. S.: Circulation and metabolism of the human brain in health and disease, Am. J. Med. 8:205, 1950.

25. Korner, P. J.: Circulatory adaptations in hypoxia, Physiol. Rev. 39:687, 1959.

26. Lindo, C. L., and Doctor, L. R.: Electrocardiogram in sickle cell anemia, Am. Heart J. 50:218, 1955.

27. Marshall, R. A.: Review of lesions of the optic fundus in various diseases of the blood, Blood 14:882, 1959.

28. Mendlowitz, M.: Effect of anemia and polycythemia on digital intravascular blood viscosity, J. Clin. Invest. 27:565, 1948.

29. Murray, J. F., Gold, P., and Johnson, B. L., Jr.: Systemic oxygen transport in induced normovolemic anemia and polycythemia, Clin. Rev. 9:93, 1961.

30. Myers, J. D.: Effects of anemia on hepatic blood flow and splanchnic metabolism, Am. J. Med. 11:248, 1951.

31. Pickering, G. W., and Wayne, E. J.: Observations on angina pectoris and intermittent claudication in anemia, Clin. Sc. 1:305, 1934.

32. Porter, W. B., and James, G. W., III: The heart in anemia, Circulation 8:111, 1953.

33. Rankin, J., McNeill, R. S., and Forster, R. E.: Effect of anemia on the alveolar-capillary exchange of carbon monoxide in man, J. Clin. Invest. 40:1323, 1961.

34. Richardson, T. Q., and Guyton, A. C.: Effects of polycythemia and anemia on cardiac output and other circulatory factors, Am. J. Physiol. 197:1167, 1959.

35. Rodman, T., Close, H. P., Cathcart, R., and Purcell, M. K.: Oxyhemoglobin dissociation curve in the common hemoglobinopathies, Am. J. Med. 27:558, 1959.

36. Rodman, T., Close, H. P., and Purcell, M. K.: Oxyhemoglobin dissociation curve in anemia, Ann. Int. Med. 52:295, 1960.

37. Romano, J., and Evans, J. W.: Symptomatic psychosis in a case of secondary anemia, Arch. Neurol. & Psychiat. 39:1295, 1938.

38. Ryan, J. M., and Hickan, J. B.: Alveolar-arterial oxygen pressure gradient in anemia, J. Clin. Invest. 31:188, 1952.

39. Sanghvi, L. M., Sharma, R., and Misra, S. N.: Cardiovascular disturbance in chronic severe anemia, Circulation 15:373, 1957.

40. Sanghvi, L. M., Misra, S. N., Banerjee, K., and Gupta, K. D.: Electrocardiogram in chronic severe anemia, Am. Heart J. 56:79, 1958.

41. Sanghvi, L. M., Misra, S. N., and Banerjee, K.: Cardiac enlargement in chronic anemia, Circulation 22:412, 1960.

42. Scheinberg, P.: Effects of postural change, stellate ganglion block and anemia on the cerebral circulation, J. Clin. Invest. 28:808, 1949.

43. Scheinberg, P.: Cerebral blood flow and metabolism in pernicious anemia, Blood 6:213, 1951.

44. Schilling, R. F., and Harris, J. W.: Liver function in untreated Addisonian pernicious anemia, J. Lab. & Clin. Med. 40:718, 1952.

45. Sharpey-Schafer, E. P.: Cardiac output in severe anemia, Clin. Sc. 5:125, 1944.
46. Siekert, R. G., Whisnant, J. P., and Millikan, C. H.: Anemia and intermittent focal cerebral arterial insufficiency, Arch. Neurol. 3:351, 1960.
47. Sproule, B. J., Holden, E. F., and Miller, W. F.: Study of cardiopulmonary alterations in patients with sickle cell disease and its variants, J. Clin. Invest. 37:486, 1958.
48. Sproule, B. J., Mitchell, J. H., and Miller, W. F.: Cardiopulmonary physiologic responses to heavy exercise in patients with anemia, J. Clin.. Invest. 39:378, 1960.
49. Strauss, M. B., and Fox, H. J.: Anemia and water retention, Am. J. M. Sc. 200:454, 1940.
50. Tandon, O. P., and Katiyar, B. C.: Ballistocardiographic changes in severe anaemia, Circulation 23:195, 1961.
51. Tybjaerg, H. A.: Osmotic pressure effect of the red blood cells: Possible physiological significance, Nature 190:504, 1961.
52. Valtis, D. J., and Baikie, A. G.: Influence of red cell thickness on the oxygen dissociation curve of blood, Brit. J. Haemat. 1:146, 1955.
53. Whitaker, W.: Some effects of severe chronic anaemia on the circulatory system, Quart. J. Med. 25:175, 1956.
54. Whyte, H. M.: Plasma and blood volume in anaemia and the effect of transfusion, Australasian Ann. Med. 5:192, 1956.
55. Wintrobe, M. M.: The cardiovascular system in anemia, with a note on the particular abnormalities of sickle cell anemia, Blood 1:121, 1946.
56. Zamcheck, M., Chalmers, T. C., White, F. W., and Davidson, C. S.: Bromsulfulein test in early diagnosis of liver disease in gross upper gastrointestinal hemorrhage, Gastroenterology 14:343, 1950.
57. Zoll, P. M., Wessler, S., and Blumgart, H. L.: Angina pectoris: A clinical and pathologic correlation, Am. J. Med. 11:331, 1951.

CHAPTER SIX

NORMAL RED CELL PRODUCTION

1. Alpen, E. L., and Cranmore, D.: Observations on the regulation of erythropoiesis and on cellular dynamics by Fe^{59} autoradiography, *in* Stohlman, F., Jr. (ed.), Kinetics of Cellular Proliferation, p. 290, Grune & Stratton, New York, 1959.
2. Alpen, E. L., and Cranmore, D.: Cellular kinetics and iron utilization in bone marrow as observed by Fe^{59} radioautography, Ann. New York Acad. Sc. 77:753, 1959.
3. Bessis, M., and Breton Gorius, J.: Diapédèse des réticulocytes et des érythroblasts, Compt. rend. Acad. sc. 251:465, 1960.
4. Bialestock, D.: Anaemia of renal origin, studied by micro-dissection of the kidney, Australasian Ann. Med. 9:44, 1960.
5. Bjorkman, S. E.: Method for determining absolute reticulocyte count, Scandinav. J. Clin. & Lab. Invest. 10:1435, 1958.
6. Bonsdorff, E., and Jalavisto, E.: Humoral mechanism in anoxic erythrocytosis, Acta physiol. scandinav. 16:150, 1948.
7. Bothwell, T. H., Callender, S., Mallett, B., and Witts, L. J.: Study of erythropoiesis using tracer quantities of radioactive iron, Brit. J. Haemat. 2:1, 1956.
8. Brecher, G., and Stohlman, F., Jr.: Humoral factors in erythropoiesis, Progr. Hemat. 2:110, 1959.
9. Brecher, G., and Stohlman, F., Jr.: Reticulocyte size and erythropoietic stimulation, Proc. Soc. Exper. Biol. & Med. 107:887, 1961.
10. Brown, T. E., and Meineke, H. A.: Presence of an active erythropoietic factor (erythropoietin) in plasma of rats after prolonged cobalt therapy, Proc. Soc. Exper. Biol. & Med. 99:435, 1958.
11. Carnot, P., and Déflandre, C.: Sur l'activité hémopoïétique du sérum, Compt. rend. Acad. sc. 143:384, 1906.
12. Castle, W. B., and Minot, G. R.: Pathologic Physiology and Clinical Description of the Anemia, Oxford University Press, New York, 1936.
13. Castle, W. B.: Erythropoiesis: Normal and abnormal, Bull. New York Acad. Med. 30:827, 1954.
14. Cronkite, E. P., Flieder, T. M., Bond, V. P., Rusini, J. R., Brecher, G., and Quastler, H.: Dynamics of hemopoietic proliferation in man and mice studied by H^3-thymidine incorporation into DNA, Ann. New York Acad. Sc. 77:803, 1959.
15. Crosby, W. H., Finch, C. A., Haurani, F. I., Stohlman, F., and Wasserman, L.: Participants in modern methods for quantitation of red blood cell production and destruction: Erythrokinetics, Blood 18:225, 1961.
16. Crowell, J. W., Ford, R. G., and Lewis, V. M.: Oxygen transport in hemorrhagic shock as a function of the hematocrit ratio, Am. J. Physiol. 196:1033, 1959.
17. Dacie, J. V., and White, J. C.: Erythropoiesis with particular reference to its study by biopsy of human bone marrow: A review, J. Clin. Path. 2:1, 1949.

17a. DeGowin, R. L., Hofstra, D., and Gurney, C. W.: Comparison of erythropoietin bioassays, Proc. Soc. Exper. Biol. & Med. 110:48, 1962.

18. Donohue, D. M., Gabrio, B. W., and Finch, C. A.: Quantitative measurements
of hematopoietic cells of the marrow, J. Clin. Invest. 37:1564, 1958.

19. Donohue, D. M., Reiff, R. H., Hanson, M. L., Betson, Y., and Finch, C. A.:
Quantitative measurement of the erythrocytic and granulocytic cells of the
marrow and blood, J. Clin. Invest. 37:1571, 1958.

20. Erslev, A. J.: Erythropoietic function in uremic rabbits: II. Effect of nephrectomy on red cell production and iron metabolism, Acta hemat. 23:226, 1960.

21. Erslev, A. J.: Hematology: Control of red cell production, Ann. Rev. Med.
11:315, 1960.

22. Erslev, A. J., and Hughes, J. R.: Influence of environment on iron incorporation and mitotic division in a suspension of normal bone marrow, Brit. J.
Haemat. 6:414, 1960.

23. Filmanowicz, E., and Gurney, C. W.: Studies on erythropoiesis: XVI. Response to a single dose of erythropoietin in polycythemic mouse, J. Lab. &
Clin. Med. 57:65, 1961.

24. Finch, C. A., Hanson, M. L., and Donohue, D. M.: Kinetics of erythropoiesis:
A comparison of response to anemia induced by phenylhydrazine and by
blood loss, Am. J. Physiol. 197:761, 1959.

25. Finch, C. A., and Noyes, W. D.: Erythrokinetics in diagnosis of anemia,
J.A.M.A. 175: 1163, 1961.

26. Gallagher, N. I., McCarthy, J. M., and Lange, R. D.: Observations on erythropoietic-stimulating factor (ESF) in the plasma of uremic and nonuremic
anemic patients, Ann. Int. Med. 52:1201, 1960.

27. Gallagher, N. I., McCarthy, J. M., and Lange, R. D.: Erythropoietin production in uremic rabbits, J. Lab. & Clin. Med. 57:281, 1961.

28. Gallagher, N. I., Hagan, D. Q., McCarthy, J. M., and Lange, R. D.: Response
of starved rats and polycythemic rats to graded doses of erythropoietin, Proc.
Soc. Exper. Biol. & Med. 106:127, 1961.

29. Gardner, F. H., and Pringle, J. C.: Androgens and erythropoietin, A.M.A.
Arch. Int. Med. 107:486, 1961.

30. Giblett, E. R., Coleman, D. H., Pirzio-Biroli, G., Donohue, D. M., Motulsky,
A. G., and Finch, C. A.: Erythrokinetics: Quantitative measurements of red
cell production and destruction in normal subjects and patients with anemia,
Blood 11:291, 1956.

31. Gley, P.: Double aspects of the hematopoietic hormone of serum, *in* Proceedings, Sixth Congress of the International Society of Hematology, p. 785,
Grune & Stratton, New York, 1958.

32. Goldwasser, E., Jacobson, L. O., Fried, W., and Plzak, L.: Mechanism of the
erythropoietic effect of cobalt, Science 125:1085, 1957.

33. Goldwasser, E., Fried, W., and Jacobson, L. O.: Studies on erythropoiesis:
VIII. Effect of nephrectomy on response to hepatic anoxia, J. Lab. & Clin.
Med. 52:375, 1958.

34. Gordon, A. S.: Hemopoietine, Physiol. Rev. 39:1, 1959.

35. Grant, W. C., and Root, W. S.: Fundamental stimulus for erythropoiesis,
Physiol. Rev. 32:449, 1952.

36. Grant, W. C., Linkenheimer, W. H., Patterson, E. L., and Berger, H.: Partial
purification of erythropoietin by alcoholic fractions, Proc. Soc. Exper. Biol.
& Med. 107:221, 1961.

37. Gray, D. F., and Erslev, A. J.: Reticulocytosis induced by serum from hypoxic
animals, Proc. Soc. Exper. Biol. & Med. 94:283, 1957.

38. Gurney, C. W., Jacobson, L. O., and Goldwasser, E.: Physiologic and clinical
significance of erythropoietin, Ann. Int. Med. 49:363, 1958.

39. Gurney, C. W., and Pan, C.: Studies on erythropoiesis: IX. Mechanism of decreased erythropoiesis in experimental polycythemia, Proc. Soc. Exper. Biol. & Med. 98:789, 1958.

40. Gurney, C. W., and Pan, C.: Studies on erythropoiesis: XIII. A comparison of methods of bio-assay of erythropoietin in human plasma, J. Lab. & Clin. Med. 55:67, 1960.

41. Gurney, C. W., Wackman, N., and Filmanowicz, E.: Studies on erythropoiesis: XVII. Some quantitative aspects of the erythropoietic response to erythropoietin, Blood 17:531, 1961.

41a. Harrison, W. J.: Total cellularity of the bone marrows in man, J. Clin. Path. 15: 254, 1962.

42. Haurani, F. I., and Tocantins, L. M.: Ineffective erythropoiesis, Am. J. Med. 31:519, 1961.

43. Hematopoietic mechanisms, Ann. New York Acad. Sc. 77:407, 1959.

44. Hodgson, G., Fischer, S., Perretta, M., Eskuche, I., Araya, G., and Dinamarca, M.: Separation and properties of urinary hemopoietin, Blood 16:1398, 1960.

45. Hodgson, G., Eskuche, I., Fischer, S., and Perretta, M.: Effects of urinary hemopoietine on Fe^{59} distribution in rats studied while plasma Fe^{59} is high, Proc. Soc. Exper. Biol. & Med. 104:441, 1960.

46. Isaacs, R.: Physiologic histology of bone marrow: The mechanism of the development of blood cells and their liberation into the peripheral circulation, Folia haemat. 40:395, 1930.

47. Jacobson, L. O., Goldwasser, E., Plzak, L. F., and Fried, W.: Studies on erythropoiesis: IV. Reticulocyte response of hypophysectomized and polycythemic rodents to erythropoietin, Proc. Soc. Exper. Biol. & Med. 94:243, 1957.

48. Jacobson, L. O., and Goldwasser, E.: Dynamic equilibrium of erythropoiesis: Homeostatic mechanisms, Brookhaven Symp. Biol. 10:110, 1957.

49. Jacobson, L. O., Gurney, C. W., and Goldwasser, E.: Control of erythropoiesis, Advances Int. Med. 10:297, 1960.

50. Jandl, J. H.: Agglutination and sequestration of immature red cells, J. Lab. & Clin. Med. 55:663, 1960.

51. Jones, B., and Klingberg, W. G.: Study of erythropoietin in two types of hemolytic anemia—erythroblastosis fetalis and sickle cell anemia, J. Pediat. 56:752, 1960.

52. Keighley, G., Lowy, P. H., Borsook, H., Goldwasser, E., Gordon, A. S., Prentice, T. C., Rambach, W. A., Stohlman, F., Jr., and Van Dyke, D. C.: Cooperative assay of a sample with erythropoietic stimulating activity, Blood 16:1424, 1960.

53. Kennedy, B. J., and Gilbertsen, A. S.: Increased erythropoiesis induced by androgenic-hormone therapy, New England J. Med. 256:719, 1957.

53a. Kirashima, K., and Takaku, F.: Experimental studies on erythropoietin: II. The relationship between juxtaglomerular cells and erythropoietin, Blood 20:1, 1962.

54. Krzymowski, T., and Krzymowska, H.: Studies on the erythropoiesis inhibiting factor in the plasma of animals with transfusion polycythemia, Blood 19:38, 1962.

55. Lajtha, L. G.: Bone marrow cell metabolism, Physiol. Rev. 37:50, 1957.

56. Lajtha, L. G.: Autoradiography in bone marrow studies, in University of London, British Postgraduate Medical Federation, The Scientific Basis of Medicine, Annual Reviews, Athlone Press, London, 1961.

57. Lange, R. D., McCarthy, J. M., and Gallagher, N. I.: Plasma and urinary erythropoietin in bone marrow failure, A.M.A. Arch. Int. Med. 108:94, 1961.

58. Levy, H., Levison, V., and Schade, A. L.: Effect of cobalt on the activity of certain enzymes in homogenates of rat tissue, Arch. Biochem. 27:34, 1950.

59. Linkenheimer, W. H., Grant, W. C., and Berger, H.: Erythropoietin and known erythropoietic stimuli, Proc. Soc. Exper. Biol. & Med. 104:230, 1960.

60. Linman, J. W., and Bethell, F. H.: Effect of irradiation on the plasma erythropoietic stimulating factor, Blood 12:123, 1957.

61. Linman, J. W., Bethell, F. H., and Long, M. J.: Studies on the nature of the plasma erythropoietic factor(s), J. Lab. & Clin. Med. 51:8, 1958.

62. Linman, J. W., Long, M. J., Korst, D. R., and Bethell, F. H.: Studies on the stimulation of hemopoiesis by batyl alcohol, J. Lab. & Clin. Med. 54:335, 1959.

63. Linman, J. W., and Bethell, F. H.: Factors Controlling Erythropoiesis, Charles C. Thomas, Springfield, Ill., 1960.

64. Linman, J. W.: Factors controlling hemopoiesis: Erythropoietic effects of "anemic" plasma, J. Lab. & Clin. Med. 59:249, 1962.

65. Lochte, H. L., Jr., Ferrebee, J. W., and Thomas, E. D.: Effect of heparin and EDTA on DNA synthesis by marrow *in vitro,* J. Lab. & Clin. Med. 55:435, 1960.

66. Lowy, P. H., Keighley, G., and Borsook, H.: Question of purity of erythropoietic factor concentrates, Proc. Soc. Exper. Biol. & Med. 99: 668, 1958.

67. Lowy, P. H., Keighley, G., Borsook, H., and Graybiel, A.: On the erythropoietic principle in the blood of rabbits made severely anemic with phenylhydrazine, Blood 14:262, 1959.

68. Matoth, Y., Ben-Porath, E. (Arkin), and Menzer, E.: Effect of erythropoietin on the mitotic rate of erythroblasts in bone marrow cultures, J. Lab. & Clin. Med. 54: 722, 1959.

69. Miescher, F.: Über die Beziehungen zwischen Meereshohe und Beshaffen heit des Blutes, Cor.-Bl. schweiz. Ärtze 23:809, 1893.

70. Mirand, E. A., and Prentice, T. C.: Presence of plasma erythropoietin in hypoxic rats with or without kidney(s) and/or spleen, Proc. Soc. Exper. Biol. & Med. 96:49, 1957.

71. Misrahy, G. A., Hardwick, D. F., Brooks, C. J., Garwood, V. P., and Hall, W. P.: Bone, bone marrow, and brain oxygen, Am. J. Physiol. 202:225, 1962.

72. Naets, J. P.: Erythropoietic factor in kidney tissue of anemic dogs, Proc. Soc. Exper. Biol. & Med. 103:129, 1960.

73. Naets, J. P.: Role of the kidney in erythropoiesis, J. Clin. Invest. 39:102, 1960.

74. Naets, J. P.: Role of the kidney in the production of the erythropoietic factor, Blood 16:1770, 1960.

75. Nakao, K., Takaku, F., and Hirashima, K.: Clinical studies on erythropoietic factor in plasma, Proc. Soc. Exper. Biol. & Med. 103:47, 1960.

75a. Noyes, W. D., Domm, B. M., and Willis, L. C.: Regulation of erythropoiesis: I. Erythropoietin assay as a clinical tool, Blood 20:9, 1962.

76. Osnes, S.: Experimental study of an erythropoietic principle produced in the kidney, Brit. M. J. 2:650, 1959.

77. Pease, D. C.: Electron microscopic study of red bone marrow, Blood 11:501, 1956.

78. Powsner, E. R., and Berman, L.: Correlation of radioactive hemin formation with morphologic alterations in cultures of human bone marrow, Blood 14:1213, 1959.

79. Prentice, T. C., and Mirand, E. A.: Studies of plasma erythropoietic factor in anemic human patients, Blood 12:993, 1957.

80. Red cell regulators, Lancet 1:810, 1960.

81. Reichlin, M., and Harrington, W. J.: Studies on erythropoietin: I. Demonstration of erythropoietin in normal plasma, Blood 16:1298, 1960.

82. Reiff, R. H., Nutter, J. Y., Donohue, D. M., and Finch, C. A.: Relative number of marrow reticulocytes, Am. J. Clin. Path. 30:199, 1958.

83. Reissmann, K. R.: Studies on the mechanisms of erythropoietic stimulation in parabiotic rats during hypoxia, Blood 5:372, 1950.

84. Reissmann, K. R., Nomura, T., Gunn, R. W., and Brosius, F.: Erythropoietic response to anemia or erythropoietin injection in uremic rats with or without functioning renal tissue, Blood 16:1411, 1960.

85. Reynafarje, C.: Influence of high altitude on erythropoietic activity, Brookhaven Symp. Biol. 10:132, 1957.

86. Rosse, W. F., and Gurney, C. W.: Studies on erythropoiesis: X. The use of bone marrow tissue culture in demonstrating erythropoietin, J. Lab. & Clin. Med. 53:446, 1959.

87. Rosse, W. F., and Waldmann, T. A.: Role of the kidney in the erythropoietic response to hypoxia in parabiotic rats, Blood 19:75, 1962.

88. Sacks, M. S.: Erythropoietin, Ann. Int. Med. 48:207, 1958.

89. Slaunwhite, W. R., Jr., Mirand, E. A., and Prentice, T. C.: Probable polypeptidic nature of erythropoietin, Proc. Soc. Exper. Biol. & Med. 96:616, 1957.

90. Stickney, J. C., and Van Liere, E. J.: Acclimatization to low oxygen tension, Physiol. Rev. 33:13, 1953.

91. Stohlman, F., Jr., and Brecher, G.: Humoral regulation of erythropoiesis: III. Effect of exposure to simulated altitude, J. Lab. & Clin. Med. 49:890, 1957.

92. Stohlman, F., Jr., and Brecher, G.: Humoral regulation of erythropoiesis: IV. Relative heat stability of erythropoietin, Proc. Soc. Exper. Biol. & Med. 95:797, 1957.

93. Stohlman, F., Jr. (ed.): Kinetics of Cellular Proliferation, Grune & Stratton, New York, 1959.

94. Stohlman, F., Jr., and Brecher, G.: Humoral regulation of erythropoiesis: V. Relationship of plasma erythropoietine level to bone marrow activity, Proc. Soc. Exper. Biol. & Med. 100:40, 1959.

95. Stohlman, F., Jr.: Observations on the changes in the kinetics of red cell proliferation following irradiation and hypertransfusion, Blood 16:1777, 1960.

96. Stohlman, F., Jr.: Humoral regulation of erythropoiesis: VI. Mechanism of action of erythropoietine in the irradiated animal, Proc. Soc. Exper. Biol. & Med. 107:751, 1961.

97. Stohlman, F., Jr.: Humoral regulation of erythropoiesis: VII. Shortened survival of erythrocytes produced by erythropoietine or severe anemia, Proc. Soc. Exper. Biol. & Med. 107:884, 1961.

98. Stohlman, F., Jr.: Use of Fe^{59} and Cr^{51} for estimating red cell production and destruction: An interpretive review, Blood 18:236, 1961.

99. Suki, W., and Grollman, A.: Role of the kidney in erythropoiesis, Am. J. Physiol. 199:629, 1960.

100. Swann, M. M.: Control of cell divisions: A review: I. General mechanisms, Cancer Res. 17:727, 1957.

101. Swann, M. M.: Control of cell divisions: II. Special mechanisms, Cancer Res. 18:1118, 1958.

102. Szur, L., and Smith, M. D.: Red cell production and destruction in myelosclerosis, Brit. J. Haemat. 7:147, 1961.

103. Tei, Y.: Production of hematopoietic substance in serum, J. Chosen M.A. 28:179, 1938.

104. Van Dyke, D. C., and Berlin, N. I.: Production of normal-lived erythrocytes with erythropoietin, Proc. Soc. Exper. Biol. & Med. 104:573, 1960.

105. Van Dyke, D. C., Layrisse, M., Lawrence, J. H., Garcia, J. F., and Pollycove, M.: Relation between severity of anemia and erythropoietin titer in human beings, Blood 18:187, 1961.

106. Waldmann, T. A., Weissman, S. M., and Berlin, N.: Effect of splenectomy on erythropoiesis in the dog, Blood 15:873, 1960.
107. Weiss, L.: Electron microscopic study of the vascular sinuses of the bone marrow of the rabbit, Bull. Johns Hopkins Hosp. 108:171, 1961.
108. White, W. F., Gurney, C. W., Goldwasser, E., and Jacobson, L. O.: Studies on erythropoietin, Progr. Hormone Res. 16:219, 1960.
109. Winkert, J., Gordon, A. S., Medici, P. T., Piliero, S. J., Luhby, A. L., and Tannenbaum, M.: Erythropoietic stimulating activity of urine from anemic human subjects, Proc. Soc. Exper. Biol. & Med. 97:191, 1958.
110. Wolstenholme, G. E. W., and O'Connor, M. (ed.): Symposium on Haemopoiesis: Cell Production and Its Regulation (Ciba Foundation Symposium), Little, Brown, Boston, 1960.
111. Zamboni, L., and Pease, D. C.: Vascular bed of red bone marrow, J. Ultrastructure Res. 5:65, 1961.

CHAPTER SEVEN

PERNICIOUS ANEMIA AND THE
NON-ADDISONIAN MEGALOBLASTIC ANEMIAS

1. Abeles, R. H., and Lee, H. A., Jr.: Intramolecular oxidation reduction requiring a vitamin B_{12} coenzyme, J. Biol. Chem. 236:1, 1961.
2. Abels, J., Vegter, J. J. M., Woldring, M. G., Hans, J. H., and Nieweg, H. O.: Physiologic mechanism of vitamin B_{12} absorption, Acta med. scandinav. 165:105, 1959.
3. Adams, J. F.: Therapeutic effect, utilization, and fate of injected vitamin B_{12} in man, Brit. M. J. 1:1735, 1961.
4. Adams, J. F.: Urinary excretion of assayable vitamin B_{12} and radioactivity after parenteral ^{58}Co B_{12} in man, J. Clin. Path. 14:351, 1961.
5. Adams, R. D., and Kubik, C. S.: Subacute degeneration of the brain in pernicious anemia, New England J. Med. 231:1, 1944.
6. Adlersberg, D. (ed.): The Malabsorption Syndrome, Grune & Stratton, New York, 1957.
7. Allcock, E.: Absorption of vitamin B_{12} in man following extensive resection of the jejunum, ileum and colon, Gastroenterology 40:81, 1961.
8. Anderson, B., Belcher, E. H., Chanarin, I., and Mollin, D. L.: Urinary and faecal excretion of radioactivity after oral doses of ^{3}H-folic acid, Brit. J. Haemat. 6:439, 1960.
9. Anemia after gastrectomy, Lancet 1:147, 1959.
10. Badenoch, J.: Blind loop syndrome, Proc. Roy. Soc. Med. 53:657, 1960.
11. Baker, S. J., Mackinnon, N. L., and Vasudeva, P.: Site of absorption of orally administered vitamin B_{12} in dogs, Indian J. M. Res. 46:812, 1958.
12. Baldwin, J. N., and Dalessio, D. J.: Folic acid therapy and spinal-cord degeneration in pernicious anemia, New England J. Med. 264:1339, 1961.
13. Barker, H. A., Smyth, R. D., Weissbach, H., Munch-Petersen, A., Toohey, J. I., Ladd, J. N., Volcani, B. E., and Wilson, R. M.: Assay, purification and properties of the adenylcobamide coenzyme, J. Biol. Chem. 235:181, 1960.
14. Barker, H. A., Smyth, R. D., Weissbach, H., Toohey, J. I., Ladd, J. N., and Volcani, B. E.: Isolation and properties of crystalline cobamide coenzymes containing benzimidazole or 5, 6-dimethylbenzimidazole, J. Biol. Chem. 235:480, 1960.
15. Barker, H. A.: Structure and function of cobamide coenzymes, Fed. Proc. 20:956, 1961.
16. Beck, W. S.: Metabolic functions of vitamin B_{12}, New England J. Med. 266:708, 1962.
17. Berkson, J., Comfort, M. W., and Butt, H. R.: Occurrence of gastric cancer in persons with achlorhydria and with pernicious anemia, Proc. Staff Meet. Mayo Clin. 31:583, 1956.
18. Berlin, R., Berlin, H., Brante, G., and Sjoberg, S. G.: Refractoriness to intrinsic factor-B_{12} preparations abolished by massive doses of intrinsic factor, Acta med. scandinav. 162:317, 1958.
19. Berlyne, G. M., Liversedge, L. A., and Emery, E. W.: Radioactive vitamin B_{12} in the diagnosis of neurological disorders, Lancet 1:294, 1957.

20. Boddington, M. M., and Spriggs, A. I.: Epithelial cells in megaloblastic anemias, J. Clin. Path. 12:228, 1959.

21. Bok, J., Faber, J. G., DeVries, J. A., Kroese, W. F. S., and Nieweg, H. O.: Effect of pteroylglutamic acid administration on the serum vitamin B_{12} concentration in pernicious anemia in relapse, J. Lab. & Clin. Med. 51:667, 1958.

22. Booth, C. C., and Mollin, D. L.: Site of absorption of vitamin B_{12} in man, Lancet 1:18, 1959.

23. Booth, C. C., and Mollin, D. L.: Blind loop syndrome, Proc. Roy. Soc. Med. 53:658, 1960.

24. Brante, G., and Ernberg, T.: In vitro uptake of vitamin B_{12} by *Diphyllobothrium latum* and its blockage by intrinsic factor, Scandinav. J. Clin. & Lab. Invest. 9:313, 1957.

25. Brodine, C., Friedman, B. I., Saenger, E. L., and Will, J. J.: Absorption of vitamin B_{12} labeled with radioactive cobalt-60 following subtotal gastrectomy, J. Lab. & Clin. Med. 53:220, 1959.

26. Brody, E. A., Estren, S., and Wasserman, L. R.: Treatment of pernicious anemia by oral administration of vitamin B_{12} without added intrinsic factor, New England J. Med. 260:361, 1959.

27. Brody, E. A., Estren, S., and Wasserman, L. R.: Kinetics of intravenously injected radioactive vitamin B_{12}: Studies on normal subjects and patients with chronic myelocytic leukemia and pernicious anemia, Blood 15:646, 1960.

28. Broquist, H. P., and Luhby, A. L.: Detection and isolation of formiminoglutamic acid from urine in folic acid deficiency in humans, Proc. Soc. Exper. Biol. & Med. 100:349, 1959.

29. Buchanan, J. M., Hartman, S. C., Herrmann, R. L., and Day, R. A.: Reactions involving the carbon-nitrogen bond: Heterocyclic compounds, J. Cell. & Comp. Physiol. 54:139 (Suppl. 1) 1959.

30. Bunge, M. B., Schloesser, L. L., and Schilling, R. F.: Intrinsic factor studies: IV. Selective absorption and binding of cyanocobalamin by gastric juice in the presence of excess pseudovitamin B_{12} or 5, 6-dimethylbenzimidazole, J. Lab. & Clin. Med. 48:735, 1956.

31. Bunge, M. B., and Schilling, R. F.: Intrinsic factor studies: VI. Competition for vitamin B_{12} binding sites offered by analogues of the vitamin, Proc. Soc. Exper. Biol. & Med. 96:587, 1957.

32. Callender, S. T., and Evans, J. R.: Observations on the relationship of intrinsic factor to the absorption of labelled vitamin B_{12} from the intestine, Clin. Sc. 14:387, 1955.

33. Callender, S. T., and Denborough, M. A.: Family study of pernicious anaemia, Brit. J. Haemat. 3:88, 1957.

34. Callender, S. T., Retief, F. P., and Witts, L. J.: Augmented histamine test with special reference to achlorhydria, Gut 1:326, 1960.

35. Callender, S. T., Witts, L. J., Allison, P. R., and Ganning, A.: Some metabolic and haematologic effects of oesophago-jejunostomy with by-pass of the stomach, Gut 2:150, 1961.

36. Castle, W. B.: Present status of the etiology of pernicious anemia, Ann. Int. Med. 34:1053, 1951.

37. Castle, W. B.: Development of knowledge concerning the gastric intrinsic factor and its relation to pernicious anemia, New England J. Med. 249:603, 1953.

38. Castle, W. B.: Factors involved in the absorption of vitamin B_{12}, Gastroenterology 37:377, 1959.

39. Castle, W. B.: Advances in physiology derived from the study of anemia in

man, *in* Beecher, H. K. (ed.), Disease and the Advancement of Basic Science, p. 132, Harvard University Press, Cambridge, Mass., 1960.

40. Castro, Z., Herbert, V., and Wasserman, L. R.: Blocking of hog intrinsic factor by human gastric juice and certain mucopolysaccharides, including blood group substance, J. Clin. Invest. 40:66, 1961.

41. Causes of pernicious anaemia, Brit. M. J. 2:282, 1960.

42. Chanarin, I., Elmes, P. C., and Mollin, D. L.: Folic-acid studies in megaloblastic anaemia due to primidone, Brit. M. J. 2:80, 1958.

43. Chanarin, I., and Bennett, M.: Disposal of small doses of intravenously injected folic acid, Brit. J. Haemat. 8:28, 1962.

43a. Chanarin, I., Bennett, M. C., and Berry, V.: Urinary excretion of histidine derivatives in megaloblastic anemia and other conditions and a comparison with the folic acid clearance test, J. Clin. Path. 15: 269, 1962.

44. Citrin, Y., DeRosa, C., and Halsted, J. A.: Sites of absorption of vitamin B_{12}, J. Lab. & Clin. Med. 50:667, 1957.

45. Clement, D. H., Nichol, C. A., and Welch, A. D.: A case of juvenile pernicious anemia: Study of the effects of folic acid and vitamin B_{12}, Blood 17:618, 1961.

46. Colle, E., Greenberg, L., and Krivit, W.: Studies of a patient with selective deficiency in absorption of vitamin B_{12}, Blood 18:48, 1961.

47. Conley, C. L., and Krevans, J. R.: Development of neurologic manifestations of pernicious anemia during multivitamin therapy, New England J. Med. 245:529, 1951.

48. Cooper, B. A., and Castle, W. B.: Sequential mechanisms in the enhanced absorption of vitamin B_{12} by intrinsic factor in the rat, J. Clin. Invest. 39:199, 1960.

49. Cooper, B. A., and Lowenstein, L.: Evaluation of assessment of folic acid deficiency by serum folic acid activity measured with *L. casei*, Canad. M.A.J. 18:987, 1961.

50. Cooperman, J. M., Lubb, A. L., Taller, D. N., and Marley, J. F.: Distribution of radioactive and nonradioactive vitamin B_{12} in the dog, J. Biol. Chem. 235:191, 1960.

51. Cox, E. V., Meynell, M. J., Cooke, W. T., and Gaddie, R.: Folic acid and cyanocobalamin in pernicious anemia, Clin. Sc. 17:693, 1958.

52. Cox, E. V., Meynell, M. J., Cooke, W. T., and Gaddie, R.: Scurvy and anemia, Am. J. Med. 32:240, 1962.

53. Dacie, J. V., and White, J. C.: Erythropoiesis with particular reference to its study by biopsy of human bone marrow: A review, J. Clin. Path. 2:1, 1949.

54. Darby, W. J., Bridgforth, E. B., LeBrocquy, J., Clark, S. I., Dutra de Oliveira, J., Kevany, J., and McGanity, W. J.: Vitamin B_{12} requirement of adult man, Am. J. Med. 25:726, 1958.

55. Darby, W. J., Jones, E., Clark, S. L., McGanity, W. J., Dutra de Oliveira, J., Perez, C., Kevany, J., and LeBrocquy, J.: Development of vitamin B_{12} deficiency by untreated patients with pernicious anemia, Am. J. Clin. Nutrition 6:513, 1958.

56. Davidson, C. S., Murphy, J. C., Watson, R. J., and Castle, W. B.: Comparison of the effects of massive blood transfusions and of liver extract in pernicious anemia, J. Clin. Invest. 25:858, 1946.

57. Davidson, L. S. P., Davis, L. J., and Innes, J.: Effect of liver therapy on erythropoiesis as observed by serial sternal punctures in twelve cases of pernicious anemia, Quart. J. Med. 11:19, 1942.

58. Davidson, L. S. P.: Thirty years' experience of the megaloblastic anemias, Edinburgh M. J. 59:315, 1952.

59. Davidson, Sir Stanley: Clinical picture of pernicious anaemia prior to introduction of liver therapy in 1926 and in Edinburgh subsequent to 1944, Brit. M. J. 1:241, 1957.

60. Davis, L. J., and Brown, A.: The Megaloblastic Anaemias, Blackwell, Oxford, 1953.

61. Deller, D. J., Germar, H., and Witts, L. J.: Effect of food on absorption of radioactive vitamin B_{12}, Lancet 1:574, 1961.

62. Deller, D. J., and Witts, L. J.: Changes in the blood after partial gastrectomy with special reference to vitamin B_{12}: I. Quart. J. Med. 31:71, 1962.

63. Deller, D. J., Richards, W. C. D., and Witts, L. J.: Changes in the blood after partial gastrectomy with special reference to vitamin B_{12}: II. Quart. J. Med. 31:89, 1962.

64. Denny-Brown, D.: Combined system disease, *in* Cecil, R. L., and Loeb, R. F. (ed.), Textbook of Medicine, ed. 10, p. 1505, Saunders, Philadelphia, 1959.

65. Doscherholmen, A., and Hagen, P. S.: Dual mechanism of vitamin B_{12} plasma absorption, J. Clin. Invest. 36:1551, 1957.

66. Doscherholmen, A., and Hagen, P. S.: Delay of absorption of radiolabeled cyanocobalamin in the intestinal wall in the presence of intrinsic factor, J. Lab. & Clin. Med. 54:434, 1959.

67. Doscherholmen, A., Finley, P. R., and Hagen, P. S.: Distribution of radioactivity in man after the oral ingestion of small test doses of radiolabeled cyanocobalamin, J. Lab. & Clin. Med. 56:547, 1960.

68. Downey, H.: The megaloblast-normoblast problem, J. Lab. & Clin. Med. 39:837, 1952.

69. Eilenberg, M. D.: Psychiatric illness and pernicious anaemia: A clinical re-evaluation, J. Ment. Sc. 106:1939, 1960.

70. Ellenbogen, L., Burson, S. L., and Williams, W. L.: Purification of intrinsic factor, Proc. Soc. Exper. Biol. & Med. 97:760, 1958.

71. Enoksson, P., and Norden, A.: Vitamin B_{12} deficiency affecting the optic nerve, Acta med. scandinav. 167:199, 1960.

72. Estren, S., and Wasserman, L. R.: Pernicious anemia: I. Remission by small oral doses of purified vitamin B_{12}, Proc. Soc. Exper. Biol. & Med. 91:499, 1956.

73. Estren, S., Brody, E. A., and Wasserman, L. R.: Metabolism of vitamin B_{12} in pernicious and other megaloblastic anemias, Advances Int. Med. 9:11, 1958.

74. Estren, S., Brody, E. A., and Wasserman, L. R.: Disappearance of intravenously administered vitamin B_{12}: Studies in normal subjects and in patients with pernicious anemia, Am. J. Clin. Nutrition 8:259, 1960.

75. Exfoliative cytology in pernicious anaemia, Lancet 2:591, 1960.

76. Farrant, P. C.: Nuclear changes in oral epithelium in pernicious anaemia, Lancet 1:830, 1958.

77. Finch, C. A., Coleman, D. H., Motulsky, A. G., Donohue, D. M., and Reiff, R. H.: Erythrokinetics in pernicious anemia, Blood 11:807, 1956.

78. Flexner, J. M., and Hartmann, R. C.: Megaloblastic anemia associated with anticonvulsant drugs, Am. J. Med. 28:386, 1960.

79. Folic acid cycle in methionine biosynthesis established (editorial), Chem. & Engin. News 40:36, 1962.

80. Follis, R. H.: Deficiency Disease, Charles C. Thomas, Springfield, Ill., 1958.

81. Fone, D. J., Cooke, W. T., Meynell, M. J., and Harris, E. L.: Co^{58} B_{12} absorption (hepatic surface count) after gastrectomy, ileal resection, and in coeliac disorders, Gut 2:218, 1961.

82. Fowler, D., Cox, E. V., Cooke, W. T., and Meynell, M. J.: Aminoaciduria and megaloblastic anaemia, J. Clin. Path. 13:230, 1960.

83. Fox, M. R. S., and Ludwig, W. J.: Excretion of formiminoglutamic acid as an index of vitamin B_{12}, folic acid, and methionine deficiencies, Proc. Soc. Exper. Biol. & Med. 108:703, 1961.

84. Fox, M. R. S., Ludwig, W. J., and Baroody, M. C.: Effects of vitamin B_{12} and methionine on excretion of formiminoglutamic acid by the chick, Proc. Soc. Exper. Biol. & Med. 107:723, 1961.

85. Fraser, T. N.: Cerebral manifestations of Addisonian pernicious anemia, Lancet 2:458, 1960.

86. Frost, J. W., Goldwein, M. I., and Kaufman, B. D.: Studies of B_{12} Co^{60} absorption in malabsorption syndrome: Results before and during specific therapy, Am. Int. Med. 47:293, 1957.

87. Fudenberg, H., and Estren, S.: Non-Addisonian megaloblastic anemia, Am. J. Med. 25:198, 1958.

88. Gardner, F. H.: Gastrointestinal flora and the red cells, Am. J. Digest. Dis. 2:175, 1957.

89. Gardner, F. H.: Tropical sprue, New England J. Med. 258:835, 1958.

90. Gehrmann, G.: Histaminrefraktäre Anazidität und Perniciosa: Resorptionsstudien mit radioaktiven Vitamin B_{12}, Deutsche med. Wchnschr. 85:2233, 1960.

91. Girdwood, R. H.: Megaloblastic anaemias, Quart. J. Med. 25:87, 1956.

92. Girdwood, R. H.: Folic acid, its analogs and antagonists, Advances Clin. Chem. 3:236, 1960.

93. Glass, G. B. J., Boyd, L. J., Rubinstein, M. A., and Svigals, C. S.: Relationship of glandular mucoprotein from human gastric juice to Castle's intrinsic antianemia factor, Science 115:101, 1952.

94. Glass, G. B. J., Boyd, L. J., Stephanson, L., and Jones, E. L.: Metabolic interrelations between intrinsic factor and vitamin B_{12}: III. B_{12} absorption at varied intrinsic factor doses, Proc. Soc. Exper. Biol. & Med. 88:1, 1955.

95. Glass, G. B. J., Goldbloom, A., Boyd, L. J., Laughton, R., Rosen, S., and Rich, M.: Intestinal absorption and hepatic uptake of radioactive vitamin B_{12} in various age groups and the effect of intrinsic factor preparations, Am. J. Clin. Nutrition 4:124, 1956.

96. Glass, G. B. J.: Radioactive vitamin B_{12} in the liver: III. Hepatic storage and discharge of Co^{60} B_{12} in pernicious anemia, J. Lab. & Clin. Med. 52:875, 1958.

97. Glass, G. B. J., Lee, D. H., and Hardy, W. W.: Hydroxocobalamin: II. Absorption from the site of injection and uptake by the liver and calf muscle in man, Blood 18:522, 1961.

98. Glass, G. B. J., Skeggs, H. R., Lee, D. H., Jones, E. L., and Hardy, W. W.: Hydroxocobalamin: I. Blood levels and urinary excretion of vitamin B_{12} in man after a single parenteral dose of aqueous hydroxocobalamin, aqueous cyanocobalamin and cyanocobalamin zinc-tannate complex, Blood 18:511, 1961.

99. Glazer, H. S., Mueller, J. F., Jarrold, T., Sakurei, K., Will, J. J., and Vilter, R. W.: Effect of vitamin B_{12} and folic acid on nucleic acid composition of the bone marrow of patients with megaloblastic anemia, J. Lab. & Clin. Med. 43:905, 1954.

100. Graham, R. M.: Characteristic cellular changes in epithelial cells in pernicious anemia, J. Lab. & Clin. Med. 43:235, 1954.

101. Grasbeck, R., Nyberg, W., and Reizenstein, P.: Biliary and fecal vitamin B_{12} excretion in man, Proc. Soc. Exper. Biol. & Med. 97:780, 1958.

102. Grasbeck, R.: Physiology and pathology of vitamin B_{12} absorption, distribution, and excretion, Advances Clin. Chem. 3:299, 1960.

103. Grasbeck, R., Bjorksten, F., and Nyberg, W.: Urinary excretion of formimino-glutamic acid in folic-acid deficiency, Nord. med. 66:1343, 1961.

104. Grasbeck, R., Nyberg, W., Saarni, M., and Von Bonsdorff, B.: Lognormal distribution of serum vitamin B_{12} levels and dependence of blood values on the B_{12} level in a large population heavily infected with *Diphyllobothrium latum*, J. Lab. & Clin. Med. 59:419, 1962.

104a. Grossowicz, N., Rachmilewitz, M., Izak, G., and Zan, S.: Determination of folic acid metabolites in normal subjects and in patients with nutritional megaloblastic anemia, Proc. Soc. Exper. Biol. & Med. 109:770, 1962.

105. Gydell, K.: Megaloblastic anemia in patients treated with diphenylhydantoin and primidone, Acta haemat. 17:1, 1957.

106. Hall, C. A.: Plasma disappearance of intravenously administered cobalt[58] vitamin B_{12}, J. Clin. Invest. 39:1312, 1960.

107. Hall, C. A.: Plasma disappearance of radioactive vitamin B_{12} in myeloproliferative diseases and other blood disorders, Blood 18:717, 1961.

108. Halsted, J. A., Briggs, J. D., and Gasster, M.: Nutritional problems after total gastrectomy, New York J. Med. 57:223, 1957.

109. Halsted, J. A., Carroll, J., and Rubert, S.: Serum and tissue concentrations of vitamin B_{12} in certain pathological states, New England J. Med. 260:575, 1959.

110. Hamilton, H. E., Sheets, R. F., and DeGowin, E. L.: Studies with inagglutinable erythrocyte counts: VII. Further investigation of the hemolytic mechanism in untreated pernicious anemia and the demonstration of a hemolytic property in the plasma, J. Lab. & Clin. Med. 51:942, 1958.

111. Hamilton, H. E., Ellis, P. P., and Sheets, R. F.: Visual impairment due to optic neuropathy in pernicious anemia: Report of a case and review of the literature, Blood 14:378, 1959.

112. Harrison, R. J., Booth, C. C., and Mollin, D. L.: Vitamin B_{12} deficiency due to defective diet, Lancet 1:727, 1956.

113. Hawkins, C. F., and Meynell, M. J.: Macrocytosis and macrocytic anaemia caused by anticonvulsant drugs, Quart. J. Med. 27:45, 1958.

114. Heaton, J. M., McCormick, A. J. A., and Freeman, A. G.: Tobacco amblyopia: A clinical manifestation of vitamin B_{12} deficiency, Lancet 1:286, 1958.

115. Hedbom, A.: A native cobalamin-polypeptide complex from liver: Isolation and characterization, Biochem. J. 74:307, 1960.

116. Hedbom, A.: A native cobalamin-polypeptide complex from liver: Amino-acid composition and terminal amino acid analyses of the peptide part, Biochem. J. 79:469, 1961.

117. Heinrich, H. C. (ed.), Vitamin B_{12} und intrinsic Factor, Enke, Stuttgart, 1957.

118. Herbert, V.: Mechanism of intrinsic factor action in everted sacs of rat small intestine, J. Clin. Invest. 38:102, 1959.

119. Herbert, V.: Studies on the role of intrinsic factor in vitamin B_{12} absorption, transport, and storage, Am. J. Clin. Nutrition 7:433, 1959.

120. Herbert, V.: The Megaloblastic Anemias: Modern Medical Monographs, Grune & Stratton, New York, 1959.

121. Herbert, V.: Mechanism of absorption of vitamin B_{12}, Fed. Proc. 19:884, 1960.

122. Herbert, V., Baker, H., Frank, O., Pasher, I., Sobotka, H., and Wasserman, L. R.: Measurement of folic acid activity in serum: A diagnostic aid in the differentiation of the megaloblastic anemias, Blood 15:228, 1960.

123. Herbert, V.: Assay and nature of folic acid activity in human serum, J. Clin. Invest. 40:81, 1961.

124. Herbert, V., and Castle, W. B.: Divalent cation and pH dependence of rat intrinsic factor action in everted sacs and mucosal homogenates of rat small intestine, J. Clin. Invest. 40:1978, 1961.

125. Herbert, V., and Kaplan, M. E.: Studies suggesting the presence of intrinsic factor in bile, Proc. Soc. Exper. Biol. & Med. 107:900, 1961.

125a. Herbert, V., Larrabee, A. R., and Buchanan, J. M.: Studies on the identification of a folate compound of human serum, J. Clin. Invest. 41:1134, 1962.

126. Hitchcock, C. R., MacLean, L. D., and Sullivan, W. A.: Secretory and clinical aspects of achlorhydria and gastric atrophy as precursors of gastric cancer, J. Nat. Cancer Inst. 18:795, 1957.

127. Horrigan, D., Jarrold, T., and Vilter, R. W.: Direct action of vitamin B_{12} upon human bone marrow, J. Clin. Invest. 30:31, 1951.

128. Huguley, C. M., Jr., Bain, J. A., Rivers, S. L., and Scoggins, R. B.: Refractory megaloblastic anemia associated with excretion of orotic acid, Blood 14:615, 1959.

129. Huguley, C. M., and Bain, J. A.: Oroticaciduria, in Stanbury, J. B., Wyngaarden, J. B., and Fredrickson, D. S. (ed.), Metabolic Basis of Inherited Disease, p. 776, McGraw-Hill, New York, 1960.

130. Hyland, H. H., Watts, G. O., and Farquharson, R. F.: Course of subacute combined degeneration of the spinal cord, Canad. M.A.J. 65:295, 1951.

131. Israels, L. G., and Zipursky, A.: Primary shunt hyperbilirubinaemia, Nature 193:73, 1962.

132. Jacobs, A.: Pernicious anemia, 1822–1929, A.M.A. Arch. Int. Med. 103:329, 1959.

132a. Jeffries, G. H., Hoskins, D. W., and Sleisenger, M. H.: Antibody to intrinsic factor in serum from patients with pernicious anemia, J. Clin. Invest. 41:1106, 1962.

133. Johns, D. G., Sperti, S., and Burgen, A. S. V.: Disposal of tritiated folic acid injected intravenously in man, Canad. M.A.J. 84:77, 1961.

134. Johns, D. G., Sperti, S., and Burgen, A. S. V.: Metabolism of tritiated folic acid in man, J. Clin. Invest. 40:1684, 1961.

135. Jones, O. P.: Influence of disturbed metabolism on the morphology of blood cells, in MacFarlane, R. G., and Ross-Smith, A. H. T. (ed.), Functions of the Blood, p. 172, Academic Press, New York, 1961.

136. Kaplan, H. S., and Rigler, L. G.: Pernicious anemia and carcinoma of the stomach: Autopsy studies concerning their interrelationships, Am. J. M. Sc. 209:339, 1945.

137. Keeley, K. J., and Politzer, W. M.: Amino-aciduria in the megaloblastic anaemias, J. Clin. Path. 9:142, 1956.

138. Keuning, F. J., Arends, A., Mandema, E., and Nieweg, H. O.: Observations on the site or production of Castle's intrinsic factor in the rat, J. Lab. & Clin. Med. 53:127, 1959.

139. Killander, A.: Oral treatment of pernicious anaemia with vitamin B_{12} and purified intrinsic factor: II. Studies on the reduced effect of prolonged treatment, Acta Soc. med. upsalien. 63:1, 1958.

140. Killander, A.: Subacute combined degeneration of the spinal cord: The diagnostic value of serum vitamin B_{12} assay, Acta med. scandinav. 60:75, 1958.

141. Killander, A., and Schilling, R. F.: Studies on hydroxo-cobalamin: I. Excretion and retention of massive doses in control subjects, J. Lab. & Clin. Med. 57:553, 1961.

142. Knowles, J. P., Prankerd, T. A. J., and Westall, R. G.: Simplified method for detecting FIGLU in urine as a test of folic-acid deficiency, Lancet 2:340, 1960.

143. Kohn, J., Mollin, D. L., and Rosenbach, L. M.: Conventional voltage electrophoresis for formiminoglutamic acid determination of folic acid deficiency,
J. Clin. Path. 14:345, 1961.

144. Lambert, H. P., Prankerd, T. A. J., and Smellie, J. M.: Pernicious anaemia in
childhood, Quart. J. Med. 30:71, 1961.

145. Larrabee, A. R., Rosenthal, S., Cathon, R., and Buchanan, J. M.: A methyl-
ated derivative of tetrahydrofolate as an intermediate of methionine biosynthesis, J. Am. Chem. Soc. 83:4094, 1961.

146. Latner, A. L., Merrills, R. J., and Raine, L.: Preparation of highly potent
intrinsic factor mucoprotein, Biochem. J. 63:501, 1956.

147. Latner, A. L.: Intrinsic factor and vitamin B_{12} absorption, Brit. M. J. 2:278,
1958.

148. Lear, A. A., Harris, J. W., Castle, W. B., and Fleming, E. M.: Serum vitamin
B_{12} concentration in pernicious anemia, J. Lab. & Clin. Med. 44:715, 1954.

149. Lear, A. A.: Effect of folic acid on serum vitamin B_{12} concentrations in pernicious anemia, J. Clin. Invest. 34:948, 1955.

150. Lee, D. H., and Glass, G. B. J.: Hepatic uptake and intestinal absorption of
Co^{58}-labelled 5, 6-dimethylbenzimidazolyl cobamide coenzyme, Proc. Soc.
Exper. Biol. & Med. 107:293, 1961.

151. Leikin, S. L.: Pernicious anemia in childhood, Pediatrics 25:91, 1960.

152. Lengyel, P., Mazumder, R., and Ochoa, S.: Mammalian methylmalonyl
isomerase and vitamin B_{12} coenzymes, Proc. Nat. Acad. Sc. 46:1312, 1960.

153. Lenhert, P. G., and Hodgkin, D. C.: Structure of 5, 6-dimethylbenzimidazolyl
cobamide coenzyme, Nature 192:937, 1961.

154. Lerman, S., and Feldmahn, A. L.: Centrocecal scotomata as presenting sign
in pernicious anemia, A.M.A. Arch. Ophth. 65:381, 1961.

155. Lewis, U. J., Register, U. D., Thompson, H. T., and Elvehjem, C. A.: Distribution of vitamin B_{12} in natural materials, Proc. Soc. Exper. Biol. & Med.
72:479, 1949.

156. Limarzi, L.: Effect of argenic (Fowler's solution) on erythropoiesis: A contribution to the megaloblast-normoblast problem, Am. J. M. Sc. 206:339,
1943.

157. Loewenstein, F.: Absorption of cobalt[60]-labeled vitamin B_{12} after subtotal
gastrectomy, Blood 13:339, 1958.

158. London, I. M., and West, R.: Formation of bile pigments in pernicious
anemia, J. Biol. Chem. 184:359, 1950.

159. London, I. M., West, R., Shemin, D., and Rittenberg, D.: On the origin of
bile pigment in normal man, J. Biol. Chem. 184:351, 1950.

160. Lous, P., and Schwartz, M.: Absorption of vitamin B_{12} following partial gastrectomy, Acta med. scandinav. 164:407, 1959.

161. Lowenstein, L., Cooper, B. A., Brunton, L., and Gartha, S.: Immunologic
basis for acquired resistance to oral administration of hog intrinsic factor
and vitamin B_{12} in pernicious anemia, J. Clin. Invest. 40:1656, 1961.

162. Luhby, A. L., Cooperman, J. M., and Teller, D. N.: Histidine metabolic loading test to distinguish folic acid deficiency from vitamin B_{12} in megaloblastic
anemias, Proc. Soc. Exper. Biol. & Med. 101:350, 1959.

163. Luhby, A. L., Cooperman, J. M., and Teller, D. N.: Urinary excretion of
formiminoglutamic acid, Am. J. Clin. Nutrition 7:397, 1959.

164. Lustberg, A., Goldman, D., and Dreskin, O.: Megaloblastic anemia due to
dilantin therapy, Ann. Int. Med. 54:153, 1961.

165. MacIntyre, H. W., and Stent, L.: Anaemia following partial gastrectomy:
A review of 100 cases, Brit. J. Surg. 44:150, 1956.

166. MacLean, L. D., and Sandberg, R. D.: Incidence of megaloblastic anemia
after total gastrectomy, New England J. Med. 254:885, 1956.

167. MacLean, L. D.: Incidence of megaloblastic anemia after subtotal gastrectomy, New England J. Med. 257:262, 1957.
168. Magnus, H. A.: Re-assessment of the gastric lesion in pernicious anemia, J. Clin. Path. 11:289, 1958.
169. Magnus, H. A.: The stomach in pernicious anemia, Acta haemat. 24:6, 1960.
170. Mallarmet, J.: Study of the myelogram in pernicious anemia and the problem of the megaloblast, Blood 3:103, 1948.
171. Marshall, R. A., and Jandl, J. H.: Responses to "physiologic" doses of folic acid in megaloblastic anemias, A.M.A. Arch. Int. Med. 105:352, 1960.
172. Mason, J. D., Jr., and Leavell, B. S.: Effect of transfusions of erythrocytes on untreated pernicious anemia, Blood 11:632, 1956.
173. McIntyre, P. A., Hahn, R., Conley, C. L., and Glass, B.: Genetic factors in predisposition to pernicious anemia, Bull. Johns Hopkins Hosp. 104:309, 1959.
174. McIntyre, P. A., Hahn, R., Masters, J. M., and Krevans, J. R.: Treatment of pernicious anemia with orally administered cyanocobalamin (vitamin B_{12}), A.M.A. Arch. Int. Med. 106:280, 1960.
175. Meyer, L. M., Meyer, R. M., Bertcher, R. W., Cronkite, E. P., Suarez, R. M., Miller, I. F., Mulzac, C. W., and Olvaretta, S. T.: Co^{60} vitamin B_{12} binding capacity of serum in persons with hematologic disorders, various medical diseases, and neoplasms, Acta med. scandinav. 169:557, 1961.
176. Milhaud, G.: Intestinal absorption of vitamin B_{12} and of vitamin B_{12} peptide complex in normal subjects and in patients with partial gastrectomy, Nature 189:33, 1961.
177. Miller, O. N., and Hunter, F. M.: Stimulation of vitamin B_{12} uptake in tissue slices by intrinsic factor concentrate, Proc. Soc. Exper. Biol. & Med. 96:39, 1957.
178. Minot, G. R., and Murphy, W. P.: Treatment of pernicious anemia by special diet, J.A.M.A. 87:470, 1926.
179. Minot, G. R., and Castle, W. B.: Interpretation of reticulocyte reactions: Their value in determining the potency of therapeutic materials, especially in pernicious anemia, Lancet 2:319, 1935.
180. Mollin, D. L., Baker, S. J., and Doniach, I.: Addisonian pernicious anaemia without gastric atrophy in a young man, Brit. J. Haemat. 1:278, 1955.
181. Mollin, D. L., Booth, C. C., and Baker, S. J.: Absorption of vitamin B_{12} in control subjects, in Addisonian pernicious anemia and in malabsorption syndrome, Brit. J. Haemat. 3:412, 1957.
182. Mollin, D. L.: The megaloblastic anemias, in University of London, British Postgraduate Medical Federation, Lectures on the Scientific Basis of Medicine, vol. 7, p. 94, Athlone Press, London, 1959.
183. Mooney, F. S., and Heathcote, J. G.: Oral treatment of pernicious anaemia with low doses of H.P.P./1, Lancet 2:291, 1960.
184. Mooney, F. S., and Heathcote, J. G.: Oral treatment of pernicious anaemia: Further studies, Brit. M. J. 1:232, 1961.
185. Mosbech, J.: Heredity in Pernicious Anemia: A Proband Study of the Heredity and Relationship to Cancer of the Stomach, Munksgaard, Copenhagen, 1953.
186. Mueller, J. F., Glazer, H. S., and Vitter, R. W.: Preliminary studies on the purine and pyrimidine bases of human bone marrow as determined by paper chromatography: I. Variations in pernicious anemia in response to therapy, J. Clin. Invest. 31:651, 1952.
187. Mueller, J. F., and Will, J. J.: Interrelationships of folic acid, vitamin B_{12} and ascorbic acid in patients with megaloblastic anemia, Am. J. Clin. Nutrition 3:30, 1955.

188. Nieweg, H. O., Shen, S. C., and Castle, W. B.: Mechanism of intrinsic factor action in the gastrectomized rat, Proc. Soc. Exper. Biol. & Med. 94:223, 1957.

189. Nyberg, W.: Absorption and excretion of vitamin B_{12} in subjects infected with *Diphyllobothrium latum* and in non-infected subjects following oral administration of radioactive B_{12}, Acta haemat. 19:90, 1958.

190. Nyberg, W., and Reizenstein, P.: Intestinal absorption of radiovitamin B_{12} bound in pig liver, Lancet 2:832, 1958.

191. Okuda, K., Grasbeck, R., and Chow, B. F.: Bile and vitamin B_{12} absorption, J. Lab. & Clin. Med. 51:17, 1958.

192. Okuda, K., Wider, J. A., and Chow, B. F.: Effect of intrinsic factor on the hepatic uptake of vitamin B_{12} following intravenous injection, J. Lab. & Clin. Med. 54:535, 1959.

193. Okuda, K.: Excretion into bile of intrinsic factor and its vitamin B_{12} complex following intravenous injection, Proc. Soc. Exper. Biol. & Med. 108:737, 1961.

194. Paulson, M., and Harvey, J. C.: Hematological alterations after total gastrectomy: Evolutionary sequences over a decade, J.A.M.A. 156:1556, 1954.

195. Payne, R. W.: Pernicious anaemia and gastric cancer in England and Wales, Brit. M. J. 1:1807, 1961.

196. Pederson, J., and Ebbesen, I.: Radioactive vitamin B_{12} tests in pernicious anaemia after oral maintenance therapy, Acta med. scandinav. 161:413, 1958.

197. Peel, J. L.: Vitamin B_{12} derivatives and the Co_2-pyruvate exchange reaction: A reappraisal, J. Biol. Chem. 237:263, 1962.

198. Pitney, W. R., and Onesti, P.: Vitamin B_{12} and folic acid concentrations of human liver with reference to the assay of needle biopsy material, Australian J. Exper. Biol. & M. Sc. 39:1, 1961.

199. Pollycove, M., and Apt, L.: Absorption, elimination and excretion of orally administered vitamin B_{12} in normal subjects and in patients with pernicious anemia, New England J. Med. 255:207, 1956.

200. Pollycove, M., Apt, L., and Colbert, M. J.: Pernicious anemia due to dietary deficiency of vitamin B_{12}, New England J. Med. 255: 164, 1956.

201. Rabiner, S. F., Lichtman, H. C., Messite, J., Watson, J., Ginsberg, V., Ellenbogen, L., and Williams, W. L.: Urinary excretion test in the diagnosis of Addisonian pernicious anemia, Ann. Int. Med. 44:437, 1956.

202. Rabinowitz, J. C.: Factor B and other compounds related to vitamin B_{12} in pyruvic acid–Co_2 exchange, J. Biol. Chem. 235:50, 1960.

203. Rabinowitz, J. C.: Folic acid, *in* Boyer, P. D. et al. (ed.), The Enzymes, ed. 2, vol. 2, p. 185, Academic Press, New York, 1960.

204. Rabinowitz, J. C., and Hines, R. H.: Folic acid coenzymes, Fed. Proc. 19:963, 1960.

205. Rabinowitz, J. C., and Allen, E. H.: Role of vitamin B_{12} derivatives in reactions of pyruvate, Fed. Proc. 20:962, 1961.

206. Rath, C. E., McCurdy, P. R., and Duffy, B. J., Jr.: Effect of renal disease on the Schilling test, New England J. Med. 256:111, 1957.

207. Reisner, E. H., Jr.: Nature and significance of megaloblastic blood formation, Blood 13:313, 1958.

208. Reizenstein, P. G.: Excretion, enterohepatic circulation and retention of radiovitamin B_{12} in pernicious anemia and in controls, Proc. Soc. Exper. Biol. & Med. 101:703, 1959.

209. Reizenstein, P. G., and Nyberg, W.: Intestinal absorption of liver-bound radiovitamin B_{12} in patients with pernicious anaemia and in controls, Lancet 2:248, 1959.

210. Reizenstein, P. G., Cronkite, E. P., Meyer, L. M., and Usenik, E. A.: Lymphatics in intestinal absorption of vitamin B_{12} and iron, Proc. Soc. Exper. Biol. & Med. 105:233, 1960.

211. Reizenstein, P. G., Cronkite, E. P., and Cohn, S. H.: Measurement of absorption of vitamin B_{12} by whole-body gamma spectrometry, Blood 18:95, 1961.

212. Rhodes, M. B., Feeney, R. E., and Miller, O. N.: Fractions with high activity for intrinsic factor and combining vitamin B_{12} with receptor substances, Proc. Soc. Exper. Biol. & Med. 101:70, 1959.

213. Richmond, J., and Davidson, S.: Subacute combined degeneration of the spinal cord in non-Addisonian megaloblastic anaemia, Quart. J. Med. 27:517, 1958.

214. Rodriguez-Rosado, A. L., and Sheehy, T. W.: Role of calcium in the intestinal absorption of vitamin B_{12} in tropical sprue, Am. J. M. Sc. 242:548, 1961.

215. Ross, G. I. M.: Vitamin B_{12} assay in body fluids, Nature 166:270, 1950.

216. Ross, G. I. M.: Vitamin B_{12} assay in body fluids using *Euglena gracilis*, J. Clin. Path. 5:250, 1952.

217. Rothenberg, S. P.: Assay of serum vitamin B_{12} concentration using Co^{57}-B_{12} and intrinsic factor, Proc. Soc. Exper. Biol. & Med. 108:45, 1961.

218. Rundles, R. W.: Prognosis in the neurologic manifestations of pernicious anemia, Blood 1:209, 1946.

219. Rundles, R. W., and Brewer, S. S., Jr.: Hematologic responses in pernicious anemia to orotic acid, Blood 13:99, 1958.

220. Sakami, W., and Ukstins, I.: Enzymatic methylation of homocysteine by a synthetic tetrahydrofolate derivative, J. Biol. Chem. 236: 50, 1961.

221. Schilling, R. F., Clatanoff, D. V., and Korst, D. R.: Intrinsic factor studies: III. Further observations utilizing the urinary radioactivity test in subjects with achlorhydria, pernicious anemia or a total gastrectomy, J. Lab. & Clin. Med. 45:926, 1955.

222. Schloesser, L. L., Deshpande, P., and Schilling, R. F.: Biologic turnover rate of cyanocobalamin (vitamin B_{12}) in human liver, A.M.A. Arch. Int. Med. 101:306, 1958.

223. Schwartz, M., Lous, P., and Meulengracht, E.: Reduced effect of heterologous intrinsic factor, Lancet 1:751, 1957.

224. Schwartz, M.: Intrinsic-factor-inhibiting substance in serum of orally treated patients with pernicious anaemia, Lancet 1:61, 1958.

225. Schwartz, M., Lous, P., and Meulengracht, E.: Absorption of vitamin B_{12} in pernicious anaemia, Lancet 2:1200, 1958.

226. Schwartz, M.: Intrinsic factor antibody in serum from patients with pernicious anaemia, Lancet 2:1263, 1960.

227. Schwartz, S. O., Kaplan, S. R., and Armstrong, B. E.: Long-term evaluation of folic acid in the treatment of pernicious anemia, J. Lab. & Clin. Med. 35:894, 1950.

228. Sheehy, T. W.: How much folic acid is safe in pernicious anemia? Am. J. Clin. Nutrition 9:708, 1961.

229. Sheehy, T. W., Perez-Santiago, E., and Haddock, J.: Tropical sprue and vitamin B_{12}, New England J. Med. 265:1232, 1961.

230. Sheehy, T. W., Rubini, M. E., Perez-Santiago, E., Santini, R., Jr., and Haddock, J.: Effect of "minute" and "titrated" amounts of folic acid on the megaloblastic anemia of tropical sprue, Blood 18:623, 1961.

231. Shinton, N. K.: Oral treatment of pernicious anemia with vitamin B_{12} peptide, Brit. M. J. 1:1579, 1961.

232. Smith, A. D. M.: Megaloblastic madness, Brit. M. J. 2:1840, 1960.

233. Smith, E. L.: Biological activities of anti-vitamin B_{12} substances, Acta haemat. 24:9, 1960.

234. Smith, E. L.: Vitamin B_{12}, *in* Peters, Sir Rudolph, and Young, F. J. (ed.), Methuen Monographs on Biochemical Subjects, Wiley, New York, 1960.

235. Smith, L. H., Sullivan, M., and Huguley, C. M., Jr.: Pyrimidine metabolism in man: IV. The enzymatic defect of orotic aciduria, J. Clin. Invest. 40:656, 1961.

236. Spray, G. H., and Witts, L. J.: Thymidine in megaloblastic anaemia, Lancet 2:869, 1958.

237. Stevenson, T. D., Little, J. A., and Langley, L.: Pernicious anemia in childhood, New England J. Med. 255:1219, 1956.

238. Stomach in pernicious anaemia, Lancet 2:1051, 1958.

239. Swendseid, M. E., Gasster, M., and Halsted, J. A.: Limits of absorption of orally administered vitamin B_{12}: Effect of intrinsic factor sources, Proc. Soc. Exper. Biol. & Med. 86:834, 1954.

240. Swendseid, M. E., Hvolboll, E., Schick, G., and Halsted, J. A.: Vitamin B_{12} content of human liver tissue and its nutritional significance, Blood 12:24, 1957.

241. Taylor, K. B., Mallett, B. J., and Spray, G. H.: Observations on the inhibitory effects of intrinsic factor preparations on vitamin B_{12} absorption, Clin. Sc. 17:647, 1958.

242. Taylor, K. B., and Morton, J. A.: An antibody to Castle's intrinsic factor, J. Path. & Bact. 77:117, 1959.

243. Taylor, W. H., Mallett, B. J., and Taylor, K. B.: Intrinsic factor: Active and inhibitory components from the mitochondria of human gastric mucosal cells, Biochem. J. 80:342, 1961.

244. Thomas, E. D., and Lochte, H. L., Jr.: Studies on the biochemical defect of pernicious anemia: I. In vitro observations on oxygen consumption, heme synthesis and deoxyribonucleic acid synthesis by pernicious anemia bone marrow, J. Clin. Invest. 37:166, 1958.

245. Todd, D.: Observations on the amino-aciduria in megaloblastic anaemia, J. Clin. Path. 12:238, 1959.

246. Toohey, J. I., and Barker, H. A.: Isolation of coenzyme B_{12} from liver, J. Biol. Chem. 236:560, 1961.

247. Toporek, M.: Vitamin B_{12} intrinsic factor studies with isolated perfused rat liver, Am. J. Physiol. 200:557, 1961.

248. Victor, M., and Lear, A. A.: Subacute combined degeneration of the spinal cord: Current concepts of the disease process: Value of serum vitamin B_{12} determinations in clarifying some of the common clinical problems, Am. J. Med. 20:896, 1956.

249. Vilter, R. W., Horrigan, D., Mueller, J. F., Jarrold, T., Vilter, C. F., Hawkins, V., and Seamon, A.: Studies on the relationships of vitamin B_{12}, folic acid, thymine, uracil and methyl group donors in persons with pernicious anemia and related megaloblastic anemias, Blood 5:695, 1950.

250. Vilter, R. W., and Mueller, J. F.: Growth and maturation of the erythrocyte, *in* Bean, W. B. (ed.), Monographs in Medicine, series I, p. 519, Williams & Wilkins, Baltimore, 1952.

251. Von Bonsdorff, B.: *Diphyllobothrium latum* as a cause of pernicious anemia, Exper. Parasitol. 5:207, 1956.

252. Waters, A. H., and Mollin, D. L.: Studies on the folic acid activity of human serum, J. Clin. Path. 14:335, 1961.

253. Watson, G. M., and Florey, H. W.: Absorption of vitamin B_{12} in gastrectomised rats, Brit. J. Exper. Path. 36:479, 1955.

254. Weinstein, I. B., Weissman, S. M., and Watkin, D. M.: The plasma vitamin B_{12} binding substance, J. Clin. Invest. 38:1904, 1959.

255. Weinstein, I. B., and Watkin, D. M.: Co[59] B_{12} absorption, plasma transport,

and excretion in patients with myeloproliferative disorders, solid tumors, and non-neoplastic diseases, J. Clin. Invest. 39:1667, 1960.

256. Welbourn, R. B., Nelson, M. G., and Zacharias, F. J.: Megaloblastic anemia following gastric resection: Report of ten cases, Brit. J. Surg. 43:422, 1956.

257. Wenger, J., Backerman, I., and Gendel, B. R.: Augmented histamine test in the diagnosis of pernicious anemia, Clin. Res. 10:28, 1962.

258. White, J. C., Leslie, I., and Davidson, J. M.: Nucleic acids of bone marrow cells with special reference to pernicious anaemia, J. Path. & Bact. 64:291, 1953.

259. Wilkinson, J. F.: Pernicious anaemia and gastric carcinoma, Brit. M. J. 2:576, 1950.

260. Will, J. J., Mueller, J. F., Brodine, C., Kiely, C. E., Friedman, B., Hawkins, V. R., Dutra, J., and Vilter, R. W.: Folic acid and vitamin B_{12} in pernicious anemia, J. Lab. & Clin. Med. 53:22, 1959.

261. Williams, A. W., Coghill, N. F., and Edwards, F.: Gastric mucosa in pernicious anaemia: Biopsy studies, Brit. J. Haemat. 4:457, 1958.

262. Williams, J. F.: Diseases associated with pernicious anaemia (in a study of 370 cases), Quart. J. Med. 2:281, 1933.

263. Williams, R. T. (ed.), Biochemistry of Vitamin B_{12}, Biochemical Society Symposia, No. 13, Cambridge University Press, London, 1955.

264. Williams, W. L., Ellenbogen, L., Rabiner, S. F., and Lichtman, H. C.: Improved urinary excretion test as an assay for intrinsic factor: III. Comparison of results of this method with the classical clinical method, J. Lab. & Clin. Med. 48:511, 1956.

265. Wintrobe, M. W.: Search for an experimental counterpart of pernicious anemia, A.M.A. Arch. Int. Med. 100:862, 1957.

266. Witts, L. J.: Development of pernicious anaemia, Acta haemat. 24:1, 1960.

267. Witts, L. J.: Some aspects of the pathology of anaemia: I. Theory of maturation arrest; II. Investigation of Castle's hypothesis, Brit. M. J. 2:5248, 1961.

268. Wong, V. G., LaCombe, M., Beizer, L., Okuda, K., and Chow, B. F.: Effect of hog intrinsic factor on the absorption of the coenzyme form of vitamin B_{12} (5, 6-dimethylbenzimidazolyl cobamide), Am. J. Clin. Nutrition 10:134, 1962.

269. Woolf, A. L.: Changes in the nervous system in vitamin B_{12} deficiency, J. Clin. Path. 9:388, 1956.

270. Zalusky, R., and Herbert, V.: Megaloblastic anemia in scurvy, with response to fifty micrograms of folic acid daily, New England J. Med. 265:1033, 1961.

271. Zalusky, R., Herbert, V., and Castle, W. B.: Cyanocobalamin therapy effect in folic acid deficiency, A.M.A. Arch. Int. Med. 109:545, 1962.

272. Zamchek, N., Grable, E., Ley, A., and Norman, L.: Occurrence of gastric cancer among patients with pernicious anemia at the Boston City Hospital, New England J. Med. 252:1103, 1955.

CHAPTER EIGHT
RED CELL METABOLISM AND METHEMOGLOBINEMIA

1. Abrahmov, A., and Diamond, L. K.: Erythrocyte glycolysis in erythroblastic newborns, A.M.A. Am. J. Dis. Child. 99:202, 1960.
2. Allison, A. C., and Burn, G. P.: Enzyme activity as a function of age in the human erythrocyte, Brit. J. Haemat. 1:291, 1955.
3. Altman, K. I., and Swisher, S. N.: Incorporation of acetate–2–^{14}C into human erythrocyte stroma as a function of storage, Nature 174:459, 1954.
4. Altman, K. I.: Some enzymologic aspects of the human erythrocyte, Am. J. Med. 27:936, 1959.
5. Anderson, H. M., and Turner, J. C.: Relation of hemoglobin to the red cell membrane, J. Clin. Invest. 39:1, 1960.
6. Bartlett, G. R.: Organization of red cell glycolytic enzymes: Cell coat phosphorous transfer, Ann. New York Acad. Sc. 75:110, 1958.
7. Bartlett, G. R.: Human red cell glycolytic intermediates, J. Biol. Chem. 234:445, 1959.
8. Bartlett, G. R.: Influence of glucose and nucleoside metabolism on viability of erythrocytes during storage, A.M.A. Arch. Int. Med. 106:889, 1960.
9. Bateman, J. B., Hsu, S. S., Knudsen, J. P., and Yudovitch, K. L.: Hemoglobin spacing in erythrocytes, Arch. Biochem. 45:411, 1953.
10. Behrendt, H.: Chemistry of Erythrocytes, Charles C. Thomas, Springfield, Ill. 1957.
11. Benesch, R. E., and Benesch, R.: Relation between erythrocyte integrity and sulfhydryl groups, Arch. Biochem. 48:38, 1954.
12. Berger, H., Zuber, C., and Miescher, P.: Reduction of methaemoglobin to haemoglobin in the ageing red cell, Gerontologia 4:220, 1960.
13. Bernstein, R. E.: Rates of glycolysis in human red cells in relation to energy requirements for cation transport, Nature 172:911, 1953.
14. Bernstein, R. E.: Alterations in metabolic energetics and cation transport during aging of red cells, J. Clin. Invest. 38:1572, 1959.
15. Bertles, J. F.: Sodium transport across the surface membrane of red blood cells in hereditary spherocytosis, J. Clin. Invest. 36:816, 1957.
16. Bessis, M.: Cytology of the Blood and Blood Forming Organs (tr. by E. Ponder), Grune & Stratton, New York, 1956.
17. Bessis, M.: Blood cells and their formation, in Brachet, J., and Mirsky, A. E. (ed.), The Cell, vol. V, part 2, p. 163, Academic Press, New York, 1961.
18. Betke, K., Baltz, A., Kleihauer, E., and Scholz, P.: Methämoglobingehalt, Methämoglobin-Reduktion und Sauerstoffverbrauch in jungen und alter Erythrozyten, Blut 6:203, 1960.
19. Betke, K., Gröschner, E., and Bock, K.: Properties of a further variant of haemoglobin M, Nature 188:864, 1960.
20. Beutler, E., and Mikus, B. J.: Effect of sodium nitrite and para-amino-propriophenone administration on blood methemoglobin levels and red blood cell survival, Blood 18:455, 1961.

21. Bischoff, F., and Bryson, G.: Estradiol transport by human red cells, J. Appl. Physiol. 15:515, 1960.

22. Bodansky, O., and Gutmann, H.: Treatment of methemoglobinemia, J. Pharmacol. & Exper. Therap. 90:46, 1947.

23. Bond, V. P., Fliedner, T. M., Cronkite, E. P., Rubini, J. R., and Robertson, J. S.: Cell turnover in blood and blood-forming tissues studied with tritiated thymidine, *in* Stohlman, F. (ed.), The Kinetics of Cellular Proliferation, p. 188, Grune & Stratton, New York, 1959.

24. Boran, E. R., Figuerra, W. G., and Perry, S. M.: Distribution of Fe^{59} tagged human erythrocytes in centrifuged specimens as a function of cell age, J. Clin. Invest. 36:676, 1957.

25. Boszormenyi-Nagy, I., and Blackford, D.: Effect of methylene blue on the metabolism of adenine nucleotides in human erythrocytes, Arch. Biochem. 65:580, 1956.

26. Brandenburg, R. O., and Smith, H. L.: Sulfhemoglobinemia: Study of sixty-two clinical cases, Am. Heart J. 42:582, 1951.

27. Breakug, V. K. St. G., Gibson, H., and Harrison, D. C.: Familial idiopathic methaemoglobinemia, Lancet 1:935, 1951.

28. Brewer, G. J., Tarlov, A. R., Kellermeyer, R. W., and Alving, A. S.: Hemolytic effect of primaquine: XV. The role of methemoglobin, J. Lab. & Clin. Med. 59:905, 1962.

29. Brill, A. S., and Williams, R. J. P.: Absorption spectra, magnetic moments and the binding of iron in some haemoproteins, Biochem. J. 78:246, 1961.

30. Brown, E. A.: Adsorption of serum albumin by human erythrocytes, J. Cell. & Comp. Physiol. 47: 167, 1956.

31. Buchanan, A. A.: Lipid synthesis by human leukocytes in vitro, Biochem. J. 74:25, 1960.

32. Bucklin, R., and Myint, M. K.: Fatal methemoglobinemia due to well water nitrates, Ann. Int. Med. 52:703, 1960.

33. Carlsen, E., and Comroe, J. H.: Rate of gas uptake by intact human erythrocytes, Am. J. Physiol. 187:590, 1956.

34. Carlsen, E., and Comroe, J. H.: Rate of uptake of carbon monoxide and of nitric oxide by normal human erythrocytes and experimentally produced spherocytes, J. Gen. Physiol. 42:83, 1958.

35. Carson, P. E.: Glucose–6–phosphate dehydrogenase deficiency in hemolytic anemia, Fed. Proc. 19:995, 1960.

36. Chalfin, D.: Differences between young and mature rabbit erythrocytes, J. Cell. & Comp. Physiol. 47:215, 1956.

36a. Chapman, R. G., Hennessey, M. A., Waltersdorph, A. M., Huennekens, F. M., and Gabrio, B. W.: Erythrocyte metabolism: V. Levels of glycolytic enzymes and regulation of glycolysis, J. Clin. Invest. 41:1249, 1962.

37. Clarkson, E. M., and Maizels, M.: Distribution of phosphatases in human erythrocytes, J. Physiol. 116:112, 1952.

38. Crosby, W.: Diseases of the reticuloendothelial system and hematology: The red cell and some of its problems, Ann. Rev. Med. 8:151, 1957.

39. Dalziel, K., and O'Brien, J. R. P.: Kinetics of deoxygenation of human haemoglobin, Biochem. J. 78: 236, 1961.

40. Danon, D.: Osmotic hemolysis by a gradual decrease in the ionic strength of the surrounding medium, J. Cell. & Comp. Physiol. 57:111, 1961.

41. Darling, R. C., and Roughton, F. J. W.: Effect of methemoglobin on the equilibrium between oxygen and hemoglobin, Am. J. Physiol. 137:56, 1942.

42. DeGruchy, G. C.: Red cell metabolism: Fundamental and clinical aspects, Australasian Ann. Med. 9:237, 1960.

43. Dimant, E., Landsberg, E., and London, I. M.: Metabolic behavior of re-

duced glutathione in human and avian erythrocytes, J. Biol. Chem. 213:769, 1955.

44. Drabkin, D. L.: Metabolism of the hemin chromoproteins, Physiol. Rev. 31:345, 1951.

45. Eder, H. A., Finch, C. A., and McKee, R. W.: Congenital methemoglobinemia: A clinical and biochemical study of a case, J. Clin. Invest. 28:265, 1949.

46. Edwards, M. J., Koler, R. D., Rigas, D. A., and Pitcairn, D. M.: Effect of in vivo aging of normal human erythrocytes and erythrocyte macromolecules upon oxyhemoglobin dissociation, J. Clin. Invest. 40:636, 1961.

47. Enzymes in blood: II: Enzymes in red blood cells, Ann. New York Acad. Sc. 75:71, 1958.

48. Evans, A. S., Enzer, N., Eder, H. A., and Finch, C. A.: Hemolytic anemia with paroxysmal methemoglobinemia and sulphemoglobinemia: Two cases. Arch. Int. Med. 86:22, 1950.

49. Evelyn, K. A., and Malloy, H. T.: Microdetermination of oxyhemoglobin: Methemoglobin and sulfhemoglobin in a single blood sample, J. Biol. Chem. 126:655, 1938.

50. Falk, J. E., and Phillips, J. M.: Binding of haem to protein in haemoglobin and myoglobin, Nature 184:1651, 1959.

51. Finch, C. A.: Methemoglobinemia and sulfhemoglobinemia, New England J. Med. 239:470, 1948.

52. Gabrio, B. W., Finch, C. A., and Huennekens, F. M.: Erythrocyte preservation: A topic in molecular biochemistry, Blood 11:103, 1956.

53. George, P.: On the nature of haemoprotein reactions, *in* Green, D. E. (ed.), Currents in Biochemical Research, p. 338, Interscience, New York, 1956.

54. Gerald, P. S.: Electrophoretic and spectroscopic characterization of hemoglobin M, Blood 13:936, 1958.

55. Gerald, P. S., and George, P.: Second spectroscopically abnormal methemoglobin associated with hereditary cyanosis, Science 129:393, 1959.

56. Gerald, P. S.: The hereditary methemoglobinemias, *in* Stanbury, J. B., Wyngaarden, J. B., and Fredrickson, D. S. (ed.), The Metabolic Basis of Inherited Disease, p. 1068, McGraw-Hill, New York, 1960.

57. Gerald, P. S., Efron, M. L., and Pease, M. T.: Presence of an altered amino acid sequence in hemoglobin M (Boston type), J. Clin. Invest. 39:989, 1960.

58. Gibson, Q. H., and Harrison, D. C.: Familial idiopathic methemoglobinemia: Five cases in one family, Lancet 2:941, 1947.

59. Gibson, Q. H.: Reduction in methaemoglobin in red blood cells and studies on the cause of idiopathic methaemoglobinemia, Biochem. J. 42:13, 1948.

60. Gibson, Q. H.: Methaemoglobin and sulfhaemoglobin, Biochemical Society Symposia, No. 12, p. 55, Cambridge University Press, London, 1954.

61. Gibson, Q. H., Kreuzer, F., Meda, E., and Roughton, F. J. W.: Kinetics of human haemoglobin in solution and in the red cell at 37°C, J. Physiol. 129:68, 1955.

62. Gibson, Q. H.: Kinetics of reactions between hemoglobin and gases, *in* Butler, J. A. V., and Katz, B. (ed.), Progress in Biophysics and Biophysical Chemistry, p. 2, Pergamon Press, New York, 1959.

63. Glynn, I. M.: Sodium and potassium movements in nerve, muscle and red cell, Internat. Rev. Cytol. 8:449, 1959.

64. Gold, G. L., and Solomon, A. K.: Transport of sodium into human erythrocytes in vivo, J. Gen. Physiol. 38:389, 1955.

65. Goldstein, D. A., and Solomon, A. K.: Determination of equivalent pore radius for human red cells by osmotic pressure measurement, J. Gen. Physiol. 44:1, 1960.

66. Goluboff, N., and Wheaton, R.: Methylene blue induced cyanosis and acute

hemolytic anemia complicating the treatment of methemoglobinemia, J. Pediat. 58:86, 1961.

67. Granick, S.: Chemistry and functioning of the mammalian erythrocytes in vivo, Blood 4:404, 1949.

68. Griggs, R. C., and Harris, J. W.: Susceptibility to immune hemolysis as related to age of human and dog red blood cells, Blood 18:806, 1961.

69. Gross, R. T., and Hurwitz, R. E.: The pentose phosphate pathway in human erythrocytes, Pediatrics 22:453, 1958.

70. Harris, E. J., and Prankerd, T. A. J.: Rate of sodium extrusion from human erythrocytes, J. Physiol. 121:470, 1953.

71. Harris, H.: Some abnormalities of amino acid and haemoglobin metabolism, in Thompson, R. H. J., and King, F. J. (ed.), Biochemical Disorders of Human Diseases, p. 578, Academic Press, New York, 1957.

72. Heller, P., Weinstein, H. G., West, M., and Zimmerman, H. J.: Glycolytic, citric acid cycle, and hexosemonophosphate shunt enzymes of plasma and erythrocytes in megaloblastic anemia, J. Lab. & Clin. Med. 55:425, 1960.

73. Hemmingsen, E., and Scholander, P. F.: Specific transport of oxygen through hemoglobin solutions, Science 132:1379, 1960.

74. Hillier, J., and Hoffman, J. F.: On the ultrastructure of the plasma membrane as determined by the electron microscope, J. Cell. & Comp. Physiol. 42:203, 1953.

75. Hoffman, J. F.: On the relationship of certain erythrocyte characteristics to their physiological age, J. Cell. & Comp. Physiol. 51:415, 1958.

76. Hoffman, J. F.: Physiological characteristics of human red blood cell ghosts, J. Gen. Physiol. 42:9, 1958.

77. Hoffman, J. F., Eden, M., Barr, J. S., Jr., and Bedell, R. H. S.: Hemolytic volume of human erythrocytes, J. Cell. & Comp. Physiol. 51:405, 1958.

78. Hoffman, J. F.: Link between metabolism and the active transport of Na in human red cell ghosts, Fed. Proc. 19:127, 1960.

79. Hokin, L. E., and Hokin, M. R.: Phosphatidic acid on a carrier for Na$^+$ ions, Fed. Proc. 19:130, 1960.

80. Hokin, L. E., and Hokin, M. R.: Studies on the carrier function of phosphatidic acid in sodium transport: I. The turnover of phosphatidic acid and phosphorinositide in the avian salt gland on stimulation of secretion, J. Gen. Physiol. 44:61, 1960.

81. Hörlein, H., and Weber, G.: Über chronische familiäre Methämoglobinämie und eine neue Modifikation des Methämoglobins, Deutsche med. Wchnschr. 73:476, 1948.

82. Huennekens, F. M., Caffrey, R. W., Basford, R. E., and Gabrio, B. W.: Erythrocyte metabolism: IV. Isolation and properties of methemoglobin reductase, J. Biol. Chem. 227:261, 1957.

83. Huennekens, F. M., Caffrey, R. W., and Gabrio, B. W.: Electron transport sequence of methemoglobin reductase, Ann. New York Acad. Sc. 75:167, 1958.

84. Hunter, F. R.: Effect of n-butyl alcohol on the permeability of erythrocytes to non-electrolytes, J. Cell. & Comp. Physiol. 3:203, 1961.

85. Hurley, T. H., Weisman, R., Jr., and Pasquariello, A. E.: Determination of the survival of transfused red cells by a method of differential hemolysis, J. Clin. Invest. 33:835, 1954.

86. Ingram, D. J. E., Gibson, J. F., and Perutz, M. F.: Orientation of the four haem groups in haemoglobin, Nature 178:906, 1956.

87. Israels, L. G., Chutorian, A., Delory, G. E., and Israels, E.: Effect of sulph-

haemoglobin on red cell viability, Canad. J. Biochem. & Physiol. 35:1171, 1957.

88. Itano, H. A., and Robinson, E.: Demonstration of intermediate forms of carbonmonoxy- and ferrihemoglobin by moving boundary electrophoresis, J. Am. Chem. Soc. 78:6415, 1956.

88a. Jacob, H. S., and Jandl, J. H.: Effects of sulfhydryl inhibition on red blood cells: I. Mechanism of hemolysis, J. Clin. Invest. 41:779, 1962.

89. Jacobs, M. H.: Measurement of cell permeability with particular reference to the erythrocyte, *in* Barron, E. S. G. (ed.), Modern Trends in Physiology and Biochemistry, p. 145, Academic Press, New York, 1952.

90. Jacobs, M. H.: Blood (formed elements), Ann. Rev. Physiol. 20:405, 1958.

91. Jaffé, E. R., Vanderhoff, G. A., Lowy, B. A., and London, I. M.: Effect of nucleosides on osmotic resistance of mammalian erythrocytes in relation to the age of the cells, J. Clin. Invest. 36:903, 1957.

92. Jaffé, E. R., Vanderhoff, G. A., Lowy, B. A., and London, I. M.: Relationship of the age of rabbit erythrocytes to the effects of inosine on their osmotic resistance, J. Clin. Invest. 37:1293, 1958.

93. Jaffé, E. R.: Reduction of methemoglobin in human erythrocytes incubated with purine nucleosides, J. Clin. Invest. 38:1555, 1959.

94. Jaffé, E. R., and Gordon, E. E.: Incorporation of nicotinic acid into pyridine nucleotides of erythrocytes of rabbits in vitro, Fed. Proc. 20:64, 1961.

95. Jalavisto, E., and Solantera, L.: Methaemoglobin reduction rate of nitrite treated red cells as a function of cell age, Acta physiol. scandinav. 46:273, 1959.

96. James, A. T., Lovelock, J. E., and Webb, J.: The lipids in whole blood: I. The lipid biosynthesis in human blood in vitro, Biochem. J. 73:106, 1959.

97. Jope, E. M.: Disappearance of sulphaemoglobin from circulating blood in relation to red cell destruction, Proc. Phys. Soc. Med. 39:760, 1946.

98. Josephson, A. M., Wienstein, H. G., Yakulis, B. S., Singer, L., and Heller, P.: A new variant of hemoglobin M disease—Hemoglobin $M_{Chicago}$, J. Lab. & Clin. Med. 59:918, 1962.

99. Joyce, C. R. B.: Uptake of potassium and sodium by parts of packed human blood cell column, Quart. J. Exper. Physiol. 43:299, 1958.

100. Jung, F.: Alter hämolytishe Resistenz und Methämoglobingehalt der Erythrozyten, Deutsches Arch. klin. Med. 195:454, 1949.

101. Keilin, J.: Nature of the haem-binding groups in native and denatured haemoglobin and myoglobin, Nature 187:365, 1960.

102. Keohane, K. W., and Metcalf, W. K.: Investigation of the differing sensitivity of juvenile and adult erythrocytes to methaemoglobinization, Phys. Med. Biol. 5:27, 1960.

103. Kiese, M.: Die Reduktion des Hämoglobins, Biochem. J. 316:264, 1944.

104. Kiese, M., and Waller, H. D.: Kinetic der Hämoglobinbildung: Die Stoffwechselvorgange in roten Zellen bei der Hämoglobinbildung durch den Kreisprogess Phenylhydroxylamin-nitrosobenzol, Arch. exper. Path. u. Pharmakol. 211:345, 1950.

105. Kiese, M., Kurz, H., and Schneider, C.: Chronische Hämoglobinämie durch pathologischen Blutfarbstoff, Klin. Wchnschr. 34:957, 1956.

106. Kiese, M., Schneider, C., and Waller, H. D.: Hämoglobinreduktase, Arch. exper. Path. u. Pharmakol. 231:158, 1957.

107. Kravitz, H., Elegant, L. D., Kaiser, E., and Kagan, B. M.: Methemoglobin values in premature and mature infants and children, A.M.A. Am. J. Dis. Child. 91:1, 1956.

108. Lajtha, L. G.: On DNA labeling in the study of the dynamics of bone marrow

cell population, *in* Stohlman, F. (ed.), The Kinetics of Cellular Proliferation, p. 173, Grune & Stratton, New York, 1959.

109. Laris, P. C.: Permeability and utilization of glucose in mammalian erythrocytes, J. Cell. & Comp. Physiol. 51:273, 1958.

109a. Laris, P. C., Ewers, A., and Novinger, G.: Comparison of stromal adenosine triphosphatase and inhibition of sugar permeability in erythrocytes, J. Cell. & Comp. Physiol. 59:145, 1962.

110. Lathem, W., and Worley, W. E.: Distribution of extracorpuscular hemoglobin in circulating plasma, J. Clin. Invest. 38:474, 1959.

111. Lecks, H. I.: Methemoglobinemia in infancy, Am. J. Dis. Child. 79:117, 1950.

112. LeFevre, P. G.: Molecular structural factors in competitive inhibition of sugar transport, Science 130:104, 1959.

113. LeFevre, P. G.: Penetration of glucose into the human red cell: The recent attack on the carrier hypothesis, J. Cell. & Comp. Physiol. 56:163, 1959.

114. LeFevre, P. G., and McGinniss, G. F.: Tracer exchange vs. net uptake of glucose through human red cell surface: New evidence for carrier-mediated diffusion, J. Gen. Physiol. 44:87, 1960.

115. LeFevre, P. G.: Sugar transport in the red blood cell: Structure-activity relationship in substrates and antagonists, Pharmacol. Rev. 13:39, 1961.

116. Lehmann, H., and Huntsman, R. G.: Why are red cells the shape they are? The evolution of the human red cell, *in* MacFarlane, R. G., and Robb-Smith, A. H. T. (ed.), Functions of the Blood, p. 173, Academic Press, New York, 1961.

117. Löhr, G. W., Waller, H. D., Karges, O., Schlegel, B., and Müller, A. A.: Zur Biochemie der Alterung menschlicher Erythrocyten, Klin. Wchnschr. 36:1008, 1958.

118. Löhr, G. W., and Waller, H. D.: Enzyme-deficiency haemolytic anaemia, German Med. Monthly 6:37, 1961.

119. London, I. M., and Schwartz, H.: Erythrocyte metabolism: Metabolic behavior of the cholesterol of human erythrocytes, J. Clin. Invest. 32:1248, 1953.

120. London, I. M.: Metabolism of the mammalian erythrocyte, Bull. New York Acad. Med. 36:79, 1960.

121. London, I. M.: Metabolism of the erythrocyte, Harvey Lectures, p. 151, Academic Press, New York, 1961.

122. Lovelock, J. E.: Physical instability of the human red blood cells, Biochem. J. 60:692, 1955.

123. Lovelock, J. E.: Physical instability of human red blood cells and its possible importance in their senescence, *in* Wolstenholme, G. E. W., and Millar, E. C. P. (ed.), Ciba Foundation Colloquia on Aging, vol. 2, p. 215, Little, Brown, Boston, 1956.

124. Lovelock, J. E., James, A. T., and Rowe, C. E.: Lipids of whole blood: II. The exchange of lipids between the cellular constituents and the lipoproteins of human blood, Biochem. J. 74:137, 1960.

125. Lowenstein, L. M.: Studies on reticulocyte division, Exper. Cell Res. 17:336, 1959.

126. Lowenstein, L. M.: The mammalian reticulocyte, Internat. Rev. Cytol. 8:135, 1959.

127. Lowy, B. A., Ramot, B., and London, I. M.: Adenosine triphosphate metabolism in the rabbit erythrocyte in vivo, Nature 181:324, 1958.

128. Lowy, B. A., and Williams, M. K.: Presence of a limited portion of the pathway of *de novo* purine nucleotide biosynthesis in rabbit erythrocytes in vitro, J. Biol. Chem. 235: 2924, 1960.

129. Lowy, B. A., Cook, J. L., and London, I. M.: Biosynthesis of purine nucleotides *de novo* in the rabbit reticulocyte in vitro, J. Biol. Chem. 236:1442, 1961.

130. Lowy, B. A., Williams, M. K., and London, I. M.: Utilization of purines and their ribosyl derivatives for the formation of adenosine triphosphate and guanosine triphosphate in the mature rabbit erythrocyte, J. Biol. Chem. 236:1439, 1961.

131. Ludewig, S.: Carbohydrate constituents of human red cell stroma, Proc. Soc. Exper. Biol. & Med. 104:250, 1960.

132. Mactet, D. I., and Hurden, W. C.: Toxicology and assay of methylene blue, Ann. Int. Med. 71:738, 1933.

133. Maizels, M.: Anion and cation contents of normal and anaemic bloods, Biochem. J. 30:821, 1936.

134. Maizels, M.: Cation control in human erythrocytes, J. Physiol. 108:247, 1949.

135. Maizels, M.: Factors in the active transport of cations, J. Physiol. 112:59, 1951.

136. Mangelsdorff, A. F.: Treatment of methemoglobinemia, A.M.A. Arch. Indust. H. 14:148, 1956.

137. Marks, P. A.: Relationship between human erythrocyte aging in vivo and the activities of glucose–6–phosphate and 6–phosphogluconic dehydrogenases, J. Clin. Invest. 36:913, 1957.

138. Marks, P. A., and Johnson, A. B.: Relationship between the age of human erythrocytes and their osmotic resistance: A basis for separating young and old erythrocytes, J. Clin. Invest. 37:1542, 1958.

139. Marks, P. A., Johnson, A. B., and Hirschberg, E.: Effect of age on the enzyme activity in erythrocytes, Proc. Nat. Acad. Sc. 44:529, 1958.

140. Marks, P. A., Johnson, A. B., Hirschberg, E., and Banks, J.: Studies on the mechanism of aging of human red blood cells, Ann. New York Acad. Sc. 75:95, 1958.

141. Marks, P. A., Gelhorn, A., and Kidson, C.: Lipid synthesis in human leukocytes, platelets, and erythrocytes, J. Biol. Chem. 235:2579, 1960.

142. Matthies, H.: Methämoglobinrackbildung in Reticulocyten, Arch. exper. Path. u. Pharmakol. 229:331, 1956.

143. Mendelsohn, D.: Metabolism of the human red cell: I. Interrelationships of carbohydrate and lipid metabolism in the human erythrocyte in vivo, a comparison between diabetic patients and normal subjects, South African J. M. Sc. 26:15, 1961.

144. Mendelsohn, D.: Metabolism of the human red cell: II. Interrelationships of carbohydrate and lipid metabolism in the human erythrocyte in vitro, a comparison between diabetic and normal subjects, South African J. M. Sc. 26:24, 1961.

145. Metcalf, W. K.: Sensitivity of intracorpuscular haemoglobin in oxidation by nitrite ions: I. The effect of growth, starvation, and diet, Phys. Med. Biol. 6:427, 1962.

146. Metcalf, W. K.: Sensitivity of intracorpuscular haemoglobin in oxidation by nitrite ions: II. Observations on pregnant women and in some pathological states, Phys. Med. Biol. 6:437, 1962.

147. Meyering, C. A., Israels, A. L. M., Sebens, T., and Huisman, T. H. J.: Studies on the heterogeneity of hemoglobin: II. The heterogeneity of different human hemoglobin types in carboxymethylcellular and Amberlite IRC-50 chromatography: quantitative aspects, Clin. chim. acta 5:208, 1960.

148. Michel, H. O.: Study of sulfhemoglobin, J. Biol. Chem. 128:323, 1938.

149. Miller, A. A.: Congenital sulfhemoglobinemia, J. Pediat. 51:233, 1957.

150. Mills, G. C.: Hemoglobin catabolism: I. Glutathione peroxidase, an erythrocyte enzyme which protects hemoglobin from oxidative breakdown, J. Biol. Chem. 229:189, 1957.

151. Mills, G. C., and Randall, H. P.: Hemoglobin catabolism: II. The protection

of hemoglobin from oxidative breakdown in the intact erythrocyte, J. Biol. Chem. 232:589, 1958.

152. Mollison, P. L., and Robinson, M. A.: Observations on the effects of purine nucleosides on red-cell preservation, Brit. J. Haemat. 5:331, 1959.

153. Moore, C. V.: Long-term preservation of blood (editorial), J.A.M.A. 173:1668, 1960.

154. Moskowitz, M., and Calvin, M.: On the components and structure of the human red cell membrane, Exper. Cell Res. 3:33, 1952.

155. Munn, J. I.: Studies of lipids in human red cells, Brit. J. Haemat. 4:344, 1958.

156. Murphy, J. R.: Erythrocyte metabolism: I. The equilibrium of glucose-C^{14} between serum and erythrocytes, J. Lab. & Clin. Med. 55:281, 1960.

157. Murphy, J. R.: Erythrocyte metabolism: II. Glucose metabolism and pathways, J. Lab. & Clin. Med. 55:286, 1960.

158. Nadler, J. E., Green, H., and Rosenbaum, A.: Intravenous injection of methylene blue in man with reference to the toxic symptoms and effect on the electrocardiogram, Am. J. M. Sc. 188:15, 1934.

159. Nakao, M., Nakao, T., and Yamazoe, S.: Adenosine triphosphate and maintenance of shape of the human red cells, Nature 187:945, 1960.

160. Nakao, M., Nakao, T., Yamazoe, S., and Yoshikawa, H.: Adenosine triphosphate and shape of erythrocytes, J. of Biochem. (Japan) 49:487, 1961.

161. Necheles, T., and Beutler, E.: Effect of triiodothyronine on the oxidative metabolism of erythrocytes: I. Cellular studies, J. Clin. Invest. 38:788, 1959.

162. Nevo, A.: On the estimation of the thickness of the red cell membrane from ultracentrifuge studies, Exper. Cell Res. 21:286, 1960.

163. Nikkila, E. A., Pitkanen, E., Vuopio, P., and Forsell, O.: Erythrocyte enzymes in anemias of different etiology, Ann. med. int. Fenniae 49:187, 1960.

164. Olmstead, E. G.: Efflux and influx of erythrocyte water, J. Gen. Physiol. 44:235, 1960.

165. Olmstead, E. G.: Extracellular and metabolic factors affecting the efflux and influx of erythrocyte water, J. Gen. Physiol. 45:59, 1961.

166. Park, C. R., Post, R. C., Kalmon, C. F., Wright, J. H., Johnson, L. H., and Morgan, H. E.: Transport of glucose and other sugars across cell membranes and the effect of insulin, in Wolstenholme, G. E. W., and O'Connor, C. M. (ed.), Ciba Foundation Colloquia on Endocrinology, vol. 9, p. 240, Little, Brown, Boston, 1956.

167. Parpart, A. K., and Ballentine, R.: Molecular anatomy of the red cell plasma membrane, in Barron, E. S. G. (ed.), Modern Trends in Physiology and Biochemistry, p. 135, Academic Press, New York, 1952.

168. Perutz, M. F., Rossmann, M. G., Cullis, A. F., Muirhead, H., Will, G., and North, A. C. T.: Structure of haemoglobin: A three-dimensional fourier synthesis at 5.5 Å resolution, obtained by x-ray analysis, Nature 185:416, 1960.

169. Phillips, G. B., and Roome, N. S.: Phospholipids of human red blood cells, Proc. Soc. Exper. Biol. & Med. 100:489, 1959.

170. Pisciotta, A. V., Ebbe, S. N., and Hinz, J. E.: Clinical and laboratory features of two variants of methemoglobin M disease, J. Lab. & Clin. Med. 54:73, 1959.

171. Ponder, E.: Hemolysis and Related Phenomena, Grune & Stratton, New York, 1948.

172. Ponder, E.: Red cell structure and its breakdown, Protoplasmalogia 10:1, 1955.

173. Ponder, E.: The red blood cell, Scient. American 196:95, 1957.

174. Post, R. L., and Jolly, P. C.: Linkage of sodium, potassium and ammonium active transport across the human erythrocyte membrane, Biochim. et biophys. acta 25:118, 1957.

175. Post, R. L.: Relationship of an ATPase in human erythrocyte membranes to the active transport of sodium and potassium, Fed. Proc. 18:121, 1959.

176. Post, R. L., Merritt, C. R., Kinselving, C. R., and Albright, C. D.: Membrane adenosine triphosphatase as a participant in the active transport of sodium and potassium in the human erythrocyte, J. Biol. Chem. 235:1796, 1960.

177. Prankerd, T. A. J.: The aging of red cells, J. Physiol. 143:325, 1958.

178. Prankerd, T. A. J.: Red-cell structure and metabolism in haemolytic anaemia, Brit. M. Bull. 15:54, 1959.

179. Prankerd, T. A. J.: Viability and survival of red cells, *in* University of London, British Postgraduate Medical Federation, Lectures on the Scientific Basis of Medicine, vol. 8, p. 269, Athlone Press, London, 1960.

180. Prankerd, T. A. J.: The Red Cell: An Account of Its Chemical Physiology and Pathology, Blackwell, Oxford, 1961.

181. Prankerd, T. A. J.: Metabolic aberrations of erythrocytes: Clinical and patho-physiological considerations, Progr. Hemat. 3:53, 1962.

182. Preiss, J., and Handler, P.: Synthesis of diphosphopyridine nucleotide from nicotinic acid by human erythrocytes in vitro, J. Am. Chem. Soc. 79:1514, 1957.

183. Rapport, S.: Dimensional, osmotic, and chemical changes of erythrocytes in stored blood: I. Blood preserved in sodium citrate, neutral and acid-citrate-glucose (ACD) mixtures, J. Clin. Invest. 26:591, 1947.

184. Reed, C. F.: Studies of in vivo and in vitro exchange of erythrocytes and plasma phospholipid, J. Clin. Invest. 38:1032, 1959.

185. Reissman, K. R., Ruth, W. E., and Nomura, T.: A human hemoglobin with lowered oxygen affinity and impaired heme-heme interactions, J. Clin. Invest. 40:1826, 1961.

186. Rigas, D. A., and Koler, R. D.: Erythrocyte enzymes and reduced glutathione in hemoglobin H disease, J. Lab. & Clin. Med. 58:417, 1961.

187. Rigas, D. A., and Koler, R. D.: Ultracentrifugal fractionation of human eryth-rocytes on the basis of cell age, J. Lab. & Clin. Med. 58:242, 1961.

188. Rodman, T., Close, P., and Purcell, M. K.: Oxyhemoglobin dissociation curve in anemia, Ann. Int. Med. 52:295, 1960.

189. Rooth, G., and Caligara, F.: Influence of metabolic acid base variation on the oxygen dissociation curve, Clin. Sc. 21:393, 1961.

190. Ross, J. D., and Desforges, J. F.: Erythrocyte glucose–6–phosphate dehydro-genase activity and methemoglobin reduction, J. Lab. & Clin. Med. 54:450, 1959.

191. Rossi-Fanelli, A., Antonini, E., and Mondovi, B.: Ferrihemoglobin reduction in normal and methemoglobinemic subjects, Clin. chim. Acta 2:476, 1957.

192. Roueché, B.: Eleven Blue Men, p. 64, Berkley, New York, 1955.

193. Roughton, F. J. W.: Average time spent by the blood in the human lung capillary and its relation to the rates of CO uptake and elimination in man, Am. J. Physiol. 143:621, 1945.

194. Roughton, F. J. W., and Rupp, T. C.: Problems concerning the kinetics of the reaction of oxygen, carbon monoxide, and carbon dioxide in the intact red cell, Ann. New York Acad. Sc. 75:156, 1958.

195. Roughton, F. J. W.: Diffusion and simultaneous chemical reaction velocity in haemoglobin solutions and red cell suspensions, *in* Butler, J. A. V., and Katz, B. (ed.), Progress in Biophysics and Biophysical Chemistry, p. 56, Pergamon Press, New York, 1959.

196. Rowe, C. E.: Biosynthesis of phospholipids by human blood cells, Biochem. J. 73:438, 1959.

197. Rowe, C. E., Allison, A. C., and Lovelock, J. E.: Lipid biosynthesis in human

blood: The incorporation of acetate in lipids by different types of human blood cells, Biochem. J. 74:26, 1960.

198. Rubinstein, D., and Denstedt, O. F.: Metabolism of the erythrocyte: XIV. Metabolism of nucleosides by the erythrocyte, Canad. J. Biochem. & Physiol. 34:927, 1956.

199. Ruch, T. C., and Fulton, J. F.: Medical Physiology and Biophysics, ed. 18, Saunders, Philadelphia, 1960.

200. Sabine, J. C.: Erythrocyte cholinesterase titers in hematologic disease states, Am. J. Med. 27:81, 1959.

201. Schatzmann, H. J.: Herzglykoside als Hemmstoffe für den aktiven Kalium- und Natriumtransport durch die Erythrocytenmembran, Helvet. physiol. et pharmacol. acta 11:346, 1953.

202. Schlegel, B., and Kappest, P.: Untersuchungen zur intravitalen Erythrocytolyse, Klin. Wchnschr. 34:805, 1956.

203. Scholander, P. F.: Oxygen transport through hemoglobin solutions, Science 131:589, 1960.

204. Scott, E. M., and Hoskins, D. D.: Hereditary methemoglobinemia in Alaskan Eskimos and Indians, Blood 13:795, 1958.

205. Scott, E. M., and Griffith, I. V.: Enzymatic defect of hereditary methemoglobinemia: Diaphorase, Biochim. et biophys. acta 34:584, 1959.

206. Scott, E. M.: Erythrocyte diaphorase: The enzymatic defect of hereditary methemoglobinemia, Fed. Proc. 19:194, 1960.

207. Scott, E. M.: Relation of diaphorase of human erythrocytes to inheritance of methemoglobinemia, J. Clin. Invest. 39:1176, 1960.

208. Scott, E. M., and McGraw, J. C.: Purification and properties of diphosphopyridine nucleotide diaphorase of human erythrocytes, J. Biol. Chem. 237:249, 1962.

209. Seamon, G. V. F., and Heard, D. H.: Surface of the washed human erythrocyte as a polyanion, J. Gen. Physiol. 44:251, 1960.

210. Shafer, A. W., and Bartlett, G. R.: Phosphorylated carbohydrate intermediates of the human erythrocyte during storage in acid citrate dextrose: I. Effect of the addition of inosine at the beginning of storage, J. Clin. Invest. 40:1178, 1961.

211. Shafer, A. W., and Bartlett, G. R.: Phosphorylated carbohydrate intermediates of the human erythrocyte during storage in acid citrate dextrose: II. Effect of the addition of inosine late in storage, J. Clin. Invest. 40:1185, 1961.

211a. Shafer, A. W., and Bartlett, G. R.: Phosphorylated carbohydrate intermediates of the human erythrocyte during storage in acid citrate dextrose: III. Effect of incubation at 37°C with inosine, inosine plus adenine, and adenosine after storage for 6, 10, 14, and 18 weeks, J. Clin. Invest. 41:690, 1962.

212. Sheets, R. F., and Hamilton, H. E.: Reversible effect on the metabolism of human erythrocytes by p-chloromercuribenzoic acid and N-ethyl maleimide, J. Lab. & Clin. Med. 52:138, 1958.

213. Shibata, S., Tamura, A., Inchi, I., and Takahashi, H.: Hemoglobin M_1: Demonstration of a new abnormal hemoglobin in hereditary nigremia, Acta haemat. jap. 23:96, 1960.

214. Silver, D., Brown, I. W., and Eadie, G. S.: Studies of experimental sulfhemoglobinemia, J. Lab. & Clin. Med. 48:79, 1956.

215. Simon, E. R., and Topper, Y. J.: Fractionation of human erythrocytes on the basis of their age, Nature 180:1211, 1957.

216. Simon, E. R., Chapman, R. G., and Finch, C. A.: Adenine in red cell preservation, J. Clin. Invest. 41:351, 1962.

217. Solomon, A. K., and Gold, G. L.: Potassium transport in human erythrocytes: Evidence for a three-compartment system, J. Gen. Physiol. 38:371, 1955.

218. Solomon, A. K., Gill, T. J., and Gold, G. L.: K transport in human erythrocytes: Evidence for a three-compartment system, J. Gen. Physiol. 40:327, 1956.

219. Solomon, A. K.: Permeability of red cells to water and ions, Ann. New York Acad. Sc. 75:175, 1958.

220. Solomon, A. K.: Pores in the cell membrane, Scient. American 203:146, 1960.

221. Solomon, A. K.: Red cell membrane structure and ion transport, J. Gen. Physiol. 43:1, 1960.

222. Spicer, S. J., and Reynolds, H.: Individual and age variation in methemoglobin formation and reduction in rabbit erythrocytes, Am. J. Physiol. 159:47, 1949.

223. Staub, N. C., Bishop, J. M., and Forster, R. E.: Velocity of O_2 uptake by human red blood cells, J. Appl. Physiol. 16:511, 1961.

224. Strumia, M. M., Colwell, L. S., and Strumia, P. V.: Preservation of blood for transfusion: IV. In vitro recovery after freezing and thawing of red cells modified with sugars, J. Lab. & Clin. Med. 56:576, 1960.

225. Strumia, M. M., Colwell, L. S., and Strumia, P. V.: Preservation of blood for transfusion: V. Posttransfusion survival of red cells modified with sugars, frozen, and stored in the frozen state, J. Lab. & Clin. Med. 56:587, 1960.

226. Szeinberg, A., and Marks, P. A.: Substances stimulating glucose catabolism by the oxidative reactions of the pentose phosphate pathway in human erythrocytes, J. Clin. Invest. 40:914, 1961.

227. Takahara, S., Hamilton, H. B., Neel, J. V., Kobara, T. Y., Ogura, Y., and Nishimura, E. T.: Hypocatalasemia: A new genetic carrier state, J. Clin. Invest. 39:610, 1960.

228. Thorell, B.: Studies with microspectrography, Advances Biol. & Med. Phys. 6:95, 1958.

229. Tiepperman, J., Bodansky, O., and Jandorf, B. J.: Effect of para-aminopropriophenone induced methemoglobinemia on oxygenation of working muscle in human subjects, Am. J. Physiol. 146:702, 1946.

230. Tosteson, D. C.: Sodium and potassium transport in red blood cells, *in* Shanes, A. M. (ed.), Electrolytes in Biological Systems, p. 123, American Physiological Society, Washington, D.C., 1955.

231. Tosteson, D. C.: Halide transport in red blood cells, Acta physiol. scandinav. 46:19, 1959.

232. Tosteson, D. C., and Hoffman, J. F.: Regulation of cell volume by active cation transport in high and low potassium sheep cells, J. Gen. Physiol. 44:169, 1960.

233. Townes, P. L., and Lovell, G. R.: Hereditary methemoglobinemia: A new variant exhibiting dominant inheritance of methemoglobin A, Blood 18:18, 1961.

234. Townes, P. L., and Morrison, M.: Investigation of the defect in a variant of hereditary methemoglobinemia, Blood 19:60, 1962.

235. Valentine, W. N., Tanaka, K. R., and Fredricks, R. E.: Erythrocyte acid phosphatase in health and disease, Am. J. Clin. Path. 36:328, 1961.

236. Valtis, D. J.: Influence of red cell thickness on the oxygen dissociation curve of blood, Brit. J. Haemat. 1:46, 1955.

237. Waisman, H. A., Bain, J. A., Richmond, J. B., and Munsey, F. A.: Laboratory and clinical studies in congenital methemoglobinemia, Pediatrics 10:293, 1952.

238. Walker, J.: Human foetal dissociation curve for oxygen, Scottish M. J. 4:405, 1959.

239. Waller, H. D., Schlegel, B., Müller, A. A., and Löhr, G. W.: Der Hämiglobingehalt in alternden Erythrocyten, Klin. Wchnschr. 37:898, 1959.

240. Warburg, O., Kubowitz, F., and Christian, W.: Über die katalytische Wirkung von Methylenblau in lebenden Zellen, Biochem. Ztschr. 227:245, 1930.

241. Weed, R., Eber, J., and Rothstein, A.: Interaction of mercury with human erythrocytes, J. Gen. Physiol. 45:395, 1962.

242. Whittam, R.: Potassium movements and ATP in human red cells, J. Physiol. 140:479, 1958.

243. Wilbrandt, W., and Schatzmann, H. T.: Changes in the passive cation permeability of erythrocytes in low electrolyte media, in Wolstenholme, G. E. W., and O'Connor, C. M. (ed.), Regulation of the Inorganic Ion Content of Cells (Ciba Foundation Study Group No. 5), p. 34, Little, Brown, Boston, 1960.

244. Wiley, J. S., and Whittan, R.: Some aspects of inosine metabolism in red cells, Biochem. J. 78:27, 1961.

245. Wolstenholme, G. E. W., and O'Connor, C. M. (ed.): Regulation of the Inorganic Ion Content of Cells (Ciba Foundation Study Group No. 5), Little, Brown, Boston, 1960.

CHAPTER NINE
RED CELL DESTRUCTION AND THE HEMOLYTIC DISORDERS

1. Alber, G. M., and Rowe, D. S.: Binding of haematin by serum proteins, Brit. J. Haemat. 6:160, 1960.
2. Alber, G. M., and Rowe, D. S.: Electrophoresis of haemoglobin with serum proteins, Brit. J. Haemat. 6:166, 1960.
3. Allen, D. W., and Jandl, J. H.: Oxidative hemolysis and precipitation of hemoglobin: II. Role of thiols in oxidant drug action, J. Clin. Invest. 40:454, 1961.
4. Allison, A. C.: Acute haemolytic anaemia with distortion and fragmentation of erythrocytes in children, Brit. J. Haemat. 3:1, 1957.
5. Allison, A. C., Kates, J., and James, A. T.: An abnormality of blood lipids in hereditary spherocytosis, Brit. M. J. 2:1766, 1960.
6. Allison, A. C., and Clyde, D. F.: Malaria in African children with deficient erythrocyte glucose-6-phosphate dehydrogenase, Brit. M. J. 1:1346, 1961.
7. Astaldi, G., Rondanelli, E. G., Bernerdelli, E., and Strosseli, E.: Abnormal substance present in the erythroblasts of thalassemia major: Cytochemical investigations, Acta hemat. 12:145, 1954.
8. Bailey, I. S., and Prankerd, T. A. J.: Studies in thalassemia, Brit. J. Haemat. 4:150, 1958.
9. Baker, S. J., Jacob, E., Rajan, K. T., and Gault, E. W.: Hereditary haemolytic anaemia associated with elliptocytosis: A study of three families, Brit. J. Haemat. 7:210, 1961.
10. Bannerman, R. M., Grinstein, M., and Moore, C. V.: Haemoglobin synthesis in thalassaemia: In vitro studies, Brit. J. Haemat. 5:102, 1959.
11. Bannerman, R. M.: Thalassemia: A Survey of Some Aspects, Grune & Stratton, New York, 1961.
12. Barry, R. M.: Phospholipid distribution in the erythrocyte in paroxysmal nocturnal haemoglobinuria, Brit. J. Haemat. 5:212, 1959.
13. Bates, G. C., and Brown, C. H.: Incidence of gall bladder disease in chronic hemolytic anemia (spherocytosis), Gastroenterology 21:104, 1952.
14. Bearn, A. G.: Genetical variations in the serum proteins of man, Bull. New York Acad. Med. 37:593, 1961.
15. Beaven, G. H., and White, J. C.: Oxidation of phenyl-hydrazines in the presence of oxyhaemoglobin and the origin of Heinz bodies in erythrocytes, Nature 173:389, 1954.
16. Beaven, G. H., Ellis, M. J., and White, J. C.: Studies on human foetal haemoglobin: III. The hereditary haemoglobinopathies and thalassaemias, Brit. J. Haemat. 7:169, 1961.
17. Beinhauer, L. G., and Gruhn, J. G.: Dermatologic aspects of congenital spherocytic anemia, A.M.A. Arch. Dermat. 75:642, 1957.
18. Benesch, R. E., Ranney, H. M., Benesch, R., and Smith, G. M.: Chemistry of the Bohr effect: II. Some properties of hemoglobin H, J. Biol. Chem. 236:2926, 1961.

428]   REFERENCES

19. Berlin, N. I., Beeckmans, M., Elmlinger, P. J., and Lawrence, J. H.: Comparative study of the Ashby differential agglutination, carbon 14 and iron 59 methods for the determination of red cell life span, J. Lab. & Clin. Med. 50:558, 1957.

20. Berlin, N. I., Waldmann, T. A., and Weissman, S. M.: Life span of the red blood cell, Physiol. Rev. 39:577, 1959.

21. Bertles, J. F.: Sodium transport across the surface membrane of red blood cells in hereditary spherocytosis, J. Clin. Invest. 36:816, 1957.

22. Bessis, M.: Cytology of the Blood and Blood-forming Organs (tr. by E. Ponder), Grune & Stratton, New York, 1956.

23. Beutler, E.: Hemolytic effect of primaquine and related compounds: A review, Blood 14:103, 1959.

24. Beutler, E.: Drug-induced hemolytic anemia (primaquine sensitivity), *in* Stanbury, J. B., Wyngaarden, J. B., and Fredrickson, D. S. (ed.), The Metabolic Basis of Inherited Disease, p. 1031, McGraw-Hill, New York, 1960.

25. Beutler, E., Yeh, M., and Fairbanks, V. F.: Normal human female as a mosaic of x-chromosome activity: Studies using the gene for G-6-PD deficiency as marker, Proc. Nat. Acad. Sc. 48:9, 1962.

26. Bianco, I., Montalenti, G., Silvestroni, E., and Siniscalco, M.: Further data on genetics of microcythaemia or thalassaemia minor or Cooley's disease or thalassaemia major, Ann. Eugenics 16:299, 1952.

27. Bjorkman, S. E.: Splenic circulation, with special reference to the function of the spleen sinus wall, Acta med. scandinav., Suppl. 191, 1947.

28. Bradley, T. B., Jr., Brawner, J. M., III, and Conley, C. L.: Further observations on an inherited anomaly characterized by persistence of fetal hemoglobin, Bull. Johns Hopkins Hosp. 108:242, 1961.

29. Brenner, S., and Allison, A. C.: Catalase inhibition: A possible mechanism for the production of Heinz bodies in erythrocytes, Experientia 9:381, 1953.

30. Brewer, G. J., Tarlov, A. R., and Kellermeyer, R. W.: Hemolytic effect of primaquine: XII. Shortened erythrocyte life span in primaquine-sensitive male Negroes in the absence of drug administration, J. Lab. & Clin. Med. 58:217, 1961.

31. Brewer, G. J., Tarlov, A. R., Kellermeyer, R. W., and Alving, A. S.: Hemolytic effect of primaquine: XV. The role of methemoglobin, J. Lab. & Clin. Med. 59:905, 1962.

32. Brewer, G. J., Tarlov, A. R., and Powell, R. D.: Genetic implications of diisopropyl fluorophosphate (DFP)[32]: Erythrocyte survival studies in Negro females heterozygous for glucose-6-phosphate dehydrogenase deficiency, J. Clin. Invest. 41:1348, 1962.

33. Broberger, O., Gyulai, G., and Hirschfeldt, J.: Splenectomy in childhood: A clinical and immunological study of forty-two children splenectomized in the years 1951–58, Acta paediat. 49:679, 1960.

34. Brock, M. A.: Production and life span of erythrocytes during hibernation in the golden hamster, Am. J. Physiol. 198: 1181, 1960.

35. Brus, I., and Lewis, S. M.: Haptoglobin content of serum in haemolytic anaemia, Brit. J. Haemat. 5:348, 1959.

36. Burman, D.: Congenital spherocytosis in infancy, Arch. Dis. Childhood 33:335, 1958.

37. Burnet, M.: Auto-immune disease: I. Modern immunological concepts, Brit. M. J. 2:645, 1959.

38. Burnet, M.: Auto-immune disease: II. Pathology of the immune response, Brit. M. J. 2:720, 1959.

39. Burris, M. B., and Barzilai, R.: Thalassemia minor: Experience with fifty consecutive patients, J. Florida M. A. 43:1204, 1957.

40. Caffey, J.: Cooley's anemia: A review of roentgenographic findings in the skeleton, Am. J. Roentgenol. 78:381, 1957.

41. Callender, S. T., and Mallett, B. J.: Thalassaemia in Britain, Brit. J. Haemat. 7:1, 1961.

42. Carruthers, M. F.: Mild hereditary spherocytosis: A family study, Brit. M. J. 2:1845, 1960.

43. Carson, P. E.: Glucose-6-phosphate dehydrogenase deficiency in hemolytic anemia, Fed. Proc. 19:995, 1960.

44. Castle, W. B., and Daland, G. A.: Susceptibility of mammalian erythrocytes to hemolysis with hypotonic solutions, Arch. Int. Med. 60:949, 1937.

45. Castle, W. B., Ham., T. H., and Shen, S. C.: Observations on the mechanism of hemolytic transfusion reactions occurring without demonstrable hemolysis, Tr. A. Am. Physicians 63:161, 1950.

46. Caviles, A., Bergren, W. R., and Sturgeon, P.: Hemoglobin A_2 in thalassemia trait, Clin. Res. 10:107, 1962.

47. Chanarin, I., Dacie, J. V., and Mollin, D. L.: Folic acid deficiency in haemolytic anaemia, Brit. J. Haemat. 5:245, 1959.

47a. Chanarin, I., Burman, D., and Bennett, M. C.: Familial aplastic crisis in hereditary spherocytosis: Urocanic acid and formiminoglutamic acid excretion studies in a case with megaloblastic arrest, Blood 20:33, 1962.

48. Chaplin, H., Jr., Cassell, M., and Hanks, G. E.: Stability of the plasma hemoglobin level in the normal human subject, J. Lab. & Clin. Med. 57:612, 1961.

49. Chatterjea, J. B., and Ray, R. M.: Hereditary spherocytosis, J. Indian M. A. 33:1, 1959.

50. Chatterjea, J. B.: Splenectomy for thalassemia, J. Indian M. A. 37:1, 1961.

51. Chernoff, A. I.: Distribution of the thalassemia gene: A historical review, Blood 14:899, 1959.

52. Chernoff, A. I.: Chromium-51 tagging of the a-chain of human haemoglobin, Nature 192:327, 1961.

53. Childs, B., Zinkham, W., Browne, E. A., Kimbro, E. L., and Torbert, J. V.: Genetic study of a defect in glutathione metabolism of the erythrocyte, Bull. Johns Hopkins Hosp. 102: 21, 1958.

54. Choremis, C., Zannos-Mariolea, L., and Kattamis, C.: Frequency of glucose-6-phosphate dehydrogenase deficiency in certain highly malarial areas of Greece, Lancet 1:17, 1962.

55. Christenson, W. N., and Dacie, J. V.: Serum proteins in acquired haemolytic anaemia (auto-antibody type), Brit. J. Haemat. 3:153, 1957.

56. Cohen, A. S., Weiss, L., and Calkins, E.: Electron microscopic observations of the spleen during the induction of experimental amyloidosis in the rabbit, Am. J. Path. 37:413, 1960.

57. Coleman, H. D., and Finch, C. A.: Effect of adrenal steroids in hereditary spherocytic anemia, J. Lab. & Clin. Med. 47:602, 1956.

58. Comandon, J., and DeFonbrune, P.: Contribution à l'étude du mechanisme de l'hémolyse, Arch. Anat. Micr. 25:555, 1929.

59. Conrad, M. E., Crosby, W. H., and Howie, D. L.: Hereditary non-spherocytic hemolytic disease, Am. J. Med. 29:811, 1960.

60. Cooley, T. B., and Lee, P.: A series of cases of splenomegaly in children with anemia and peculiar bone changes, Tr. Am. Pediat. Soc. 37:29, 1925.

61. Crosby, W. H.: Paroxysmal nocturnal hemoglobinuria: A classical description by Paul Strübing in 1883 and a bibliography of the disease, Blood 6:270, 1951.

62. Crosby, W. H., and Dameshek, W.: Significance of hemoglobinuria and associated hemosiderinuria, with particular reference to various types of hemolytic anemia, J. Lab. & Clin. Med. 38:829, 1951.

63. Crosby, W. H., and Akeroyd, J. H.: Limit of hemoglobin synthesis in hereditary hemolytic anemia, Am. J. Med. 13:273, 1952.

64. Crosby, W. H.: Metabolism of hemoglobin and bile pigment in hemolytic disease, Am. J. Med. 18:112, 1955.

65. Crosby, W. H., and Rappaport, H.: Reticulocytopenia in auto-immune hemolytic anemia, Blood 11:929, 1956.

66. Crosby, W. H., and Conrad, M. E.: Hereditary spherocytosis: Observations on hemolytic mechanisms and iron metabolism, Blood 15:662, 1960.

67. Cutbush, M., and Mollison, P. L.: Relation between characteristics of blood-group antibodies in vitro and associated patterns of red-cell destruction in vivo, Brit. J. Haemat. 4:115, 1958.

68. Dacie, J. V.: Presence of cold hemolysins in sera containing cold hemagglutinins, J. Path. & Bact. 62:241, 1950.

69. Dacie, J. V., Mollison, P. L., Richardson, N., Selwyn, J. G., and Shapiro, L.: Congenital hemolytic anemia, Quart. J. Med. 22:79, 1953.

70. Dacie, J. V.: The auto-immune haemolytic anaemias, Am. J. Med. 18:810, 1955.

71. Dacie, J. V.: Acquired haemolytic anaemia, in University of London, British Postgraduate Medical Federation, Lectures on the Scientific Basis of Medicine, vol. 2, p. 59, Athlone Press, London, 1959.

72. Dacie, J. V.: The Haemolytic Anaemias, Congenital and Acquired: Part I. The Congenital Anaemias, ed. 2, Grune & Stratton, New York, 1960; Part II. The Auto-Immune Haemolytic Anaemias, ed. 2, Grune & Stratton, New York, 1962.

73. Dacie, J. V., Lewis, S. M., and Tills, D.: Comparative sensitivity of the erythrocytes in paroxysmal nocturnal haemoglobinuria to haemolysis by acidified normal serum and by high-titre cold antibody, Brit. J. Haemat. 6:362, 1960.

74. Dacie, J. V., and Lewis, S. M.: Paroxysmal nocturnal haemoglobinuria: Variations in chemical severity and association with bone marrow hypoplasia, Brit. J. Haemat. 7:442, 1961.

75. Dameshek, W.: Hemolytic anemia, Am. J. Med. 18:315, 1955.

76. Danon, D., Nevo, A., and Marikovsky, Y.: Preparation of erythrocyte ghosts by gradual hemolysis in hypotonic aqueous solution, Bull. Res. Council Israel 6E:36, 1956.

77. Danon, D.: Osmotic hemolysis by a gradual decrease in the ionic strength of the surrounding medium, J. Cell. & Comp. Physiol. 57:111, 1961.

78. Danon, D., Sheba, C., and Ramot, B.: Morphology of glucose-6-phosphate dehydrogenase deficient erythrocytes: Electron-microscopic studies, Blood 27:229, 1961.

79. Das Gupta, C. R., Chatterjea, J. B., Ghosh, S. K., and Rayn, R. N.: Plasma hemoglobin in Cooley's anemia, Indian J. M. Sc. 10:517, 1956.

80. Dausset, J., and Colombani, J.: Serology and the prognosis of 128 cases of auto-immune hemolytic anemia, Blood 12:1280, 1959.

81. Davidson, R. J. L., and Strauss, W. T.: Hereditary elliptocytic anaemia, J. Clin. Path. 14:615, 1961.

82. DeGruchy, G. C., Santamaria, J. N., Parsons, I. E., and Crawford, H.: Non-spherocytic congenital hemolytic anemia, Blood 16:1371, 1960.

83. DeSandre, G., and Ghiotto, G.: An enzymic disorder in the erythrocytes of paroxysmal nocturnal haemoglobinuria: A deficiency in acetylcholinesterase activity, Brit. J. Haemat. 6:39, 1960.

84. Desforges, J. F., Kalaw, E., and Gilchrist, P.: Inhibition of glucose-6-phosphate dehydrogenase by hemolysis-inducing drug, J. Lab. & Clin. Med. 55:757, 1960.

85. Dimant, E., Landsberg, E., and London, I. M.: Metabolic behavior of reduced glutathione in human and avian erythrocytes, J. Biol. Chem. 213:769, 1955.

86. Donath, J., and Landsteiner, K.: Über paroxysmale Haemoglobinuria, München med. Wchnschr. 512:590, 1904.

87. Ebaugh, F. G., Jr., Emerson, C. P., and Ross, J. F.: Use of radioactive chromium 51 as an erythrocyte tagging agent for the determination of red cell survival in vivo, J. Clin. Invest. 32:1260, 1953.

88. Eernisse, J. G., and Van Rood, J. J.: Erythrocyte survival-time determinations with the aid of DF^{32}P, Brit. J. Haemat. 3:382, 1961.

89. Ehrenstein, G. V., and Lockner, D.: Sites of physiological breakdown of the red blood corpuscles, Nature 181:911, 1958.

90. Emanuel, B., and Schoenfeld, A.: Favism in a nursing infant, J. Pediat. 58:263, 1961.

91. Emerson, C. P.: Influence of the spleen on the osmotic behavior and the longevity of red cells in hereditary spherocytosis (congenital hemolytic jaundice): A case study, Boston Med. Quart. 5:65, 1954.

92. Emerson, C. P., Shen, S. C., Ham, T. H., Fleming, E. M., and Castle, W. B.: Studies on the destruction of red blood cells: IX. Quantitative methods for determining the osmotic and mechanical fragility of red cells in the peripheral blood and spleen pulp; the mechanism of increased hemolysis in hereditary spherocytosis as related to the functions of the spleen, A.M.A. Arch. Int. Med. 97:1, 1956.

93. Emery, J. L., and Lemmon, D. W.: Crises in congenital spherocytic anaemia (acholuric jaundice), Brit. M. J. 1:737, 1954.

94. Engstedt, L.: Endogenous formation of carbon monoxide in hemolytic disease, Acta med. scandinav., Suppl. 332, 1957.

95. Erlandson, M. E., Schulman, I., Stern, G., and Smith, C. H.: Studies on congenital hemolytic syndromes: I. Rates of destruction and production of erythrocytes in thalassemia, Pediatrics 22:910, 1958.

96. Erlandson, M. E., Schulman, I., and Smith, C. H.: Studies on congenital hemolytic syndromes: II. Rates of destruction and production of erythrocytes in hereditary spherocytosis, Pediatrics 23:462, 1959.

97. Erlandson, M. E., Wehman, J., Stern, G., Hilgartner, M., and Smith, C. H.: Heme synthesis in thalassemia: Defect in conversion of glycine to δ-aminolevulinic acid, Am. J. Dis. Child. 102:590, 1961.

98. Evans, R. S., and Weiser, R. S.: Serology of auto-immune hemolytic disease, A.M.A. Arch. Int. Med. 100:371, 1957.

99. Evans, R. S., Binghan, M., and Boehni, P.: Autoimmune hemolytic disease: Antibody dissociation and activity, A.M.A. Arch. Int. Med. 108:338, 1961.

100. Fairley, N. H.: Methaemalbumin, Quart. J. Med. 10:95, 1941.

100a. Faulstick, D. A., Lowenstein, J., and Yiengst, M. J.: Clearance kinetics of haptoglobin-hemoglobin complex in the human, Blood 20:65, 1962.

101. Fertman, M. H., and Fertman, M. B.: Toxic anemias and Heinz bodies, Medicine 34:131, 1955.

102. Fessas, P., Stamatoyannopoulos, G., and Karaklis, A.: Hemoglobin "Pylos": Study of a hemoglobinopathy resembling thalassemia in the heterozygous, homozygous, and double heterozygous state, Blood 19:1, 1962.

103. Finland, M.: Serious infections in splenectomized children, Pediatrics 27:689, 1961.

104. Frick, P. G., Hitzig, W. H., and Stauffer, U.: Das Hämoglobin-Zürich-syndrome, Schweiz. med. Wchnschr. 91:1203, 1961.

105. Fudenberg, H., Barry, I., and Dameshek, W.: Erythrocyte-coating substance in auto-immune hemolytic disease: Its nature and significance, Blood 13:201, 1958.

106. Garby, L.: Analysis of red-cell survival curves in clinical practice and the use of di-isopropylfluorophosphonate ($DF^{32}P$) as a label for red cells in man, Brit. J. Haemat. 8:15, 1962.

107. Gasser, C.: Erythroblastopénie aiguë dans les anémies hémolytiques, Sang 21:237, 1950.

108. Gehrmann, G., and Grobel, P.: Site of red cell breakdown in haemolytic anaemia, German Med. Monthly 7:5, 1962.

109. Gerald, P. S., and Diamond, L. K.: Diagnosis of thalassemia trait by starch block electrophoresis of hemoglobin, Blood 13:61, 1958.

110. Gerald, P. S.: The abnormal haemoglobins, in Penrose, L. S., and Brown, H. L. (ed.), Recent Advances in Human Genetics, Churchill, London, 1961.

111. Giblett, E. R.: Haptoglobin: A review, Vox sang. 6:513, 1961.

112. Gilbertsen, A. S., Lowry, P. T., Hawkinson, V., and Watson, C. J.: Studies of the dipyrrylmethene ("Fuscin") pigments: I. The anabolic significance of the fecal mesobilifuscin, J. Clin. Invest. 38:1166, 1959.

113. Gilbertsen, A. S., Hawkinson, V., and Watson, C. J.: Studies of the dipyrryl-methene ("Fuscin") pigments: II. The contrasting ratios and significance of the fecal urobilinogen and mesobilifuscin in certain anemias, J. Clin. Invest. 38:1175, 1959.

114. Ginsburg, S. M.: Acute erythroid aplasia (erythroblastopenia) and vascular purpura in an otherwise hematologically normal child, Ann. Int. Med. 55:317, 1961.

115. Glenn, F., Cornell, G. N., Smith, C. H., and Schulman, I.: Splenectomy in children with idiopathic thrombocytopenic purpura, hereditary spherocytosis and Mediterranean anemia, Surg. Gynec. & Obst. 99:689, 1954.

116. Gordon, R. J., Jr.: Preparation and properties of cold hemagglutinin, J. Immunol. 71:220, 1953.

117. Gray, C. H.: Bile Pigments in Health and Disease, Charles C. Thomas, Springfield, Ill., 1961.

118. Green, H., Barrow, P., and Goldberg, B.: Effect of antibody and complement on permeability control of ascites tumor cells and erythrocytes, J. Exper. Med. 110:699, 1959.

119. Griggs, R. C., Weisman, R., Jr., and Harris, J. W.: Alterations in osmotic and mechanical fragility related to in vivo erythrocyte aging and splenic sequestration in hereditary spherocytosis, J. Clin. Invest. 39:89, 1960.

120. Grinstein, M., Bannerman, R. M., Vavra, J. D., and Moore, C. V.: Hemoglobin metabolism in thalassemia: In vivo studies, Am. J. Med. 29:18, 1960.

121. Guest, G. M.: Osmometric behavior of normal and abnormal erythrocytes, Blood 3:541, 1948.

122. Gustafsson, B. E., and Lanke, L. S.: Site of urobilin production, J. Exper. Med. 112:975, 1960.

123. Ham, T. H.: Chronic hemolytic anemia with paroxysmal nocturnal hemoglobinuria, New England J. Med. 217:915, 1937.

124. Ham, T. H.: Studies on destruction of red blood cells: I. Chronic hemolytic anemia with paroxysmal nocturnal hemoglobinuria: An investigation of the mechanism of hemolysis with observations on five cases, Arch. Int. Mcd. 64:1271, 1939.

125. Ham, T. H., and Dingle, J. H.: Studies on destruction of red blood cells: II.

Chronic hemolytic anemia with paroxysmal nocturnal hemoglobinuria: Certain immunological aspects of the hemolytic mechanism with special reference to serum complement, J. Clin. Invest. 18:657, 1939.

126. Ham, T. H., Shen, S. C., Fleming, E. M., and Castle, W. B.: Studies on the destruction of red blood cells: IV. Thermal injury: Action of heat in causing increased spheroidicity, osmotic and mechanical fragilities and hemolysis of erythrocytes. Observations on the mechanisms of destruction in such erythrocytes in dogs and in a patient with a fatal thermal burn, Blood 3:373, 1948.

127. Hanks, G. E., Cassell, M., Ray, R. N., and Chaplin, H., Jr.: Further modification of the benzidine method for measurement of hemoglobin in plasma, J. Lab. & Clin. Med. 56:486, 1960.

128. Harley, J. D., and Mauer, A. M.: Studies on the formation of Heinz bodies: I. Methemoglobin production and oxyhemoglobin destruction, Blood 16:1722, 1960.

129. Harley, J. D.: Acute haemolytic anaemia in Mediterranean children with glucose-6-phosphate dehydrogenase–deficient erythrocytes, Australasian Ann. Med. 10:192, 1961.

130. Harley, J. D., and Mauer, A. M.: Studies on the formation of Heinz bodies: II. The nature and significance of Heinz bodies, Blood 17:418, 1961.

131. Harris, I. M., McAlister, J. M., and Prankerd, T. A. J.: Relationship of abnormal red cells to the normal spleen, Clin. Sc. 16:223, 1957.

132. Harris, I. M., McAlister, J. M., and Prankerd, T. A. J.: Splenomegaly and the circulating red cell, Brit. J. Haemat. 4:97, 1958.

133. Harris, J. W.: Studies on the mechanism of a drug-induced hemolytic anemia, J. Lab. & Clin. Med. 47:760, 1956.

134. Hartmann, R. C., and Auditore, J. V.: Paroxysmal nocturnal hemoglobinuria: I. Clinical studies, Am. J. Med. 27:389, 1959.

135. Haurani, F. I., and Tocantins, L. M.: Ineffective erythropoiesis, Am. J. Med. 31:519, 1961.

136. Heisterkamp, D., and Ebaugh, F. G., Jr.: Site of attachment of the chromate ion to the haemoglobin molecule, Nature 193:1253, 1962.

137. Herman, E. C., Jr.: Serum haptoglobins in hemolytic disorder: Their semiquantitative estimation by a paper electrophoretic technique, J. Lab. & Clin. Med. 57:825, 1961.

138. Hinz, C. F., Jordan, W. S., and Pillemer, L.: The properdin system and immunity: IV. The hemolysis of erythrocytes from patients with paroxysmal nocturnal hemoglobinuria, J. Clin. Invest. 35:453, 1956.

139. Hinz, C. F., Weisman, R., Jr., and Hurley, T. H.: Paroxysmal nocturnal hemoglobinuria: Relationship of in vitro and in vivo hemolysis to clinical severity, J. Lab. & Clin. Med. 48:495, 1956.

140. Hinz, C. F., Picken, M., and Lepow, I. H.: Studies on immune hemolysis: I. The kinetics of the Donath-Landsteiner reaction and the requirement for complement in the reaction, J. Exper. Med. 113:177, 1961.

141. Hinz, C. F., Picken, M., and Lepow, I. H.: Studies on immune hemolysis: II. The Donath-Landsteiner reaction as a model system for studying the mechanism of action of complement and the role of C'_1 and C'_1-esterase, J. Exper. Med. 113:193, 1961.

142. Hinz, C. F., and Mollner, A. M.: Initiation of the action of complement in a human autoimmune hemolytic system, the Donath-Landsteiner reaction, J. Clin. Invest. 41: 1365, 1962.

143. Hjort, P. F., Paputchis, H., and Cheney, B.: Labeling of red blood cells with radioactive diisopropylfluorophosphate (DFP[32]): Evidence for an initial release of label, J. Lab. & Clin. Med. 55:416, 1960.

144. Hoffman, J. F., Wolman, I. J., Hillier, J., and Parpart, A. K.: Ultrastructure of erythrocyte membranes in thalassemia major and minor, Blood 11:946, 1956.

145. Hoffman, J. F., Eden, M., Barr, J. S., Jr., and Bedell, R. H. S.: Hemolytic volume of human erythrocytes, J. Cell. & Comp. Physiol. 51:405, 1958.

146. Hughies-Jones, N. C., Mollison, P. L., and Veal, N.: Removal of incompatible red cells by the spleen, Brit. J. Haemat. 3:125, 1957.

147. Hutt, M. P., Reger, J. F., and Neustein, H. B.: Renal pathology in paroxysmal nocturnal hemoglobinuria, Am. J. Med. 31:736, 1961.

148. Jacob, H. S., and Jandl, J. H.: Effect of membrane sulfhydryl deficiency on the shape and survival of red cells, Clin. Res. 9:162, 1961.

148a. Jacob, H. S., and Jandl, J. H.: Effects of sulfhydryl inhibition on red blood cells: I. Mechanism of hemolysis, J. Clin. Invest. 41:779, 1962.

149. Jaffé, E. R., Lowy, B. A., Vanderhoff, G. A., Aisen, P., and London, I. M.: Effects of nucleosides on the resistance of normal human erythrocytes to osmotic lysis, J. Clin. Invest. 36:1498, 1957.

150. Jandl, J. H.: Studies on the mechanism of the anemia of liver diseases, J. Clin. Invest. 33:946, 1954.

151. Jandl, J. H., and Castle, W. B.: Agglutination of sensitized red cells by large anisometric molecules, J. Lab. & Clin. Med. 47:669, 1956.

152. Jandl, J. H., Greenberg, M. S., Yonemoto, R. H., and Castle, W. B.: Clinical determination of the sites of red cell sequestration in hemolytic anemias, J. Clin. Invest. 35:842, 1956.

153. Jandl, J. H., Jones, A. R., and Castle, W. B.: Destruction of red cells by antibodies in man: I. Observations on the sequestration and lysis of red cells altered by immune mechanisms, J. Clin. Invest. 36:1428, 1957.

154. Jandl, J. H., and Tomlinson, A. S.: Destruction of red cells by antibodies in man: II. Pyrogenic, leukocytic and dermal responses to immune hemolysis, J. Clin. Invest. 37:1202, 1958.

155. Jandl, J. H., and Greenberg, M. S.: Bone marrow failure due to relative nutritional deficiency in Cooley's hemolytic anemia, New England J. Med. 260:461, 1959.

156. Jandl, J. H.: Hereditary spherocytosis, in Stanbury, J. B., Wyngaarden, J. B., and Fredrickson, D. S. (ed.), The Metabolic Basis of Inherited Disease, p. 1015, McGraw-Hill, New York, 1960.

157. Jandl, J. H., Engle, L. K., and Allen, D. W.: Oxidative hemolysis and precipitation of hemoglobin: I. Heinz body anemias as an acceleration of red cell aging, J. Clin. Invest. 39:1818, 1960.

158. Jandl, J. H., and Kaplan, M. E.: Destruction of red cells by antibodies in man: III. Quantitative factors influencing the patterns of hemolysis in vivo, J. Clin. Invest. 39:1145, 1960.

159. Jandl, J. H., Jacob, H. S., and Daland, G. A.: Hypersplenism due to infection: Study of five cases manifesting hemolytic anemia, New England J. Med. 264:1063, 1961.

160. Jandl, J. H., Simmons, R. L., and Castle, W. B.: Red cell filtration and the pathogenesis of certain hemolytic anemias, Blood 18:133, 1961.

161. Jayle, M. F., and Moretti, J.: Haptoglobin: Biochemical, genetic, and physiopathological aspects, Progr. Hemat. 3:342, 1962.

162. Johnson, P. M., Herion, J. C., and Modring, S. L.: Scintillation scanning of the normal human spleen utilizing sensitized radioactive erythrocytes, Radiology 74:99, 1960.

163. Jordon, W. S., Prouty, R. L., Heinle, R. W., and Dingle, J. H.: Mechanism of hemolysis in paroxysmal cold hemoglobinuria: III. Erythrophagocytosis and leukopenia, Blood 4:387, 1952.

164. Josephs, H. W.: Favism, Bull. Johns Hopkins Hosp. 74:295, 1944.

165. Joske, R. A., McAlister, J. M., and Prankerd, T. A. J.: Isotope investigations of red cell production and destruction in chronic renal disease, Clin. Sc. 15:511, 1956.

166. Kantor, S. F., and Argesman, C. E.: Serologic studies on favism, J. Allergy 30:114, 1959.

167. Kaplan, E., and Zuelzer, W. W.: Erythrocyte survival in childhood: II. Studies in Mediterranean anemia, J. Lab. & Clin. Med. 36:517, 1950.

168. Kaplan, E., and Hsu, K. S.: Chromium⁵¹ erythrocyte survival in newborn, Pediatrics 27:354, 1961.

169. Katchalsky, A., Kedem, O., Klibansky, C., and DeVries, A.: Rheological considerations of the hemolysing red blood cell, *in* Copley, A. L., and Stainsby, G. (ed.), Flow Properties of Blood and Other Biological Systems, p. 155, Pergamon Press, New York, 1960.

170. Kekwick, R. A., and Mollison, P. L.: Blood group antibodies associated with the 19S and 7S components of human sera, Vox sang. 6:398, 1961.

171. Kellermeyer, R. W., Tarlov, A. R., Schrier, S. L., Carson, P. E., and Alving, A. S.: Hemolytic effect of primaquine: XIII. Gradient susceptibility to hemolysis of primaquine-sensitive erythrocytes, J. Lab. & Clin. Med. 58:225, 1961.

172. Kellermeyer, R. W., Carson, P. E., Schrier, S. L., Tarlov, A. R., and Alving, A. S.: Hemolytic effect of primaquine: XIV. Pentose metabolism in primaquine-sensitive erythrocytes, J. Lab. & Clin. Med. 58:715, 1961.

173. Kellermeyer, R. W., Tarlov, A. R., Brewer, G. J., Carson, P. E., and Alving, A. S.: Hemolytic effect of therapeutic drugs, J.A.M.A. 180:388, 1962.

174. Kellner, G.: Splenic lymph passages, J.A.M.A. 178:777, 1961.

175. Keohane, K. W., and Metcalf, W. K.: Sensitivity of blood cells to light of different wavelengths, Phys. Med. Biol. 4:140, 1959.

176. Kiese, M., and Waller, H. D.: Kinetic der Hämiglobinbildung: Die Stoffwechselvorgange in roten Zellen bei der Hämiglobinbildung durch den Kreisprogess phenylhydroxylamin-nitrosobenzol, Arch. exper. Path. u. Pharmakol. 231:158, 1957.

177. Kirkman, H. N., Riley, H. D., Jr., and Crowell, B. B.: Different enzymatic expressions of mutants of human glucose-6-phosphate dehydrogenase, Proc. Nat. Acad. Sc. 46:938, 1960.

178. Kirkman, H. N., and Riley, H. D., Jr.: Congenital nonspherocytic hemolytic anemia: Studies on a family with a qualitative defect in glucose-6-phosphate dehydrogenase, A.M.A. Am. J. Dis. Child. 102:313, 1961.

179. Kissmeyer-Nielsen, F., Jensen, K. B., and Ersbak, J.: Severe haemolytic transfusion reactions caused by apparently compatible red cells, Brit. J. Haemat. 7:36, 1961.

180. Klatskin, G.: Bile pigment metabolism, Ann. Rev. Med. 12:21, 1961.

181. Koler, R. D., and Rigas, D. A.: Genetics of haemoglobin H, Ann. Human Genet. 25:95, 1961.

182. Laski, B., and MacMillan, A.: Incidence of infection in children after splenectomy, Pediatrics 24:523, 1959.

183. Lathem, W., and Worley, W. E.: Distribution of extracorpuscular hemoglobin in circulating plasma, J. Clin. Invest. 38:474, 1959.

184. Lathem, W., and Worley, W. E.: Renal excretion of hemoglobin: Regulatory mechanisms and the differential excretion of free and protein-bound hemoglobin, J. Clin. Invest. 38:652, 1959.

185. Lathem, W., Davis, B. B., Zweig, P. H., and Dew, R.: Demonstration and localization of renal tubular reabsorption of hemoglobin by stop flow analysis, J. Clin. Invest. 39:840, 1960.

186. Lathem, W., and Jensen, W. N.: Renal excretion of hemoglobin in sickle cell anemia, with observations on spontaneously occurring hemoglobinemia and methemalbuminemia, J. Lab. & Clin. Med. 59:137, 1962.

187. Leddy, J. P., Trabold, N. C., Vaughn, J. H., and Swisher, S. N.: Unitary nature of "complete" and "incomplete" pathologic cold hemagglutinins, Blood 19:379, 1962.

188. Lee, C. L., Takahushi, T., and Davidson, I.: Electrophoretic separation of certain in vitro and in vivo reactions of rabbit anti-mouse erythrocyte serum, Nature 187:157, 1960.

189. Lehmann, H., and Ager, J. A. M.: The hemoglobinopathies and thalassemia, in Stanbury, J. B., Wyngaarden, J. B., and Fredrickson, D. S. (ed.), The Metabolic Basis of Inherited Disease, p. 1086, McGraw-Hill, New York, 1960.

190. Leibetseder, F., and Ahrens, E. H., Jr.: Fatty-acid composition of red cells in paroxysmal nocturnal haemoglobinuria, Brit. J. Haemat. 5:356, 1959.

191. Lester, R., and Schmid, R.: Enterohepatic circulation of bilirubin, J. Lab. & Clin. Med. 58:938, 1962.

192. Lewis, S. M., Dacie, J. V., and Szur, L.: Mechanism of haemolysis in the cold-haemagglutinin syndrome, Brit. J. Haemat. 6:154, 1960.

193. Lewis, S. M., Szur, L., and Dacie, J. V.: Pattern of erythrocyte destruction in haemolytic anaemia, as studied with radioactive chromium, Brit. J. Haemat. 6:122, 1960.

194. Lewis, S. M., Dacie, J. V., and Tills, D.: Comparison of the sensitivity to agglutination and haemolysis by a high-titre cold antibody of the erythrocytes of normal subjects and of patients with a variety of blood diseases including paroxysmal nocturnal haemoglobinuria, Brit. J. Haemat. 7:64, 1961.

195. Little, H. N., and Neilands, J. B.: Binding of haematin by human serum albumin, Nature 188:913, 1960.

196. Lock, S. P., and Dormandy, K. M.: Red-cell fragmentation syndrome: A condition of multiple etiology, Lancet 1:1020, 1961.

197. Lock, S. P., Smith, R. S., and Hardisty, R. M.: Stomatocytosis: A hereditary red cell anomaly associated with haemolytic anaemia, Brit. J. Haemat. 7:303, 1961.

198. Löhr, G. W., and Waller, H. D.: The enzyme-deficiency haemolytic anaemias, German Med. Monthly 6:37, 1961.

199. London, I. M.: Metabolism of hemoglobin and of bile pigment, Bull. New York Acad. Med. 30:509, 1954.

200. Lowdon, A. G. R., Walker, J. H., and Walker, W.: Infection following splenectomy in childhood, Lancet 1:499, 1962.

201. Lowenstein, J., Faulstick, D. A., Yiengst, M. J., and Shock, N. W.: Glomerular clearance and renal transport of hemoglobin in adult males, J. Clin. Invest. 40:1172, 1961.

202. Luisada, A.: Favism: A singular disease chiefly affecting the red blood cells, Medicine 20:229, 1941.

203. MacGibbon, B. H., Loughridge, L. W., Hourehane, D. O'B., and Boyd, D. W.: Auto-immune haemolytic anaemia with acute renal failure due to phenacetin and p-aminosalicylic acid, Lancet 1:7, 1960.

204. MacIver, J. E., Went, L. N., and Irvine, R. A.: Hereditary persistence of foetal haemoglobin: A family study suggesting allelism of the F gene to the S and C haemoglobin genes, Brit. J. Haemat. 7:373, 1961.

205. MacKenzie, G. M.: Paroxysmal hemoglobinuria: A review, Medicine 8:159, 1929.

206. MacKinney, A. A., Jr., Morton, N. E., Kosower, N. S., and Schilling, R. F.: Ascertaining genetic carriers of hereditary spherocytosis by statistical analysis of multiple laboratory tests, J. Clin. Invest. 41:554, 1962.

207. Malamos, B., Belcher, E. H., Cyftaki, E., and Binopoulos, D.: Simultaneous radioactive tracer studies of erythropoiesis and red-cell destruction in thalassemia, Brit. J. Haemat. 7:411, 1961.

208. March, H. W., Schlyen, S. M., and Schwartz, S. E.: Mediterranean hemopathic syndromes (Cooley's anemia) in adults, Am. J. Med. 13:46, 1952.

209. Marks, P. A., and Gross, R. T.: Erythrocyte glucose-6-phosphate dehydrogenase deficiency: Evidence of differences between Negroes and Caucasians with respect to this genetically determined trait, J. Clin. Invest. 38:2253, 1959.

210. Marks, P. A., Szeinberg, A., and Banks, J.: Erythrocyte glucose-6-phosphate dehydrogenase of normal and mutant human subjects: Properties of the purified enzymes, J. Biol. Chem. 236:10, 1961.

211. McClellan, J. E., Donegan, C., Thorup, O., and Leavell, B. S.: Survival time of the erythrocyte in myxedema and hyperthyroidism, J. Lab. & Clin. Med. 51:91, 1958.

212. McCrea, P. C.: Latent haemolysis in rheumatoid arthritis, Lancet 1:402, 1957.

213. McFarland, W., Galbraith, R. G., and Miale, A.: Heparin therapy in autoimmune hemolytic anemia, Blood 15:741, 1960.

214. Metz, J., Bradlow, B. A., Lewis, S. M., and Dacie, J. V.: Acetylcholinesterase activity of the erythrocytes in paroxysmal noctural haemoglobinuria in relation to the severity of the disease, Brit. J. Haemat. 6:372, 1960.

215. Metz, J., Stevens, K., Van Rensburg, N. J., and Hart, D.: Failure of in vivo inhibition of acetylcholinesteral to affect erythrocyte life-span: The significance of the enzyme defect in paroxysmal nocturnal haemoglobinuria, Brit. J. Haemat. 7:458, 1961.

216. Meyer, L. M., and Bertcher, R. W.: Acquired hemolytic anemia and transient erythroid hypoplasia of bone marrow, Am. J. Med. 28:606, 1960.

217. Mohler, D. N., and Williams, W. J.: Effect of phenylhydrazine on the adenosine triphosphate content of normal and glucose-6-phosphate dehydrogenase–deficient human blood, J. Clin. Invest. 40:1735, 1961.

218. Mollison, P. L.: Blood-group antibodies and red-cell destruction, Brit. M. J. 2:1035, 1959.

219. Mollison, P. L.: Measurement of survival and destruction of red cells in haemolytic syndromes, Brit. M. Bull. 15:59, 1959.

220. Mollison, P. L.: Further observations on the normal survival curve of ^{51}Cr-labelled red cells, Clin. Sc. 21:21, 1961.

221. Motulsky, A. G., Gabrio, B. W., Burkhardt, J., and Finch, C. A.: Erythrocyte carbohydrate metabolism in hereditary hemolytic anemias, Ann. J. Med. 19:291, 1955.

222. Muirhead, E. E., Groves, M., Guy, R., Holden, E. R., and Bass, R. K.: Acquired hemolytic anemia, exposures to insecticides and positive Coombs test dependent on insecticide preparations, Vox sang. 4:277, 1959.

223. Mukherjee, A. M., Sen Gupta, P. C., and Chatterjea, J. B.: Histopathology of the liver in thalassemia syndrome, J. Indian M. A. 35:291, 1960.

224. Munn, J. I.: Studies of lipids in human red cells, Brit. J. Haemat. 4:344, 1958.

225. Munn, J. I., and Crosby, W. H.: Red-cell lipids in various abnormalities of the human red cell, Brit. J. Haemat. 7:523, 1961.

226. Murphy, J. R.: Erythrocyte metabolism: III. The relationship of energy metabolism and serum factors to the osmotic fragility following incubation, J. Lab. & Clin. Med. 60:32, 1962.

227. Myhre, E., and Flatmark, T.: Reticulocyte destruction in paroxysmal nocturnal haemoglobinuria, Brit. J. Haemat. 8:48, 1962.

228. Naylor, J., Rosenthal, I., Grossman, A., Schulman, I., and Hsia, D. Y. Y.: Activity of glucose-6-phosphate dehydrogenase in erythrocytes of patients with various abnormal hemoglobins, Pediatrics 26:285, 1960.

229. Necheles, T., and Beutler, E.: Effect of triiodothyronine on the oxidative metabolism of erythrocytes: I. Cellular studies, J. Clin. Invest. 38:788, 1959.

230. Neel, J. L.: The hemoglobin genes: A remarkable example of the clustering of related genetic functions on a single mammalian chromosome, Blood 18:769, 1961.

231. Nelson, M. G., and Marshall, R. J.: The syndrome of high-titre cold haemagglutination, Brit. M. J. 2:314, 1953.

232. Nyman, M.: Serum haptoglobins, Scandinav. J. Clin. & Lab. Invest. 11, Suppl. 39, 1959.

233. Nyman, M., Gydell, K., and Mosslin, B.: Correlations between haptoglobin, carbon monoxide and urobilinogen in hemolytic diseases, Clin. chim. acta 4:82, 1959.

234. Nyman, M.: On plasma proteins with heme or hemoglobin binding capacity, Scandinav. J. Clin. & Lab. Invest. 12:121, 1960.

235. O'Connor, W. J., Vakiener, J. M., and Watson, R. J.: Idiopathic acquired hemolytic anemia in young children, Pediatrics 17:732, 1956.

236. Olivia, J., and Myerson, R. M.: Hereditary persistence of fetal hemoglobin, Am. J. M. Sc. 241:215, 1961.

237. Oort, M., Loos, J. A., and Prins, H. K.: Hereditary absence of reduced glutathione in the erythrocytes: A new clinical and biochemical entity? Vox sang. 6:370, 1961.

238. Ostrow, J. D., Hammaker, L., and Schmid, R.: Preparation of crystalline bilirubin-C^{14}, J. Clin. Invest. 40:1442, 1961.

239. Owen, J. A., DeGruchy, G. C., and Smith, H.: Serum haptoglobin in haemolytic studies, J. Clin. Path. 13:478, 1960.

240. Owen, J. A., Padanyi, R., and Smith, H.: Serum haptoglobins and other tests in the diagnosis of hepatobiliary jaundice, Clin. Sc. 21:189, 1961.

241. Owren, P. A.: Congenital hemolytic jaundice: The pathogenesis of the "hemolytic crisis," Blood 3:231, 1948.

242. Panizon, F., and Vullo, C.: Mechanism of haemolysis in favism: Researches on the role of noncorpuscular factors, Acta haemat. 26:337, 1961.

243. Paolino, W.: Variations of the mean diameter in the ripening of the erythrocyte, Acta med. scandinav. 136:141, 1949.

244. Parpart, A. K., and Ballentine, R.: Molecular anatomy of the plasma membrane, in Barron, E. S. G. (ed.), Modern Trends in Physiology and Biochemistry, Academic Press, New York, 1952.

245. Pearson, H. A., McFarland, W., and Kings, E. R.: Erythro-kinetic studies in thalassemia trait, J. Lab. & Clin. Med. 56:866, 1960.

246. Pearson, H. A., and Druyan, R.: Erythrocyte glucose-6-phosphate dehydrogenase activity related to thyroid activity, J. Lab. & Clin. Med. 57:343, 1961.

247. Pearson, H. A., and Vertrees, K. M.: Site of binding of chromium[51] to haemoglobin, Nature 189:1019, 1961.

248. Pearson, H. A., and McFarland, W.: Erythrokinetics in thalassemia: II. Studies in Lepore trait and hemoglobin H disease, J. Lab. & Clin. Med. 59:147, 1962.

249. Phillips, G. B.: Quantitative chromatographic analysis of plasma and red blood cell lipids in patients with acanthocytosis, J. Lab. & Clin. Med. 59:357, 1962.

249a. Phillips, G. B., and Roome, N. S.: Quantitative chromatographic analysis of the phospholipids of abnormal human red blood cells, Proc. Soc. Exper. Biol. & Med. 109:360, 1962.

249b. Pierce, L. E., and Rath, C. E.: Evidence for folic acid deficiency in the genesis of anemic sickle cell crisis, Blood 20:19, 1962.

250. Pitkänen, E., and Nikkilä, E. A.: Erythrocyte enzymes in thyrotoxicosis, Ann. med. int. Fenniae 49:197, 1960.

251. Ponder, D.: Hemolysis and Related Phenomena, Grune & Stratton, New York, 1948.

252. Ponder, E.: Shape and shape transformations of heated human red cells, J. Exper. Biol. 26:35, 1949.

253. Ponder, E.: Certain hemolytic mechanisms in hemolytic anemia, Blood 6:559, 1951.

254. Ponder, E.: Volume changes and partial hemolysis in heat-fragmented red cells, as observed by interference microscopy, J. Cell. & Comp. Physiol. 51:461, 1958.

255. Po-tun Fok, F., and Schubothe, H.: Studies on various factors influencing mechanical haemolysis of human erythrocytes, Brit. J. Haemat. 6:355, 1960.

256. Prankerd, T. A. J.: Inborn errors of metabolism in red cells of congenital hemolytic anemias, Am. J. Med. 22:724, 1957.

257. Prankerd, T. A. J.: Red cell structure and metabolism in haemolytic anaemia, Brit. M. Bull. 15:54, 1959.

258. Prankerd, T. A. J.: Studies on the pathogenesis of haemolysis in hereditary spherocytosis, Quart. J. Med. 29:199, 1960.

259. Prankerd, T. A. J.: Viability and survival of red cells, *in* University of London, British Postgraduate Medical Federation, Lectures on the Scientific Basis of Medicine, vol. 8, Athlone Press, London, 1960.

260. Race, R. R.: On the inheritance and linkage relations of acholuric jaundice, Ann. Eugenics 11:365, 1942.

261. Ramot, B., Ashkenazi, I., Rimon, A., Adam, A., and Sheba, C.: Activation of glucose-6-phosphate dehydrogenase of enzyme-deficient subjects: II. Properties of the activator and the activation reaction, J. Clin. Invest. 40:611, 1961.

262. Rapaport, S. I., Reilly, E. B., Eade, N. R., and Carne, H. O.: Paroxysmal nocturnal hemoglobinuria: Case report with comments upon the urinary iron loss, Ann. Int. Med. 44:812, 1956.

263. Rappaport, H., and Crosby, W. H.: Autoimmune hemolytic anemia: II. Morphologic observations and clinicopathologic correlations, Am. J. Path. 33:492, 1957.

264. Reader, R.: Complement in acquired haemolytic anaemia, Australasian Ann. Med. 4:279, 1955.

265. Reed, C. F.: Studies of in vivo and in vitro exchange of erythrocyte and plasma phospholipids, J. Clin. Invest. 38:1032, 1959.

266. Reemtsma, K., and Elliott, R. H. E.: Splenectomy in Mediterannean anemia: An evaluation of long-term results, Ann. Surg. 144:999, 1956.

267. Reyersbach, G. C., and Butler, A. M.: Congenital hereditary hematuria, New England J. Med. 251:377, 1954.

268. Reynafarje, C., and Ramos, J.: The hemolytic anemia of human bartonellosis, Blood 17:562, 1961.

269. Rice, J. D., and Mathies, L. A.: Comparison of resistance of reticulocytes and mature erythrocytes to immune hemolysis: Studies in the guinea pig, rabbit, dog and man, A.M.A. Arch. Path. 70:435, 1960.

270. Rigas, D. A., and Koler, R. D.: Decreased erythrocyte survival in hemoglobin

H disease as a result of the abnormal properties of hemoglobin H: The benefit of splenectomy, Blood 18:1, 1961.

271. Rigas, D. A., and Koler, R. D.: Erythrocyte enzymes and reduced glutathione (GSH) in hemoglobin H disease: Relation to cell age and denaturation of hemoglobin H, J. Lab. & Clin. Med. 58:417, 1961.

272. Rimon, A., Ashkenazi, I., Ramot, B., and Sheba, C.: Activation of glucose-6-phosphate dehydrogenase of enzyme-deficient subjects: I. Activation by stroma of normal erythrocytes, Biochem. Biophys. Rev. Commun. 2:138, 1960.

273. Robinson, M. A., Loder, P. B., and DeGruchy, G. C.: Red-cell metabolism in non-spherocytic congenital haemolytic anaemia, Brit. J. Haemat. 7:327, 1961.

274. Robinson, T. W., and Sturgeon, P.: Post-splenectomy infection in infants and children, Pediatrics 25:941, 1960.

275. Rosenfield, M., and Surgenor, D. M.: Methemalbumin: Interaction between human serum albumin and ferri protoporphyrin IX, J. Biol. Chem. 183:663, 1950.

276. Ross, J. F.: Hemoglobinemia and the hemoglobinurias, New England J. Med. 233:691, 1945.

277. Roth, K. L., and Frumin, A. M.: Studies on the hemolytic principle of the fava bean, J. Lab. & Clin. Med. 56:695, 1960.

278. Rous, P.: Destruction of the red blood corpuscles in health and disease, Physiol. Rev. 3:75, 1923.

279. Rubin, D., Weisberger, A. S., and Clark, D. R.: Early detection of drug-induced erythropoietic depression, J. Lab. & Clin. Med. 56:453, 1960.

280. Rucknagel, D. L., and Neel, J. V.: The hemoglobinopathies, in Steinberg, A. G. (ed.), Progress in Medical Genetics, vol. I, Grune & Stratton, New York, 1961.

281. Rutzky, J., Cohen, F., and Zuelzer, W. W.: Anti-A agglutinins in pooled plasma as a cause of hemolytic anemia, J. Hemat. 11:403, 1956.

282. Salt, H. B., Wolff, O. H., Lloyd, J. K., Fosbrooke, A. S., Cameron, A. H., and Hubble, D. V.: On having no beta-liproprotein: A syndrome comprising a-beta-liproproteinaemia, acanthocytosis, and steatorrhoea, Lancet 2:325, 1960.

283. Schloesser, L. L., Korst, D. R., Clatanoff, D. V., and Schilling, R. F.: Radioactivity over the spleen and liver following the transfusion of chromium 51–labelled erythrocytes in hemolytic anemia, J. Clin. Invest. 36:1470, 1957.

284. Schmid, R., Brecher, G., and Clemens, T.: Familial hemolytic anemia with erythrocyte inclusion bodies and a defect in pigment metabolism, Blood 14:991, 1959.

285. Schmid, R.: Hyperbilirubinemia, in Stanbury, J. B., Wyngaarden, J. B., and Fredrickson, D. S. (ed.), The Metabolic Basis of Inherited Disease, p. 226. McGraw-Hill, New York, 1960.

286. Schrier, S. L., Kellermeyer, R. W., and Alving, A. S.: Coenzyme studies in primaquine-sensitive erythrocytes, Proc. Soc. Exper. Biol. & Med. 99:354, 1958.

287. Schroeder, W. A., Sturgeon, P., and Bergren, W. R.: Chemical investigation of haemoglobin F from an individual with persistent foetal haemoglobin, Nature 193:1161, 1962.

288. Schrumpf, A.: Life of erythrocytes in hereditary spherocytosis, Rev. hémat. 11:140, 1956.

289. Schubothe, H., and Po-tun Fok, F.: Quantitative estimation of mechanical haemolysis for clinical application, Brit. J. Haemat. 6:350, 1960.

290. Schubothe, H., and Haenle, M.: Serologishe studien über die Nichtsyphili-

tische variante des Donath-Landsteinerschen Hämolysins, Vox sang. 6:455, 1961.

291. Schwartz, R., and Dameshek, W.: Treatment of autoimmune hemolytic anemia with 6-mercaptopurine and thioguanine, Blood 19:483, 1962.

292. Schwartz, S. O., and Mason, J.: Mediterranean anemia in the Negro: A report of four cases and three families, Blood 4:736, 1949.

293. Seip, M.: Aplastic crisis in a case of immuno-hemolytic anemia, Acta med. scandinav. 153:137, 1955.

294. Shahidi, N. T., and Diamond, L. K.: Enzyme deficiency in erythrocytes in congenital nonspherocytic hemolytic anemia, Pediatrics 24:245, 1959.

295. Sharpsteen, J. R.: Physico-chemical mechanisms in the pathogenesis of certain hemolytic anemias, Am. J. M. Sc. 229:506, 1955.

296. Shen, S. C.: Hemoglobin tolerance in various types of anemia, A.M.A. Arch. Int. Med. 101:315, 1958.

297. Shen, S. C.: Urobilinogen excretion after hemoglobin infusions in patients with normal hematologic and hepatic findings, Proc. Soc. Exper. Biol. & Med. 105:264, 1960.

298. Shumway, C. N., Jr., and Miller, G.: An unusual syndrome of hemolytic anemia, thrombocytopenic purpura and renal disease, Blood 12:1045, 1957.

299. Sliwinski, A. J., and Lilienfield, L. S.: Red cell and plasma transit through spleen: The splenic hematocrit, Proc. Soc. Exper. Biol. & Med. 99:648, 1958.

300. Sliwinski, A. J., and Lilienfield, L. S.: Evidence for a functional closed circulation in the spleen, Clin. Res. 10:28, 1962.

301. Smith, C. H.: Detection of mild type of Mediterranean (Cooley's) anemia, Am. J. Dis. Child. 75:505, 1948.

302. Smith, C. H., and Morgenthau, J. E.: Cholelithiasis in severe Mediterranean (Cooley's) anemia, Blood 6:1147, 1951.

303. Smith, C. H., Erlandson, M. E., Schulman, I., and Stern, G.: Hazard of severe infections in splenectomized infants and children, Am. J. Med. 22:390, 1957.

304. Smith, C. H., Erlandson, M. E., Stern, G., and Schulman, I.: Role of splenectomy in the management of thalassemia, Blood 15:197, 1960.

305. Smith, C. H., Erlandson, M. E., Stern, G., and Hilgartner, M. W.: Postsplenectomy infection in Cooley's anemia: An appraisal of the problem in this and other blood disorders, with a consideration of prophylaxis, New England J. Med. 15:737, 1962.

306. Smith, H., and Owen, J. A.: Determination of haptoglobins in normal human serum, Biochem. J. 78:723, 1961.

307. Splenic circulation (editorial), Lancet 1:338, 1955.

308. Stamey, C. C., and Diamond, L. K.: Congenital hemolytic anemia in the newborn, A.M.A. Am. J. Dis. Child. 94:616, 1957.

309. Stefanini, M., Xefteris, E., Moschides, E., and Blumenthal, W. S.: Role of hemolytic system in human tissues in some hemolytic states, Am. J. M. Sc. 242:303, 1961.

310. Sternschuss, N., Vanderhoff, G. A., Jaffé, E. R., and London, I. M.: Metabolic changes in normal and glucose-6-phosphate dehydrogenase–deficient erythrocytes induced by acetylphenylhydrazine, J. Clin. Invest. 40:1083, 1961.

311. Sturgeon, P., and Finch, C. A.: Erythrokinetics in Cooley's anemia, Blood 12:64, 1957.

312. Swisher, S. N.: Auto-immune hemolytic disease: Some experiences and some unsolved problems, *in* Shaffer, J. H., et al. (ed.), Mechanisms of Hypersensitivity (Eighth International Symposium, Henry Ford Hospital), p. 349, Little, Brown, Boston, 1959.

313. Szeinberg, A., Sheba, C., and Adam, A.: Enzymatic abnormality in erythrocytes of a population sensitive to *Vicia fava* or hemolytic anaemia induced by drugs, Nature 181:1256, 1958.

314. Szeinberg, A., and Marks, P. A.: Substance stimulating glucose catabolism by the oxidative reactions of the pentose phosphate pathway in human erythrocytes, J. Clin. Invest. 40:914, 1961.

315. Tabechian, H., Altman, K. I., and Young, L. E.: Inhibition of P^{32}-orthophosphate exchange by sodium fluoride in erythrocytes from patients with hereditary spherocytosis, Proc. Soc. Exper. Biol. & Med. 92:712, 1956.

316. Tanaka, K. R., Valentine, W. N., and Fredricks, R. E.: Studies on leukocytic and erythrocytic enzymes in paroxysmal nocturnal hemoglobinuria, Clin. Res. 8:132, 1960.

317. Tanaka, K. R., Valentine, W. N., and Miwa, S.: Pyruvate kinase (PK) deficiency hereditary nonspherocytic hemolytic anemia, Blood 19:267, 1962.

318. Tanaka, K. R., Valentine, W. N., and Miwa, S.: Studies on hereditary spherocytosis and other hemolytic anemias, Clin. Res. 10:109, 1962.

319. Tarlov, A. R., and Kellermeyer, R. W.: Hemolytic effect of primaquine: XI. Decreased catalase activity in primaquine-sensitive erythrocytes, J. Lab. & Clin. Med. 58:204, 1961.

320. Tarlov, A. R., Brewer, G. J., Carson, P. E., and Alving, A. S.: Primaquine sensitivity: Glucose-6-phosphate dehydrogenase deficiency: An inborn error of metabolism of medical and biological significance, A.M.A. Arch. Int. Med. 109:209, 1962.

321. Theil, G. B., Brodine, C. E., and Doolan, P. D.: Red cell glutathione content and stability in renal insufficiency, J. Lab. & Clin. Med. 58:736, 1961.

322. Thomas, E. D., Lochte, H. L., Jr., Greenough, W. B., III, and Wales, M.: In vitro synthesis of foetal and adult haemoglobin by foetal haematopoietic tissues, Nature 185:396, 1960.

323. Thompson, R. B., Mitchener, J. W., and Huisman, T. H. J.: Studies on the fetal hemoglobin in the persistent high Hb-F anomaly, Blood 18:267, 1961.

324. Tisdale, W. A., Klatskin, G., and Kinsella, E. D.: Significance of the direct-reacting factor of serum bilirubin in hemolytic jaundice, Am. J. Med. 26:214, 1959.

325. Tolentine, P.: Mechanical fragility of thalassemic erythrocytes, Nature 167:905, 1951.

326. Tuffy, P., Brown, A. K., and Zuelzer, W. W.: Infantile pyknocytosis, A.M.A. Am. J. Dis. Child. 98:227, 1959.

327. Valentine, W. N., Tanaka, K. R., and Miwa, S.: Specific erythrocyte glycolytic enzyme defect (pyruvate kinase) in three subjects with congenital nonspherocytic hemolytic anemia, Tr. A. Am. Physicians 74:100, 1961.

328. Vest, M. F., and Frieder, H. R.: Erythrocyte survival in newborn infant, as measured by chromium 51 and its relation to postnatal bilirubin level, J. Pediat. 59:194, 1961.

329. Videback, A.: Auto-immune haemolytic anaemia in systemic lupus erythematosus, Acta med. scandinav. 171:187, 1962.

330. Vullo, C., and Tunioli, A. M.: Survival studies of thalassemic erythrocytes transfused into donors, into subjects with thalassemia minor and into normal and splenectomized subjects, Blood 13:803, 1958.

331. Vullo, C., and Panizon, F.: Mechanism of haemolysis in favism: Transfusion experiments with Cr^{51} tagged erythrocytes, Acta haemat. 22:146, 1959.

331a. Wagner, H. N., Jr., Razzak, M. A., Gaertner, R. A., Caine, W. P., Jr., and Feagin, O. T.: Removal of erythrocytes from the circulation, A.M.A. Arch. Int. Med. 110:90, 1962.

332. Waksman, B.: Cell lysis related phenomena in hypersensitive reactions including immuno hematologic diseases, Progr. Allergy 5:349, 1958.

333. Wasserman, L. R., Stats, D., Schwartz, L., and Fudenberg, H.: Symptomatic and hemopathic hemolytic anemia, Am. J. Med. 18:961, 1955.

334. Watson, C. J.: Importance of the fractional serum bilirubin determination in clinical medicine, Ann. Int. Med. 45:351, 1956.

335. Watson, C. J.: Pyrrol pigments and hemoglobin catabolism, Minnesota Med. 39:294, 467, 1956.

336. Watson, C. J.: Composition of the urobilin group in urine, bile, and feces and the significance of variations in health and disease, J. Lab. & Clin. Med. 54:1, 1959.

337. Weed, R., Eber, J., and Rothstein, A.: Effects of primaquine and other related compounds on the red blood cell membrane: I. Na+ and K+ permeability in normal human cells, J. Clin. Invest. 40:130, 1961.

338. Weed, R. I.: Effects of primaquine on the red blood cell membrane: II. K+ permeability in glucose-6-phosphate dehydrogenase deficient erythrocytes, J. Clin. Invest. 40:140, 1961.

339. Weiner, W.: To be or not to be an antibody: The "agent" in autoimmune hemolytic anemia, Blood 14:1057, 1959.

339a. Weintraub, A. M., Pierce, L. E., Donovan, W. T., and Rath, C. E.: Paroxysmal cold hemoglobinuria, A.M.A. Arch. Int. Med. 109:589, 1962.

340. Weisman, R., Ham, T. H., Hinz, C. F., and Harris, J. W.: Studies of the role of the spleen in the destruction of erythrocytes, Tr. A. Am. Physicians 58:181, 1955.

341. Weiss, L.: Study of the structure of splenic sinuses in man and the albino rat with the light microscope and the electron microscope, J. Biophys. & Biochem. Cytol. 3:599, 1957.

342. Weiss, L.: Experimental study of the organization of the reticuloendothelial system in the red pulp of the spleen, J. Anat. 93:465, 1959.

343. Wheby, M. S., Barrett, O'N., Jr., and Crosby, W. H.: Serum protein binding of myoglobin, hemoglobin and hematin, Blood 16:1579, 1960.

344. Whipple, A. O., Parpart, A. K., and Chang, J. J.: Study of the circulation of the blood in the spleen of the living mouse, Ann. Surg. 140:266, 1954.

345. Whitten, C. F.: Studies on serum haptoglobin: A functional inquiry, New England J. Med. 266:529, 1962.

346. Wiedermann, D., Kubikova, A., and Churg, Z. D.: Localization of cold agglutinins in electrophoretic protein spectrum, Schweiz. med. Wchnschr. 90:682, 1960.

347. Wiland, O. K., and Smith, E. B.: Morphology of the spleen in congenital hemolytic anemia (hereditary spherocytosis), Am. J. Clin. Path. 26:619, 1956.

348. Williams, T. F., Fordham, C. C., III, Hollander, W., Jr., and Welt, L. G.: Study of the osmotic behavior of the human erythrocyte, J. Clin. Invest. 38:1587, 1959.

349. Willoughby, M. L. N., Pears, M. A., Sharp, A. A., and Shields, M. J.: Megaloblastic erythropoiesis in acquired hemolytic anemia, Blood 27:351, 1961.

350. Winkelman, J. W., Wagner, H. M., McAfee, J. G., and Mozley, J. M.: Visualization of the spleen in man by radioscope scanning, Radiology 75:465, 1960.

351. Witts, L. J.: Paroxysmal haemoglobinuria, Lancet 1:115, 1936.

352. Witzleben, C. L., and Wyatt, J. P.: Effect of long survival on the pathology of thalassaemia major, J. Path. & Bact. 82:1, 1961.

353. Young, L. E.: Hereditary spherocytosis, Am. J. Med. 18:486, 1955.

354. Young, L. E., Izzo, M. J., Altman, K. I., and Swisher, S. N.: Studies on

spontaneous in vitro autohemolysis in hemolytic disorders, Blood 11:977, 1956.

355. Young, L. E., Miller, G., and Swisher, S. N.: Treatment of hemolytic disorders, J. Chronic Dis. 6:307, 1957.

356. Young, L. E.: Hemolytic disorders: Some highlights of twenty years of progress, Ann. Int. Med. 49:1073, 1958.

357. Zieve, L., Hill, E., Hanson, M., Falcone, A. B., and Watson, C. J.: Normal and abnormal variations and clinical significance of the one-minute and total serum bilirubin determinations, J. Lab. & Clin. Med. 38:446, 1951.

358. Zinkham, W. H.: An *in vitro* abnormality of glutathione metabolism in erythrocytes from normal newborns: Mechanism and clinical significance, Pediatrics 23:18, 1959.

359. Zinkham, W., and Lenhard, R. E.: Metabolic abnormalities of erythrocytes from patients with congenital non-spherocytic hemolytic anemia, J. Pediat. 55:319, 1959.

360. Zuelzer, W. W., Robinson, A. R., and Booker, C. R.: Reciprocal relationship of hemoglobins A_2 and F in beta chain thalassemia: A key to the genetic control of hemoglobin F, Blood 17:393, 1961.

361. Zuelzer, W. W., Robinson, A. R., and Ingram, V. M.: Haemoglobin F and the genetic control of protein structure, Nature 191:608, 1961.

CHAPTER TEN
POLYCYTHEMIA

1. Abraham, J. P., Ulutin, O. N., Johnson, S. A., and Caldwell, M. J.: Study of the defects in the blood coagulation mechanisms in polycythemia vera, Am. J. Clin. Path. 36:7, 1961.
2. Aggeler, P. M., Pollycove, M., Hoag, S., Donald, W. G., and Lawrence, J. H.: polycythemia vera in childhood: Studies of iron kinetics with Fe^{59} and blood clotting factors, Blood 27:345, 1961.
3. Altschule, M. D., Volk, M. C., and Henstell, H.: Cardiac and respiratory function at rest in patients with uncomplicated polycythemia vera, Am. J. M. Sc. 200:478, 1940.
4. Auchincloss, J. H., Jr., Cook, E., and Renzetti, A. D.: Clinical and physiological aspects of a case of obesity, polycythemia and alveolar hypoventilation, J. Clin. Invest. 34:1537, 1955.
5. Auchincloss, J. H., Jr., and Duggan, J. J.: Effects of venesection on pulmonary and cardiac function in patients with chronic pulmonary emphysema and secondary polycythemia, Am. J. Med. 22:74, 1957.
6. Auerback, M. L., Wolff, J. A., and Mettier, S. R.: Benign familial polycythemia in childhood, Pediatrics 21:54, 1958.
7. Berk, L., Burchard, J. H., Ward, T., and Castle, W. B.: Oxygen saturation of sternal marrow blood with special reference to pathogenesis of polycythemia vera, Proc. Soc. Exper. Biol. & Med. 69:316, 1948.
8. Berlin, N. I., Lawrence, J. H., and Lee, H. C.: Life span of the red blood cells in chronic leukemia and polycythemia, Science 114:385, 1951.
9. Bert, P.: La pression barométrique, Masson, Paris, 1878.
10. Bert, P.: Sur la richesse en hémoglobine du sang des animaux vivant sur les hautes lieux, Compt. rend. Acad. sc. 94:805, 1882.
11. Bjorkman, S. E., Laurell, C. B., and Nilsson, I. M.: Serum proteins and fibrinolysis in polycythemia vera, Scandinav. J. Clin. & Lab. Invest. 8:304, 1956.
12. Bliss, T. L.: Basal metabolism in polycythemia vera, Ann. Int. Med. 2:155, 1929.
13. Bluefarb, S. M.: Cutaneous manifestations of polycythemia vera, Quart. Bull. Northwestern Univ. M. School 29:8, 1955.
14. Blum, A. S., and Zbar, M. J.: Relative polycythemia: Alterations of red cell distribution simulating hemoconcentration, A.M.A. Arch. Int. Med. 104:385, 1959.
15. Bosenbach, L. M., and Xefteris, E. D.: Erythrocytosis associated with carcinoma of the kidney, J.A.M.A. 176:136, 1961.
16. Brody, J. I., and Rodriguez, F.: Cerebellar hemangioblastoma and polycythemia (erythrocythemia), Am. J. M. Sc. 242:579, 1961.
17. Brooks, W. D. W.: Circulatory adjustments in polycythemia rubra vera, Proc. Roy. Soc. Med. 29:1379, 1936.
18. Brumpt, L. C., and Gujar, B. J.: Treatment of polycythemia by artificial infection with *Ancylostoma duodenale,* Indian M. Gaz. 83:136, 1948.

19. Cabot, R. C.: A case of chronic cyanosis without discoverable cause, ending in cerebral hemorrhage, Boston Med. & Surg. J., Dec. 7, 1899.

20. Calabresi, P., and Meyer, O. O.: Polycythemia vera: I. Clinical and laboratory manifestations, Ann. Int. Med. 50:1182, 1959.

21. Calabresi, P., and Meyer, O. O.: Polycythemia vera: II. Course and therapy, Ann. Int. Med. 50:1203, 1959.

22. Cassels, D. E., and Morse, M.: Arterial blood gases, the oxygen dissociation curve and the acid-base balance in polycythemia vera, J. Clin. Invest. 32:52, 1951.

23. Cherniack, R. M., Ewart, W. B., and Hildes, J. A.: Polycythemia secondary to respiratory disturbances in poliomyelitis, Ann. Int. Med. 46:720, 1957.

24. Christensen, B. C., and Probst, J. H.: Studies on polycythemia idiopathica or vera: I. Symptoms and course, Ugesk. laeger 119:1227, 1957.

25. Christensen, B. C., and Probst, J. H.: Studies on polycythemia idiopathica or vera: II. Treatment with radioactive phosphorus (P^{32}), Ugesk. laeger 119:1236, 1957.

26. Cobb, L. A., Kramer, R. J., and Finch, C. A.: Circulatory effects of chronic hypervolemia in polycythemia vera, J. Clin. Invest. 39:1722, 1960.

27. Cross, R. J.: Polycythemia, Am. J. Med. 24:132, 1958.

28. Dahl, J. D., Blaisdell, R. K., and Beutler, E.: Gastric ulceration in rats with experimentally-induced polycythemia, Proc. Soc. Exper. Biol. & Med. 101:622, 1959.

29. Dameshek, W.: Physiopathology and course of polycythemia vera related to therapy, J.A.M.A. 142:790, 1950.

30. Dameshek, W.: Stress erythrocytosis, Blood 8:282, 1953.

31. Damon, A., and Holub, D. A.: Host factors in polycythemia vera, Ann. Int. Med. 49:43, 1958.

32. de Wardener, H. E., McSwiney, R. R., and Miles, B. E.: Renal hemodynamics in primary polycythemia, Lancet 2:204, 1951.

33. de Wardener, H. E., and Young, I. M.: Oxygen consumption of polycythemic blood in vitro with a note on the arterial O_2 saturation of primary polycythemia, Clin. Sc. 10:497, 1951.

34. Eder, H. A., Finch, C. A., and McKee, R. W.: Congenital methemoglobinemia: A clinical and biochemical study of a case, J. Clin. Invest. 28:265, 1949.

35. Elwood, J. S., and de Wardener, H. E.: Survival of transfused erythrocytes from patients with polycythemia vera, J. Clin. Path. 4:218, 1951.

36. Erf, L. A.: Radioactive phosphorus in treatment of primary polycythemia vera, Progr. Hemat. 1:153, 1956.

37. Fisher, J. M., Bedell, G. N., and Seebohm, P. M.: Differentiation of polycythemia vera and secondary polycythemia by arterial oxygen saturation and pulmonary function tests, J. Lab. & Clin. Med. 50:455, 1957.

38. Frost, J. W., Jones, R., and Jonsson, U.: Pyrimethamine in the treatment of polycythemia, South. M. J. 51:1260, 1958.

39. Gardner, F. H., and Freymann, J. G.: Erythrocythemia (polycythemia) and hydronephrosis, New England J. Med. 259:323, 1958.

40. Goldsmith, G.: Cardiac output in polycythemia vera, Arch. Int. Med. 58:1041, 1936.

41. Grant, W. C., and Root, W. J.: Fundamental stimulus for erythropoiesis, Physiol. Rev. 32:449, 1952.

42. Halbertsma, T.: Polycythemia in childhood, Am. J. Dis. Child. 46:1356, 1933.

43. Hecht, H. H., and Samuels, A. J.: Observations on the oxygen content of sternal bone marrow with reference to polycythemic states, Fed. Proc. 11:68, 1952.

44. Hewlett, J. S., Hoffman, G. C., Senhauser, D. A., and Battle, J. D.: Hypernephroma with erythrocythemia: Report of a case and assay of the tumor for an erythropoietic-stimulating substance, New England J. Med. 262:1058, 1960.

45. Houston, C. S., and Riley, R. L.: Respiratory and circulatory changes during acclimatization to high altitude, Am. J. Physiol. 149:565, 1947.

46. Huff, R. L., Lawrence, J. H., Siri, W. E., Wasserman, L. R., and Hennessy, T. G.: Effects of changes in altitude on hematopoietic activity, Medicine 30:197, 1951.

47. Hurtado, A., Merino, C., and Delgado, E.: Influence on anoxemia or the hemopoietic activity, Arch. Int. Med. 75:284, 1945.

48. Hurtado, A., Valasquez, T., et al.: Mechanisms of natural acclimatization, USAF Report No. 56–1, School of Aviation Medicine, March 1956.

49. Hurtado, A.: Some clinical aspects of life at high altitudes, Ann. Int. Med. 53:247, 1960.

50. Isaacs, R.: Pathologic physiology of polycythemia vera, Arch. Int. Med. 31:285, 1923.

51. James, T. N., Johnson, S. A., and Monto, R. A.: Physiology and morphology of blood coagulation in polycythemia vera, J. Appl. Physiol. 15:1049, 1960.

52. Johnson, P. C., Hughes, W. L., Bird, R. M., and Patrick, D.: Diagnosis of hemolysis by a simplified Cr^{51} determination, A.M.A. Arch. Int. Med. 100:415, 1957.

53. Josephs, B. N., Robbins, G., and Levine, A.: Polycythemia secondary to hamartoma of the liver, J.A.M.A. 179:867, 1962.

54. Kaltreider, M. L., Hurtado, A., and Brooks, W. D. W.: Study of the blood in chronic respiratory diseases, with special reference to the volume of the blood, J. Clin. Invest. 13:999, 1934.

55. Kety, S. S.: Circulation and metabolism of the human brain in health and disease, Am. J. Med. 8:205, 1950.

56. Killmann, S. A., and Cronkite, E. P.: Treatment of polycythemia vera with Myleran, Am. J. M. Sc. 241:218, 1961.

57. Knock, H. L., and Githens, J. H.: Primary erythrocytosis of childhood, A.M.A. Am. J. Dis. Child. 100:189, 1960.

58. Lawrence, J. H., and Goetsch, A. T.: Familial occurrence of polycythemia and leukemia, California Med. 73:361, 1950.

59. Lawrence, J. H., Elmlinger, P. J., and Fulton, G.: Oxygen and the control of red cell production in primary and secondary polycythemia: Effects on the iron turnover patterns with Fe^{59} as tracer, Cardiologia 21:337, 1952.

60. Lawrence, J. H.: Polycythemia: Physiology, Diagnosis and Treatment, Grune & Stratton, New York, 1955.

61. Lawrence, J. H., and Donald, W. G.: Polycythemia and hydronephrosis or renal tumors, Ann. Int. Med. 50:959, 1959.

62. Leigh, T. F., Corley, C. C., Jr., Huguley, C. M., Jr., and Rogers, J. V., Jr.: Myelofibrosis: The general and radiologic findings in 24 proved cases, Am. J. Roentgenol. 82:183, 1959.

63. Lemon, W. S.: Study of the effect of chronic pulmonary disease on the volume and composition of the blood, Arch. Int. Med. 3:430, 1929.

64. Limarzi, L. R., Keeton, R. W., and Seed, L.: Early effect of total thyroidectomy in a case of polycythemia vera (Vaquez-Osler syndrome), Proc. Soc. Exper. Biol. & Med. 36:353, 1937.

65. Linman, J. W., Bethell, F. H., and Long, M. J.: Factors controlling hemopoiesis: Experimental observations on their role in polycythemia vera, Ann. Int. Med. 51:1003, 1959.

66. Linman, J. W., Long, M. J., Korst, D. R., and Bethell, F. H.: Studies on the stimulation of hemopoiesis by batyl alcohol, J. Lab. & Clin. Med. 54:335, 1959.

67. Linman, J. W.: Factors controlling hemopoiesis: Thrombopoietic and leuko-poietic effects of "anemic" plasma, J. Lab. & Clin. Med. 59:262, 1962.

68. London, I. M., Shemin, D., West, R., and Rittenberg, D.: Heme synthesis and red blood cell dynamics in normal humans and in subjects with polycythemia vera, sickle-cell anemia and pernicious anemia, J. Biol. Chem. 179:463, 1949.

69. Marlow, A. A., and Fairbanks, V. F.: Polycythemia vera in an eleven-year-old girl, New England J. Med. 263:950, 1960.

70. Martt, J. M., Sayman, A., and Neal, M. P.: Polycythemia and hydronephrosis, Ann. Int. Med. 54:790, 1961.

71. Masoaredis, S. P., and Lawrence, J. H.: Problem of leukemia in polycythemia vera, Am. J. M. Sc. 233:268, 1957.

72. McCurdy, P. R.: Effect of hyperoxia on the plasma iron turnover rate, Clin. Res. 8:18, 1960.

73. McKeen, S. F.: A case of marked cyanosis difficult to explain, Boston Med. & Surg. J., June 20, 1901.

74. Merskey, C.: Red cell fragility, endogenous uric acid and red cell survival in polycythemia vera, South African J. M. Sc. 14:1, 1949.

75. Minot, G. R., and Buckman, T. E.: Erythremia (polycythemia rubra vera): The development of anemia, the relation to leukemia, consideration of the basal metabolism blood formation and destruction and fragility of the red cells, Am. J. M. Sc. 166:469, 1923.

76. Mitus, W. J., Mednicoff, I. B., and Dameshek, W.: Alkaline phosphatase of mature neutrophils in various "polycythemias," New England J. Med. 260:1131, 1959.

77. Murray, J. F., Gold, P., and Johnson, B. J., Jr.: Systemic oxygen transport in induced normovolemic anemia and polycythemia, Clin. Res. 9:164, 1961.

78. Murray, J. F., Gold, P., and Johnson, B. L., Jr.: Blood volume effects in poly-cythemia and anemia, Clin. Res. 10:102, 1962.

79. Myrhe, J., and Wallace, F.: Hookworm treatment of polycythemia vera, Min-nesota Med. 39:99, 1959.

80. Nadler, S. B., and Cohn, I.: Familial polycythemia, Am. J. M. Sc. 198:41, 1937.

81. Nelson, D., and Fazekas, J. F.: Cerebral blood flow in polycythemia vera, A.M.A. Arch. Int. Med. 98:328, 1956.

82. Newman, W., Feltman, J. A., and Devlin, B.: Pulmonary function studies in polycythemia vera: Results in five probable cases, Am. J. Med. 11:706, 1951.

82a. Noyes, W. D., Domm, B. M., and Willis, L. C.: Regulation of erythropoiesis: I. Erythropoietin assay as a clinical tool, Blood 20:9, 1962.

83. Osler, W.: Chronic cyanosis with polycythemia and enlarged spleen: A new clinical entity, Am. J. M. Sc. 126:187, 1903.

84. Pare, P., and Lowenstein, L.: Polycythemia associated with disturbed func-tion of the respiratory center, Blood 11:1077, 1956.

85. Parker, R. G. F.: Hepatic vein occlusion, Medicine 38:369, 1959.

86. Parl, J. T., Limarzi, L. R., and Seed, L.: Effect of myxedema upon hemopoie-sis in leukemia and related disorders, Am. J. M. Sc. 206:625, 1943.

87. Pike, G. M.: Polycythemia vera, New England J. Med. 258:1250, 1297, 1958.

88. Ralston, L. A., Cobb, L. A., and Bruce, R. A.: Role of blood volume in regula-tion of cardiac output: The effects of arterial bleeding in normal subjects, Clin. Res. 8:124, 1960.

89. Ratto, O., Brescoe, W. A., Morton, J. W., and Comroc, J. H., Jr.: Anoxemia

secondary to polycythemia and polycythemia secondary to anoxemia, Am. J. Med. 19:958, 1955.

90. Reinhard, E. H., and Hahneman, B.: Treatment of polycythemia vera, J. Chronic Dis. 6:332, 1957.

91. Reynafarje, C.: Influence of high altitude on erythropoietic activity, Brookhaven Symp. Biol. 10:132, 1957.

92. Reynafarje, C., Lozano, R., and Valdivieso, J.: The polycythemia of high altitudes: Iron metabolism and related aspects, Blood 14:433, 1959.

93. Reznikoff, P., Fost, N. C., and Bethea, J. M.: Etiologic and pathologic factors in polycythemia vera, Am. J. M. Sc. 189:753, 1935.

94. Richardson, T. Q., and Vogel, J. A.: Effects of polycythemia and anemia on cardiac output and other circulatory factors, Am. J. Physiol. 197:1167, 1959.

95. Richter, K., and Bruschke, G.: Die Erythrocytenlebendauer bei der Polycythemia vera, Klin. Wchnschr. 37:150, 1959.

96. Rigby, P. G., and Leavell, B. S.: Polycythemia vera: A review of fifty cases with emphasis on the risk of surgery, A.M.A. Arch. Int. Med. 106:622, 1960.

97. Rosenthal, N., and Bassen, F. A.: Course of polycythemia, Arch. Int. Med. 62:903, 1938.

98. Rotta, A., and Lopez, A.: Electrocardiographic patterns in man at high altitudes, Circulation 19:719, 1959.

99. Saunby, R., and Russell, J. W.: Unexplained condition of chronic cyanosis, with a report of a case, Lancet 1:515, 1902.

100. Schmid, R., and French, L. A.: Cerebellar hemangioblastoma with polycythemia, Schweiz. med. Wchnschr. 85:1274, 1955.

101. Schmid, R., and Gilbertsen, A. S.: Fundamental observations on the production of compensatory polycythemia in a case of patent ductus arteriosus with reversed blood flow, Blood 10:247, 1955.

102. Schonfeld, A., Babbott, D., and Gundersen, K.: Hypoglycemia and polycythemia associated with primary hepatoma, New England J. Med. 265:231, 1961.

103. Schwartz, B. M., and Stats, D.: Oxygen saturation of sternal marrow blood in polycythemia vera, J. Clin. Invest. 28:736, 1949.

104. Schwartz, S. O., and Ehrlich, L.: Relationship of polycythemia to leukemia: Critical review, Acta haemat. 4:129, 1950.

105. Sharney, L., Schwartz, L., Wasserman, L. R., Port, S., and Leavitt, D.: Pool systems in iron metabolism, with special reference to polycythemia vera, Proc. Soc. Exper. Biol. & Med. 87:489, 1954.

106. Shaw, D. B., and Simpson, T.: Polycythemia in emphysema, Quart. J. Med. 30:135, 1961.

107. Shepard, R. J.: Influence of age on the hemoglobin level in congenital heart disease, Brit. Heart J. 18:49, 1956.

108. Singmaster, L.: Uterine fibroids associated with polycythemia, J.A.M.A. 163:363, 1957.

109. Sleversky, N., Mendell, T. H., and Framm, A. H.: Polycythemia vera terminating in acute leukemia: Report of case and review of literature, A.M.A. Arch. Int. Med. 96:565, 1955.

110. Stecher, G., Wolfers, H., and Nettesheim, P.: Polycythemia vera, Deutsche med. Wchnschr. 86:1861, 1961.

111. Stroebel, C. F., and Fowler, W. S.: Secondary polycythemia, Med. Clin. North America 40:1061, 1956.

112. Stroebel, C. F., and Hanlon, D. G.: Prognostic value of leukocyte studies in polycythemia vera treated with radiophosphorus, Minnesota Med. 42:10, 1959.

113. Talbott, J. H.: Gout and blood dyscrasias, Medicine 38:173, 1959.
114. Tappan, D. V., and Reynafarje, B.: Mechanisms of natural acclimatization: Tissue pigment studies in altitude adaptation, USAF Report No. 56–97, School of Aviation Medicine, October 1956.
115. Theilen, E. O., Gregg, D. E., and Rotta, A.: Exercise and cardiac work response at high altitude, Circulation 12:383, 1955.
116. Thiede, T., and Chievitz, E.: Increase in cell volume and pulmonary changes in polycythemia vera, Acta med. scandinav. 170:443, 1961.
117. Tinney, W. S., Polley, H. F., Hall, B. E., and Griffin, H. Z.: Polycythemia vera and gout: A report of eight cases, Proc. Staff Meet. Mayo Clin. 20:49, 1945.
118. Valtis, D. J., and Kennedy, A. C.: Effect of therapeutic radiophosphorus on the affinity of haemoglobin for oxygen in patients with polycythemia vera, J. Clin. Path. 7:284, 1954.
119. Verel, D.: Blood volume changes in cyanotic congenital heart disease and polycythemia rubra vera, Circulation 23:749, 1961.
120. Videbaek, A.: Polycythemia vera: Course and prognosis, Acta med. scandinav. 138:179, 1950.
121. Wasserman, L. R., Dobson, R. L., and Lawrence, J. H.: Blood O_2 studies in patients with polycythemia and in normal subjects, J. Clin. Invest. 28:60, 1949.
122. Wasserman, L. R., Lawrence, J. H., Berlin, N. I., Dobson, R. L., and Estren, S.: Bone marrow picture in polycythemia vera before and after treatment with radioactive phosphorus, Acta med. scandinav. 143:442, 1952.
123. Wasserman, L. R.: Polycythemia vera: Its course and treatment: Relation to myeloid metaplasia and leukemia, Bull. New York Acad. Med. 30:343, 1954.
124. Wasserman, L. R., and Bassen, F.: Polycythemia, J. Mt. Sinai Hosp. 26:1, 1959.
125. Weiner, A. A.: Polycythemia vera and its sequelae, Am. Pract. & Digest. Treat. 12:889, 1961.
126. Wells, R. E., Jr., and Merrill, E. W.: Variability of blood viscosity (editorial), Am. J. Med. 31:505, 1961.
127. Wennesland, R., Brown, E., Hopper, J., Jr., Hodges, J. L., Jr., Guttentag, O. E., Scott, K. G., Tucker, I. N., and Bradley, B.: Red cell, plasma and blood volume in healthy men measured by radio-chromium (Cr^{51}) cell tagging and hematocrit: Influence of age, somatotype and habits of physical activity on the variance after regression of volume to height and weight combined, J. Clin. Invest. 38:1065, 1959.
128. Wilson, S. J., Heath, H. E., and Larsen, W. E.: Polycythemia vera: Study of coagulation abnormalities, both thrombotic and hemorrhagic, J. Kansas M. Soc. 58:90, 1958.
129. Wiseman, B. K., Rohn, R. J., Bouroncle, B. A., and Myer, W. G.: Treatment of polycythemia vera with radioactive phosphorus, Ann. Int. Med. 34:311, 1951.
130. Yu, T. F., Weissmann, B., Sharney, L., Kupfer, S., and Gutman, A. B.: On the biosynthesis of uric acid from glycine-N^{15} in primary and secondary polycythemia, Am. J. Med. 21:901, 1956.

CHAPTER ELEVEN
THE ANEMIAS OF BONE MARROW FAILURE

1. Abelmann, W. H., Kramer, G. E., Verstraeten, J. M., Gravallese, M. A., and McNeely, W. F.: Cirrhosis of the liver and decreased arterial oxygen saturation, A.M.A. Arch. Int. Med. 108:34, 1961.
2. Adams, E. B.: Aplastic anemia: Review of twenty-seven cases, Lancet 1:657, 1951.
3. Aherne, W. A.: The "burr" red cell and azotemia, J. Clin. Path. 10:252, 1957.
4. Alexander, W. R. M., Richmond, J., Roy, L. M. H., and Duthie, J. J. R.: Nature of anaemia in rheumatoid arthritis: II. Survival of transfused erythrocytes in patients with rheumatoid arthritis, Ann. Rheumat. Dis. 15:12, 1956.
5. Allen, D. M., and Diamond, L. K.: Congenital (erythroid) hypoplastic anemia: Cortisone treated, A.M.A. Am. J. Dis. Child. 102:416, 1961.
6. Allen, F. A., Carr, M. H., and Klotz, A. P.: Decreased red blood cell survival time in patients with portal cirrhosis, J.A.M.A. 164:955, 1957.
7. Allison, A. C.: Acute haemolytic anaemia with distortion and fragmentation of erythrocytes in children, Brit. J. Haemat. 3:1, 1957.
8. Altman, K. I., and Miller, G.: Disturbance of tryptophan metabolism in congenital hypoplastic anaemia, Nature 172:868, 1953.
9. Altschule, M.: Symposium on anemia: IV. Anemia in uremia, Am. Pract. & Digest Treat. 4:215, 1953.
10. Anaemia in rheumatoid arthritis, Brit. M. J. 1:509, 1957.
11. Axelrod, A. R., and Berman, L.: Bone marrow in hyperthyroidism and hypothyroidism, Blood 6:436, 1951.
12. Bayrd, E. D., and Bernatz, P. E.: Benign thymoma and agenesis of erythrocytes, J.A.M.A. 163:723, 1957.
13. Bellanti, J. A., and Pinkel, D.: Idiopathic aplastic anemia treated with methyltestosterone and fresh platelets, J.A.M.A. 178:70, 1961.
14. Berman, L., Axelrod, A. R., Horan, T. M., Jacobson, S. D., Sharp, E. A., and von der Heide, E. C.: Blood and bone marrow in patients with cirrhosis and other disorders of the liver, Blood 4:511, 1949.
15. Bernard, J., Mathe, G., and Majean, Y.: Contribution à l'étude clinique et physiopathologique de la maladie de Fanconi, Rev. franç. étude clin. biol. 3:599, 1958.
16. Biechl, A., Stapleton, J. E., Woodbury, J. F. L., and Read, H. C.: Anemia in rheumatoid arthritis: I. Red cell survival studies, Canad. M.A.J. 86:401, 1962.
17. Bingham, J.: Macrocytosis of hepatic disease: I. Thin macrocytosis, Blood 14:694, 1959.
18. Bingham, J.: Macrocytosis of hepatic disease: II. Thick macrocytosis in blood, Blood 15:244, 1960.
19. Bishop, R. C., and Bethell, F. H.: Hereditary hypochromic anemia with transfusion hemosiderosis treated with pyridoxine, New England J. Med. 261:486, 1959.
20. Bjorkman, S. E.: Chronic refractory anemia with sideroblastic bone marrow: A study of 4 cases, Blood 11:250, 1956.

21. Block, M., Jacobson, L. O., and Bethard, W. F.: Preleukemic acute human leukemia, J.A.M.A. 152:1018, 1953.
22. Bloom, W., and Jacobson, L. O.: Some hematologic effects of irradiation, Blood 3:586, 1948.
23. Bomford, R.: Anaemia in myxoedema and the role of the thyroid gland in erythropoiesis, Quart. J. Med. 7:495, 1938.
24. Bomford, R. R., and Rhoades, C. P.: Refractory anemia, Quart. J. Med. 10:235, 1941.
25. Boon, T. H., and Walton, J. M.: Aplastic anemia, Quart. J. Med. 20:75, 1951.
26. Bowman, W. D., Jr.: Abnormal ("ringed") sideroblasts in various hematologic and non-hematologic disorders, Blood 18:662, 1961.
27. Braverman, M. M.: The anemia of pulmonary tuberculosis, Am. Rev. Tuberc. 38:466, 1938.
28. Brown, G. M.: Pathogenesis of secondary anaemia, Canad. M.A.J. 62:472, 1951.
29. Burgest, E. O., Kennedy, R. L. J., and Pease, G. L.: Congenital hypoplastic anemia, Pediatrics 13:218, 1954.
30. Bush, J. A., Ashenbrucker, H., Cartwright, G. E., and Wintrobe, M. M.: The anemia of infection: XX. The kinetics of iron metabolism in the anemia associated with chronic infection, J. Clin. Invest. 35:89, 1956.
31. Byrd, R. B., and Cooper, T.: Hereditary iron-loading anemia with secondary hemochromatosis, Ann. Int. Med. 55:103, 1961.
32. Callen, I. R., and Limarzi, L. R.: Blood and bone marrow studies in renal disease, Am. J. Clin. Path. 20:3, 1950.
33. Cartwright, G. E., and Wintrobe, M. M.: The anemia of infection: XVII. A review, Advances Int. Med. 5:165, 1952.
34. Cawein, M. J., Hagedorn, A. B., and Owen, C. A.: Cause of anemia accompanying hepatic disease, Gastroenterology 38:324, 1960.
35. Chaplin, H., Jr., and Mollison, P. L.: Red cell life span in nephritis and in hepatic cirrhosis, Clin. Sc. 12:351, 1953.
36. Chodos, R. B., Denton, J., Ferguson, B., and Ross, J. F.: Clinical significance of the blood volume in the anemia of portal cirrhosis, Clin. Res. Proc. 1:111, 1953.
37. Clarkson, B., and Prockop, D. J.: Aregenerative anemia associated with benign thymoma, New England J. Med. 259:253, 1958.
38. Cooper, W.: Pancytopenia associated with disseminated tuberculosis, Ann. Int. Med. 50:1497, 1959.
39. Cotton, H. B., and Harris, J. W.: Familial pyridoxine-responsive anemia, J. Clin. Invest. 41:1352, 1962.
40. Court-Brown, W. B., and Doll, R.: Leukaemia and aplastic anaemia in patients irradiated for ankylosing spondylitis, Medical Research Council, Special Report, p. 295, Her Majesty's Stationery Office, London, 1957.
41. Cristoffanini, A. P.: Transplantation of bone marrow, Progr. Hemat. 3:360, 1962.
42. Crosby, W. H.: Siderocytes and the spleen, Blood 12:165, 1957.
43. Crosby, W. H., Feinstein, F. E., Heilmeyer, L., Kawakita, Y., Whitby, L., and Dameshek, W.: Panels in therapy: XII. Hypoplastic-aplastic anemia, Blood 12:193, 1957.
44. Crosby, W. H., and Sheehy, T. W.: Hypochromic iron-loading anaemia: Studies of iron and haemoglobin metabolism by means of vigorous phlebotomy, Brit. J. Haemat. 6:56, 1960.
45. Custer, R. P.: Aplastic anemia in soldiers treated with atabrine (quinacrine), Am. J. M. Sc. 212:211, 1946.
46. Dacie, J. V., Smith. M. D., White, J. C., and Mollin, D. L.: Refractory

normoblastic anaemia: A clinical and haematological study of 7 cases, Brit. J. Haemat. 5:56, 1959.

47. Daughaday, W. H., Williams, R. H., and Daland, G. A.: Effect of endocrinopathies on the blood, Blood 3:1342, 1948.
48. Davidson, L. S. P.: Refractory megaloblastic anemia, Blood 3:107, 1948.
49. Davis, L. J., and Davidson, L. S. P.: Proteolysed liver in the treatment of refractory anaemias, Quart. J. Med. 13:53, 1944.
50. Dawborn, J. K., and Cowling, D. C.: Disseminated tuberculosis and bone marrow dyscrasias (abstract), Australasian Ann. Med. 10:230, 1961.
51. Dawson, J. P.: Congenital pancytopenia associated with multiple congenital anomalies (Fanconi type), Pediatrics 15:325, 1955.
52. Desforges, J. F., and Dawson, J. P.: The anemia of renal failure, A.M.A. Arch. Int. Med. 101:326, 1958.
53. Desforges, J. F., Ross, J. D., and Moloney, W. C.: Mechanisms of anemia in leukemia and malignant lymphoma, Am. J. Med. 28:69, 1960.
54. Diamond, L. K., Allen, D. M., and Magill, F. B.: Congenital (erythroid) hypoplastic anemia: A twenty-five-year study, A.M.A. Am. J. Dis. Child. 102:403, 1961.
55. Ebaugh, F. G., Jr.: The anemia of rheumatoid arthritis, *in* Wallerstein, R. O., and Mettier, S. R. (ed.), Iron in Clinical Medicine, p. 261, University of California Press, Berkeley, 1958.
56. Ehrlich, P.: Ueber einen Fall von Anämie mit Bemerkungen über Regenerative Veränderungen des Knochenmarks, Charité-Ann. 13:300, 1888.
57. Eisenberg, S.: Blood volume in patients with Laennec's cirrhosis of liver as determined by radioactive chromium–tagged red cells, Am. J. Med. 20:189, 1956.
58. Emerson, C. P.: Pathogenesis of anemia in acute glomerulonephritis: Estimate of blood production and blood destruction in a case receiving massive transfusions, Blood 3:363, 1948.
59. Engle, M. A., Stern, G., Master, J., Goldberg, H. P., and Smith, C. H.: Late cardiac complications of severe refractory anemia, A.M.A. Am. J. Dis. Child. 100:729, 1960.
60. Erslev, A. J., Iverson, C. K., and Lawrason, F. D.: Cortisone and ACTH in hypoplastic anemia, Yale J. Biol. &. Med. 28:44, 1952.
61. Evans, T. S., DeLuca, V. A., and Waters, L. L.: Association of miliary tuberculosis of the bone marrow and pancytopenia, Ann. Int. Med. 37:1044, 1952.
62. Ferrebee, J. W., and Thomas, E. D.: Transplantation of marrow in man, A.M.A. Arch. Int. Med. 106:523, 1960.
63. Finch, C. A., Gibson, J. C., II, Peacock, W. C., and Fluharty, R. G.: Iron metabolism: Utilization of intravenous radioactive iron, Blood 4:905, 1949.
63a. Finkelstein, A., Kwok, G., Hall, A. P., and Bayles, T. B.: The erythrocyte in rheumatoid arthritis: I. A method for the detection of an abnormal globulin coating, New England J. Med. 264:270, 1961.
64. Fliedmer, T. M., Cronkite, E. P., Bond, V. P., Rubini, J. R., and Andrews, G.: Mitotic index of human bone marrow in healthy individuals and irradiated human beings, Acta haemat. 22:65, 1959.
65. Fountain, J. R.: Blood changes associated with disseminated tuberculosis: Report of four fatal cases and review, Brit. M. J. 2:76, 1954.
66. Foy, H., and Kondi, A.: A case of true red cell aplastic anemia successfully treated with riboflavin, J. Path. & Bact. 65:559, 1953.
67. Francis, R. C., Moir, R. A., and Swift, P. N.: Value of splenectomy in Fanconi's anemia, Arch. Dis. Childhood 30:439, 1955.
68. Freireich, E. J., Miller, A., Emerson, C. P., and Ross, J. F.: Effect of inflam-

mation on the utilization of erythrocyte and transferrin bound radioiron for red cell production, Blood 12:972, 1957.

69. Freireich, E. J., Ross, J. F., Bayler, T. B., Emerson, C. P., and Finch, S. C.: Radioactive iron metabolism and erythrocyte survival studies of the mechanism of the anemia associated with rheumatoid arthritis, J. Clin. Invest. 36:1043, 1957.

70. Garby, L., Sjolin, S., and Vahlquist, B.: Chronic refractory hypochromic anaemia with disturbed haem-metabolism, Brit. J. Haemat. 3:55, 1957.

71. Gardner, F. H.: Use of cobaltous chloride in the anemia associated with chronic renal disease, J. Lab. & Clin. Med. 41:56, 1953.

72. Gardner, F. H., and Pringle, J. C., Jr.: Androgens and erythropoiesis, A.M.A. Arch. Int. Med. 107:846, 1961.

73. Garriga, S., and Crosby, W. H.: Incidence of leukemia in families of patients with hypoplasia of the marrow, Blood 14:1008, 1959.

74. Garvin, R. O., and Bargen, J. A.: Hematologic picture of chronic ulcerative colitis: Its relation to prognosis and treatment, Am. J. M. Sc. 193:744, 1937.

75. Gasser, C., Gautier, E., Steck, A., Siebermann, R. E., and Dehslin, R.: Hämolytisch-urämische Syndrome: Bilaterale Nierenrindennekrosen bei akuten erworbenen hämolytischen Anämien, Schweiz. med. Wchnschr. 85:905, 1955.

76. Gasser, C.: Aplasia of erythropoiesis: Acute and chronic erythroblastopenia or pure (red cell) aplastic anaemias in childhood, Pediat. Clin. North America, p. 449, May 1957.

77. Gelpi, A. P., and Ende, N.: An hereditary anemia with hemochromatosis, Am. J. Med. 25:303, 1958.

78. Gevirtz, N. R., and Berlin, N. I.: Erythrokinetic studies in severe bone marrow failure of diverse etiology, Blood 18:637, 1961.

79. Giblett, E. R., Coleman, D. H., Pirzio-Biroli, G., Donohue, D. M., Motulsky, A. G., and Finch, C. A.: Erythrokinetics: Quantitative measurements of red cell production and destruction in normal subjects and patients with anemia, Blood 11:291, 1956.

80. Gordon, A. S.: Endocrine influences upon the formed elements of blood and blood forming organs, Progr. Hormone Res. 10:339, 1954.

80a. Greendyke, R. M.: Congenital refractory normoblastic anemia with jaundice and ineffective erythropoiesis, Am. J. Med. 32:611, 1962.

81. Gussoff, B. D., Lee, S. L., and Lichtman, H. C.: Erythropoietic changes during therapy with chloramphenicol, A.M.A. Arch. Int. Med. 109:176, 1962.

82. Hall, C. A.: The macrocytosis of liver disease, J. Lab. & Clin. Med. 48:345, 1956.

83. Hall, C. A.: Erythrocyte dynamics in liver disease, Am. J. Med. 28:541, 1960.

84. Harris, J. W., Whittington, R. M., Weisman, R., Jr., and Horrigan, D. L.: Pyridoxine responsive anemia in the human adult, Proc. Soc. Exper. Biol. & Med. 91:427, 1956.

85. Hasselback, R. C., and Thomas, J. W.: Aplastic anemia, Canad. M. A. J. 82:1253, 1960.

86. Hathaway, W. E., and Githens, J. H.: Pancytopenia with hyperplastic marrow, A.M.A. Am. J. Dis. Child. 102:135, 1961.

87. Havard, C. W. H., and Scott, R. B.: Thymic tumour and erythroblastic aplasia, Brit. J. Haemat. 6:178, 1960.

88. Havard, C. W. H.: An investigation of refractory anemias, Quart. J. Med. 31:21, 1962.

89. Heaton, L. D., Crosby, W. H., and Cohen, A.: Splenectomy in the treatment of hypoplasia of the bone marrow, with a report of 12 cases, Ann. Surg. 146:637, 1957.

90. Heilmeyer, L., Keiderling, W., Merker, H., Clotten, R., and Schubothe, H.: Die Anaemie refractoria sideroblastica und ihre Beziehungen zur Leber-siderose und Hämochromatose, Acta haemat, 23:1, 1960.

91. Heilmeyer, L.: Splenectomy for panmyelopathy, Med. Klin. 56:617, 1961.

92. Horrigan, D. L., Whittington, R. M., Weisman, R., Jr., and Harris, J. W.: Hypochromic anemia with hyperferricemia responding to oral crude liver extract, Am. J. Med. 22:99, 1957.

93. Huang, K., and Wang, H.: Anemia associated with cirrhosis of the liver: Study of 32 cases, Arch. Int. Med. 84:958, 1949.

94. Hubbard, J. P., and McKee, M. H.: Anemia of rheumatic fever, J. Pediat. 14:66, 1939.

95. Hyman, G. A., and Southworth, H.: Hemolytic anemia associated with liver disease, Am. J. M. Sc. 221:448, 1951.

96. Hyman, G. A., and Harvey, J. E.: Pathogenesis of anemia in patients with carcinoma, Am. J. Med. 19:350, 1955.

97. Hyman, G. A., Gellhorn, A., and Harvey, J. L.: Studies on anemia of dis-seminated malignant neoplastic disease: I. Study of life-span of erythrocyte, Blood 11:618, 1956.

98. Israels, M. C. G., and Wilkinson, J. F.: New observations on aetiology and prognosis of achrestic anaemia, Quart. J. Med. 9:163, 1940.

99. Israels, M. C. G., and Wilkinson, J. F.: Idiopathic aplastic anaemia: In-cidence and management, Lancet 1:63, 1961.

100. Jacobs, E. M., Hutter, R. V. P., Pool, J. L., and Ley, A. B.: Benign thymoma and selective erythroid aplasia of the bone marrow, Cancer 12:47, 1959.

101. Jacobson, L. O., Marks, E. K., and Lorenz, E.: Hematologic effects of ionizing radiations, Radiology 52:371, 1949.

102. Jandl, J. H.: The anemia of liver disease: Observations on its mechanism, J. Clin. Invest. 34:390, 1955.

103. Jandl, J. H., and Lear, A. A.: Metabolism of folic acid in cirrhosis, Ann. Int. Med. 45:1027, 1956.

104. Jandl, J. H., Jacob, H. S., and Daland, G. A.: Hypersplenism due to infection: Study of five cases manifesting hemolytic anemia, New England J. Med. 264:1063, 1961.

105. Jarrold, T., and Vilter, R. W.: Hematologic observations in patients with chronic hepatic insufficiency: Sternal bone marrow morphology and bone marrow plasmacytosis, J. Clin. Invest. 38:286, 1949.

106. Javett, S. N., and Senior, B.: Syndrome of hemolysis, thrombopenia, and nephropathy in infancy, Pediatrics 29:209, 1962.

107. Jeffrey, M. R.: Some observations on anemia in rheumatoid arthritis, Blood 8:502, 1953.

108. Jeffrey, M. R., Freundlich, H. F., Jackson, E. B., and Watson, D.: Absorption and utilization of radioiron in rheumatoid disease, Clin. Sc. 14:395, 1955.

109. Jeffrey, M. R.: Hemodilution in rheumatoid disease, Ann. Rheumat. Dis. 15:151, 1956.

110. Jones, P. N., Weinstein, I. M., Ettinger, R. H., and Capps, R. B.: Decreased red cell survival associated with liver disease, A.M.A. Arch. Int. Med. 95:93, 1955.

111. Joske, R. A., McAlister, J. M., and Prankerd, T. A. J.: Isotope investigations of red cell production and destruction in chronic renal disease, Clin. Sc. 15:511, 1956.

112. Josse, J. W., and Zacks, S. I.: Thymoma and pancytopenia: Report of a case and review of the literature, New England J. Med. 259:113, 1958.

113. Kaye, M.: The anemia associated with renal disease, J. Lab. & Clin. Med. 52:83, 1958.

113a. Kessel, L.: Acute transient hyperlipemia due to hepatopancreatic damage in chronic alcoholics (Zieve's syndrome), Am. J. Med. 32:747, 1962.

114. Keys, A., and Snell, A. M.: Respiratory properties of arterial blood in normal man and in patients with disease of liver, J. Clin. Invest. 17:59, 1938.

115. Krakoff, I. H., Karnofsky, D. A., and Burchenal, J. H.: Effects of large doses of chloramphenicol in human subjects, New England J. Med. 253:7, 1955.

116. Krasnow, S. E., Walsh, J. R., Zimmerman, H. J., and Heller, P.: Megaloblastic anemia in "alcoholic" cirrhosis, A.M.A. Arch. Int. Med. 100:870, 1957.

117. Kuroyanagi, T.: Anemia associated with chronic renal failure, with special reference to kinetics of the erythron, Acta haemat. jap. 24:156, 1961.

118. Kyser, F. A., and Danforth, D. N.: Reversible refractory anemia in pregnancy, J.A.M.A. 174:485, 1960.

119. Lamvik, J. O.: Acute glomerulonephritis with hemolytic anemia in infants: Report of three fatal cases, Pediatrics 29:224, 1962.

120. Lange, R. D., Wright, S. W., Tomonaga, M., Kurasaki, H., Matsuoke, S., and Matsunaga, H.: Refractory anemia occurring in survivors of the atomic bombing of Nagasaki, Japan, Blood 10:312, 1955.

121. Lange, R. D., McCarthy, J. M., and Gallagher, N. I.: Plasma and urinary erythropoietin in bone marrow failure, A.M.A. Arch. Int. Med. 108:850, 1961.

122. Lassen, H. C. A., Henrikson, E., Neukirch, F., and Kristensen, H. S.: Treatment of tetanus: Severe bone marrow depression after prolonged nitrous-oxide anaesthesia, Lancet 1:527, 1956.

123. Leavell, B. S., Thorup, O. A, and McClellan, J. E.: Observations on the anemia in myxedema, Tr. Am. Clin. & Climatol. A. 68:137, 1956.

124. Lehnhoff, H. J., Jr.: Androgen therapy for refractory anemia: Report of a case associated with thymoma, Ann. Int. Med. 53:1059, 1960.

125. Leithold, S. L., David, D., and Best, W. R.: Hypothyroidism with anemia demonstrating abnormal vitamin B_{12} absorption, Am. J. Med. 24:535, 1958.

126. Lescher, F. G., and Hubble, D.: Idiopathic aplastic anaemia with an analysis of four cases, Lancet 1:239, 1933.

127. Levin, J., Andrews, J. R., and Berlin, N. I.: Effects of total body irradiation on some aspects of human iron metabolism, J. Clin. Invest. 40:649, 1961.

128. Lewis, S. M., and Porter, I. H.: Erythrocyte survival in rheumatoid arthritis, Ann. Rheumat. Dis. 19:54, 1960.

129. Ley, A. B., and Ellison, R. R.: Management of disseminated neoplastic disease: Hematological problems, Bull. New York Acad. Med. 33:693, 1957.

130. Lock, S. P., and Dormady, K. M.: Red cell fragmentation syndrome: A condition of multiple etiology, Lancet 1:1020, 1961.

131. Loeb, V., Jr., Moore, C. V., and Dubach, R.: Physiologic evaluation and management of chronic bone marrow failure, Am. J. Med. 15:499, 1953.

132. Loge, J. P., Lange, R. D., and Moore, C. V.: Characterization of anemia associated with chronic renal insufficiency, J. Lab. & Clin. Med. 51:91, 1958.

133. Maier, C.: Anaemia refractoria sideroblastica, Schweiz. med. Wchnschr. 89:1074, 1959.

134. Manganaro, F. J.: Aplastic anemia preceding acute myeloblastic (histiocytic) leukemia, J.A.M.A. 173:1559, 1960.

135. Marver, H. S.: Studies on tryptophan metabolism: I. Urinary tryptophan metabolites in hypoplastic anemias and other hematologic disorders, J. Lab. & Clin. Med. 58:425, 1961.

136. Mauer, A. M.: Early anemia of acute rheumatic fever, Pediatrics 27:707, 1961.

137. McClellan, J. E., Donegan, C., Thorup, O., and Leavell, B. S.: Survival time of the erythrocyte in myxedema and hyperthyroidism, J. Lab. & Clin. Med. 51:91, 1958.

138. McCrea, P. C.: Latent haemolysis in rheumatoid arthritis, Lancet 1:402, 1957.

139. McCurdy, P. R., Pierce, L. E., and Rath, C. E.: Abnormal bone marrow morphology in acute alcoholism, New England J. Med. 266:505, 1962.

140. McFarland, W., Granville, N., Schwartz, R., Oliner, H., Misra, D. K., and Dameshek, W.: Therapy of hypoplastic anemia with bone marrow transplantation, A.M.A. Arch. Int. Med. 108:23, 1961.

141. Meacham, G. C., and Weisberger, A. J.: Early atypical manifestations of leukemia, Ann. Int. Med. 41:780, 1954.

142. Medd, W. E., and Hayhoe, F. G. J.: Tuberculous miliary necrosis with pancytopenia, Quart. J. Med. 24:351, 1955.

143. Meulengracht, E., and Gormsen, H.: Blood and bone marrow in infective subacute and chronic atrophy of the liver, Blood 3:1416, 1948.

144. Miesch, D. C., Baxter, R., and Levin, W. C.: Acute erythroblastopenia: Pathogenesis, manifestations, management, A.M.A. Arch. Int. Med. 99:461, 1957.

145. Miescher, P., Gsell, O., and Fust, B.: Pathogenesis of anemia in tuberculosis, Schweiz. med. Wchnschr. 85:917, 1955.

146. Miller, A., Chodos, R. B., Emerson, C. P., and Ross, J. F.: Studies of the anemia and iron metabolism in cancer, J. Clin. Invest. 35:1248, 1956.

147. Minot, G. R., and Sparling, R. G.: Effect on blood of irradiation, especially short wave length roentgen ray therapy, Am. J. M. Sc. 168:215, 1924.

148. Mohler, D. N., and Leavell, B. S.: Aplastic anemia: An analysis of 50 cases, Ann. Int. Med. 49:326, 1958.

149. Mohler, D. N., Smith, D. E., and Leavell, B. S.: Exogenous hemochromatosis occurring in aplastic anemia: An autopsy study on fourteen patients, Clin. Res. Proc. 6:116, 1958.

150. Moore, C. V.: Concept of relative bone marrow failure, Am. J. Med. 23:1, 1957.

151. Moore, C. V.: Treatment of refractory anemia or bone marrow failure, J. Chronic Dis. 6:324, 1957.

152. Mouitt, E. R.: Megaloblastic erythropoiesis in patients with cirrhosis of the liver, Blood 5:468, 1950.

153. Muldowney, F. P., Crooks, J., and Wayne, E. J.: Total red cell mass in thyrotoxicosis and myxoedema, Clin. Sc. 16:309, 1957.

154. Naets, J. P.: Role of the kidney in erythropoiesis, J. Clin. Invest. 39:102, 1960.

155. Najean, Y., Meeus-Bith, L., Bernard, C., Boiron, M., Bousser, J., and Bernard, J.: Isotopic study of erythrokinetics in 31 cases of chronic idiopathic pancytopenia with histologically normal or rich marrow, Sang 30:101, 1959.

156. Nilssen, F.: Anaemia problems in rheumatoid arthritis, Acta med. scandinav. 130, Suppl. 210, 1948.

157. Nunnally, R. M., and Levine, I.: Macronormoblastic hyperplasia of the bone marrow in hepatic cirrhosis, Am. J. Med. 30:972, 1961.

158. Osgood, E. E.: Drug induced hypoplastic anemias and related syndromes, Ann. Int. Med. 39:1173, 1953.

159. Ozer, F. L., Truax, W. E., and Levin, W. C.: Erythroid hypoplasia associated with chloramphenicol therapy, Blood 16:997, 1960.

160. Palmen, K., and Vahlquist, B.: Stationary hypoplastic anemia, Acta haemat. 4:273, 1950.

161. Parson, W. B., Jr., Cooper, T., and Scheifley, C. H.: Anemia in bacterial endocarditis. J.A.M.A. 153:14, 1953.

162. Pearson, H. A., and Cone, T. E., Jr.: Congenital hypoplastic anemia, Pediatrics 19:192, 1957.

163. Peters, J. T.: Equine infectious anemia transmitted to man, Ann. Int. Med. 23:271, 1945.

164. Peterson, R. E.: The serum iron in acute hepatitis, J. Lab. & Clin. Med. 39:225, 1952.

165. Pisciotta, A. V.: Clinical and pathologic effects of space-occupying lesions of the bone marrow, Am. J. Clin. Path. 20:915, 1950.

166. Pritchard, J. A., and Adams, R. H.: Erythrocyte production and destruction during pregnancy, Am. J. Obst. & Gynec. 79:750, 1960.

167. Rachmilewitz, M., Aronovitch, J., and Grossowicz, N.: Serum concentrations of vitamin B_{12} in acute and chronic liver disease, J. Lab. & Clin. Med. 48:339, 1956.

168. Ragen, P. A., Hagedorn, A. B., and Owen, C. A.: Radioisotopic study of anemia in chronic renal disease, A.M.A. Arch. Int. Med. 105:518, 1960.

169. Rankin, A. M.: A review of twenty cases of aplastic anaemia, M. J. Australia 2:95, 1961.

170. Reinhold, J.: Survival of transfused red cells in acute rheumatic fever with reference to a latent hemolytic mechanism, Arch. Dis. Childhood 29:201, 1954.

171. Rhoads, C. P., and Barker, W. H.: Refractory anemia: Analysis of one hundred cases, J.A.M.A. 110:794, 1938.

172. Richet, G., Alagille, D., and Fournier, E.: Acute erythroblastopenia due to anuria, Presse méd. 62:50, 1954.

173. Richmond, J., Gardner, D. L., Roy, L. M. H., and Duthie, J. J. R.: Nature of anaemia in rheumatoid arthritis: III. Changes in the bone marrow and their relation to other features of the disease, Ann. Rheumat. Dis. 15:217, 1956.

174. Richmond, J., Alexander, W. R. M., Potter, J. L., and Duthie, J. J. R.: Nature of anemia in rheumatoid arthritis: V. Red cell survival measured by radioactive chromium, Ann. Rheumat. Dis. 20:133, 1961.

175. Robins, M. M., and Noyes, W. D.: Aplastic anemia treated with bone-marrow transfusion from identical twin, New England J. Med. 265:974, 1961.

176. Rohr, K.: Familial panmyelopthisis: Fanconi syndrome in adults, Blood 4:130, 1949.

177. Roscoe, M. H.: Anaemia and nitrogen retention in patients with chronic renal failure, Lancet 1:444, 1952.

178. Ross, J. F., Crockett, C. L., Jr., and Emerson, C. P.: Mechanism of anemia in leukemia and lymphoma, J. Clin. Invest. 30:668, 1951.

179. Rovinsky, J. J.: Primary refractory anemia complicating pregnancy, Obst. & Gynec. Surv. 14:149, 1959.

180. Roy, L. M. H., Alexander, W. R. M., and Duthie, J. J. R.: Nature of anaemia in rheumatoid arthritis: I. Metabolism of iron, Ann. Rheumat. Dis. 14:63, 1955.

181. Rubin, D., Botti, R. E., Storaasli, J. P., and Weisberger, A. S.: Changes in iron metabolism in early chloramphenicol toxicity, J. Lab. & Clin. Med. 50:947, 1957.

182. Saidi, P., Wallerstein, R. O., and Aggeler, P. M.: Effect of chloramphenicol on erythropoiesis, J. Lab. & Clin. Med. 57:247, 1961.

183. Saiti, M. F., and Vaughn, J. M.: The anaemia associated with infection, J. Path. & Bact. 56:189, 1944.

184. Sakol, M. J.: Red cell aplasia, A.M.A. Arch. Int. Med. 94:481, 1954.

185. Schwartz, S. O., and Motto, S. A.: Diagnostic significance of "burr" red blood cells, Am. J. M. Sc. 218:563, 1949.

186. Scott, J. L., Cartwright, G. E., and Wintrobe, M. M.: Acquired aplastic anemia: An analysis of thirty-nine cases and review of the pertinent literature, Medicine 38:119, 1959.

187. Scott, R. B., Matthias, J. Q., Constandoulakis, M., Kay, H. E. M., Lucas, P. F., and Whiteside, J. D.: Hypoplastic anaemia treated by transfusion of foetal haemopoietic cells, Brit. M. J. 2:1385, 1961.

188. Seaman, A. J., and Koler, R. D.: Acquired erythrocytic hypoplasia: A recovery during cobalt therapy: Report of two cases with review of the literature, Acta haemat. 9:153, 1953.

189. Seip, M.: Aplastic anemia treated with anabolic steroids and corticosteroids, Acta pediat. 50:561, 1961.

190. Shahidi, N. T., and Diamond, L. K.: Testosterone-induced remission in aplastic anemia, A.M.A. Am. J. Dis. Child. 98:293, 1959.

191. Shahidi, N. T., and Diamond, L. K.: Testosterone-induced remission in aplastic anemia of both acquired and congenital types: Further observations in twenty-four cases, New England J. Med. 264:953, 1961.

192. Shahidi, N. T., Gerald, P. S., and Diamond, L. K.: Alkali-resistant hemoglobin in aplastic anemia of both acquired and congenital types, New England J. Med. 266:117, 1961.

193. Sheehy, T. W., and Berman, A.: The anemia of cirrhosis, J. Lab. & Clin. Med. 56:72, 1960.

194. Shen, S. C., and Homburger, F.: The anemia of cancer patients and its relation to metastases to the bone marrow, J. Lab. & Clin. Med. 37:182, 1951.

195. Simms, E., Pfeiffenberger, M., and Heinbecker, P.: Neuro-endocrine and endocrine influences on the circulating blood elements, Endocrinology 49:45, 1951.

196. Sinclair, R. J. G., and Duthie, J. J. R.: Intravenous iron in hypochromia: Anemia associated with rheumatoid arthritis, Lancet 2:646, 1949.

197. Smith, C. H.: Hypoplastic and aplastic anemias of infancy and childhood with a consideration of the syndrome of non-hemolytic anemia of the newborn, J. Pediat. 43:487, 1953.

198. Smith, N. J., Price, J. M., Brown, R. R., and Moon, R. L.: Urinary excretion of tryptophan metabolites by patients with congenital hypoplastic anemia, A.M.A. Am. J. Dis. Child. 100:752, 1960.

199. Stevenson, T. D., and Beard, M. F.: Serum vitamin B_{12} content in liver disease, New England J. Med. 260:206, 1959.

200. Straus, B.: Aplastic anemia following exposure to carbon tetrachloride, J.A.M.A. 155:737, 1954.

201. Summers, V. K.: The anaemia of hypopituitarism, Brit. M. J. 1:787, 1952.

202. Swan, R. S., and Merrill, J. P.: Clinical course of acute renal failure, Medicine 32:215, 1953.

203. Theil, G. B., Brodine, C. E., Doolan, P. D., and Martinez, E.: Red cell glutathione content and stability in renal insufficiency, J. Lab. & Clin. Med. 58:736, 1961.

204. Thomas, E. D.: Treatment of refractory anemia with cobalt, Ann. Int. Med. 44:412, 1956.

205. Tsai, S. Y., and Levin, W. C.: Chronic erythrocytic hypoplasia in adults, Am. J. Med. 22:322, 1957.

206. Tudhope, G. R., and Wilson, G. M.: Anaemia in hypothyroidism: Incidence, pathogenesis, and response to treatment, Quart. J. Med. 29:513, 1960.

206a. Tudhope, G. R., and Wilson, G. M.: Deficiency of vitamin B_{12} in hypothyroidism, Lancet 1:703, 1962.

207. Vaughn, J. M., and Saiti, M. F.: Hemoglobin metabolism in chronic infections, J. Path. & Bact. 49:69, 1939.

208. Vaughn, J.: Anaemia associated with trauma and sepsis, Brit. M. J. 1:35, 1948.

209. Verel, D., Turnbull, A., Tudhope, G. R., and Ross, J. H.: Anaemia in Bright's disease, Quart. J. Med. 28:491, 1959.
210. Videbaek, A., and Kofod, O.: On the treatment of so-called aplastic anemia, Acta haemat. 6:147, 1951.
211. Vilter, R. W., Jarrold, T., Will, J. J., Mueller, J. F., Friedman, B. I., and Hawkins, V. R.: Refractory anemia with hyperplastic bone marrow, Blood 15:1, 1960.
211a. Wagner, H. P., and Smith, N. J.: Study of detoxification mechanisms in children with aplastic anemia, Blood 19:676, 1962.
212. Warren, S.: Pathology of Ionizing Radiation, Charles C. Thomas, Springfield, Ill., 1961.
213. Watson, C. J.: Studies on urobilinogen: III. The per diem excretion of urobilinogen in the common form of jaundice and disease of the liver, Arch. Int. Med. 59:206, 1937.
214. Watson, R. J., Lichtman, H. C., Messite, J., Ellison, R. R., Conrad, H., and Ginsberg, V.: Clinical studies with the citrovorum factor in megaloblastic anemia, Am. J. Med. 17:17, 1954.
215. Wayne, E. J.: Clinical and metabolic studies in thyroid disease, Brit. M. J. 1:1, 1960.
216. Weinstein, I. M.: A correlative study of the erythrokinetics and disturbances in iron metabolism associated with the anemia of rheumatoid arthritis, Blood 14:950, 1959.
217. Welch, H., Lewis, C. N., and Kerlan, I.: Blood dyscrasias: A nationwide survey, Antibiotics & Chemotherapy 4:607, 1954.
218. Wilson, P., Martin, F. I. R., and Last, P. M.: Bone marrow depression in tetanus, Lancet 2:442, 1956.
219. Wold, N., Thoma, G., Jr., and Brown, G. O., Jr.: Hematologic manifestations of radiation exposure in man, Progr. Hemat. 3:1, 1962.
220. Wolff, J. A.: Anemias caused by infection and toxins, idiopathic aplastic anemia and anemia caused by renal disease, Pediat. Clin. North America, p. 469, May 1957.
221. Zieve, L.: Jaundice, hyperlipemia and hemolytic anemia: A heretofore unrecognized syndrome associated with alcoholic fatty liver and cirrhosis, Ann. Int. Med. 48:471, 1958.

INDEX

INDEX